Seven AVMs

Tenets and Techniques for Resection

Thieme

Seven AVMs

Tenets and Techniques for Resection

Michael T. Lawton, MD
Professor of Neurological Surgery
Chief of Vascular and Skull Base Neurosurgery Program
Vice-Chairman, Department of Neurological Surgery
Tong-Po Kan Endowed Chair
University of California, San Francisco

Illustrations by Xavier Studio: Kenneth Xavier Probst, MA, CMI

Thieme
New York • Stuttgart

Thieme Medical Publishers, Inc.
333 Seventh Ave.
New York, NY 10001

Executive Editor: Kay Conerly
Managing Editor: Judith Tomat and Barbara A. Chernow
Editorial Assistant: Sara D'Emic
Senior Vice President, Editorial and Electronic Product Development: Cornelia Schulze
Production Editor: Sean Woznicki
Illustrations by Xavier Studio: Kenneth Xavier Probst, MA, CMI
International Production Director: Andreas Schabert
Vice President, Finance and Accounts: Sarah Vanderbilt
President: Brian D. Scanlan
Printer: Beltz Grafische Betriebe

Library of Congress Cataloging-in-Publication Data

Lawton, Michael T., author.
Seven AVMs : tenets and techniques for resection / Michael T. Lawton ; illustrations by Kenneth Xavier Probst.
p. ; cm.
Seven arteriovenous malformations
Includes bibliographical references and index.
ISBN 978-1-60406-875-7 — ISBN 978-1-60406-876-4 (eISBN)
I. Title. II. Title: Seven arteriovenous malformations.
[DNLM: 1. Intracranial Arteriovenous Malformations—surgery. 2. Neurosurgical Procedures—methods. 3. Vascular Surgical Procedures—methods. WL 355]
RD593
617.48—dc23 2014000129

Important note: Medical knowledge is ever-changing. As new research and clinical experience broaden our knowledge, changes in treatment and drug therapy may be required. The authors and editors of the material herein have consulted sources believed to be reliable in their efforts to provide information that is complete and in accord with the standards accepted at the time of publication. However, in view of the possibility of human error by the authors, editors, or publisher of the work herein or changes in medical knowledge, neither the authors, editors, nor publisher, nor any other party who has been involved in the preparation of this work, warrants that the information contained herein is in every respect accurate or complete, and they are not responsible for any errors or omissions or for the results obtained from use of such information. Readers are encouraged to confirm the information contained herein with other sources. For example, readers are advised to check the product information sheet included in the package of each drug they plan to administer to be certain that the information contained in this publication is accurate and that changes have not been made in the recommended dose or in the contraindications for administration. This recommendation is of particular importance in connection with new or infrequently used drugs.

Printed in Germany.
5 4 3 2 1
ISBN 978-1-60406-875-7

Also available as an e-book:
eISBN 978-1-60406-876-4

FSC
www.fsc.org
MIX
Papier aus verantwortungsvollen Quellen
FSC® C089473

To William L. Young, my wingman in all things AVM related.
Although this extraordinary man of insight, creativity, and musical gifts could not develop his life's symphony further, he inspired so many others to ask challenging research questions, "dare to know," and enjoy the adventure.

Acknowledgments

The author thanks the following companies for their generous support of this book:

Carl Zeiss Meditec, Inc.
Dublin, California

Mizuho America, Inc.
Union City, California

Aesculap, Inc.
Center Valley, Pennsylvania

Contents

Foreword I

Dr. Michael Lawton is one of the most outstanding academic and clinical cerebrovascular surgeons of our time. This book, based on his experience with more than 600 arteriovenous malformations (AVMs), stands as a tribute to his dedication to excellence in operative neurosurgery. *Seven AVMs*, based on his years of intensive clinical study of vascular anatomy and pathology, provides the basis for making the management of the most dangerous, complicated, and multifaceted lesions involving the brain as accurate, gentle, and safe as possible. I view this book on AVMs as the angry twin of Dr. Lawton's other excellent book, *Seven Aneurysms*. In a beautiful and well-written preface to *Seven AVMs*, one of the most eloquent pieces of medical writing I have seen, he contrasts the difference between aneurysm and AVM surgery. He describes aneurysm surgery as ballet, while AVM surgery is war. He points out that AVM surgery is more difficult than aneurysm surgery, requires more approaches, involves more locations, and necessitates more frequent intrusion into the brain. He notes that aneurysms are much more predictable than AVMs, because of the AVMs' complex of feeding arteries, draining veins, nidus sizes, and variable locations. He concludes that no two AVMs are alike. However, recognizable types and subtypes with definable anatomy occur over and over again, with minor variations. The seven types of AVMs are divided into 32 subtypes in developing a plan for the management battle. He likens preoperative embolization and radiosurgery to airstrikes and bombing raids on the AVM, but notes that hand-to-hand combat with a neurosurgeon is usually necessary. This twin set of books, *Seven Aneurysms* and *Seven AVMs,* should be on the bookshelf of every neurosurgical trainee and practitioner and should be required reading by everyone dealing with stroke. These books contain a wealth of information in a concise, well-organized format. Neurosurgeons of the world are fortunate to have access to these books by one of our greatest masters of cerebrovascular surgery.

Albert L. Rhoton, Jr., MD
R.D. Keene Professor and Chairman Emeritus
University of Florida
Gainesville, Florida
January 2014

Foreword II

In my long acquaintance with Michael Lawton, I have never known him to produce work that is anything less than excellent. In *Seven AVMs*, he surpasses even himself. As with his previous book, *Seven Aneurysms*, Michael has again given us an outstanding neurosurgical resource. *Seven AVMs* is a beautiful example of Michael's strategic thinking and surgical expertise. As he mentions in his *Preface*, arteriovenous malformations (AVMs) are both "stunningly beautiful and fearsome" and thus hold a supreme challenge to neurosurgeons, calling us to be particularly resourceful in our approach to treating patients with AVMs. The challenge in our field has long been the extreme diversity and complexity of AVMs. Each time we approach a patient with one of these lesions, regardless of the pathology, size, or location, we must develop a unique strategy that may involve expertise in open, endovascular, and radiosurgical techniques.

Because of these challenges, it would seem difficult to develop a single volume that adequately describes treatment approaches to such divergent and complex anatomical lesions. But Michael has built upon the Spetzler-Martin classification to guide surgical approaches by organizing AVMs into finite categories and subtypes. A thorough, strategic approach to the complex anatomy of AVMs and treatment decisions is clearly communicated both in words and in illustrations. The illustrations nicely emphasize the essence of the three-dimensional anatomy that the surgeon must comprehend to treat AVMs successfully.

The surgical techniques required to treat patients with AVMs are diabolically challenging and require patience, precision, and experience. Michael is someone in whom I take considerable paternal pride, as he did his residency training at the Barrow Neurological Institute. My personal interaction with him then and during our subsequent years as colleagues give me the confidence that this work comes from the hands of a superb surgeon. By sharing his skills and honest experience, he has provided a practical template to the principles guiding AVM resection and technical details to performing surgery. As with his previous book *Seven Aneurysms,* which has become the reference for the management of aneurysms, this current volume will become a must-have book for both the neurosurgeon in training as well as the experienced practitioner. They, along with the teams of endovascular and radiological surgeons with whom they work, will find gems of information to treat these complex and difficult lesions that will ultimately benefit the patients who entrust their lives into our care. I congratulate Dr. Lawton on this excellent work.

Robert F. Spetzler, MD
Barrow Neurological Institute
Phoenix, Arizona
January 2014

Preface

An arteriovenous malformation (AVM) is a spectacular freak of nature, an explosion of hemodynamic energy and red fury. Dilated arteries converge from all directions and dive into adjacent sulci like angry snakes. Engorged veins twist and throb with the swirling turbulence of shunted blood flow. A veil of glistening arachnoid conceals the tangled beast within. There is nothing like it in neurosurgery, at once so stunningly beautiful and fearsome that it is almost untouchable.

Arteriovenous malformation surgery is difficult—much more difficult than aneurysm surgery. Aneurysms concentrate around the circle of Willis, and most are exposed with just four approaches: pterional, orbitozygomatic, anterior interhemispheric, and far lateral. Saccular aneurysm anatomy, as well as the anatomy of parent and branch arteries, is simple and consistent. Aneurysm dissection is confined to subarachnoid spaces and surgical triangles, and can be choreographed into steps that secure proximal and distal control, define the neck anatomy, identify perforators, and permanently clip the aneurysm. The cleanliness of aneurysm surgery made my earlier book, *Seven Aneurysms: Tenets and Techniques for Clipping*, relatively easy to write.

Whereas aneurysm clipping is "white collar" surgery, AVM resection is "blue collar" surgery. Arteriovenous malformations are not concentrated around the circle of Willis, but scattered throughout the brain. They require a multitude of approaches, each one tailored to specific AVM anatomy. That anatomy, as well as the anatomy of feeding arteries and draining veins, varies with location, size, and prior intervention. Arteriovenous malformation dissection is not confined to subarachnoid spaces; it requires pial transgression, circumferential dissection in brain parenchyma, and deep dissection to ependymal planes. The resection of an AVM is far more difficult to choreograph. The complexity of AVM surgery makes this book, *Seven AVMs: Tenets and Techniques for Resection*, a major challenge.

The prevailing metaphor in *Seven Aneurysms* was ballet: aneurysm surgery is a dance that can be choreographed, practiced, and performed as an elegant art. In contrast, the prevailing metaphor in *Seven AVMs* is, with some misgivings, war: AVM surgery is a battle that can be strategized, planned, and waged victoriously. Although not violent or deliberately bloody, AVM surgery can be a dangerous engagement that warrants this military perspective. Diagnoses are established, patients are examined, and management options are evaluated like the diplomacy before a clash. An AVM can be surveyed radiographically, and then typed and subtyped based on its location in the brain and the surface on which it resides, the way a general sizes up his enemy. Like a battlefield, the brain harboring an AVM can be mapped anatomically for the eloquent cortex and tracts that are landmines and traps during the dissection. Like a battle plan, steps for AVM resection can be defined and executed. Arterial feeders, like enemy supply lines, are destroyed early; draining veins, like critical runways and bridges, are preserved throughout the campaign; and circumferential AVM dissection in brain parenchyma is like flanking maneuvers on multiple fronts in enemy territory. With the description of seven AVM types and 32 AVM subtypes, a unique surgical strategy for each AVM can be developed in preparation for battle. Although adjunctive support like preoperative embolization or radiosurgery can be ordered like air strikes or bombing raids, defeating an AVM usually requires hand-to-hand combat by the neurosurgeon, the soldier in battle. The neurosurgeon must elicit surrender with clear surgical strategy, meticulous execution, and an iron will to resect the AVM.

My personal surgical series now exceeds 600 AVMs (**Table P.1**), and throughout most of this experience, I viewed each AVM as unique. The mixture of feeding arteries, draining veins, nidus anatomy, size, and patient variables seemed to make each AVM different from the last. Although no two AVMs are alike, patterns emerge. Operating on AVMs is so challenging that the learning process demands a new perspective. Therefore, a central concept in the book is that the number of AVMs is finite; recognizable subtypes with definable anatomy occur over and over again, with minor variations, and these subtypes can be systematically analyzed from a surgical perspective. The title *Seven AVMs* refers to the types of AVMs in the lobes and deep regions of the brain: frontal, temporal, and parieto-occipital lobes; ventricles; deep central core; brainstem; and cerebellum. Within each type, four to six subtypes are defined that further categorize the AVMs based on brain surface (lateral, medial, basal, etc.) or other specific anatomy (e.g., midbrain, pons, and medulla). With this perspective, the broad spectrum of brain AVMs is simplified to 32 different AVM subtypes, each

Table P.1 Summary of Arteriovenous Malformation (AVM) Cases from Author's Consecutive 16-Year Experience with 600 AVMs, According to Type and Subtype

Type	Subtype	*n*	Percent
Frontal AVMs		**135**	**22.5**
	Lateral frontal	48	8.0
	Medial frontal	21	3.5
	Paramedian frontal	24	4.0
	Basal frontal	21	3.5
	Sylvian frontal	21	3.5
Temporal AVMs		**112**	**18.7**
	Lateral temporal	76	12.7
	Basal temporal	12	2.0
	Medial temporal	17	2.8
	Sylvian temporal	7	1.2
Parieto-occipital AVMs		**108**	**18.0**
	Lateral parieto-occipital	52	8.7
	Medial parieto-occipital	17	2.8
	Paramedian parieto-occipital	29	4.8
	Basal occipital	10	1.7
Ventricular/periventricular AVMs		**42**	**7.0**
	Callosal	23	3.8
	Ventricular body	5	0.8
	Atrial	9	1.5
	Temporal horn	5	0.8
Deep AVMs		**56**	**9.3**
	Pure sylvian	8	1.3
	Insular	25	4.2
	Basal ganglial	10	1.7
	Thalamic	13	2.2
Brainstem AVMs		**26**	**4.3**
	Anterior midbrain	1	0.2
	Posterior midbrain	6	1.0
	Anterior pontine	6	1.0
	Lateral pontine	7	1.2
	Anterior medullary	1	0.2
	Lateral medullary	5	0.8
Cerebellar AVMs		**82**	**13.7**
	Suboccipital Cerebellar	18	3.0
	Tentorial cerebellar	16	2.7
	Vermian cerebellar	25	4.2
	Tonsillar cerebellar	7	1.2
	Petrosal cerebellar	16	2.7
Mixed AVMs		**39**	**6.5**
Total AVMs		**600**	

characterized by its own arterial supply, draining veins, eloquent structures, surgical approach, and resection strategy. Categorization of AVMs is meant to inform the learning process and guide surgical resection, not account for every existing AVM. Some AVMs may be mixed subtypes, some giant in size, and others different beyond these subtypes. However, as with the previous book, *Seven Aneurysms*, this book is meant to be a summary of common AVMs encountered in practice, rather than an encyclopedia of all AVMs.

The book is organized into three sections: tenets, the seven arteriovenous malformations, and selection. The tenets establish eight steps for AVM resection that comprise the phases of battle, as follows: step 1, exposure; step 2, subarachnoid dissection; step 3, defining the draining vein; step 4, defining the feeding arteries; step 5, pial dissection; step 6, parenchymal dissection; step 7, ependymal or deep dissection; and step 8, finally resection. Critical concepts for dissection and resection are covered in the tenets section.

In the section on the seven arteriovenous malformations, the anatomical battlefields for the lobes and deep regions are reviewed, 32 subtypes are described, and a resection strategy is presented for each subtype, step by step. Ken Probst's color illustrations depict AVM subtypes and stepwise resection strategy, a format that worked well in describing aneurysm dissection in *Seven Aneurysms*. The "battle plans" illustrate the seven steps leading to AVM resection. Exposures are shown from the surgeon's perspective, and AVMs are shown schematically as boxes with a cortical surface (depicted with a circle on its base side and that side's label underlined), an axis (depicted with a line through the box), and arterial and venous anatomy superimposed on the box (red inflow arrows and blue outflow arrows, respectively). Subarachnoid dissection is depicted with a thick, white arrow showing the approach (No. 2). Draining veins (No. 3) and feeding arteries (No. 4) are numbered. Pial dissection across arterial fronts is depicted with dashed black lines (No. 5), parenchymal circumdissection with encircling white arrows (No. 6), and ependymal dissection with half of a sphere scooping across the deep side of the AVM (No. 7). Abbreviations used in these figures and throughout the book are summarized in **Tables P.2, P.3, P.4,** and **P.5**. As in *Seven Aneurysms*, this book is designed as a cross between a textbook and an atlas, and this section is loaded with demonstrative cases and intraoperative pictures.

The selection section addresses the secret to successful AVM surgery, which has nothing to do with surgical strategy or technique; rather, it is choosing your battles wisely. Good patient outcomes depend on discriminating patient selection, often telling patients not to have surgery. Grading scales are critical to patient selection, but modifications to the Spetzler-Martin system and supplementary grading scales can improve surgical risk estimation and patient selection. Selection of other therapies in a multimodality management can decimate an AVM preoperatively or address residual AVM that proved formidable or risky intraoperatively.

Learning to resect AVMs is challenging. As a resident at the Barrow Neurological Institute, I participated in 40 AVM operations with Dr. Robert Spetzler but did only three by myself. As with basilar apex aneurysms, residents and young neurosurgeons would learn AVM surgery if they performed more of these cases in their entirety as residents, yet residents

Table P.2 Abbreviations for Arteries

Abbreviation	Artery	Abbreviation	Artery
ACA	anterior cerebral artery	OphA	ophthalmic artery
AChA	anterior choroidal artery	OrbFrA	orbitofrontal artery (ACA)
ACoA	anterior communicating artery	OrbFrA	orbitofrontal artery (MCA)
AICA	anterior inferior cerebellar artery	ParaCenA	paracentral artery
AIFA	anterior internal frontal artery	ParOccA	parieto-occipital artery
An	aneurysm	PCA	posterior cerebral artery
AngA	angular artery	PcaA	pericallosal artery
AntParA	anterior parietal	PCoA	posterior communicating artery
AntSpA	anterior spinal artery	PedP	peduncular perforators
AntThaP	anterior thalamoperforator	PICA	posterior inferior cerebellar artery
ATA	anterior temporal artery	PIFA	posterior internal frontal artery
BA	basilar artery	PosParA	posterior parietal artery
CalcA	calcarine artery	PosTempA	posterior temporal artery (MCA)
CenA	central artery	PosTempA	posterior temporal artery (PCA)
CirP	circumflex perforator	PosThaP	thalamoperforators
CmaA	callosomarginal artery	PreCenA	precentral artery
FrPolA	frontopolar artery	PreFrA	prefrontal artery
HippoA	hippocampal artery	RAH	recurrent artery of Heubner
ICA	internal carotid artery	SCA	superior cerebellar artery
InfParA	inferior parietal artery	SHA	superior hypophyseal artery
InfTr	inferior trunk of MCA	SplenA	splenial artery
InsP	insular perforators	SupParA	superior parietal artery
lLSA	lateral lenticulostriate artery	SupTr	superior trunk of MCA
lPChA	lateral posterior choroidal artery	TempOccA	temporo-occipital artery
MCA	middle cerebral artery	TempPolA	temporopolar artery
MidTempA	middle temporal artery	ThaP	thalamoperforator
MidTr	middle trunk of MCA	ThGenP	thalamogeniculate perforator
MIFA	middle internal frontal artery	VA	vertebral artery
mLSA	medial lenticulostriate artery	VBJ	vertebrobasilar junction
mPChA	medial posterior choroidal artery		

Table P.3 Abbreviations for Arterial Segments

Abbreviation	Arterial Segment	Abbreviation	Arterial Segment
C1	ICA, cervical segment	P2	PCA, postcommunicating segment
C2	ICA, petrous segment	P2A	PCA, crural segment
C3	ICA, lacerum segment	P2P	PCA, ambient segment
C4	ICA, cavernous segment	P3	PCA, quadrigeminal segment
C5	ICA, clinoidal segment	P4	PCA, calcarine segment
C6	ICA, ophthalmic segment	s1	SCA, anterior pontomesencephalic segment
C7	ICA, communicating segment	s2	SCA, lateral pontomesencephalic segment
A1	ACA, precommunicating or horizontal segment	s3	SCA, cerebellomesencephalic segment
A2	ACA, postcommunicating or infracallosal segment	s4	SCA, cortical segment
		a1	AICA, anterior pontine segment
A3	ACA, precallosal segment	a2	AICA, lateral pontine segment
A4	ACA, supracallosal segment	a3	AICA, flocculopeduncular segment
A5	ACA, postcallosal segment	a4	AICA, cortical segment
M1	MCA, sphenoidal segment	p1	PICA, anterior medullary segment
M2	MCA, insular segment	p2	PICA, lateral medullary segment
M3	MCA, opercular segment	p3	PICA, tonsillomedullary segment
M4	MCA, cortical segment	p4	PICA, telovelotonsillar segment
P1	PCA, precommunicating segment	p5	PICA, cortical segment

Table P.4 Abbreviations for Veins and Venous Sinuses

Abbreviation	Vein	Abbreviation	Vein
AHemV	anterior hemispheric vein	PedV	peduncular vein
AntCalcV	anterior calcarine vein (internal occipital vein)	PosCalcV	posterior calcarine vein
AntFrV	anterior frontal vein	PosCenV	postcentral vein
AntParV	anterior parietal vein	PosFrV	posterior frontal vein
AntTempV	anterior temporal vein	PosParV	posterior parietal vein
AtrV	atrial vein (medial, lateral)	PosTempV	posterior temporal vein
BVR	basal vein of Rosenthal	PreCenCblV	precentral cerebellar vein
CauV	caudate vein (anterior, posterior)	PreCenV	precentral vein
CavS	cavernous sinus	ReOlvV	retro-olivary veins
CenV	central vein	ReTonsV	retrotonsillar vein
ChorV	choroidal vein (superior, inferior)	SepV	septal vein (anterior, posterior)
DeepSylV	deep sylvian vein	SHemV	superior hemispheric vein (anterior, posterior)
FrPolV	frontopolar vein	SigmS	sigmoid sinus
FrSylV	frontosylvian vein	SPetrV	superior petrosal vein
HippoV	anterior hippocampal vein	SphBasS	sphenobasal sinus
ICV	internal cerebral vein	SphParS	sphenoparietal sinus
IHemV	inferior hemispheric vein	SphPetS	sphenopetrosal sinus
IPetrV	inferior petrosal vein	SplenV	splenial vein
IPS	inferior petrosal sinus	SPS	superior petrosal sinus
ISS	inferior sagittal sinus	SSS	superior sagittal sinus
IVerV	inferior vermian vein	StrS	straight sinus
Labbé	vein of Labbé	SupSylV	superficial sylvian vein
LAMedV	lateral anterior medullary vein	SVerV	superior vermian vein
LAPonMesV	lateral anterior pontomesencephalic vein	TecV	tectal vein
LMedV	lateral medullary vein	TempBasV	temporal basal vein (anterior, middle, posterior)
LMesV	lateral mesencephalic vein	TentS	tentorial sinus
MAMedV	median anterior medullary vein	ThaStrV	thalamostriate vein
MAPonMesV	median anterior pontomesencephalic vein	TonsV	tonsillar vein
MedFrV	medial frontal veins (anterior, central, posterior)	Torc	torcular
MedParV	medial parietal veins (anterior, posterior)	TrMedV	transverse medullary vein
MedTempV	medial temporal vein	Trolard	vein of Trolard
MidFrV	middle frontal vein	TrPonV	transverse pontine vein
MidTempV	middle temporal vein	TrvS	transverse sinus
MPMedV	median posterior medullary vein	UncV	uncal vein
OccBasV	occipital basal vein	VCMedF	vein of cerebellomedullary fissure
OccV	occipital vein	VCMesF	vein of cerebellomesencephalic fissure
OlfV	olfactory vein	VCPonF	vein of cerebellopontine fissure
OrbFrV	orbitofrontal vein (anterior, posterior)	VoG	vein of Galen
ParaCenV	paracentral vein	VPonMedS	vein of the pontomedullary sulcus
PcaV	pericallosal vein (anterior, posterior)	VPonMesS	vein of the pontomesencephalic sulcus
PComV	posterior communicating vein		

do not perform many of these cases in their entirety because they are technically demanding and dangerous. In notes from my final AVM case as a resident, I commented that I felt tentative, slow, and unready to do AVM surgery, particularly compared to Dr. Spetzler's quickness, aggressivity, and confidence. Experience with over 600 cases has developed these traits, but AVM experience is hard to come by, because AVMs are only one tenth as common as aneurysms; even in an academic, subspecialized vascular neurosurgery practice, I operate on just 40 to 50 AVM patients annually. Therefore, experience with AVMs is more precious than with aneurysms, which compels me to write this book. I never found a book that helped me conceptualize and systematize AVM surgery when I was developing my skills. This book is my attempt to make AVMs a little more understandable and their resections a little easier, as well as to help maintain our high surgical standards.

The earlier book, *Seven Aneurysms*, was rewarding for me because so many neurosurgeons told me that it helped them in surgery. Even in this endovascular heyday when aneurysm

Table P.5 Abbreviations for Brain, Nerves, Cisterns, and Miscellaneous

Approaches	
AIA	anterior interhemisperic approach
ATcA	anterior transcallosal approach
ATcTchA	anterior transcallosal-transchoroidal approach
ATiA	anterior transinsular approach
ExRS	extended retrosigmoid approach
FL	far lateral approach
OZ	orbitozygomatic-pterional approach
PIA	posterior interhemispheric approach
PTcA	posterior transcallosal approach
PTiA	posterior transinsular approach
SCIF	supracarotid-infrafrontal approach
SCIT	supracerebellar-infratentorial approach
SPL	superior parietal lobule approach
STIO	supratentorial-infraoccipital approach
SubOcc	suboccipital-transventricular approach
TF	transfrontal approach
TO	transoccipital approach
TP	transparietal approach
TSyl	lateral transsylvian approach
TT	transtemporal approach
Brain	
AOG	anterior orbital gyrus
Cau	caudate nucleus
Cbl	cerebellum
CC	corpus callosum
ChPl	choroid plexus
ChFis	choroidal fissure
Clau	claustrum
EC	external capsule
FoM	foramen of Monro
GPe	globus pallidus, pars external
GPi	globus pallidus, pars internal
IC	internal capsule
IFG	inferior frontal gyrus
InfCP	inferior cerebellar peduncle
IOG	inferior occipital gyrus
IPL	inferior parietal lobule
ITG	inferior temporal gyrus
Lent	lentiform nucleus
LGB	lateral geniculate body
LOG	lateral orbital gyrus
MFG	middle frontal gyrus
MidCP	middle cerebellar peduncle
MOG	medial orbital gyrus
MTG	middle temporal gyrus
OTG	occipitotemporal gyrus
POG	posterior orbital gyrus
Put	putamen
SFG	superior frontal gyrus
SOG	superior occipital gyrus
SPL	superior parietal lobule
STG	superior temporal gyrus
SupCP	superior cerebellar peduncle
Tha	thalamus
Vent	ventricle
Cisterns	
AmbC	ambient cistern
AntSpC	anterior spinal cistern
CallC	callosal cistern
CarC	carotid cistern
CbMedC	cerebellomedullary cistern
CbPonC	cerebellopontine cistern
ChiC	chiasmatic cistern
CruC	crural cistern
IpC	interpeduncular cistern
LTC	lamina terminalis cistern
MagnC	cisterna magna
MedC	premedullary cistern
OlfC	olfactory cistern
PonC	prepontine cistern
PosSpC	posterior spinal cistern
QuadC	quadrigeminal cistern
SylC	sylvian cistern
Miscellaneous	
A#B#C#	age, bleeding, and compactness in supplementary grading scale
ACP	anterior clinoid process
AVM	arteriovenous malformation
CSF	cerebrospinal fluid
CT	computed tomography
EAC	external auditory canal
EEG	electroencephalogram
ICG	indocyanine green
IHT	infra-hypoglossal triangle
L	left
MEP	motor evoked potentials
PCP	posterior clinoid process
R	right
RAG	radial artery graft
S#V#E#	size, venous drainage, eloquence in Spetzler-Martin grading scale
SAH	subarachnoid hemorrhage
SHT	supra-hypoglossal triangle
SOF	superior orbital fissure
SSEP	somatosensory evoked potentials
Tent	tentorium
Nerves	
CN1, or I	olfactory nerve
CN2, or II	optic nerve
CN3, or III	oculomotor nerve
CN4, or IV	trochlear nerve
CN5, or V	trigeminal nerve
CN6, or IX	abducens nerve
CN7, or VII	facial nerve
CN8, or VIII	vestibulocochlear nerve
CN9, or IX	glossopharyngeal nerve
CN10, or X	vagus nerve
CN11, or XI	spinal accessory nerve
CN12, or XII	hypoglossal nerve

surgery is decreasing and aneurysm surgeons are dwindling, there was enough interest for the book to have an impact. *Seven AVMs* is aimed at a less common disease and a smaller audience, but it is important to remember that AVM surgery is alive and well. Whereas endovascular therapies compete with aneurysm surgery, they complement and enhance AVM surgery. Endovascular cures are uncommon with AVMs, even with improving embolic agents and catheter technology. Consequently, endovascular and surgical techniques join synergistically against a common foe. Similarly, radiosurgical cures can be achieved with small AVMs but are unlikely with larger AVMs. Radiation-induced arterial thickening, flow reduction, and surrounding gliosis make incompletely obliterated AVMs some of my favorite surgical lesions. Therefore, these other modalities are surgical adjuncts, and a steady need for AVM surgeons remains. Arteriovenous malformation surgery is more difficult than aneurysm surgery, and AVM surgeons must be skillful, strategic, and strong. This surgery can be exhausting, but after battling for hours, capturing elusive bleeders, surrounding deep portions of nidus, darkening the draining vein, and pulling the AVM out of its resection cavity, it feels more satisfying than completing a tough operation; it feels like winning a war.

I The Tenets

1 Arteriovenous Malformation Exposure

The Box

Arteriovenous malformations (AVMs) come in many shapes: spheres, ellipses, cylinders, and, classically, cones. The cone is based on the cortical surface and tapers to a tip at the ependyma. Although AVMs are never cube shaped, it is useful to conceptualize them as a box with six sides: one top (or superficial side), four sides, and a bottom (or deep side). This orthogonal conceptualization applies structure to an otherwise amorphous tangle, giving the AVM definable sides that are medial and lateral, anterior and posterior, superior and inferior.

These distinct sides can then be characterized by relationships to dural structures, cortical landmarks, feeding arteries, draining veins, fissures, and cranial anatomy. When preparing for surgery, I study computed tomography (CT) scans, magnetic resonance (MR) images, and angiograms scan by scan, sequence by sequence, and run by run, to familiarize myself with the AVM in ways that are not possible in surgery. Angiograms can replay forward and backward to see relationships between arteries and veins, to analyze bifurcations or tortuosities that may be buried in a sulcus, and to identify embolic agents that might serve as landmarks intraoperatively. Magnetic resonance images can be scrolled up and down to localize the motor strip or Broca's area, to identify clean pial planes in a fissure, or to map out the adjacent clot as a route of access. The box enables the neurosurgeon to organize AVM anatomy as this information is gathered. A side can be "hot" or "cold" depending on its arterial input; a side can be eloquent or non-eloquent depending on its proximity to critical neurologic structures; a side can be pial, parenchymal, or ependymal, depending on its depth in the brain; and a side can be ruptured or unruptured depending on the presence or absence of an adjacent hematoma.

The box concept also organizes microsurgical dissection. Hot sides are confronted early to de-arterialize the AVM, whereas eloquent sides are confronted late when the nidus is quiet. Ruptured sides are also dissected early when hematoma evacuation accesses the nidus or relaxes the brain. The box localizes specific arterial feeders. For example, paramedian parietal AVMs receive anterior cerebral artery (ACA) input on its anterior side, middle cerebral artery (MCA) input on its lateral side, and posterior cerebral artery (PCA) input on its inferior side. Similarly, the box localizes draining veins, deep tracts, and ventricles, and the box paces progress as dissection advances from top to the four sides to bottom.

Surfaces

Most AVMs are based on a cortical surface, and this cortical surface defines the AVM subtypes. A simple example is the lateral frontal AVM based on the superior, middle, or inferior frontal gyrus. Cortical, cerebellar, and brainstem surfaces have been detailed thoroughly by Albert Rhoton and colleagues, and the names for AVM subtypes are derived from this magnificent body of work. A surface perspective generates an intuitive nomenclature that is descriptive, practical, and not overwhelming (32 subtypes). Like characterizing plants or animals by genus and species, each AVM can be characterized by type and subtype, the former based on brain location and the latter based on brain surface (**Table 1.1**).

Arteriovenous malformation exposures access this defining surface. The lateral frontal AVM is exposed with a unilateral convexity craniotomy, and the dural opening immediately exposes the top of the box. The top side of the AVM box comes to the cortical surface and, in a sense, is already separated from the brain. "Free" surfaces require no parenchymal dissection, only the craniotomy and dural opening (free convexity surfaces, **Table 1.2**). They may still require the release of arachnoid adhesions or division of meningeal feeding arteries, but not the pial and parenchymal invasion required for other bound sides. Some free surfaces may not be exposed with craniotomy and dural opening alone (free fissure surfaces, **Table 1.2**); for example, the basal temporal AVM has a free surface inferiorly that requires subtemporal dissection for access, and the medial frontal AVM has a free surface medially that requires interhemispheric dissection for access. Most AVMs have one free surface, but some may have two or three or more, and others buried in brain parenchyma may have no free surfaces (**Fig. 1.1**).

Table 1.1 Summary of AVM Exposures

Type	Subtype	Craniotomy	Angle of Attack	Gravity Retraction	Free Surfaces
Frontal AVMs					
	Lateral frontal	Frontal	Parallel	No	1
	Medial frontal	Bifrontal	Perpendicular	Yes	1
	Paramedian frontal	Bifrontal	Parallel	No	2
	Basal frontal	Orbital-pterional	Perpendicular	Yes	1
	Sylvian frontal	Pterional	Parallel	Yes	1
Temporal AVMs					
	Lateral temporal	Temporal	Parallel	No	1
	Basal temporal	Temporal	Perpendicular	No	1
	Medial temporal	Orbitozygomatic	Perpendicular	Yes	1
	Sylvian temporal	Pterional	Parallel	Yes	1
Parieto-occipital AVMs					
	Lateral parieto-occipital	Parieto-occipital	Parallel	No	1
	Medial parieto-occipital	Torcular	Perpendicular	Yes	1
	Paramedian parieto-occipital	Biparieto-occipital	Parallel	No	2
	Basal occipital	Torcular	Perpendicular	No	1
Ventricular/Periventricular AVMs					
	Callosal	Bifrontal	Parallel	Yes	2
	Ventricular body	Bifrontal	Perpendicular	Yes	2
	Atrial	Parietal	Parallel	No	2
	Temporal horn	Temporal	Perpendicular	No	2
Deep AVMs					
	Pure sylvian	Pterional	Parallel	No	1
	Insular	Pterional	Parallel	No	1
	Basal ganglial	Pterional	Perpendicular	No	0
	Thalamic	Bifrontal	Perpendicular	Yes	1
Brainstem AVMs					
	Anterior midbrain	Orbitozygomatic	Perpendicular	Yes	1
	Posterior midbrain	Torcular	Perpendicular	Yes	1
	Anterior pontine	Retrosigmoid	Perpendicular	No	1
	Lateral pontine	Retrosigmoid	Perpendicular	No	1
	Anterior medullary	Suboccipital	Perpendicular	No	1
	Lateral medullary	Far Lateral	Perpendicular	No	1
Cerebellar AVMs					
	Suboccipital cerebellar	Suboccipital	Parallel	No	1
	Tentorial cerebellar	Torcular	Perpendicular	No	1
	Vermian cerebellar	Torcular	Perpendicular	No	1
	Tonsillar cerebellar	Suboccipital	Parallel	No	3
	Petrosal cerebellar	Retrosigmoid	Perpendicular	No	1

Table 1.2 Summary of Free Surfaces

Free Convexity Surface	AVM Subtype
Supratentorial	
Frontal convexity	Lateral frontal AVM
	Paramedian frontal AVM
Temporal convexity	Lateral temporal AVM
Parieto-occipital convexity	Lateral parieto-occipital AVM
	Paramedian parieto-occipital AVM
Infratentorial	
Cerebellar convexity	Suboccipital cerebellar AVM
Free Fissure Surface	**AVM subtype**
Supratentorial	
Subfrontal plane	Basal frontal AVM
Subtemporal plane	Basal temporal AVM
	Medial temporal AVM (posterior)
Sylvian fissure	Frontal sylvian AVM
	Temporal sylvian AVM
	Pure sylvian AVM
	Insular AVM
Interhemispheric fissure	Medial frontal AVM
	Paramedian frontal AVM
	Medial parieto-occipital AVM
	Paramedian parieto-occipital AVM
	Callosal AVM
	Ventricular body AVM
	Basal ganglial AVM
Choroidal fissure	Ventricular body AVM
	Thalamic AVM
Supratentorial-infraoccipital	Basal occipital AVM
Infratentorial	
Sylvian fissure	Anterior midbrain AVM
Supracerebellar-infratentorial fissure	Vermian cerebellar AVM
	Tentorial cerebellar AVM
	Posterior midbrain AVM
Cerebellomesencephalic fissure	Tentorial cerebellar AVM
	Posterior midbrain AVM
Cerebellopontine fissure	Petrosal cerebellar AVM
	Lateral pontine AVM
	Anterior pontine AVM
Cerebellomedullary fissure	Tonsillar cerebellar AVM
	Lateral medullary AVM

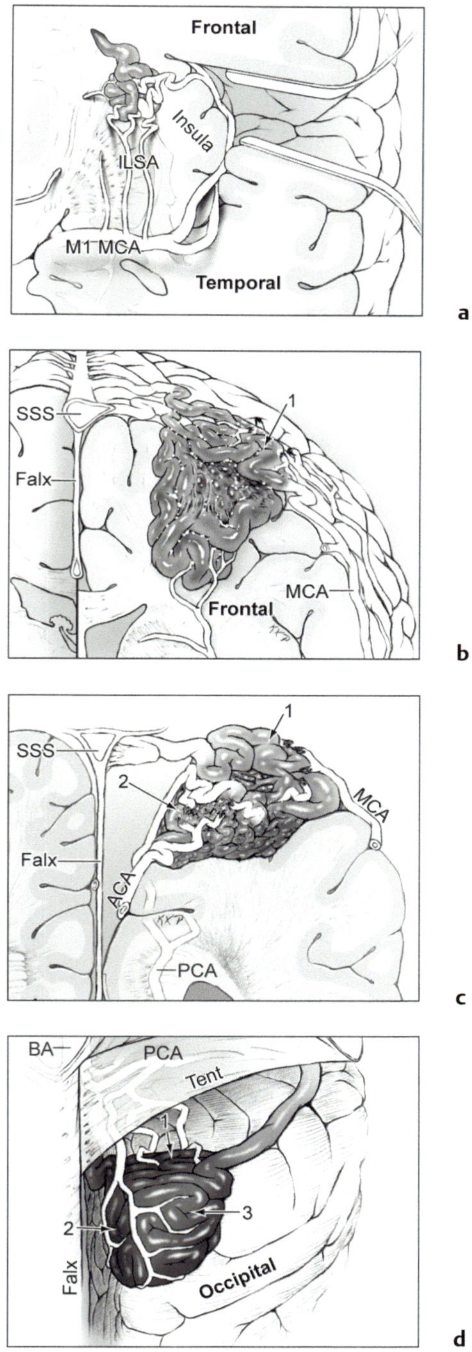

Fig. 1.1 Arteriovenous malformations (AVMs) are based on a cortical surface that defines its type and subtype, and the craniotomy exposes this surface. An AVM presenting on this surface has a free surface that requires no parenchymal dissection. Most AVMs have one free surface, but can have multiple free surfaces or none. (**a**) Basal ganglial AVM with no free surface (coronal cross-sectional view); (**b**) lateral frontal AVM with one free surface (lateral surface, coronal cross-sectional view); (**c**) paramedian parieto-occipital AVM with two free surfaces (lateral and medial surfaces, coronal cross-sectional view); and (**d**) occipital pole AVM with three free surfaces (lateral, medial, and basal surfaces, posterior view).

Bilateral Craniotomy

- Medial frontal AVM
- Paramedian frontal AVM
- Medial parieto-occipital AVM
- Paramedian parieto-occipital AVM
- Callosal AVM
- Ventricular body AVM
- Basal ganglial AVM (caudate)
- Thalamic AVM
- Posterior midbrain AVM
- Anterior medullary AVM
- Tentorial cerebellar AVM
- Vermian cerebellar AVM
- Tonsillar cerebellar AVM

Gravity Retraction

- Medial frontal AVM
- Basal frontal AVM
- Sylvian frontal AVM
- Medial temporal AVM (anterior)
- Sylvian temporal AVM
- Medial parieto-occipital AVM
- Callosal AVM
- Ventricular body AVM
- Basal ganglial AVM (caudate)
- Thalamic AVM
- Anterior midbrain AVM
- Posterior midbrain AVM

Craniotomy

An AVM's defining surface dictates surgical exposure, and the craniotomy should expose this surface. AVM craniotomies are big; these are not cases for minimally invasive approaches. Some periphery is needed to survey the course of feeding arteries and draining veins as they travel to and from the AVM. The craniotomy should open room to dissect the subarachnoid spaces and accommodate brain shift as tissues relax. Only one third of AVM craniotomies are unilateral convexity craniotomies; nearly one half are bilateral, crossing the midline and associated venous sinuses to expose medial surfaces through fissures like the interhemispheric fissure, supracerebellar-infratentorial plane, and cisterna magna (see text box). Midline access requires careful management of adherent dural sinuses. Paramedian veins are often variceal and can notch the inner table of the skull; epidural dissection under direct visualization preserves dura and protects these veins during elevation of the bone flap. Skull base craniotomies are required in approximately one fifth of AVM craniotomies to access basal surfaces, widen deep exposures, or address brainstem AVMs. When it comes to craniotomy, bigger is better. Small craniotomies can cover portions of an AVM, create an obstructive ledge of bone, force dissection into an incorrect plane, constrain the instruments, and force unnecessary errors.

Angle of Attack

Angle of attack is an aerodynamics term that describes the angle between the wing of an airplane and the oncoming air flow, but it can also describe the angle at which one attacks an AVM (**Fig. 1.2**). An AVM has an axis that runs through the center of the box. When the exposure aligns with the AVM's axis, the top and all four sides are accessible circumferentially, with feeding arteries, draining veins, and dissection planes clearly visible and squarely confronted at the margins. This direct angle of attack is best described as "parallel": the axis of the AVM aligns with or parallels the trajectory of the exposure. Parallel exposures allow circumdissection without significant brain retraction, corticectomy, or AVM manipulation. Examples of parallel angle of attack include convexity AVMs in the lateral frontal, lateral temporal, and lateral parieto-occipital lobes (**Table 1.1**).

In contrast, other AVM exposures have a "perpendicular" angle of attack, meaning that the axis of the AVM box intersects with the trajectory of the exposure. Perpendicular approaches are used with deeper AVMs where surgical corridors are long and limited, and cannot be adapted to the AVM. Perpendicular approaches access one side of the AVM box directly but the other four sides indirectly. Circumdissection proceeds off the axis of exposure, requiring compensatory maneuvers such as brain retraction, corticectomy, or AVM manipulation to visualize the AVM or mobilize it into the surgical corridor. Such maneuvers are more invasive, can be injurious, and might aggravate the AVM. Examples of perpendicular exposure include the transsylvian approach to medial temporal AVMs, the supracerebellar-infratentorial approach to vermian cerebellar AVMs, and retrosigmoid approaches to lateral pontine AVMs. These elegant approaches reach deep AVMs through fissures and subarachnoid spaces that avoid direct transcortical routes through normal brain tissue, but perpendicularity limits visualization and reduces maneuverability around the AVM. These difficulties make perpendicular exposures more dangerous, so they are reserved for smaller AVMs or those with an associated hematoma, encephalomalacia, or an adjacent ventricle, fissure, or cistern.

It should be noted that this terminology differs from what is published in the literature. Bennett Stein used "perpendicular" and "tangential" to describe "parallel" and "perpendicular" exposures, respectively. Whereas he used perpendicularity to describe the relationship between the neurosurgeon

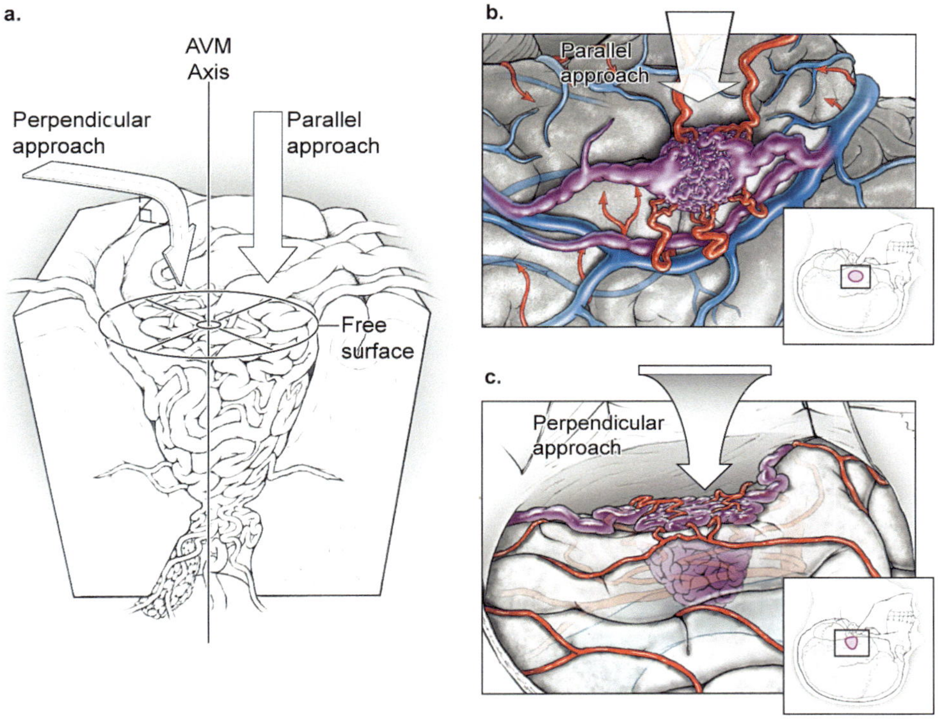

Fig. 1.2 (**a**) The angle of AVM attack may be parallel or perpendicular to the AVM's axis. (**b**) When the exposure's trajectory and the AVM's axis align, the nidus can be circumdissected directly (parallel; lateral temporal AVM). (**c**) When the exposure's trajectory intersects the AVM's axis, brain retraction, AVM mobilization, and/or corticectomy are required to circumdissect the nidus (perpendicular; subtemporal approach to basal temporal AVM). Perpendicular attack avoids transcortical routes through normal brain but is more difficult and is reserved for smaller AVMs in deep locations.

and the arteries intersecting with the AVM, I prefer parallelism to describe the coaxial alignment between the neurosurgeon and the AVM. Whereas Stein used tangential to describe the skiving view of just one AVM surface, I prefer perpendicularity to describe veering off-axis into less accessibility areas. I have used Stein's terminology in previous publications, but the "parallel-perpendicular" terminology seems more intuitive.

■ Gravity

The lateral convexity is the most common surface on which AVMs are based, and these AVMs require no opening of deep planes. Consequently, patient positioning is straightforward. However, medial, basal, and deep AVMs require deep openings and some brain shifting, which is facilitated by gravity retraction. Gravity retraction opens anatomic planes for surgical access through a combination of patient and head position, a generous craniotomy, cerebrospinal fluid (CSF) release, and extensive subarachnoid dissection that enables the brain to sag. Gravity retraction also requires help from dural structures like the falx or tentorium to hold back some brain and prevent it from shifting. Examples include the anterior interhemispheric approach with the midline oriented horizontally and the frontal lobe in the dependent position; the posterior interhemispheric approach with the midline oriented horizontally and the occipital lobe in the dependent position; the transsylvian approach with the head extended and the frontal and temporal lobes in the dependent position; and the supracerebellar-infratentorial approach with the patient sitting and the cerebellum in the dependent position. In these approaches, gravity retraction exposes the free surface on which the AVM is based, but the angle of attack is perpendicular and circumdissection of parenchymal sides is off-axis. Approaches that use gravity retraction facilitate deep incursions into subarachnoid recesses and ventricles without brain transgression and without additional fixed retraction, but sacrifice a parallel angle of attack.

The application of gravity retraction requires planning at the earliest stages of a case. Placing the patient in the sitting position requires preoperative screening for a patent foramen ovale with an echocardiogram and bubble test. Mannitol and some hyperventilation are essential. The patient and head are positioned to align dependent brain tissue in gravity's pull. The craniotomy extends beyond the fissure or surface of interest to open space for the dependent brain to descend. CSF drainage catheters are rarely used; I prefer instead early microsurgical dissection of arachnoid cisterns and direct drainage with suction. The key to the success of gravity retraction is extensive subarachnoid dissection. The surgical corridor is widened well beyond the boundaries of the nidus, particularly at the mouth to the corridor. Arachnoid sheets, bands, and trabeculae that maintain the brain's natural structure are thoroughly disrupted for gravity to have its way with the tissues. Deep corridors opened with gravity retraction are so exquisite in the way they exploit natural tissue planes, but are particularly challenging when an AVM waits at the end of the tunnel.

2 Subarachnoid Dissection

Reconnaissance

Subarachnoid dissection is the calm before the clash, when the arteriovenous malformation (AVM) is approached, encountered, and surveyed under the microscope without salvo. The labyrinth of subarachnoid spaces around the AVM is splayed, deconstructing arachnoid membranes, disconnecting interlobular trabeculae, and intercommunicating cisternal compartments. Cerebrospinal fluid (CSF) drainage slackens and shifts the cerebral terrain. Misshapen feeding arteries and distorted draining veins are inspected, with their unusual features offering clues to their angiographic identity. Subarachnoid dissection transforms the brain's natural landscape into the surgical field, a battlefield, with AVM surfaces laid bare, fissures opened widely, and anatomic landmarks in sight. This phase of AVM surgery is like aneurysm surgery, with microdissection that is clean and extrapial, and that can be savored as a time of reconnaissance without confrontation.

Approaches

The subarachnoid approach can be short with superficial AVMs on a cortical surface or long with deep AVMs in central or ependymal locations (**Fig. 2.1**). Superficial approaches to convexity AVMs require minimal subarachnoid dissection because the AVM is based right on the cortical surface (transfrontal, transtemporal, and transparieto-occipital approaches, **Table 2.1**). Intermediate approaches require more subarachnoid dissection down a fissure such as the sylvian and interhemispheric fissures or along a basal or dural plane (transsylvian, medial interhemispheric, and basal approaches, **Table 2.1**). Deep approaches are forays to the bottom of these fissures and beyond, through the corpus callosum, ventricles, and choroidal fissures, and along the skull base or tentorial planes (transcallosal, transchoroidal, and posterior fossa approaches, **Table 2.1**).

Although superficial AVMs are easily localized on their free surface, they are often concealed in arachnoid thickened by microhemorrhages, chronic inflammation, radiosurgery, or prior embolization. An opaque white veil must first be opened to reveal the AVM's anatomy. Distended veins are freed from their arachnoidal investments and peeled back to expose AVM margins. Hemorrhage, both new and old, stains adjacent surfaces with hemosiderin and presents a trail to fresh clot, liquefied hematoma, or encephalomalacia. Hemorrhage can create extra-anatomic cavities that often connect with subarachnoid spaces. Some AVM margins separate from adjacent brain as a subarachnoidal plane, often following gyral contours into a sulcus. An example is the pure sylvian AVM, which sits entirely in the sylvian fissure without invading frontal, temporal, or insular parenchyma, and can be circumdissected completely with subarachnoid dissection and without subpial invasion.

Other than these cerebral and cerebellar convexity AVMs that are superficial and immediately apparent on brain surface, the rest require more dissection to expose the AVM. Transsylvian approaches expose eight lateral and deep AVM subtypes; interhemispheric approaches expose eight medial and deep subtypes; skull base approaches expose eight basal, brainstem, and cerebellar subtypes; and transtorcular approaches expose six posterior, cerebellar, and brainstem subtypes (**Table 2.2**). All of these AVMs have their base on a surface buried in a fissure that must be opened, or along a basal plane that does not face the axis of the approach. The initial survey of the brain after dural opening may reveal only an arterialized vein or nothing abnormal at all. Consequently, these AVMs require bilateral craniotomies, gravity retraction, or transventricular access. These buried AVMs are localized by following arterialized veins around corners

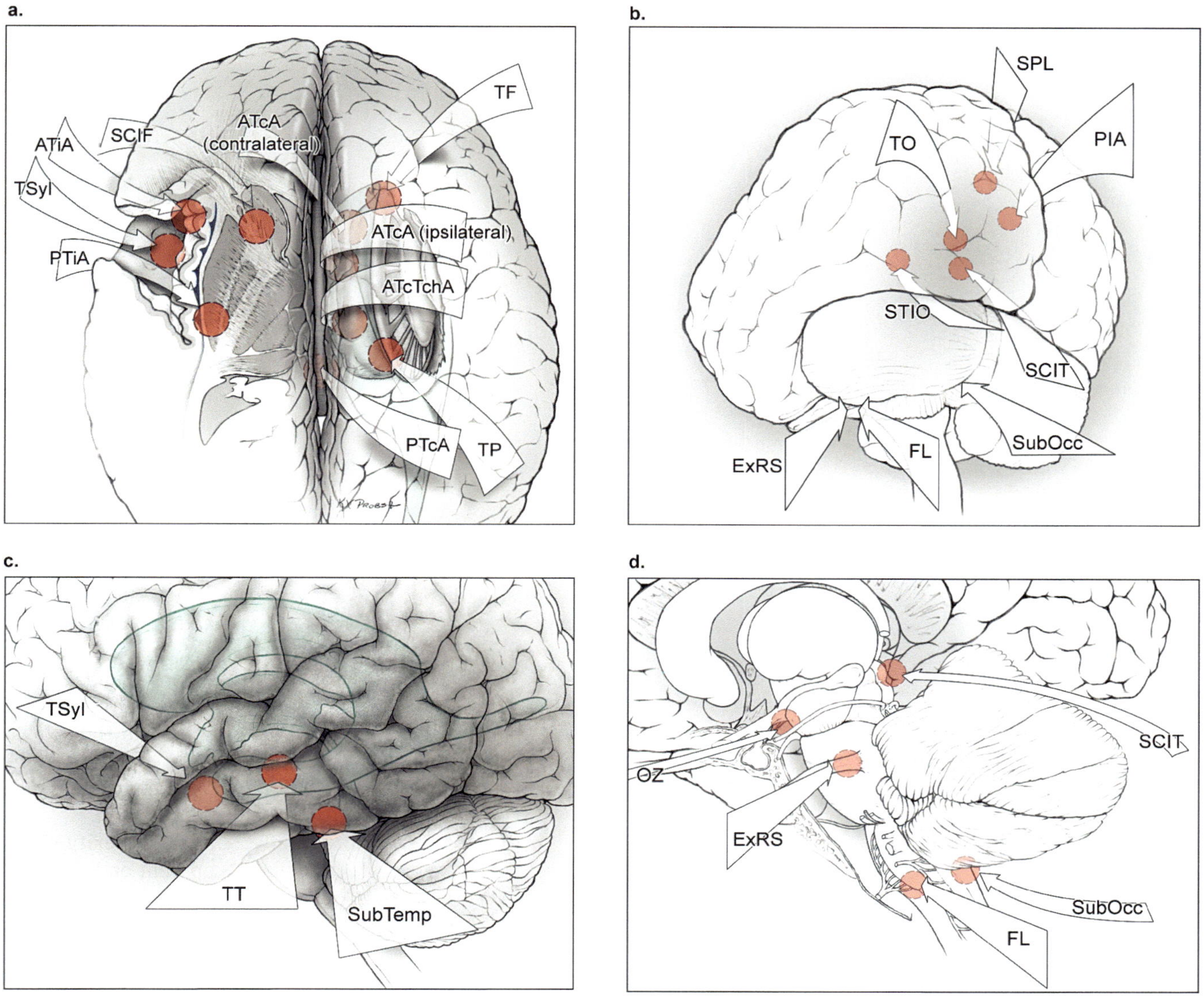

Fig. 2.1 Summary of surgical approaches to brain AVMs. (**a**) Medial interhemispheric and lateral transsylvian approaches to supratentorial AVMs (superior view). (**b**) Posterior and posterolateral approaches to supra- and infratentorial AVMs (posterior oblique view). (**c**) Lateral approaches to temporal AVMs (lateral view). (**d**) Approaches to brainstem AVMs (lateral view). Medial interhemispheric approaches include the anterior interhemispheric approach (AIA); posterior interhemispheric approach (PIA); anterior transcallosal approach (ATcA, ipsilateral and contralateral); anterior transcallosal-transchoroidal approach (ATcTchA); and posterior transcallosal approach (PTcA). Lateral transsylvian approaches include the transsylvian approach (TSyl), anterior transinsular approach (ATiA), posterior transinsular approach (PTiA), and supracarotid-infrafrontal approach (SCIF). Transcortical approaches are used instead of subarachnoid and transventricular routes when hematomas or encephalomalacia create direct, nonanatomic corridors to deep AVMs and include transfrontal (TF), transtemporal (TT), transparietal (TP), transoccipital (TO), and superior parietal lobule (SPL) approaches. Brainstem approaches include the orbitozygomatic-pterional approach (OZ), supracerebellar-infratentorial approach (SCIT), extended retrosigmoid approach (ExRS), far lateral approach (FL), and suboccipital-transventricular approach (SubOcc). Additional posterior approaches include the supratentorial-infraoccipital approach (STIO).

Table 2.1 Summary of Subarachnoid Approaches and Cisternal Dissection

Type	Subtype	Approach	Cisterns
Frontal AVMs			
	Lateral frontal	Transfrontal	None
	Medial frontal	Anterior interhemispheric	CallC
	Paramedian frontal	Transfrontal and anterior interhemispheric	CallC
	Basal frontal	Subfrontal	CarC, ChiC, OlfC
	Sylvian frontal	Transsylvian	SylC
Temporal AVMs			
	Lateral temporal	Transtemporal	None
	Basal temporal	Subtemporal	AmbC
	Medial temporal	Transsylvian or transtemporal	CarC, CruC, SylC
	Sylvian temporal	Transsylvian	SylC
Parieto-occipital AVMs			
	Lateral parieto-occipital	Transparieto-occipital	None
	Medial parieto-occipital	Posterior interhemispheric	QuadC, CallC
	Paramedian parieto-occipital	Transparieto-occipital and posterior interhemispheric	QuadC, CallC
	Basal occipital	Supratentorial-infraoccipital	QuadC
Ventricular/Periventricular AVMs			
	Callosal	Transcallosal	CallC, lateral ventricle
	Ventricular body	Transcallosal-transchoroidal fissure	CallC, lateral, IIIrd ventricles
	Atrial	Superior parietal lobule-transventricular	Lateral ventricle
	Temporal horn	Transtemporal-transventricular	Lateral ventricle
Deep AVMs			
	Pure sylvian	Transsylvian	SylC
	Insular	Transsylvian	SylC
	Basal ganglial	Transsylvian	SylC
	Thalamic	Transcallosal-transchoroidal fissure	CallC, lateral, IIIrd ventricles
Brainstem AVMs			
	Anterior midbrain	Transsylvian-interpeduncular	SylC, CarC, CruC, IpC
	Posterior midbrain	Supracerebellar-infratentorial	QuadC, AmbC
	Anterior pontine	Retrosigmoid-transcisternal	CbPonC, PonC
	Lateral pontine	Retrosigmoid-transcisternal	CbPonC
	Anterior medullary	Transventricular	MagnC, IVth ventricle, MedC
	Lateral medullary	Far lateral-transcisternal	CbMedC, MagnC
Cerebellar AVMs			
	Suboccipital cerebellar	Transcerebellar	MagnC
	Tentorial cerebellar	Supracerebellar-infratentorial	QuadC, MagnC
	Vermian cerebellar	Supracerebellar-infratentorial	QuadC, MagnC
	Tonsillar cerebellar	Transtonsillar	MagnC
	Petrosal cerebellar	Retrosigmoid	CbPonC, CbMedC

and into fissures, maneuvering around and deep to these dilating veins, and separating adhesions to the falx, tentorium, or skull base. For the deepest approaches, subarachnoid dissection extends further into ventricles or deep cisterns around the brainstem to reach the AVM base and optimize the angle of attack. At such depths, the AVM axis and angle of attack are often perpendicular, and expanding the surgical corridor with extensive dissection can improve visualization and maneuverability in the working channel.

Table 2.2 Summary of Subarachnoid Approaches and Their AVM Subtypes

Approaches	AVM Subtypes
Lateral approaches	
Transfrontal	Lateral frontal AVM
Transtemporal	Lateral temporal AVM
	Temporal horn AVM
Transparieto-occipital	Lateral parieto-occipital AVM
	Atrial AVM
	Thalamic AVM (transcortical)
Transsylvian approaches	
Anterior transsylvian	Sylvian frontal AVM
	Sylvian temporal AVM
	Medial temporal AVM (anterior)
	Pure sylvian AVM
Posterior transsylvian	Insular AVM
	Basal ganglial AVM (putamen)
Supracarotid-infrafrontal	Basal ganglial AVM (pallidum)
Transsylvian-interpeduncular	Anterior midbrain AVM
Basal approaches	
Subfrontal	Basal frontal AVM
Subtemporal	Basal temporal AVM
	Medial temporal AVM (posterior)
Supratentorial-infraoccipital	Basal occipital AVM
Medial approaches, supratentorial	
Anterior interhemispheric	Medial frontal AVM
	Paramedian frontal AVM
Posterior interhemispheric	Medial parieto-occipital AVM
	Paramedian parieto-occipital AVM
Anterior transcallosal	Callosal AVM
	Ventricular body AVM
	Thalamic AVM (superior)
Posterior transcallosal	Callosal AVM (splenium)
Contralateral transcallosal	Basal ganglial AVM (caudate)
Transcallosal-transchoroidal fissure	Thalamic AVM (medial)
Medial approaches, infratentorial	
Supracerebellar-infratentorial	Posterior midbrain AVM
	Tentorial cerebellar AVM
	Vermian cerebellar AVM
Transcerebellar	Suboccipital cerebellar AVM
Transtonsillar	Tonsillar cerebellar AVM
Transventricular	Anterior medullary AVM
Skull base approaches	
Orbital-pterional	Basal frontal AVM
Orbitozygomatic-pterional	Medial temporal AVM (anterior)
	Anterior midbrain AVM
Extended retrosigmoid	Anterior pontine AVM
	Lateral pontine AVM
	Petrosal cerebellar AVM
Far lateral	Lateral medullary AVM
	Anterior medullary AVM

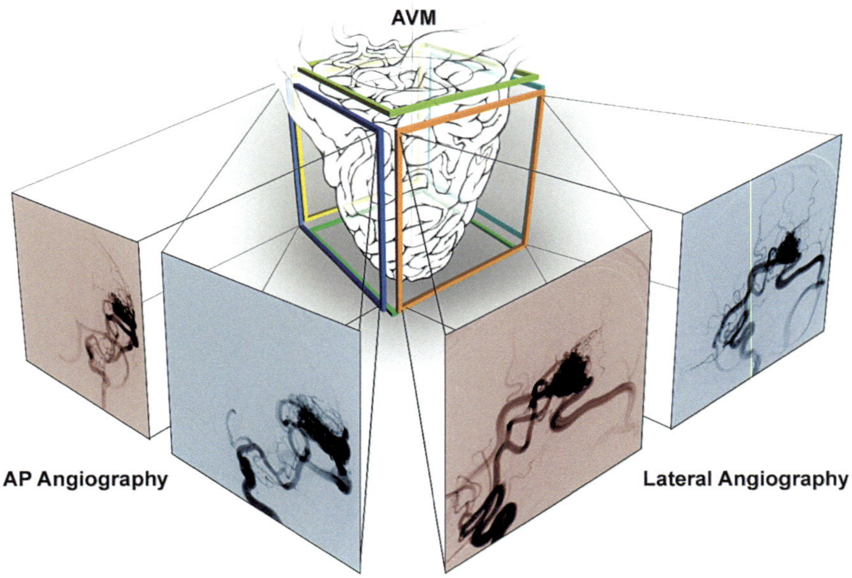

Fig. 2.2 Subarachnoid dissection translates angiographic anatomy onto the surgical field. The angiogram is studied to the point that the intraoperative survey is no longer a process of discovery but one of recognition, allowing the neurosurgeon to anticipate, react, and execute reflexively. AP, anteroposterior.

Translation of Angiographic Anatomy

Beyond AVM exposure, subarachnoid dissection is a translation of angiographic anatomy onto the surgical field. Nothing is more informative about AVMs than the preoperative angiogram, and the anatomic information that was collected preoperatively is transferred during subarachnoid dissection (**Fig. 2.2**). Arteries form the most striking angiographic impressions. Feeding arteries are identified, named, sized, and counted. Their branches, tortuosities, dilatations, and aneurysms are studied for identifying clues and safe points of occlusion. The panorama and clarity of an angiogram are lost intraoperatively where there are only glimpses of arterial anatomy. Angiography shows every anatomic detail and, when scrolled on a computer display, controls perspective, magnification, and hemodynamics. Anteroposterior, lateral, and oblique views define arterial inputs; the velocity of the injected bolus of dye can be slowed and replayed to separate arterial and venous phases of flow; and carotid and vertebral artery injections tease apart contributions from the anterior and posterior circulations and from the right and left sides. This interpretation of arterial hemodynamics is superimposed on the surgical field as fissures are split and anatomy around the AVM is explored.

As striking as arteries are angiographically, the veins are the best landmarks. They sit on the brain surface and are encountered first in the dissection. Their trunks, secondary branches, and varices are so much larger in caliber than arteries, and they conceal the arteries that travel with them. Rewinding the angiogram reverses time and flow supernaturally on a computer, juxtaposing artery and vein on the computer screen as they are in the surgical field. This technology reveals the clues and landmarks that inform the dissection.

Angiography shows normal anatomy better than direct inspection, like the distal course of a transit artery that supplies the AVM but also continues en passage to normal brain. Similarly, normal bystander arteries that do not contribute to the AVM at all are distinguished from other feeders by tracing their course alongside the AVM, which is easier angiographically than microsurgically. Normal anatomy noted in advance is correlated with vascular structures as they are revealed in the subarachnoid dissection. Angiography demonstrates margins that are compact and diffuse better than direct inspection. Preoperative embolization offers additional insights through selective injections that resolve the anatomy of branches, through flow reduction that demonstrates the remaining arterial supply, with postembolization runs that show the extent of AVM occlusion, and with coils or glue casts that offer identifying markers intraoperatively.

Angiography and the ability to translate its information to the surgical field is a skill akin to reading a map in the wilderness; when used wisely, angiograms and maps will guide the journey and prevent getting lost. An investment of time and attention to both the angiographic review preoperatively and the subarachnoid dissection phase intraoperatively is essential. I study the angiogram to the point that the intraoperative survey is no longer a process of discovery but one of recognition. Things in the surgical field happen quickly and under pressure with many visual and anatomic limitations, and I cannot expect to "figure out" an AVM as I am operating. Thorough preparation and extensive subarachnoid dissection give the neurosurgeon the ability to anticipate, react, and execute reflexively.

3 Draining Veins

Absolute Preservation

The most basic and important tenet of arteriovenous malformation (AVM) surgery is that the draining vein must be preserved until the very end of the resection. It seems counterintuitive in the presence of ferocious arterial afferents to place efferent veins at the center of the AVM dissection strategy. It also seems contrary to aneurysm surgery, which places afferent arteries at the center of the dissection strategy. Aneurysms originate from the afferent artery and are controlled by proximal temporary occlusion. When an aneurysm ruptures intraoperatively, the catastrophe is managed by tamponading the dome, suctioning the field, and occluding afferent and efferent arteries with temporary clips. Gaining arterial control enables permanent clipping of the aneurysm. In contrast, AVMs rupture intraoperatively when venous outflow is occluded prematurely by mistake. Intranidal pressure increases, the AVM distends, and before long it ruptures and torrential bleeding floods the surgical field. There is no orderly sequence of winning maneuvers as there is with aneurysm rupture. Tamponade is ineffective because there are multiple bleeding sites, suction may not clear the field, and afferent arteries are too numerous to control quickly or completely. Therefore, absolute preservation of the efferent vein must always be the first priority in AVM surgery. Arterial afferents may be the source of nasty bleeding during the resection, but they are not the cause of AVM rupture. Although they must all be isolated, occluded, and divided eventually, they are not at the center of AVM dissection strategy.

Recognizing Veins

The secret to preserving draining veins is not mistaking them for feeding arteries. Color is usually the most striking difference between artery and vein, but AVM draining veins and feeding arteries are both bright red. Therefore, color is deceptive and cannot be trusted. Size is a more reliable distinguishing feature. Although some veins or varices are massively dilated with no question about their true identity, others are merely large and resemble a dilated artery. However, arteries dilate only so much, even when feeding a high-flow AVM with fast intranidal shunts. Thick smooth muscle cell layers and elastic laminae limit the distension of feeding arteries, such that they rarely exceed diameters of 4 mm. Veins, on the other hand, are little more than an endothelial lining of intima, a thin layer of smooth muscle cells in the tunica media, and some collagen fibers in adventitia. Veins situated on the receiving end of an arteriovenous shunt enlarge easily. Therefore, any vessel greater than 4 mm in diameter, no matter how cylindrical or "arterial" it appears, is a vein until proven otherwise.

These structural differences between arteries and veins can be detected under the illumination and magnification of the operating microscope. The muscular striations in thicker arterial wall can be visualized directly, and they mute the color of arteries to slightly pink. The lack of smooth muscle cells in thinner venous wall imparts a smooth uniformity and a brighter red color. Additionally, thin venous walls are more translucent, and the mixing of oxygenated and deoxygenated blood can be observed through them. Such mixing does not occur in arteries and cannot be observed through their thicker walls.

Following a vessel as it leaves an AVM may help determine its identity. Arteries dive into sulci and fissures as they are traced proximally, whereas veins rise to cortical surfaces en route to sinuses. An arterialized vein merges with normal venous tributaries, with mixing of darker blood at their confluence. In contrast, an artery bifurcates and sends pial branches to adjacent cortex, and there is no such mixing. Temporary "test" occlusion of a vessel with a forceps or temporary clip will darken a vein distal to the occlusion but not an artery. Embolic agents like glue, Onyx, polyvinyl alcohol particles, and coils are easy clues to a vessel's arterial nature, but they create a paradoxical color reversal that darkens feeding arteries with intraluminal thrombus while an adjacent vein remains bright red. Aggressive embolization with newer agents like Onyx may nearly occlude the AVM, to the point that even an active draining vein may be almost normal in color.

The urge to attack an AVM and subdue a big feeding artery is strong. However, that urge must be countered by scrutiny of the vessel and all its morphological nuances. Before committing to occlusion, ask, "Is it artery or is it vein?" In addition, know the veins that are in play for each AVM subtype (**Table 3.1**).

Table 3.1 Summary of Veins in the Seven AVM Locations

Abbreviation	Vein
Frontal veins	
FrPolV	Frontopolar vein
AntFrV	Anterior frontal vein
MidFrV	Middle frontal vein
PosFrV	Posterior frontal vein
PreCenV	Precentral vein
CenV	Central vein
MedFrV	Medial frontal veins (anterior, central, posterior)
PcaV	Pericallosal veins (anterior, posterior)
FrSylV	Frontosylvian vein
SupSylV	Superficial sylvian vein
DeepSylV	Deep sylvian vein
OrbFrV	Orbitofrontal vein (anterior, posterior)
OlfV	Olfactory vein
Temporal veins	
AntTempV	Anterior temporal vein
MidTempV	Middle temporal vein
PosTempV	Posterior temporal vein
Labbe	Vein of Labbé
TempBasV	Temporal basal vein (anterior, middle, posterior)
UncV	Uncal vein
HippoV	Anterior hippocampal vein
MedTempV	Medial temporal vein
BVR	Basal vein of Rosenthal
Parieto-occipital veins	
PosCenV	Postcentral vein
AntParV	Anterior parietal vein
PostParV	Posterior parietal vein
OccV	Occipital vein
Trolard	Vein of Trolard
ParaCenV	Paracentral vein
MedParV	Medial parietal veins (anterior, posterior)
AntCalcV	Anterior calcarine vein (internal occipital vein)
PosCalcV	Posterior calcarine vein
PcaV	Pericallosal veins (anterior, posterior)
SplenV	Splenial vein
OccBasV	Occipital basal vein
Ventricular and deep veins	
SepV	Septal vein (anterior, posterior)
CauV	Caudate vein (anterior, posterior)
ThaStrV	Thalamostriate vein
ICV	Internal cerebral vein
AtrV	Atrial vein (medial, lateral)
ChorV	Choroidal vein (superior, inferior)
VoG	Vein of Galen
Brainstem veins	
MAPonMesV	Median anterior pontomesencephalic vein
MAMedV	Median anterior medullary vein
LAPonMesV	Lateral anterior pontomesencephalic vein
LAMedV	Lateral anterior medullary vein
LMesV	Lateral mesencephalic vein
LMedV	Lateral medullary vein
ReOlvV	Retro-olivary veins
PedV	Peduncular vein
PComV	Posterior communicating vein
VPonMesS	Vein of the pontomesencephalic sulcus
VPonMedS	Vein of the pontomedullary sulcus
TrPonV	Transverse pontine vein
TrMedV	Transverse medullary vein
MPMedV	Median posterior medullary vein
TecV	Tectal vein
Cerebellar veins	
IHemV	Inferior hemispheric vein
SHemV	Superior hemispheric vein (anterior, posterior)
AHemV	Anterior hemispheric vein
SVerV	Superior vermian vein
IVerV	Inferior vermian vein
PreCenCblV	Precentral cerebellar vein
TonsV	Tonsillar vein
ReTonsV	Retrotonsillar vein
SPetrV	Superior petrosal vein
IPetrV	Inferior petrosal vein
VCPonF	Vein of cerebellopontine fissure
VCMedF	Vein of cerebellomedullary fissure
VCMesF	Vein of cerebellomesencephalic fissure
Sinuses	
CavS	Cavernous sinus
SphParS	Sphenoparietal sinus
SSS	Superior sagittal sinus
ISS	Inferior sagittal sinus
SPS	Superior petrosal sinus
IPS	Inferior petrosal sinus
StrS	Straight sinus
SigmS	Sigmoid sinus
TrvS	Transverse sinus
SphBasS	Sphenobasal sinus
SphPetS	Sphenopetrosal sinus
Torc	Torcular
TentS	Tentorial sinus

Compass and Odometer

Approximately one third of AVMs are beneath the cortical surface and two thirds have superficial venous drainage, which means that many of these subcortical AVMs have only an arterialized vein on the surface. The vein, therefore, becomes a compass that guides the dissection to the nidus. Dissecting along a draining vein from the outset is inherently risky; one wrong move can injure it, induce bleeding before even seeing the AVM, or compromise outflow in the process of controlling the bleeding. Distended veins are difficult to get around because of their large size, requiring gentle traction with a sucker or mobilization back and forth (dynamic retraction). As the dissection deepens, the vein can obstruct the surgical field. For example, some sylvian AVMs are covered by superficial sylvian veins and must be dissected between branches in this complex. Similarly, medial frontal and medial parieto-occipital AVMs are covered by medial veins that ascend and bridge to the superior sagittal sinus, which not only crowds the surgical corridor but also may tether the hemisphere and neutralize the benefits of gravity retraction. When superficial veins become obstacles, they are easily injured by passing instruments or fixed retractors. When attention is focused deep in the field, it is easy to lose sight of these veins. Veins are preserved by shifting the dissection to either side, connecting planes beneath the veins, keeping them irrigated and unstretched, and maintaining peripheral vision with less magnification on the microscope.

The draining vein also becomes an "odometer" that measures the progress of the resection as its color changes from red to purple to blue. The vein offers a visual signal throughout the case. Dramatic color changes do not occur until the later stages of resection, but quieting of AVM hemodynamics can sometimes be appreciated in the earlier stages through the window of the odometer. A stubbornly red vein is a clear signal that important arterial input remains. Persistent arterialization of the vein may result from incomplete circumdissection of a deep plane, deep perforating artery supply, or feeders hiding along the underbelly of the draining vein. Even small contributions from deep perforating arteries keep the draining vein of a large AVM surprisingly red. Red veins mean that the fight is still on, and blue veins are the AVM's white flag of surrender.

Secondary Veins

The tenet of absolute preservation of the draining vein applies to the primary vein, the main one that collects most of the AVM's outflow (**Fig. 3.1**). Each AVM subtype has a pre-

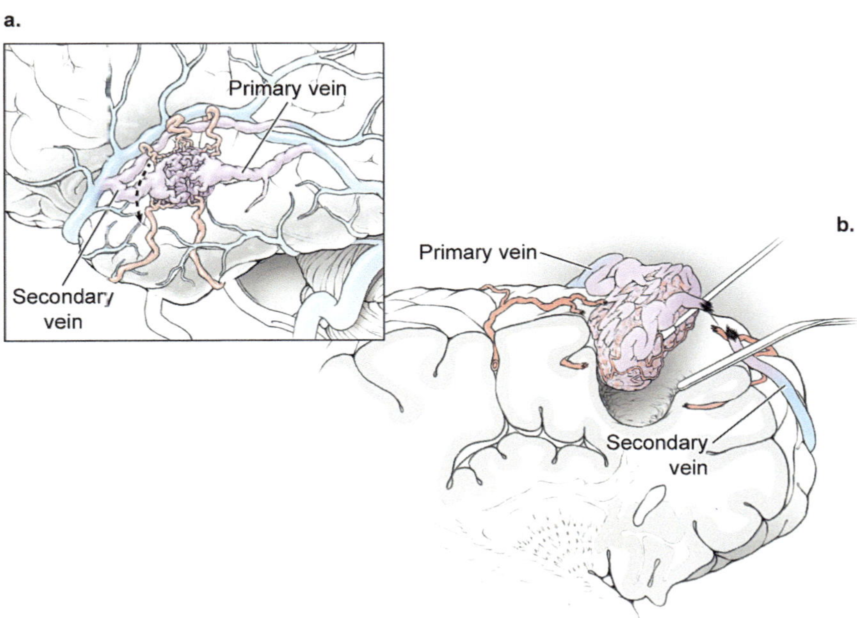

Fig. 3.1 Preservation of the draining vein is the most important tenet of AVM surgery. (**a**) The AVMs with multiple draining veins require designating a primary draining vein that must be preserved and secondary veins that may be sacrificed during the resection as arterial input is reduced. (**b**) Venous trimming de-tethers the AVM and advances circumdissection.

Table 3.2 Summary of AVM Subtypes and Their Draining Veins

Type	Subtype	Draining Veins
Frontal AVMs		
	Lateral frontal	Ascending convexity veins (FrPolV, AntFrV, MidFrV, PosFrV, PreCenV, CenV); descending convexity veins (FrSylV, SupSylV, DeepSylV)
	Medial frontal	Ascending medial veins (MedFrV); descending medial veins (PcaV)
	Paramedian frontal	Ascending convexity and medial veins; descending convexity and medial veins
	Basal frontal	Orbitofrontal veins (OrbFrV, FrPolV, OlfV)
	Sylvian frontal	Sylvian veins (FrSylV, SupSylV, DeepSylV)
Temporal AVMs		
	Lateral temporal	Descending convexity veins (AntTempV, MidTempV, PosTempV), ascending convexity veins (TempSylV)
	Basal temporal	TempBasV
	Medial temporal	UncV, HippoV, MedTempV, BVR
	Sylvian temporal	TempSylV, SupSylV, DeepSylV
Parieto-occipital AVMs		
	Lateral parieto-occipital	Ascending convexity veins (PosCenV, AntParV, PosParV, OccV)
	Medial parieto-occipital	Ascending medial veins (ParaCenV, MedParV, PosCalcV); descending medial veins (SpleV, AntCalcV)
	Paramedian parieto-occipital	Ascending convexity veins (PosCenV, AntParV, PosParV, OccV); ascending medial veins (ParaCenV, MedParV, PosCalcV)
	Basal occipital	OccBasV
Ventricular/Periventricular AVMs		
	Callosal	SepV, CauV, ThaStrV, SpleV, MedAtrV
	Ventricular body	ICV
	Atrial	MedAtrV, LatAtrV
	Temporal horn	ChorV, BVR
Deep AVMs		
	Pure sylvian	SupSylV, DeepSylV
	Insular	DeepSylV
	Basal ganglial	CauV, ThaStrV
	Thalamic	ICV, BVR
Brainstem AVMs		
	Anterior midbrain	MAPonMesV, PedV, PComV
	Posterior midbrain	TecV, SVerV, PreCenCblV
	Anterior pontine	MAPonMesV, SPetrV
	Lateral pontine	SPetrV
	Anterior medullary	MAMedV
	Lateral medullary	LMedV, MAMedV
Cerebellar AVMs		
	Suboccipital cerebellar	IVerV, IHemV, Torc, TrvS
	Tentorial cerebellar	SHemV, TentS, VoG, Torc, TrvS
	Vermian cerebellar	SVerV, VoG; IVerV, Torc
	Tonsillar cerebellar	TonsV, ReTonsV
	Petrosal cerebellar	AHemV, VCPonF, SPetrV, SPS

dictable primary vein that can be anticipated (**Table 3.2**). In addition, many AVMs and especially the large ones have multiple draining veins radiating in different directions. Arteriovenous malformation outflow distributes within the nidus and communicates with these draining veins, and preservation of every draining vein until the very end of AVM resection is not necessary. In other words, a secondary draining vein can be sacrificed safely during the resection without precipitating AVM rupture. This requires first designating the primary vein to be preserved, and second sufficiently reducing arterial input with a combination of embolization, feeding artery occlusion, and circumdissection.

The primary vein is typically the AVM's largest and lies at the far end of the trail of dissection. For example, the trail of dissection of a lateral temporal AVM is from anterior to posterior with interruption of middle cerebral artery (MCA) feeders along the anterosuperior margin. After designating the draining vein of Labbé as primary and the superficial sylvian vein as secondary, the latter is sacrificed and the nidus is mobilized posteriorly. The vein of Labbé becomes a pedicle or tail around which the dissection advances. Venous trimming, or division of secondary draining veins, de-tethers the AVM, increases access to its surgical sides, opens deep planes, and advances circumdissection toward completion.

Taking a secondary vein and reducing outflow must be proportionate to the remaining arterial inflow. One must be careful not to overestimate the extent of one's arterial occlusions or underestimate the remaining supply. As a rule of thumb, secondary veins should be sacrificed only when they are already darkening in color, or when the AVM tolerates temporary test occlusion of the vein. Veins are trimmed only after all other superficial dissection has been maximized. The concepts of secondary veins and venous trimming respect the tenet of preserving primary veins, without generalizing to other veins whose sacrifice might facilitate AVM resection.

Deep Veins

Deep draining veins are neither a "compass" nor an "odometer." They are present in approximately one third of AVMs, but hide from view until it is time to remove the AVM. They offer no feedback during the dissection, do not guide dissection, and do not measure progress like the superficial veins. Therefore, a deep draining vein adds little to surgical strategy. The importance of deep veins comes from the Spetzler-Martin grading system, where they are surrogates for deep AVM location, which is a real determinant of the risk of surgical morbidity. Deep veins sit beneath the AVM and are not surgical obstacles or at risk of injury like superficial veins. Whereas deep primary veins drain the nidus throughout the circumdissection, deep secondary veins can be divided to release the nidus and scoop it out. Deep veins indicate AVM extension to the ventricle where there will be an ependymal plane of dissection.

4 Feeding Arteries

Arterial Occlusion Techniques

Arteries are occluded at their point of contact with the arteriovenous malformation (AVM). Occlusion more proximally sacrifices intervening normal branches and infarcts adjacent brain, whereas occlusion more distally can elicit bleeding from the nidus or preserve proximal feeding branches. The point of contact may be indistinct, and branches may be difficult to differentiate as normal or afferent. Large feeding arteries on the cortical surface are welcome targets because they can be eliminated early and easily. They are cauterized with bipolar forceps along a 3- to 7-mm segment. As a general rule, arteries coagulate best after flow arrest. The bipolars are walked down the artery in a proximal-to-distal direction, coagulating a downstream artery that has no flow. Walking the bipolars up the artery from distal to proximal is less effective because the upstream artery remains under pressure and can rupture with cautery. The application of electrical current across an artery shrinks wall tissues, tapers the artery, and ultimately obliterates its lumen. Arteries and arterioles have thick elastic and smooth muscle cell layers that coagulate and occlude easily. In contrast, tiny perforating arteries have thin walls with little elastic and smooth muscle cell layers to coagulate. Consequently, they resist bipolar cautery and are difficult to occlude. Flow arrest with a proximal microclip may transform an otherwise incoagulable perforator, but if not, the perforator is closed with a distal clip and divided. At the opposite extreme, large arteries with thick walls may also be difficult to occlude with bipolar cautery. Their caliber and high flow may be too much for coagulation alone and may require permanent aneurysm clips for closure (typically 5- or 7-mm straight clips).

An artery that has been exposed to radiation during AVM radiosurgery undergoes morphological changes that enhance its coagulability. Radiation damages DNA in rapidly dividing endothelial cells, and as they attempt to regenerate, they are depleted over time. Intimal disintegration exposes smooth muscle cells and triggers a proliferative response in the medial layer. The progressive growth of the media thickens the arterial wall and constricts the lumen, which is the mechanism for radiosurgery's occlusive action. Incompletely obliterated AVMs have irradiated arteries that are thickened with morphological changes resembling atherosclerosis. These are perhaps the most coagulable of all AVM feeding arteries.

Embolized arteries are altered by intraluminal casts of embolic agents that vary greatly in their manageability. *N*-butyl cyanoacrylate (NBCA) glue forms a hard, translucent cast that is difficult to transect. Polyvinyl acetate (PVA) forms a much softer, particulate plug that can be cut, but can also crumble and reopen. Onyx forms a soft, rubbery cast that is also easily cut. Coils must be cut with heavy microscissors and may not be completely occlusive. Embolized arteries are divided to detach the AVM, and normal artery proximal to the embolic cast may need to be controlled in case flow persists around or through the embolic agent.

Terminal Feeding Arteries

Afferent arteries to and around AVMs can be categorized as terminal feeding arteries, transit arteries, perforating arteries, choroidal arteries, and bystander arteries (**Fig. 4.1**). The terminal feeding artery is dedicated to the AVM, terminates in the nidus, and has no normal territory to supply distally. It may have proximal branches that supply normal territory before it terminates. It travels in the subarachnoid space, is often large in caliber, and may have a single high-flow shunt or multiple peri- or intranidal branches. The terminal feeding artery is interrupted at the AVM margin with cautery or clips without concern for distal flow, but sometimes wraps around the nidus, transmitting normal branches before diving in. Terminal feeding arteries are quick victories.

Transit Arteries

The transit artery is treacherous. It is not dedicated to the AVM and does not terminate in the nidus, and instead has proximal branches that supply normal territories, AVM branches that supply the nidus, and distal branches that supply normal territories. It is referred to as an artery "en passage" because it continues on a course past the AVM. Occlusion of the distal trunk results in a downstream infarction postoperatively. The caliber of a transit artery is smaller than a terminal feeder but larger than a bystander artery. Branches from a transit artery are typically twigs that make a contribution to the AVM but are not major shunts. The

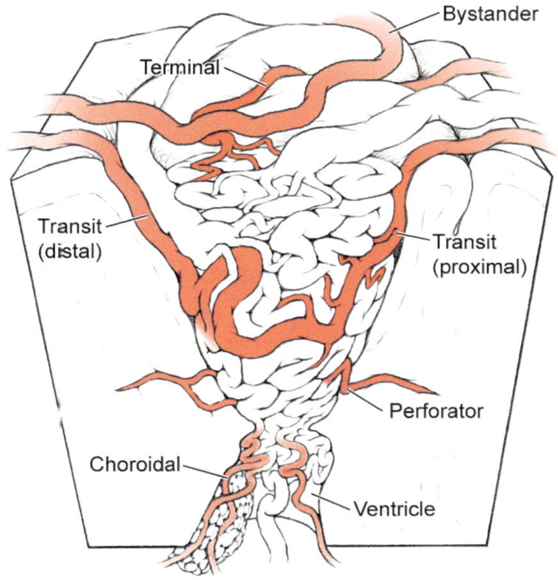

Fig. 4.1 Types of AVM arteries: terminal feeding artery, transit artery, perforating artery, choroidal artery, and bystander artery. The terminal feeding artery ends in the nidus without normal territory distally and has large caliber and high flow. The transit or "en passage" artery has AVM branches as well as proximal and distal branches to normal territories. The perforating artery is a small-caliber feeding artery that traverses deep white matter and ends in the nidus with no normal territory to supply distally. The choroidal feeding artery is also small and terminal, but traverses the ventricle to supply an ependymal AVM surface. The bystander artery is a normal artery without AVM supply that courses alongside or adjacent to the nidus.

challenge of preserving the distal artery is accomplished by skeletonization: occluding the feeding twigs one by one to prune the parent trunk and preserve its distal flow (**Fig. 4.2**). These branches are easy to coagulate and rarely require clips. Feeding twigs can be difficult to differentiate from normal branches and the distal trunk, but skeletonizing in a distal-to-proximal direction solves this problem. The distal trunk is identified past the AVM and dissected retrograde toward the nidus. Branches that can be traced to the AVM margin are interrupted, and those that can be traced to adjacent cortex are spared. Feeders are more distended, tortuous, and dysmorphic than normal branches. Retrograde skeletonization leads to the proximal side of the AVM and enables the freed transit artery to mobilize off the AVM. The pericallosal arteries and insular segments of middle cerebral artery (MCA) are examples of transit arteries that are typically skeletonized with callosal and sylvian AVMs, respectively.

Perforating Arteries

The perforating artery is a small-caliber, terminal feeding artery that traverses deep white matter and ends in the nidus

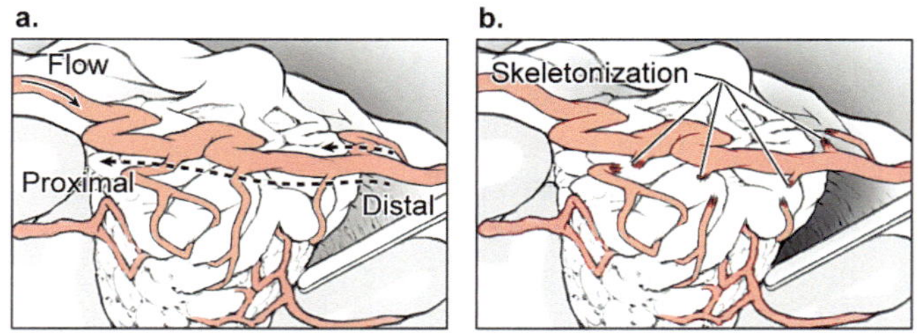

Fig. 4.2 (**a**) Skeletonization of a transit artery occludes feeding branches to the AVM and preserves flow in the distal parent artery. (**b**) The efferent trunk is protected by retrograde dissection in a distal-to-proximal direction.

with no normal territory to supply distally. Its small caliber, deep location, and input on the ependymal surface make it different from the larger terminal artery in the subarachnoid spaces. Perforators are approximately 1 mm in diameter and include the medial lenticulostriates from the A1 anterior cerebral artery (ACA), the lateral lenticulostriates from the M1 MCA, the insular perforators from the M2 MCA, thalamoperforators from the posterior communicating artery (PCoA) and the P1 posterior cerebral artery (PCA), and brainstem perforators. Although perforating arteries are small, their blood flow is vigorous. Charlie Wilson used to call these "red devils": they bleed briskly, resist cautery, course through eloquent white matter tracts, and are encountered on the deep plane of the AVM where they are hard to see. Their thin walls provide little substrate for electrocautery and they require liberal use of microclips, preferably before they start bleeding. When bleeding, they can be drawn into the sucker to dry the field and clipped proximally while suction holds the artery. An uncontrolled bleeding perforator is dangerous because it can retract into the white matter, damage brain tissue, and force pursuit deeper into vital tracts and nuclei. Red devils are more fearsome than large feeders.

Choroidal Feeding Arteries

Like the perforating artery, the choroidal feeding artery is small, terminal, and often on a deep side of the AVM, but it traverses the ventricle rather than deep white matter. Choroidal feeders supply the ependymal surface of an AVM. They originate from the anterior choroidal artery (AChA) in the temporal horn of the lateral ventricle to supply temporal AVMs; from the lateral posterior choroidal artery (PChA) in the atrium to supply atrial, thalamic, and parieto-occipital AVMs; and from the medial PChA in the velum interpositum and ventricular body to supply thalamic, basal ganglial, and ventricular body AVMs. Anastomotic interconnections between choroidal arteries enable multiple choroidal inputs. Their plexal segments swim in cerebrospinal fluid (CSF), are based in non-eloquent choroidal fissures, and only supply the choroid plexus, making them less threatening than perforating arteries. However, they too can bleed vigorously, and their deep location makes them dangerous. Bleeding can quickly fill the ventricle; the feeder can retract beneath the AVM or beyond visualization; and brain can herniate outwardly. When possible, choroidal arteries are exposed proximal to the AVM and occluded before they reach its margin. Their walls are thick and responsive to cautery.

Bystander Arteries

Uninvolved bystander arteries are normal arteries that do not supply an AVM, but course alongside or adjacent to the nidus. They are recognized best on the angiogram preoperatively and are protected intraoperatively. Their caliber is smaller than that of feeding arteries, and they have normal morphology, bifurcations, and branches. As with skeletonization of transit arteries, distal-to-proximal dissection separates bystanders safely from the AVM and identifies them as normal arteries. Once separated, they are swept aside and covered with cottonoids during AVM dissection. Insular segments of the MCA are bystander arteries with many sylvian AVMs, as are contralateral ACA vessels associated with a medial frontal AVMs and contralateral posterior inferior cerebellar artery (PICA) vessels associated with tonsillar cerebellar AVMs. With other AVMs such as insular and basal ganglial AVMs, they are central in the surgical corridor and the dissection proceeds around and deep to them.

AVM Subtype Supply

Each AVM subtype has its unique set of arterial feeders that may originate from one or more parent arteries (**Table 4.1**) and may include terminal feeders, transit arteries, perforators, and choroidal arteries. The combination of arteries that supplies a particular AVM is like a fingerprint that uniquely identifies the subtype (**Table 4.2**). Attacking and ultimately defeating an AVM comes from strangling its arterial supply. Some superficial afferents are exposed in subarachnoidal spaces and interrupted early during pial dissection; other afferents intersect the AVM's sides and are closed during parenchymal dissection; and deep afferents may not be eliminated until ependymal dissection finally accesses the remaining supply. The progressive throttling of arterial input de-pressurizes, quiets, and softens the AVM, reducing it to something more like a cavernous malformation.

Table 4.1 Summary of Intracranial Branch Arteries

Branches		Segment
Internal carotid artery branches		
OphA	Ophthalmic artery	C6
SHA	Superior hypophyseal artery	C6
PCoA	Posterior communicating artery	C7
AChA	Anterior choroidal artery	C7
Anterior cerebral artery branches		
mLSA	Medial lenticulostriate artery	A1
RAH	Recurrent artery of Heubner	A2
OrbFrA	Orbitofrontal artery (ACA)	A2
FrPolA	Frontopolar artery	A2
CmaA	Callosomarginal artery	A3
PcaA	Pericallosal artery	A4
AIFA	Anterior internal frontal artery	A2
MIFA	Middle internal frontal artery	A3
PIFA	Posterior internal frontal artery	A4
ParaCenA	Paracentral artery	A4
InfParA	Inferior parietal artery	A5
SupParA	Superior parietal artery	A5
Middle cerebral artery branches		
TempPolA	Temporopolar artery	M1
ATA	Anterior temporal artery	M1
lLSA	Lateral lenticulostriate artery	M2
InsP	Insular perforators	M2
OrbFrA	Orbitofrontal artery (MCA)	M4
PreFrA	Prefrontal artery	M4
PreCenA	Precentral artery	M4
CenA	Central artery	M4
AntParA	Anterior parietal artery	M4
PosParA	Posterior parietal artery	M4
AngA	Angular artery	M4
TempOccA	Temporo-occipital artery	M4
PosTempA	Posterior temporal artery (MCA)	M4
MidTempA	Middle temporal artery	M4
Posterior cerebral artery branches		
PosThaP	Posterior thalamoperforators	P1
CirP	Circumflex perforators	P1
PedP	Peduncular perforators	P2
ThGenP	Thalamogeniculate perforators	P2
mPChA	Medial posterior choroidal artery	P2
lPChA	Lateral posterior choroidal artery	P2
HippoA	Hippocampal artery	P2
PosTempA	Posterior temporal artery (PCA)	P2
CalcA	Calcarine artery	P4
ParOccA	Parieto-occipital artery	P4
SplenA	Splenial artery	P4
Vertebrobasilar artery branches		
PCA	Posterior cerebral artery	
SCA	Superior cerebellar artery	
AICA	Anterior inferior cerebellar artery	
PICA	Posterior inferior cerebellar artery	

Table 4.2 Summary of AVM Subtypes and Their Feeding Arteries

Type	Subtype	Feeding Arteries
Frontal AVMs		
	Lateral frontal	MCA–Sup. Trunk (OrbFrA, PreFrA, PreCenA, CenA)
	Medial frontal	ACA, PcaA, CmaA
	Paramedian frontal	MCA–Sup. Trunk; ACA, PcaA, CmaA
	Basal frontal	MCA (OrbFrA, PreFrA), ACA (A1, A2, OrbFrA, FrPolA)
	Sylvian frontal	M3 MCA–Frontal
Temporal AVMs		
	Lateral temporal	MCA–Inf. Trunk (MidTempA, PosTempA, TempOccA, AngA); TempPolA, ATA
	Basal temporal	P2 PCA (PosTempA, HippoA)
	Medial temporal	AChA, PCoA, HippoA, PosTempA, TempPolA
	Sylvian temporal	M3 MCA–Temporal
Parieto-occipital AVMs		
	Lateral parieto-occipital	MCA (CenA, AntParA, PosParA, AngA, TempOccA)
	Medial parieto-occipital	PCA (ParOccA, CalcA, SplenA); ACA (SupParA, InfParA)
	Paramedian parieto-occipital	MCA (CenA, AntParA, PosParA, AngA); PCA (ParOccA, CalcA); ACA (SupParA, InfParA)
	Basal occipital	PCA (PosTempA, CalcA)
Ventricular/Periventricular AVMs		
	Callosal	ACA, PcaA (bilateral)
	Ventricular body	mPChA
	Atrial	lPChA
	Temporal horn	AChA
Deep AVMs		
	Pure sylvian	M2 and M3 MCA
	Insular	M2 MCA, InsP
	Basal ganglial	lLSA, InsP, mLSA, RAH
	Thalamic	AntThaP, PosThaP, mPChA, lPChA
Brainstem AVMs		
	Anterior midbrain	P1 PCA, PosThaP, PedP (bilateral)
	Posterior midbrain	s3 SCA, CirP (bilateral)
	Anterior pontine	a1 AICA, s1 SCA, BA
	Lateral pontine	a2 AICA, s2 SCA
	Anterior medullary	VA
	Lateral medullary	VA, p1, p2 PICA
Cerebellar AVMs		
	Suboccipital cerebellar	s4 SCA, a4 AICA, p5 PICA
	Tentorial cerebellar	s4 SCA
	Vermian cerebellar	s4 SCA (bilateral)
	Tonsillar cerebellar	p4, p5 PICA
	Petrosal cerebellar	a4 AICA

5 Pial Dissection

■ Arterial Fronts

Previous phases of dissection—arteriovenous malformation (AVM) exposure, subarachnoid approach, definition of draining veins, and the identification of feeding arteries—are mere saber-rattling. The AVM is surveyed but not disturbed. Pial dissection is the opening salvo and the start of the battle. Early engagement is directed at surface feeding arteries on the top of the box, making the easy strikes without major effort.

Each AVM subtype has specific pial sites called arterial fronts where these superficial inputs intersect the AVM, like a line of battle where armies clash (**Fig. 5.1**). An arterial front lies on a side of the AVM box, usually an edge on the top side, and can be characterized by the side of the AVM box (anterior, lateral, superior, etc.), the cortical anatomy, and the feeding arteries. As an example, the lateral temporal AVM is based on the temporal convexity and supplied mainly by middle cerebral artery (MCA) branches from the inferior trunk of its bifurcation, like middle and posterior temporal arteries. These cortical arteries emerge from the sylvian fissure and travel across the superior temporal gyrus to reach the AVM's superior margin. Therefore, the lateral temporal AVM has a superior front of M4 arterial supply defined by the superior temporal gyrus. Arterial fronts are the initial points of attack, occluding significant input and weakening the AVM early on.

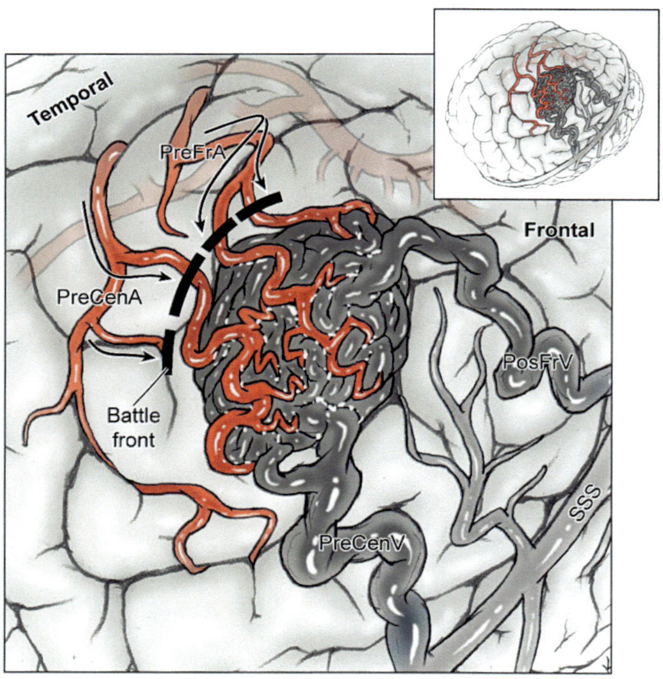

Fig. 5.1 Each AVM subtype, like this lateral frontal AVM (*inset*), has specific pial sites or arterial fronts where superficial inputs intersect the AVM like a line of battle where armies clash, defined by the AVM side, cortical anatomy, and feeding arteries. Arterial fronts are the initial points of attack (*bold dashed line*).

An arterial front can be defined for every AVM (**Table 5.1**), and these fronts inform the pial dissection. Most AVMs have one major arterial front, such as the lateral temporal AVM, but some have as many as three. The basal frontal AVM that has a lateral front of M4 MCA branches (orbitofrontal artery [OrbFrA]) arriving over the lateral orbital gyrus, a medial front of A2 anterior cerebral artery (ACA) branches (OrbFrA and frontopolar artery [FrPolA]) arriving over the gyrus rectus, and a posterior front of A1 ACA branches arriving over posterior orbital gyrus. An AVM like the lateral temporal AVM can have a major superior front and a minor inferior front of posterior cerebral artery (PCA) supply if situated low on the convexity in inferior temporal gyrus. Some AVMs have one front that receives inputs from different arteries, like the medial temporal AVM that is supplied by the internal carotid artery (ICA) (anterior choroidal artery [AChA] and posterior communicating artery [PCoA]) and PCA (hippocampal artery and posterior temporal artery).

Arterial fronts situated on pial surfaces are advantageous for their ease of attack, but some AVMs have pial fronts that are only accessible later after parenchymal dissection, like the medial front of posterior temporal arteries (P2 PCA) associated with a basal temporal AVM. Other deep AVMs have only parenchymal fronts, like the lateral front of insular perforators and the inferior front of lateral lenticulostriate arteries associated with a basal ganglial AVM.

Table 5.1 Summary of AVM Subtypes and Their Cortical Anatomy and Arterial Fronts

Type	Subtype	Cortical Anatomy	Arterial Front
Frontal AVMs			
	Lateral frontal	SFG, MFG, IFG, precentral gyrus	Inferior (IFG/M4)
	Medial frontal	SFG, paracentral lobule, cingulate gyrus	Anterior (cingulate/A3, A4)
	Paramedian frontal	SFG, precentral gyrus, paracentral lobule	Inferior (MFG, SFG/M4) and anterior (cingulate/A3, A4)
	Basal frontal	Gyrus rectus, orbital gyri	Posterolateral (LOG/M4), anteromedial (gyrus rectus/A2), and posteromedial (POG/A1)
	Sylvian frontal	Pars orbitalis, pars triangularis, pars opercularis	Inferomedial (pars orbitalis/M3)
Temporal AVMs			
	Lateral temporal	STG, MTG, ITG	Superior (STG/M4)
	Basal temporal	ITG, fusiform gyrus, parahippocampal gyrus	Medial (parahippocampus/P2)
	Medial temporal	Parahippocampal gyrus, uncus, hippocampus	Medial (uncus/ICA, P2)
	Sylvian temporal	Planum polare, planum temporale	Superomedial (planum/M3)
Parieto-occipital AVMs			
	Lateral parieto-occipital	Postcentral gyrus, SPL, IPL; SOG, IOG	Anteroinferior (supramarginal, angular gyri/M4)
	Medial parieto-occipital	Paracentral lobule, post. cingulate gyrus, precuneus; cuneus, lingula	Inferior (precuneus, cuneus, lingula/P4) and anterior (cingulate/A5)
	Paramedian parieto-occipital	Postcentral gyrus, SPL; SOG	Lateral (SPL, SOG/M4), inferior (precuneus, cuneus/P4), and anterior (cingulate/A5)
	Basal occipital	Lingula, OTG, IOG	Anterior (lingula, OTG/P4)
Ventricular/Periventricular AVMs			
	Callosal	Corpus callosum (genu, body, and splenium)	Superior (CalC/A3, A4, short callosal) and anterior (callosum/A3, A4, long callosal)
	Ventricular body	Choroid plexus, fornix, septum, velum interpositum, thalamus	Posterior (velum interpositum/mPChA) and anterior (septum/A1, A2)
	Atrial	Choroid plexus, thalamus (pulvinar), crus of fornix, caudate	Inferior (choroidal fissure/lPChA)
	Temporal horn	Choroid plexus, hippocampus, fornix	Anteromedial (choroidal fissure/AChA)
Deep AVMs			
	Pure sylvian	STG, planum polare and temporale; pars orbitalis, triangularis, opercularis	Inferomedial (limen insulae/M2, M3)
	Insular	Short gyri, long gyri	Inferolateral (limen Insulae/M2)
	Basal ganglial	Putamen, globus pallidus, caudate nucleus, internal capsule (ant. limb)	Lateral (insula/InsP) or inferior (caudate/mLSA, RAH)
	Thalamic	Thalamus (superior and medial), internal capsule (post. limb)	Superomedial (velum interpositum/mPChA, lPChA)
Brainstem AVMs			
	Anterior midbrain	Cerebral peduncle, CN3	Anterior (IpC/P1)
	Posterior midbrain	Tectum, CN4	Lateral (QuadC/CirP, s3)
	Anterior pontine	Pons, CN5, CN7/8	Inferior (CbPonC/a1), superior (CbPonC/s1), and medial (CbPonC/BA)
	Lateral pontine	Pons, MCP, CN5	Medial (CbPonC/a2, a3)
	Anterior medullary	IVth ventricular floor, CN12	Anterolateral (hematoma/VA)
	Lateral medullary	Olivary nucleus, CN9/10/11/12	Lateral (CbMedC/VA, p1, p2)
Cerebellar AVMs			
	Suboccipital cerebellar	Semilunar (sup. and inf.) lobules, biventral lobule	Superior (sup. semilunar lobule/s4), lateral (inf. semilunar lobule/a4), and inferior (biventral lobule/p5)
	Tentorial cerebellar	Quadrangular, simple, and sup. semilunar lobules	Anterior (quadrangular lobule/s4)
	Vermian cerebellar	Superior vermis, inferior vermis	Anterior (superior vermis/s4) or inferior (inferior vermis/p5)
	Tonsillar cerebellar	Tonsil	Superior (tonsil/p4, p5)
	Petrosal cerebellar	Flocculus, MidCP	Medial (flocculus/a4)

Pial Transgression and Eloquence

Pia mater is an important protective barrier that defines the boundaries of the subarachnoid domain. Microsurgical technique is most elegant when it respects this layer, as with aneurysm and bypass surgery. However, pia transgressions are inevitable requirements of AVM surgery. The pia must be incised to initiate circumdissection into brain parenchyma and advance the resection. Intact pia reassures us that brain is preserved, whereas violated pia worries us that neurologic morbidity might ensue. Therefore, pia is the anatomic link to eloquence, and the pial incision forces the neurosurgeon to confront eloquence at this phase of dissection, even though eloquence is a property of brain tissue and becomes a major factor later during parenchymal dissection.

On the one hand, eloquence is obvious, defined in the Spetzler-Martin grading system as motor cortex, somatosensory cortex, language cortex (Wernicke's and Broca's areas), visual cortex, hypothalamus, thalamus, internal capsule, brainstem (midbrain, pons, and medulla), cerebellar peduncles, and deep cerebellar nuclei. On the other hand, eloquence is vague. Where exactly does visual cortex end peripherally in the occipital lobe? What about the eloquence of tracts like the optic radiations, whose disruption in temporal white matter produces a deficit similar to that in visual cortex? Does an AVM *adjacent* to the motor strip have the same eloquence as an AVM *in* the motor strip? Do *pial* AVMs in the brainstem and sylvian fissure have the same eloquence as a brainstem and sylvian AVM in *parenchyma*? Should the areas described by Spetzler and Martin as having more subtle neurologic function, including medial temporal lobe structures in the dominant hemisphere, nondominant parietal lobe, corpus callosum, cingulate gyrus, and basal ganglia, be treated differently from areas that are clearly noneloquent, like the anterior frontal and temporal lobes and cerebellar cortex? Finally, can eloquence be graded accurately based on structural anatomy, when AVMs are known to dramatically alter functional anatomy, with shifts to an adjacent gyrus or relocations to the contralateral hemisphere? In short, eloquence is not so easy to judge intraoperatively.

The uncertainty of eloquence is dealt with in three ways. First, functional magnetic resonance imaging (fMRI) can identify some areas of eloquence preoperatively. Deoxyhemoglobin has paramagnetic properties that enable blood flow to be measured at baseline and during the execution of a specific task using blood oxygen level dependent (BOLD) imaging. Blood flow delivers oxygen to active neurons, and subtraction paradigms between these two conditions couple flow and function both spatially and temporally to identify the brain regions involved in these tasks. Therefore, fMRI can localize motor and speech areas. However, unlike normal subjects, AVM patients have such deranged blood flow and adjacent arterioles are so chronically dysautoregulated that they respond poorly to tasks, and areas of functional activation appear larger than they should. Overestimations of eloquence discourage surgery. Other functional imaging techniques such as positron emission tomography (PET) and single photon emission computed tomography (SPECT) have similar problems. Magnetic source imaging (MSI) is not dependent on blood flow and instead measures neuronal activation by detecting magnetic flux associated with depolarization during synaptic transmission and intracellular ion currents. However, the imaging output from MSI is crude. Therefore, preoperative fMRI is generally unsatisfactory in localizing eloquence and is used to screen for major reorganization of eloquent cortex.

Second, electrocortical stimulation mapping can be used intraoperatively to identify eloquent areas, specifically language and motor cortex. Ensuring patient comfort requires a coordinated team of neuroanesthesiologists, neurophysiologists, and neurosurgeons to control pain during the craniotomy, awaken the patient for language mapping, and conduct counting, naming, and reading tasks. Stimulation of language sites results in reproducible counting errors, speech arrest, or alexia. Motor and speech mapping is useful primarily for larger AVMs adjacent to these eloquent areas, below the cortical surface, or with diffuse borders. Localizing information helps protect eloquent cortex, select a dissection route to deep AVMs, perform corticectomy safely, and halt the dissection before complete resection to avoid morbidity. As important as this information is, intraoperative mapping is rarely used (3% in my experience). The AVM resection can be long, unpredictable, and uncomfortable for both the awake patient and neurosurgeon. Mapping encourages more conservative surgery, increasing our rate of incomplete resection from 2% overall to 25% with mapping, without clear proof that additional localizing data spared the patient a deficit. Therefore, mapping does not satisfactorily address the eloquence issue in most AVM patients either.

Dissection Distance

Third, rather than defining eloquence radiologically or electrophysiologically, most neurosurgeons deal with eloquence by maintaining a close dissection distance from the AVM. Eloquence is assumed based on structural anatomy and protected during dissection with tight adherence to the AVM. We begin with a pial incision that closely circumscribes the AVM, and then we develop planes that hug the nidus and pull us in to minimize brain transgression. This tact is crude and works with compact AVMs, but clean planes rarely persist. Margins often become irregular or diffuse and the dissection migrates into parenchyma. In addition, bleeding from the nidus can push back the dissection. The comfort that comes from tightly adhering to the AVM is replaced with nagging concern about assumed eloquence. There is a dynamic between tight AVM adherence on the one hand and wide dissection distance on the other, between aggravating the AVM with the former and harming the patient with the latter. The end result is a constant, unrelenting tension that comes from uncertain eloquence, beginning with the pial incision and continuing throughout circumdissection. This is the psychology of eloquence that permeates AVM resections when our measures of eloquence are inadequate.

In contrast to eloquent AVMs, non-eloquent AVMs have none of this tension or dynamic. A wider incision can be circumscribed in the pia to set a more generous course around the AVM that reduces the bleeding risk at no neurologic cost to the patient. Eloquent AVMs with both eloquent and non-eloquent sides can be managed similarly on their non-eloquent sides, but require tight adherence on their eloquent sides. Pial incisions should optimize the parallel exposure of the AVM's sides, and a cone-shaped AVM based on the cortex requires a simple circular incision. However, a spherical AVM that widens beneath the cortex might require a pial incision beyond the AVM's cortical margins (**Fig. 5.2**). Tight pial incisions create keyhole exposures with ledges of overlying brain and poorly visualized AVM margins that can be troublesome. When eloquence allows, wider pial incisions are safer for these deeper AVMs because they create funnel-shaped exposure without ledges or blind spots.

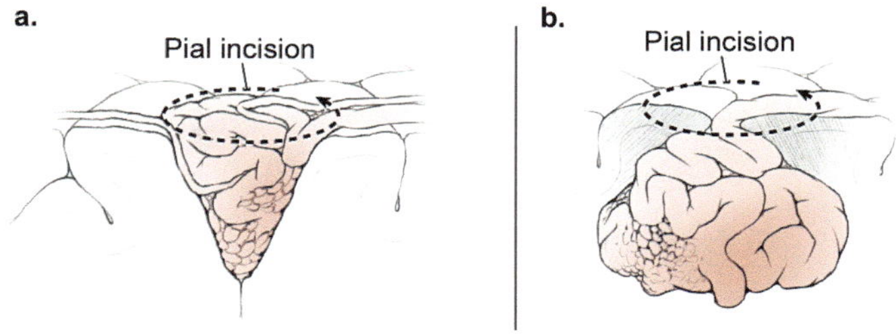

Fig. 5.2 Pial incisions should optimize the parallel exposure of AVM sides, (**a**) with tight incisions around conical AVMs, and (**b**) with wide incisions around spherical AVMs that optimize visualization of deeper planes by resecting some overlying cortex (*shaded areas*).

6 Parenchymal Dissection

Circumdissection

Parenchymal dissection detaches an arteriovenous malformation (AVM) from brain. Although pial dissection quickly exposes margins and closes superficial afferents, parenchymal dissection is lengthier and comprises two thirds of the circumdissection. Every piece of the AVM's four sides is separated from adjacent brain, every intersecting artery is interrupted, and secondary draining veins are trimmed. An AVM with reduced flow is more cooperative during circumdissection, and therefore hot sides with significant arterial input are tackled first. Circumdissection should spiral around the nidus and progressively deepen the dissection plane rather than thrusting into narrow foxholes with poor visibility. Spiraling dissection gains perspective on the AVM's shape and size, and enables retraction of the nidus. Feeding arteries in deep corners are alluring, but one should pause before engagement, zoom the microscope out, and deepen the dissection plane on other sides to optimize exposure before returning to the feeders, in case they bleed.

Parenchymal feeders tend to be smaller and less ferocious than cortical feeders, but are harder to see. Shallow parenchymal dissection is performed with dynamic retraction by the bipolar forceps or sucker on the nidus or adjacent brain, but deep parenchymal dissection may require fixed retraction with self-retaining retractors. Blades are preferentially applied to the AVM rather than brain tissue, with a small piece of Nu-Knit on the nidus at the point of contact. Fixed retraction is usually kept to one retractor; multiple retractors or circumferential retraction systems build a ring around the surgical field that deepens and obstructs it.

The tense dynamic between tight AVM adherence and wide circumdissection into brain, between aggravating the AVM and harming eloquent tissue, only increases during parenchymal dissection. Most AVM subtypes are associated with some eloquent anatomy (**Table 6.1**). Arteriovenous malformations have irregular contours formed by arterial networks, loops, veins, varicosities, and tortuosities that invite coagulation, but dissection should follow the interface plane and widen into adjacent brain. For example, with accurate interpretation of an arterial loop, dissection veers around this nidal protrusion and avoids needlessly interrupting the loop's afferent and efferent limbs or inducing bleeding. Similarly with venous loops, accurate interpretation avoids inadvertently occluding outflow. The dissection course shifts constantly as the AVM margin is explored and scrutinized, migrating to and from the nidus. Vascular structures originating from the AVM are followed into brain and resolved as artery, vein, or additional nidus. Hemosiderin stains, gliosis, and encephalomalacia are followed to redefine the interface plane. Each advancing step must avoid misinterpretations that might cause AVM bleeding, remnants, damage to eloquent brain, and new neurologic morbidity.

Rupture and Hematoma

Arteriovenous malformation hemorrhage is a significant factor that facilitates AVM resection by separating portions of the nidus from adjacent brain. The rupture performs some parenchymal dissection. Hematoma evacuation immediately accesses this dissection plane as if it were a free cortical surface. Hematomas associated with ruptured AVMs are often large, and their cortical extension localizes AVMs that are not cortically based. Hematoma that presents on the cortical surface or discolors overlying cortex, or that can be identified with ultrasonography or stereotactic navigation, can lead to deep AVMs without a superficial draining vein. By definition, clot communicates directly with a ruptured AVM and clot evacuation will reveal it. Hematoma is evacuated strategically in areas remote from the AVM, deliberately avoiding the nidus until the cavity is cleared, the brain is decompressed, and landmarks such as draining veins, feeding arteries, and ventricles are identified. Overly aggressive hematoma evacuation may re-rupture the AVM without control of afferent arteries or clear orientation within the cavity. A tenuous cap of thrombus covering the rupture site on a draining vein or varix should be left alone. Feeding arteries traversing through clot are followed to the AVM nidus which usually resides in a wall of the hematoma cavity.

The hematoma's relationship to the AVM determines its surgical advantage: hematoma adjacent to nidus dissects its parenchymal sides; hematoma beneath nidus facilitates deep dissection of its ependymal side; and hematoma above nidus

Table 6.1 Summary of AVM Subtypes and Their Cortical Anatomy and Eloquence

Type	Subtype	Cortical Anatomy	Eloquence
Frontal AVMs			
	Lateral frontal	SFG, MFG, IFG, precentral gyrus	Precentral gyrus (motor)
	Medial frontal	SFG, paracentral lobule, cingulate gyrus	Paracentral lobule (motor)
	Paramedian frontal	SFG, precentral gyrus, paracentral lobule	Precentral gyrus, paracentral lobule (motor)
	Basal frontal	Gyrus rectus, orbital gyri	None
	Sylvian frontal	Pars orbitalis, pars triangularis, pars opercularis	Broca's area (pars triangularis, pars opercularis)
Temporal AVMs			
	Lateral temporal	STG, MTG, ITG	Wernicke's area (STG)
	Basal temporal	ITG, fusiform gyrus, parahippocampal gyrus	None
	Medial temporal	Parahippocampal gyrus, uncus, hippocampus	Hippocampus (memory)
	Sylvian temporal	Planum polare, planum temporale	Heschl's gyrus (auditory)
Parieto-occipital AVMs			
	Lateral parieto-occipital	Postcentral gyrus, SPL, IPL; SOG, IOG	Postcentral gyrus (sensory), IOG (visual), angular gyrus (speech conduction)
	Medial parieto-occipital	Paracentral lobule, post. cingulate gyrus, precuneus; cuneus, lingula	Paracentral lobule (sensory), lingula (visual)
	Paramedian parieto-occipital	Postcentral gyrus, SPL; SOG	Postcentral gyrus, paracentral lobule (sensory); lingula, IOG (visual)
	Basal occipital	Lingula, OTG, IOG	None
Ventricular/Periventricular AVMs			
	Callosal	Corpus callosum (genu, body, and splenium)	None
	Ventricular body	Choroid plexus, fornix, septum, velum interpositum, thalamus	Fornix (memory)
	Atrial	Choroid plexus, thalamus (pulvinar), crus of fornix, caudate	Fornix (memory)
	Temporal horn	Choroid plexus, hippocampus, fornix	Fornix (memory)
Deep AVMs			
	Pure sylvian	STG, planum polare and temporale; pars orbitalis, triangularis, opercularis	None
	Insular	Short gyri, long gyri	None
	Basal ganglial	Putamen, globus pallidus, caudate nucleus, internal capsule (ant. limb)	Basal ganglia, internal capsule
	Thalamic	Thalamus (superior and medial), internal capsule (post. limb)	Thalamus, internal capsule
Brainstem AVMs			
	Anterior midbrain	Cerebral peduncle, CN3	Midbrain
	Posterior midbrain	Tectum, CN4	Midbrain
	Anterior pontine	Pons, CN5, CN7/8	Pons
	Lateral pontine	Pons, MCP, CN5	Pons
	Anterior medullary	IVth ventricular floor, CN12	Medulla
	Lateral medullary	Olivary nucleus, CN9/10/11/12	Medulla
Cerebellar AVMs			
	Suboccipital cerebellar	Semilunar (sup. and inf.) lobules, biventral lobule	Deep cerebellar nuclei
	Tentorial cerebellar	Quadrangular, simple, and sup. semilunar lobules	None
	Vermian cerebellar	Superior vermis, inferior vermis	Deep cerebellar nuclei; cerebellar mutism
	Tonsillar cerebellar	Tonsil	None
	Petrosal cerebellar	Flocculus, MidCP	None

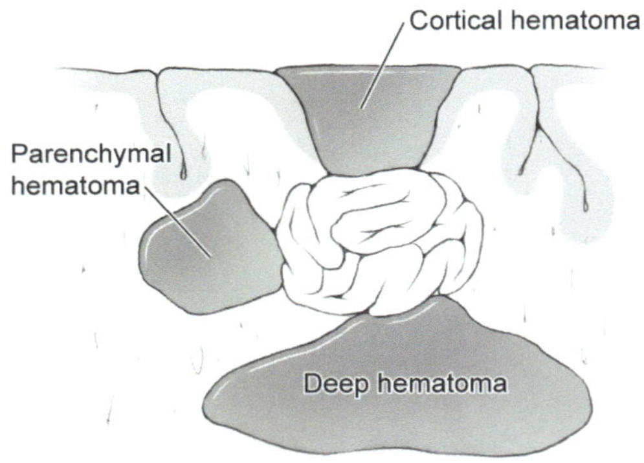

Fig. 6.1 Hemorrhage separates portions of the AVM from adjacent brain, and hematoma evacuation accesses this plane as if it were a free cortical surface. Hematoma above the nidus opens a transcortical corridor to its top side; hematoma adjacent to the nidus dissects its parenchymal sides; hematoma beneath the nidus dissects its ependymal side.

opens a transcortical corridor to its top side (**Fig. 6.1**). The latter relationship is particularly advantageous because transcortical routes to deep AVMs are nonanatomic and do not exist in patients with unruptured AVMs. Accessing an AVM through the hematoma cavity requires no corticectomy, produces no additional morbidity, and reaches AVMs in deep lobar white matter, basal ganglia, and thalamus.

Absorption of hematoma after rupture reduces, but does not eliminate, these surgical advantages. Blood is replaced with chronic inflammation, scar tissue, gliosis, and encephalomalacia. Prior surgery, including simple hematoma evacuation and incomplete AVM resection, produces similar changes in brain parenchyma. Prior radiosurgery can induce gliosis, encephalomalacia, or cysts similar to chronic hematomas. Old hemorrhage cavities can be reopened as routes of AVM access and exploited in AVM resections, but the advantages of a chronic hematoma are not as great as an acute hematoma. Therefore, surgery is performed acutely or subacutely in patients presenting with ruptured AVMs.

Rupture and Eloquence

A patient's neurologic condition at presentation after AVM rupture profoundly impacts parenchymal dissection. Rupture and ensuing hemorrhage damage brain tissues, and the destruction of eloquent brain tissues changes the surgical calculus. A patient who presents with hemiplegia from a ruptured motor strip AVM has little to lose by proceeding with surgery. The AVM has already caused the morbidity that might have been committed by the neurosurgeon. In this case, preexisting neurologic deficits and lost eloquence *simplify* parenchymal dissection. In contrast, a patient who presents in normal condition with the same motor strip AVM has much to lose by proceeding with a surgery. Normal function and critical eloquence *complicate* parenchymal dissection. Conservative observation or radiosurgery would be recommended, exposing the patient to hemorrhage risk and unpredictable sequelae from AVM rupture, but maximizing the duration of normal function. By waiting until AVM rupture to proceed with surgery, the AVM produces the morbidity, not the neurosurgeon. The stakes of circumdissection are lowered by the non-eloquence of brain that is no longer eloquent. To paraphrase the Hippocratic oath, "First let the AVM do harm."

Some preoperative deficits may be secondary effects of hemorrhage caused by cerebral edema, elevated intracranial pressure, and hydrocephalus from intraventricular extension. These factors adversely affect patients' condition at presentation, but, unlike direct brain injury from AVM rupture, can be treated and may resolve over time. Therefore, in patients who are operated on acutely with some possibility of secondary effects from hemorrhage, eloquent brain should be assumed to have some recoverability and should be handled accordingly.

Compact and Diffuse AVMs

The AVM nidus can be wound tightly or loosely (**Fig. 6.2**). A compact AVM is wound tightly with distinct margins, no intermixed brain, and separability from adjacent brain, all of which clarify parenchymal dissection. In contrast, a diffuse AVM is wound loosely, as if pulled apart or unraveled, with indistinct margins, intermixed brain, and poor separability, all of which complicate parenchymal dissection. Compact AVMs are easily deciphered and followed. Diffuse AVMs force the neurosurgeon to establish the plane of separation between AVM and brain. The margin of a diffuse AVM can be an unruly fringe that must be encircled either widely at the expense of intervening brain tissue, or closely in a way the crosses more of this arterial fringe. The interplay of eloquence and hemostasis pull in and push back the circumdissection, and challenge the neurosurgeon to find the right dissection distance. In some cases, this judgment can bring the dissection too close to the nidus and cause bleeding or leave behind an abnormal portion of nidus. In other cases, this judgment can bring the dissection too far from the nidus, resulting in complete and easier AVM resection but removing more brain tissue than is necessary.

Diffuseness comes in many variations. It may be a lacy web of small arterioles on one side of the nidus, or on all sides uniformly. It may be tentacles of large arteries on one side or multiple sides of the nidus. It may be a ragged lattice of arteries and arterioles spread across a pial surface, or a network of leptomeningeal collateral arteries in a watershed zone between vascular territories converging on the nidus.

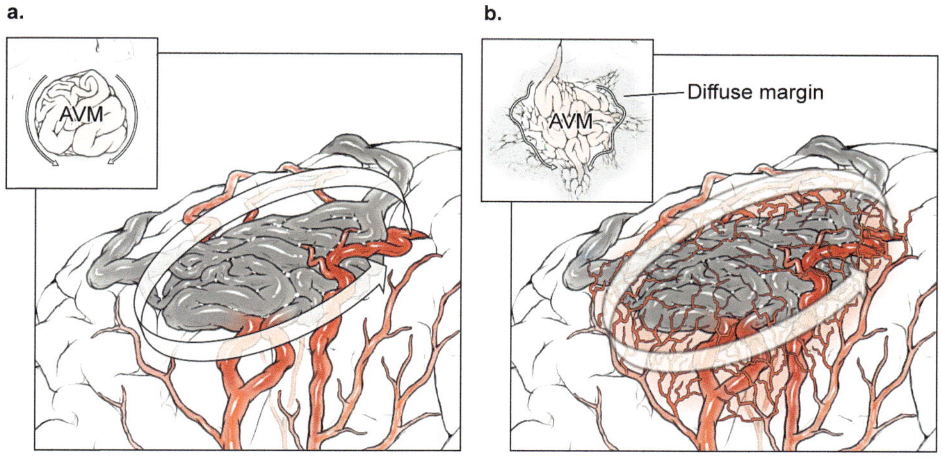

Fig. 6.2 An AVM nidus can be compact or diffuse. (**a**) A compact AVM is wound tightly with distinct margins, no intermixed brain, and separability from adjacent brain, all of which clarify parenchymal dissection and tighten the dissection distance (*inset,* cross-sectional view). (**b**) A diffuse AVM is wound loosely, as if pulled apart or unraveled, with indistinct margins, intermixed brain, and poor separability, all of which complicate parenchymal dissection and widen dissection distance (*inset,* cross-sectional view). Compact AVMs are easily deciphered and followed, whereas diffuse AVMs force the neurosurgeon to establish the plane of separation. The interplay of eloquence and hemostasis pull in and push back the circumdissection distance.

It may be wisps of perforating arteries penetrating the thalamus from below a deep or ventricular AVM, or intercommunicating choroidal arteries traversing the ventricles. These variations can make diffuseness difficult to define. As a general definition, a circle can be drawn easily around a compact AVM on an angiogram, but not so easily around a diffuse one. We developed methods using digital angiography, contour plots, and area-intensity profiles to quantitate diffuseness. At any given threshold image intensity, the computer outlined the AVM blush on angiograms and measured the area of this contour plot. As the threshold intensity was dialed down, the area of the contour plot increased linearly with compact AVMs, but exponentially with diffuse AVMs. In other words, as the AVM is outlined more generously, compact AVMs grow a little and diffuse AVMs grow a lot. Area-intensity profiling is a cumbersome research tool for defining diffuseness, but it is not difficult to recognize. Neurosurgeons familiar with AVMs develop an intuition and ability to differentiate compactness and diffuseness both radiographically and intraoperatively: "You know it when you see it."

The difficulties in circumdissecting diffuse AVMs impact patient outcomes. Patients with compact AVMs fare better than those with diffuse AVMs, with favorable outcomes in 90% and 55%, respectively. These outcomes reflect the ability to stay out of adjacent brain tissue with compact AVMs, and an inability to do so with diffuse AVMs. Dealing with dysplastic AVM vessels in adjacent parenchyma leads to tissue injury, parenchymal bleeding, contusions, postoperative edema, seizures, and delayed hemorrhagic complications.

7 Ependymal/Deep Dissection

■ The Dark Side

"Ependymal" dissection may be a confusing term because many arteriovenous malformations (AVMs) do not reach a ventricle, but it is meant to describe the deep dissection that comes at the end of the resection. In terms of the AVM box, the ependymal plane is the bottom, the sixth and final side. In terms of brain anatomy, the ependymal layer is the tip of the classic AVM cone tapering to ependyma. This phase of dissection, whether actually ependymal or not, is deep and diametrically opposite to the position of the neurosurgeon, and, as such, is inherently difficult to see, like the dark side of the moon. The ependymal plane is darkened and physically blocked by AVM nidus, making it the most challenging one. To make matters worse, this plane receives perforating and choroidal artery supply which can be troublesome.

I always anticipate some bleeding during ependymal dissection; I am prepared if it comes, and pleasantly surprised if it does not. Therefore, before beginning ependymal dissection, all of the parenchymal dissection should be completed, the other AVM sides should be free, and the nidus should be mobile. It is easy to get lured down to the ependymal plane and lose sight of unfinished parenchymal connections on another side. The resection cavity is lined circumferentially with Telfa strips to protect parenchyma from manipulation or retraction, but more importantly, to deal with deep bleeding. If bleeding fills the surgical corridor, Telfa strips provide extra-anatomic landmarks that are more orienting than bland parenchyma, and they are protective.

Retractors solve the problem of deep visualization. A self-retaining retractor placed on the AVM mobilizes the nidus from side to side, and importantly elevates it as well. Lifting an AVM enhances the view of the ependymal plane and places deep connections on traction. Although I try to limit fixed retractors to just one, a retractor on the brain may also angle the viewing trajectory across the ependymal plane when the walls of the cavity are steep and deep. Retractors and retraction pressure can inadvertently kink or tear superficial draining veins, and retractors can be bumped by passing instruments or resting hands. With attention focused at the cavity's depths, occlusions of superficial draining veins may go unrecognized with bleeding consequences. Secondary draining veins that limit deep exposure are safe to sacrifice at this stage. Deep hematomas should be found and evacuated to open up the deep plane.

■ Perforating Artery Supply

Perforating artery supply differs from cortical artery supply. Perforators traverse deep parenchyma rather than cortical surfaces, and are smaller in caliber, thin walled, fragile, and difficult to cauterize. Bleeding can draw the neurosurgeon into critical neural structures where visualization is compromised by overlying nidus, and tolerance to bleeding and electrocautery is low. Whether from lenticulostriates to a basal ganglial AVM, insular perforators to an insular AVM, thalamoperforators to a thalamic AVM, or basilar perforators to a pontine AVM, bleeding is brisk and hazardous with consequences for the surgical outcomes.

The answer to the deep perforator is, simply, the AVM microclip. Although cautery typically explodes the perforator and initiates a torrent, the microclip shuts it effectively and bloodlessly. It is almost not worth trying cautery because a bleeding perforator is so much more difficult to control. If it does bleed, the perforator is controlled by drying the field with suction on a thin cottonoid, using dynamic retraction to see into remote corners, chasing the bleeder through white matter, freeing a short perforator segment proximal to the bleeding point, drawing it into the sucker to steady it, and finally applying the microclip (**Fig. 7.1**). After microclip application and flow arrest, perforators are more responsive to cautery. They are coagulated along a segment rather than a point, and divided. Bleeding from the distal stump might require a second microclip on the nidal side if uncontrolled with cautery. Perforators are so delicate that slight manipulation or even microclip application can induce bleeding, in which case more dissection proximally exposes the perforator for additional microclips. Progressive proximal dissection leads to larger perforators with less branches and more

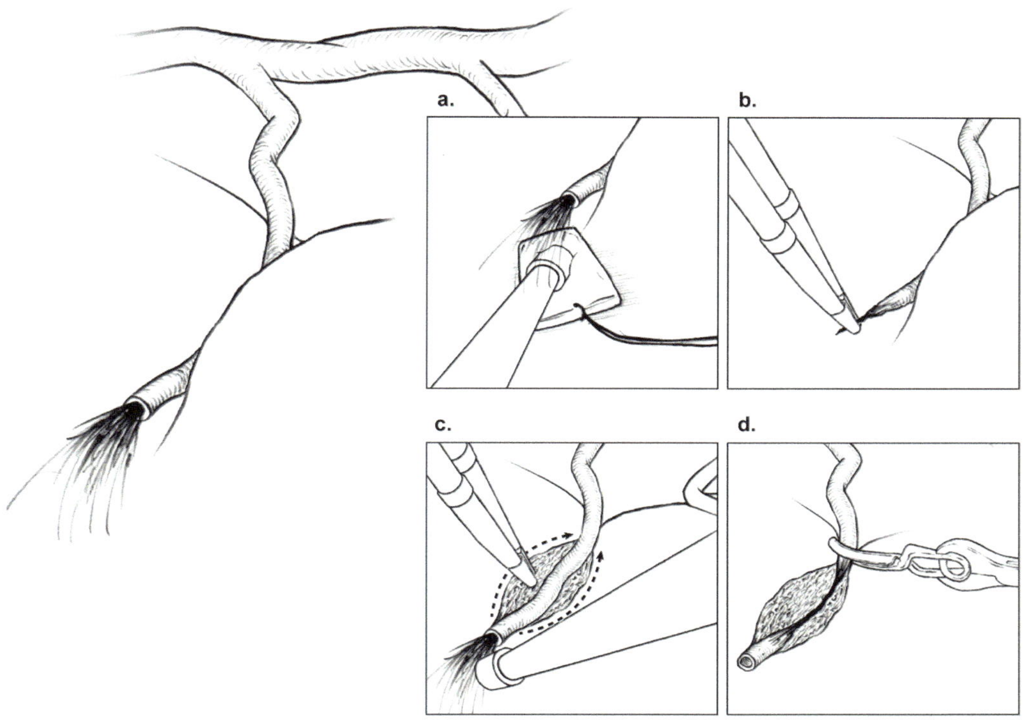

Fig. 7.1 Steps in controlling a deep perforating artery: (**a**) drying the field with suction on a thin cottonoid; (**b**) attempting to coagulate it with bipolar cautery; (**c**) proximal dissection into white matter to free a segment of artery proximal to the bleeding point, sometimes drawing it into the sucker; and (**d**) applying the microclip.

coagulability, but intrudes deeper into white matter tracts. The decision where to cross a tangle of perforators must balance the ease of a more proximal interruption with proximity to eloquence.

The battle with perforators, fortunately, is usually brief. Perforator supply is typically limited to less than five arteries, and in some cases may be just one. They coalesce at the ependymal tip or the AVM's extension into white matter. They must be controlled one by one and never packed. Thin cottonoids are very helpful to protect brain, apply suction, retract against, and define the surgical plane. However, too many cottonoids will create a tangle of strings. Perforators are difficult to see angiographically because they are small, few, and overshadowed by larger inundating arteries. However, their presence should never surprise, even with cortical, lobar, or cerebellar AVMs. Any AVM that breaches white matter can attract these perforating arteries. Furthermore, as insignificant as they might appear angiographically, they probably increase their shunt flow during the course of circumdissection as other inputs are throttled. Perforators are typically the last of the arterial supply, and I often notice that a draining vein that was bright red at the beginning of a perforator skirmish is dark blue at the end.

Choroidal Artery Supply

Choroidal supply is generally more cooperative than perforator supply because these arteries are thicker, more coagulable, and floating freely in the ventricle. Choroidal arteries run in tela choroidea and choroid plexus, making them far more visible than parenchymal perforators buried in white matter. Ventricles open widely; transcortically, transcallosally, or through a choroidal fissure; and offer anatomic orientation, working space, and proximal control. Therefore, even though they are deep, choroidal arteries are like an artery in a cistern or subarachnoid space that can be identified with clear landmarks and controlled.

Other choroidal arteries may intersect the AVM diametrically opposite to the AVM. These feeding arteries are poorly visualized, lack proximal control, and are difficult

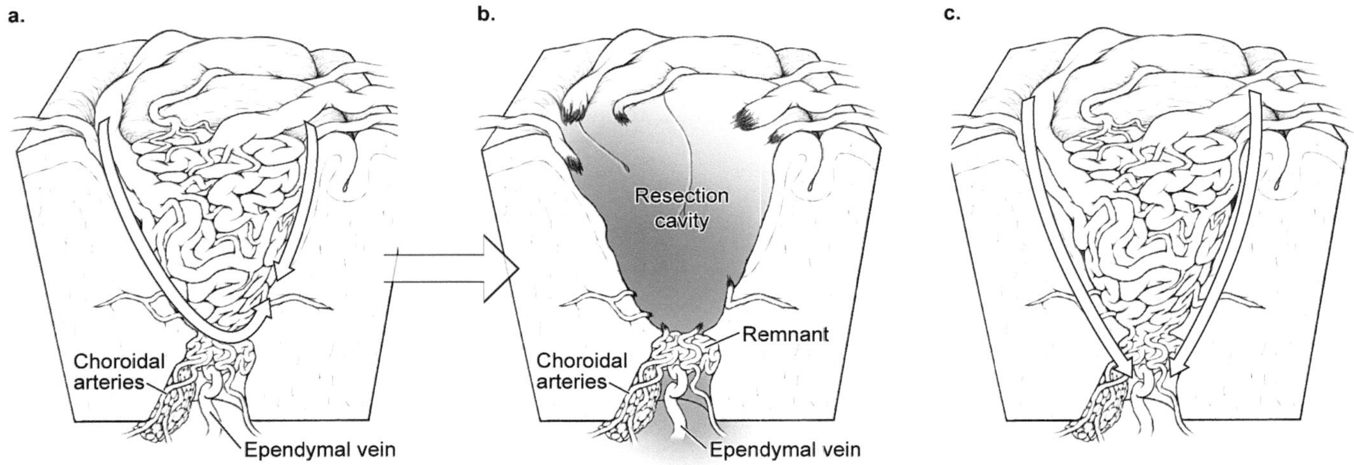

Fig. 7.2 Anatomy of an AVM's ependymal tip. (**a**) Ependymal dissection that does not enter the ventricle may truncate the AVM and (**b**) leave a remnant supplied by choroidal arteries and drained by ependymal veins with persistent arteriovenous shunting. (**c**) Additional dissection into the ventricle surrounds the AVM's tip, confirms that the draining vein is dark, and completes the circumdissection.

to access. These difficulties are encountered with bulkier AVMs that have a large ependymal surface rather than just an ependymal tip, and a network of choroidal supply from the anterior choroidal artery (AChA), medial posterior choroidal artery (mPChA), and lateral posterior choroidal artery (lPChA), rather than a single input. Bleeding from diametrically opposite arteries hides from view, causing unchecked intraventricular hemorrhage and, in the extreme, outward brain herniation. Microclips can be useful with choroidal arteries when access behind a bulky AVM makes them difficult to coagulate.

The ventricular draining vein is an important surgical landmark that helps identify choroidal arteries and ependymal portions of the AVM. If the dissection does not enter the ventricle and surround the ventricular vein, the tip of the nidus may be truncated (**Fig. 7.2**). Residual nidus with some choroidal supply and a ventricular vein will result in a remnant with persistent shunting and risk of hemorrhage. Some of my most frustrating incomplete resections resulted from not aggressively entering the ventricle and surrounding this ependymal unit. It is so easy to go the extra few millimeters, gain the panorama of the ventricle, and confirm that the ventricular vein is dark and the ependymal plane is completely circumdissected.

The presence of deep supply from choroidal or perforating arteries is one of the factors that correlate with patient outcomes. In our experience, the presence of deep perforating arteries lowered the chances of a favorable outcome by 15% and was statistically significant. This finding reflects difficulties in surgical perspective, poor accessibility and coagulability of the arteries, and their proximity to eloquent parenchymal structures (**Table 7.1**). This finding also demonstrates the importance of winning the perforator fight. Perforators are encountered at the end of the case when there may be an element of fatigue. I deliberately postpone the perforator fight until the bitter end when I am energized by the thought that this may be the final coup.

Table 7.1 Summary of AVM Subtypes and Deep Anatomy Encountered During Ependymal Dissection

Type	Subtype	Ependymal/Deep Dissection
Frontal AVMs		
	Lateral frontal	lLSA; frontal horn
	Medial frontal	PcaA; PcaV
	Paramedian frontal	PcaA, mLSA; frontal horn
	Basal frontal	Medial (A2), posterior (A1) fronts; frontal horn
	Sylvian frontal	InsP, lLSA, mLSA
Temporal AVMs		
	Lateral temporal	AChA; temporal horn
	Basal temporal	PosTempA; temporal horn
	Medial temporal	PosTempA, lPChA; BVR
	Sylvian temporal	AChA; temporal horn
Parieto-occipital AVMs		
	Lateral parieto-occipital	MCA; AtrV; occipital horn
	Medial parieto-occipital	PCA; AtrV; occipital horn
	Paramedian parieto-occipital	MCA, PCA; AtrV; occipital horn
	Basal occipital	PCA; AntCalcV; occipital horn; tentorial incisura
Ventricular/Periventricular AVMs		
	Callosal	Septal feeders; ventricular veins, SplenV
	Ventricular body	ACoA perforators, mLSA, AntThaP; ICV; fornix
	Atrial	PosThaP, lLSA; MedAtrV, LatAtrV
	Temporal horn	lPChA; ChorV, BVR; hippocampus, fornix
Deep AVMs		
	Pure sylvian	MCA (terminal feeding, transit, bystander arteries); DeepSylV
	Insular	lLSA; CauV
	Basal ganglial	mLSA, lLSA, RAH; CauV
	Thalamic	PosThaP, AntThaP; BVR
Brainstem AVMs		
	Anterior midbrain	PedP; cerebral peduncle, CN3
	Posterior midbrain	Long CirP; tectum, CN4
	Anterior pontine	BA feeders; MAPonMesV; CN6
	Lateral pontine	BA feeders; MAPonMesV; CN5, CN7/8
	Anterior medullary	VA, AntSpA; MAMedV; ventricular floor
	Lateral medullary	VA; MAMedV; CN9/10/11/12
Cerebellar AVMs		
	Suboccipital cerebellar	Deep cerebellar nuclei; perforating arteries form SCA (precerebellar arteries) and PICA
	Tentorial cerebellar	None
	Vermian cerebellar	Tectum, CN4
	Tonsillar cerebellar	Medulla, CN9/10/11
	Petrosal cerebellar	Medial AICA feeders, pons, MidCP, CN7/8

8 Arteriovenous Malformation Resection

■ Blue Tail

One of my favorite moments in an arteriovenous malformation (AVM) resection is when the venous tail turns blue, signaling that the battle has been won. According to the venous "odometer," the journey is nearly over and the finish line lies ahead. The AVM's six sides are circumscribed, the arterial supply is disconnected, and the draining tail lives only through quiet venous connections. Nothing confirms the end of an AVM resection like lifting the nidus out of its resection bed still attached to its venous tail, just in case there is any unfinished dissection or unrecognized arterial supply. This roll-out maneuver works best with superficial AVMs because they deliver without sacrificing venous drainage, whereas deep AVMs deliver only after interrupting venous drainage.

Fatigue and impatience at the end of a long dissection make it easy to ignore critical warning signs, like persistent redness in the vein, which usually indicates a hidden feeding artery underneath the draining vein, a portion of the deep dissection plane that was missed, or a deep perforator on the opposite side. An AVM whose draining vein is dark or nearly dark can be aggressively manipulated to visualize these last holes and blind spots in the bed, just like an aneurysm whose afferent artery is occluded with a temporary clip and needs one final dissection maneuver before applying the permanent clip. Any AVM bleeding at this point can be safely handled by pursuing the last trickle of input.

■ Back Bleeding

Dividing the draining vein after an AVM has been rolled out of its resection bed is almost trivial, but dilated veins require more cautery to occlude them and can rupture during the process. Large draining veins communicate freely with venous sinuses, and back-bleeding can be brisk. Aneurysm clips close this communication with the sinus and facilitate coagulation, and can sometimes be removed after it is divided. Back-bleeding from deep draining veins can fill the surgical field or spill into the ventricles. Liberal use of clips is therefore advisable with large veins.

What might appear to be the simple division of a deep ependymal vein might actually be the amputation of the tip of the nidus, with arterial feeders supplying the venous stump. Color differentiates venous back-bleeding from residual AVM bleeding: bleeding is blue with the former and red with the latter. It may be difficult to notice subtle color differences during active hemorrhaging, but these are valuable signs. Deep veins are encircled widely by entering the ventricle if necessary, visualizing the distal course of the vein, and inspecting for redness or other signs of persistent shunt flow.

■ Bleeding Bed

The resection bed should be quiet after AVM resection. The removal of Telfa strips or cottonoids can stir up minor bleeding or tweak a fragile perforator, but these are easily controlled with cautery or an additional microclip. Bleeding beyond an ooze that is difficult to control should raise suspicion for residual AVM. I pay particular attention to the ependyma, surgical blind spots, and diffuse margins that might have been truncated too close to the nidus. Ependymal bleeding may require following the ventricular vein more distally. Bleeding from a surgical blind spot may demand resecting additional cortex to better visualize the bed. Bleeding from a diffuse margin may call for resecting an additional fringe of arteries and intermixed brain. Arteries that were skeletonized may harbor feeding arteries that were mistakenly preserved as arteries en passage, and these arteries may lead to a remnant. Although there is a strong inclination to close the procedure after the nidus is removed, persistent bleeding should not be taken lightly, and never managed with packing or hemostatic agents. One needs only to think about a return to the operating in the middle of the night after the patient fails to wake up to take seriously the pursuit of persistent bleeding in the bed. It is incomparably easier to spend an extra 10 to 20 minutes exploring the hot spots before closing, even though the thought of residual AVM seems impossible.

I also worry about postoperative hemorrhage in the hours after AVM resection. Rarely, patients with large AVMs may be susceptible to normal perfusion pressure breakthrough bleeding, as vasodilated and dysautoregulated arterioles adjacent to the AVM are exposed to increased blood pressure and flow. More commonly, fragile feeding arteries that were controlled with cautery may reopen with spikes in blood pressure. Patients with many deep perforating arteries who required more than five microclips and those with an unusually bloody resections remain intubated and sedated overnight to avoid extubation, coughing, agitation, or painful stimuli that might precipitate spikes in blood pressure and perioperative bleeding. Blood pressure control in the intensive care unit is critically important.

Residual AVM

Postoperative angiography confirms complete AVM resection. One of the most humbling experiences in AVM surgery is finding residual AVM unexpectedly, particularly after declaring victory to the patient and family the day before. Residual AVM, no matter how small, has a risk of hemorrhage similar to the original AVM and therefore must be treated. I generally prefer immediate reoperation, except when the presence of perioperative brain edema necessitates a 5- to 7-day delay. The craniotomy is easily reopened perioperatively and the resection cavity is easily reentered. Microclips or aneurysm clips provide useful landmarks to identify residual AVM. As disheartening as these reoperations can be, they are enormously instructive, revealing deficiencies in surgical exposure, misinterpretations of marginal planes, and misunderstandings of the pathoanatomy. Reexplorations are generally quick and straightforward. Furthermore, immediate reoperation fulfills the patient's and family's expectations for a curative resection. Therefore, despite wounded pride, a touch of embarrassment, and the finality of the initial operation, it is always worthwhile to return a patient with residual AVM to the operating room.

Alternative treatments like radiosurgery require significant delays in curative obliteration due to scheduling another treatment and the 2- to 3-year latency period. Therefore, radiosurgery is reserved for residual nidus in highly eloquent areas deemed too risky for reoperation. Embolization is rarely able to obliterate small residual nidus, at least in our experience. After reoperation, additional angiography is again mandatory to confirm complete AVM resection. Fortunately, residual AVM is an uncommon occurrence (about 3%), and I have not had to perform more than one reoperation on a patient for residual AVM.

9 Intraoperative Arteriovenous Malformation Rupture

■ Absolute Hemostasis

Arteriovenous malformation (AVM) resection should be bloodless, with sharp dissection of subarachnoid spaces, precise occlusion of pial feeders, clean dissection of parenchymal margins, and careful occlusion of deep supply along the ependymal plane. The slightest bleeding is meticulously stopped to maintain absolute hemostasis before progressing to the next step. Ironically, AVM resections are some of the cleanest and driest dissections despite their high-charged hemodynamics. Nonetheless, some intraoperative bleeding is inevitable with AVM resection, no matter how meticulous the dissection, how skilled the neurosurgeon, or how cooperative the AVM. Cauterizing dysplastic arteries with high flow will stir up bleeding that ranges from a small trickle from a pesky perforator to a torrent from nidal rupture. The threat of intraoperative rupture permeates these cases, and when it occurs, it can transform the operation. Blood suffuses the field and visualization is lost; suction must remain on the bleeder to clear the field and the sucker hand is immobilized; the resection stalls to reestablish hemostasis; the cause and site of the bleeding may be unclear; bleeding may force technical errors and morbidity from chasing the source into eloquent white matter; and AVM bleeding can be so brisk that it overwhelms the neurosurgeon and spirals out of control. Although AVM bleeding is unnerving, it must be met with a swift response to avert catastrophe.

The technical response to intraoperative AVM rupture differs from aneurysm rupture, which progresses through an orderly sequence of tamponade, suction, proximal control with temporary clipping, distal control with temporary clipping, and permanent aneurysm clipping. There is no aneurysm dome to tamponade with AVM bleeding, and there are too many feeding arteries for proximal control. There is no temporary clipping or neck to close. The bleeding source must be pursued, exposed, and controlled. A small cottonoid is applied at or near the bleeding site and suctioned to dry the field. A jet of blood is traced back to the source, which may be arterial, venous, or nidal.

■ Arterial Bleeding

Arterial bleeding originates from the parenchymal side of the resection bed, not from the nidus itself. A cottonoid prevents suction from injuring the brain, and some retraction pressure can be applied to the cottonoid with the sucker tip, allowing the sucker to be a dynamic retractor in the hunt. Small bleeders can be controlled with bipolar forceps and suction, suctioning right at the bleeding point or even drawing the artery into the barrel of the sucker. The sucker simultaneously clears the blood and immobilizes the bleeder, while the bipolar cauterizes the artery proximally. When cautery fails, I resort to microclips for small perforating arteries and aneurysm clips for large feeding arteries. Some arteries are thin, friable, and uncontrollable, but they become more manageable as they are exposed proximally. Therefore, intractable arteries are subdued by chasing them proximally, which requires deeper transgression into brain tissue and may jeopardize eloquent tracts or cortex. The pursuit of bleeders in subarachnoid spaces is safer, but there are risks to normal branches and bystander arteries.

Arterial bleeders are points of hemorrhage that can be closed precisely. They should never be packed, covered with hemostatic agents, or left unattended because they will continue to bleed out of view, either intraparenchymally or intraventricularly. Concealed hemorrhages can also occur with arteries that reopen after they have been coagulated, cut, and retracted into brain parenchyma. These hemorrhages blossom into hematomas and fill ventricles without any apparent bleeding in the surgical field. Progressive brain fullness, narrowing of the surgical corridor, or outward herniation of brain may be the only signs of active bleeding. The hematoma may suddenly erupt into the surgical field. When there is an unexplained change in operative conditions and a concealed hemorrhage is suspected, areas with previous bleeding, persistent oozing, or friable arteries should be reexplored. A trail of edematous or hemorrhagic brain can often be followed to a clot, which is then evacuated and explored for the bleeder. Concealed ventricular hemorrhage quickly fills the system and causes outward brain herniation, demanding aggressive entry into the ventricle to control the bleeder.

Venous Bleeding

Damaging a draining vein can compromise AVM outflow with devastating consequences during AVM resection. Opportunities for venous injury occur at all phases of the operation. Large convexity veins often erode or protrude into the inner table of the calvaria and can be torn when elevating the craniotomy flap. Adherent dura in older patients can also be torn with the craniotome, bringing the drill in contact with a draining vein. The draining vein can be damaged by the dural incision or by elevating the dural flap, particularly when dense adhesions require sharp dissection. Venous injury can occur during subarachnoid dissection that follows the draining vein down to the AVM. Venous injury can occur during parenchymal dissection that progresses between bridging veins, and during ependymal dissection with retractors on the nidus that stretch, kink, or tear the vein.

Venous bleeding is managed much differently than arterial bleeding. Although a bleeding artery would be clipped or cauterized to occlusion, a bleeding vein must be controlled without occluding it. Although cauterizing a bleeding vessel may be one's natural reflex, the loss of critical drainage may pressurize the AVM and precipitate rupture. Instead, the bleeding point must be controlled while preserving outflow, particularly when there is only one draining vein or it is the primary draining vein. Small venous tears can often be controlled with Nu-Knit, a cottonoid, and gentle pressure. Tamponade and patience will stop the bleeding and often the cottonoid can be peeled away. Large veins are often so dilated that they can be remodeled with focal cautery around the bleeding point on a portion of the wall that spares the lumen. A bleeding secondary vein can be cauterized to occlusion when the primary draining vein is intact.

AVM Rupture

Arteriovenous malformation bleeding can be caused by dissecting too close to the AVM and violating its margin. Small breaches are sometimes controlled with cautery, but it can also widen the hole and aggravate bleeding. A small piece of Nu-Knit and gentle pressure with the sucker will control most minor bleeding. For more significant bleeding, a fixed retractor blade on the Nu-Knit will free the hands to continue operating. This hemostatic retraction, or "iron thumb," applies pressure, buys time, and even advances circumdissection by lifting the nidus. The retractor is released after the bleeding site has clotted. Retracting an AVM can, by itself, result in AVM bleeding if it is excessive or if the blade sticks to the AVM margin. Therefore, Nu-Knit is used to pad the blade and retraction pressure is minimized.

Frank AVM rupture is an intraoperative catastrophe that usually occurs after inadvertently occluding an AVM's venous outflow. A large red vessel is eagerly cauterized and cut, expecting drastic reduction in the AVM's arterial supply. Instead, the AVM becomes tense with increased intranidal pressure, feeding arteries become difficult to coagulate, and the nidal margins pop with scattered points of hemorrhage remote from operative site. That misinterpreted "artery" was actually a major draining vein and the AVM is now on the verge of rupture. It is no longer possible to meticulously dissect the remaining planes, or to control these random bleeding sites around the nidus. Instead, a "commando" resection must deliver the AVM before it erupts. There is an interval between the venous occlusion and rupture that is variable and unpredictable, and therefore the resection must accelerate. The occluded vein is no longer functional and is divided to mobilize the AVM. The AVM is aggressively manipulated and retracted to hunt down the remaining feeding arteries. Active bleeding requires a large sucker to maintain visualization, and excess bleeding is allowed to run out of the bed, rather than down into the bed. Attention is directed to larger, coagulable feeders. Delicate feeders that would otherwise be carefully closed with microclips may have to wait until after the AVM is removed. Typically, there are two or three last feeders on the polar opposite side of the nidus, and they are found by mobilizing the nidus out of the resection bed, even as the blood pools in it. After occluding these feeders, the AVM slackens. Arteriovenous malformation removal opens the bed and makes it easier to scour for active bleeders, typically the smaller ones that were ignored.

The commando resection is a last resort when faced with impending or frank AVM rupture. It is clearly not meant for simple arterial or venous bleeding, or for minor nidal bleeding. Arteriovenous malformation rupture calls for decisive action, and the commando resection represents a point of no return. It is a test of one's mettle, requiring the recognition of a mistake and the courage to battle on. I can think of nothing in neurosurgery more challenging than salvaging these desperate situations. One must summon skill, insight, and grit at the end of a long case. One must quiet the rush of fear, confusion, regret, stress, frustration, and excitement. One must find calm, clarity, and confidence to continue operating. One must instruct nurses passing instruments, neurosurgeons providing assistance, and anesthesiologists replenishing the blood loss. Although the orderly rhythm of a meticulous AVM resection is suddenly replaced with frenzied chaos, it need not shake one's confidence. I have always fought through the duress, always resected the AVM, and never lost a patient on the operating table. Getting through an intraoperative AVM rupture and a commando resection is an important milestone. It is inevitable for the busy AVM surgeon; it exposes technical errors that can be rectified, such as misinterpreting red veins; it establishes one's ability to manage a disaster; and it builds confidence for all subsequent AVM resections, knowing that even the worst conditions are manageable. In the end, it is just bleeding, and one must simply keep working despite bleeding. Although the amount of bleeding in these explosive situations can be shocking, it can also be ignored, fixating instead on the last arterial targets and completion of the surgical plan.

10 Surgeon Factors

The Hurt Locker

Arteriovenous malformation (AVM) resection should be an interesting and comfortable operation to perform. Nowhere else in neurosurgery will you find such a strange assortment of tangled arteries that can be dissected and then obliterated with ischemic impunity. But that interesting and comfortable operation for the surgeon can quickly turn into a "hurt locker," which is military slang for a period or place of immense, inescapable physical or emotional pain, such as trying to disarm an improvised explosive device. Resecting an AVM is like defusing a bomb, picking it apart wire by wire, artery by artery. One mistake and the AVM will detonate in front of you. The threat of explosive hemorrhage adds stress and tension to the operation. Following a draining vein to the nidus can compromise outflow or rupture it; misjudging the right dissection distance can injure eloquent brain; and perforators on the ependymal plane can be nasty. Bleeding is unavoidable, even without technical mistakes, even with a new pair of nonstick bipolars, and even when microclips are deployed correctly. Part of successful AVM surgery is not expending too much time and energy on uncontrolled bleeding.

These operations require prolonged and intense concentration. Mental sharpness and efficiency can fade, resulting in technical errors, distraction, impatience, lapses in focus, and misinterpretations of anatomy. I schedule AVMs as the day's first procedure in order to arrive at the critical moments midday, rather than at the end of the day. Running a simultaneous procedure in a second operating room is an avoidable distraction, and although I can do multiple aneurysm operations in one day, I avoid multiple AVMs in one day. I like a good night's rest, a full stomach, music in the operating room, and a break midway, if only for a few minutes to take my eyes of the AVM. If there is still significant work to be done on a large AVM late in the day, I consider staging the resection. Although staged resections are rare, I have never regretted saving the difficult final dissection for later when I was rested.

Surgeon Judgment

The tenets discussed in this section of the book focus on resection technique, and a neurosurgeon's technical skill ultimately determines patient outcomes. Technical skill encompasses many factors, such as manual dexterity, translating two-dimensional angiographic anatomy to a three-dimensional operative field, developing the right planes around the nidus, physical endurance, composure during bleeding, and experience. However, equally important is a neurosurgeon's judgment. Clinical judgment means choosing your battles wisely, and the key to sustained success in AVM surgery is discriminating patient selection. Do not pick the beasts that will break your spirit.

Determining which patients to operate on is complex. On a basic level, there is the simple comparison of natural history risk over an individual's lifetime versus treatment risks, whether microsurgical, radiosurgical, endovascular, or some multimodality combination. Risk/benefit analysis works well at the extremes, such as low Spetzler-Martin grade AVMs in young patients and high-grade AVMs in elderly patients. On a deeper level, there is an overall accounting of patient variables that include neurologic condition, hemorrhagic presentation, diffuseness, employment status, emotional concerns, expectations, and more. This calculus is the hazy but quintessential judgment that neurosurgeons exercise in selecting patients for surgery, and as subjective as it is, it clearly impacts outcomes. For example, a patient with a high-grade motor strip AVM and a prior hemorrhage and hemiparesis might be unchanged neurologically after resection with a good surgical outcome. A different patient with the same AVM presenting with a seizure and no deficits might be worse neurologically after resection with a poor surgical outcome. Therefore, judicious patient selection is as important as technical skill in achieving outcomes that patients will find satisfactory. Most reports in the literature do not detail a surgeon's selectivity, but complication rates are inversely related to it. The same AVMs that are associated with the high complication rates and poor outcomes are also the ones that are torture for the neurosurgeon in the operating room, and these are best managed nonoperatively.

The skills and judgment of the AVM surgeon are challenged most by the difficult AVMs at the outer limit of operability, namely the eloquent Spetzler-Martin grade III AVMs and high-grade AVMs. Only by operating on difficult AVMs and, in retrospect, regretting the decision, have I identified the boundaries of my skill and refined my selection criteria. As my experience has grown, I have become more discriminating. This reaction with AVMs is unlike aneurysms or other surgical lesions, where experience and skill embolden the surgeon to tackle a wider range of lesions confidently. Arteriovenous malformation experience teaches the neurosurgeon that the real art of this surgery is knowing when *not* to operate. Refusing to operate on a young, intact patient with a difficult AVM who is seeking treatment is awkward. Am I sparing him a devastating complication during surgery that might alter or ruin his life? Or am I condemning him to inevitable hemorrhage, with the hope that enough time lapses beforehand and the damage is not too debilitating? The decision not to operate goes against our nature as surgeons and requires as much courage as the decision to operate.

Each neurosurgeon should explore his or her limits to define them, meaning that inevitably there will be patients taken to the operating room who perhaps should not have been. Experience clarifies the gray zone to black and white, focusing that zone into a narrow line. Perhaps our greatest challenge is to constantly calibrate this selection line and, at the same time, not wind up in a hurt locker.

II The Seven Arteriovenous Malformations

11 Frontal Arteriovenous Malformations

■ Microsurgical Anatomy

Brain

The frontal lobe has four surfaces: lateral, medial, basal, and sylvian (**Fig. 11.1**). The lateral surface is composed of three horizontal gyri (superior, middle, and inferior frontal gyri; SFG, MFG, and IFG, respectively) that are separated by the superior and inferior frontal sulci. The posterior border of the frontal lobe is the central sulcus that courses from the midline to the sylvian fissure. Anterior and parallel to the central sulcus is its one vertical gyrus, the precentral gyrus. The sylvian surface of the frontal lobe is the continuation of IFG into operculum, and includes the pars orbitalis, pars triangularis, pars opercularis, and the end of precentral gyrus. The basal surface of the frontal lobe is composed of the gyrus rectus and the orbital gyri (medial (MOG), lateral (LOG), anterior (AOG), and posterior (POG). The medial surface of the frontal lobe is composed of the SFG's medial aspect, paracentral lobule, and cingulate gyrus, as well as a small area below the rostrum with little surgical significance, consisting of paraolfactory and paraterminal gyri. Cortical areas of eloquence include the motor strip (precentral gyrus) and Broca's speech area in the dominant hemisphere (pars trian-

a. Lateral surface

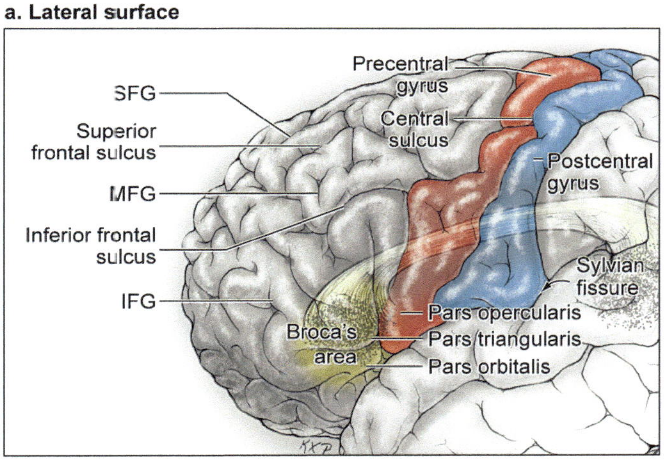

b. Medial surface

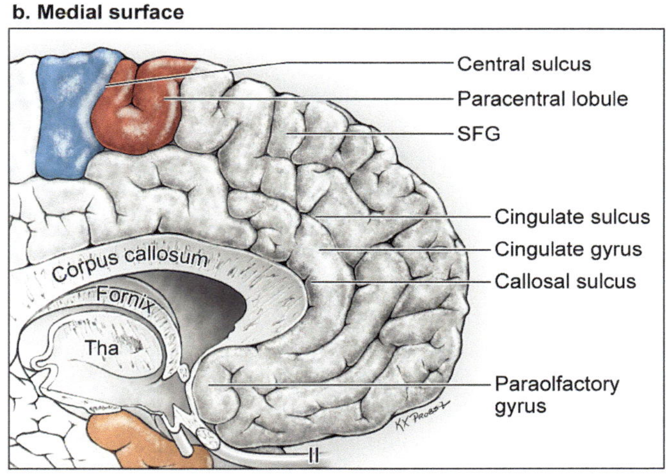

c. Basal surface

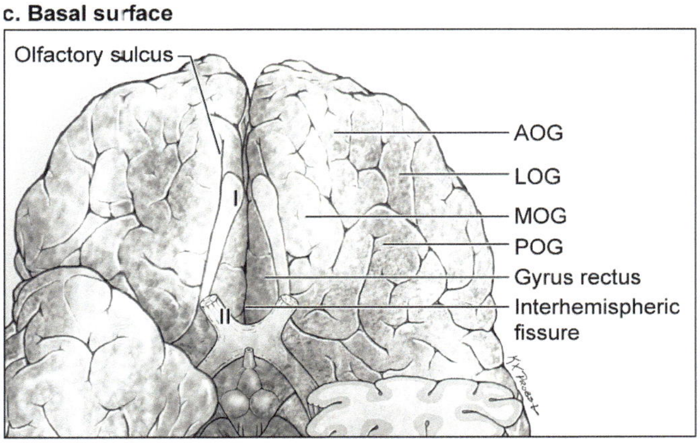

Fig. 11.1 Microsurgical anatomy of the frontal lobe. (**a**) Lateral frontal surface (lateral view). (**b**) Medial frontal surface (medial view). (**c**) Basal frontal surface (inferior view with left temporal pole removed).

gularis and opercularis). Eloquent white matter tracts include the corticospinal or pyramidal tracts, language conduction tracts, and the olfactory tracts.

Arteries

Arterial supply to frontal arteriovenous malformations (AVMs) is from middle cerebral artery (MCA) branches laterally or anterior cerebral artery (ACA) branches medially (**Fig. 11.2**). Classically, the M1 segment divides into a superior trunk that supplies the frontal lobe and an inferior trunk that supplies the temporal lobe. However, anatomic variation produces trifurcations, quadrifurcations, and asymmetrical trunks that can be superior- or inferior-trunk dominant. In general, frontal AVMs are fed by the superior trunks. The MCA trunks divide into unnamed stem arteries as they course through the insula (M2 segment) and operculum (M3 segment), on average eight per hemisphere. These stem arteries do not acquire names until they reach the cortex (M4 segment) to supply distinct territories. The frontal lobe is supplied by two to four stem arteries that then terminate in four cortical arteries: orbitofrontal (OrbFrA), prefrontal (PreFrA), precentral (PreCenA), and central arteries (CenA). The orbitofrontal artery, the most anterior and inferior branch, supplies the inferior frontal gyrus, middle frontal gyrus (anterior part), and pars orbitalis (inferior part). The prefrontal artery supplies the pars orbitalis (superior part), pars triangularis, pars opercularis, and most of the middle frontal gyrus. The precentral artery supplies the pars opercularis (posterior part), middle frontal gyrus (posterior part), and most of the precentral gyrus. The central artery supplies the precentral gyrus (superior part) and postcentral gyrus (inferior half). All four frontal arteries emerge from the sylvian fissure and course superiorly.

The ACA branches course in the interhemispheric fissure and feed the medial frontal AVMs. Eight cortical branches radiate from the ACA as it courses around the corpus callosum: orbitofrontal (OrbFrA), frontopolar (FrPolA), callosomarginal (CmaA), anterior internal frontal (AIFA), middle internal frontal (MIFA), posterior internal frontal (PIFA), paracentral (ParaCenA), and pericallosal artery (PcaA). The orbitofrontal artery is the first cortical branch of the distal ACA, arising just beyond the anterior communicating artery (ACoA) and coursing forward and down to the anterior cranial fossa floor to supply the gyrus rectus, medial orbital gyrus, and olfactory bulb/tract. Note that there are two named orbitofrontal arteries, one from the ACA and the other from the MCA. The frontopolar artery, the second branch of the distal ACA, originates from the postcommunicating or infracallosal A2 segment, courses anteriorly in the interhemispheric fissure, and supplies the frontal pole's medial and paramedian surfaces. The internal frontal arteries supply the medial and paramedian surfaces of the superior frontal gyrus, from the frontal pole anteriorly to the paracentral lobule

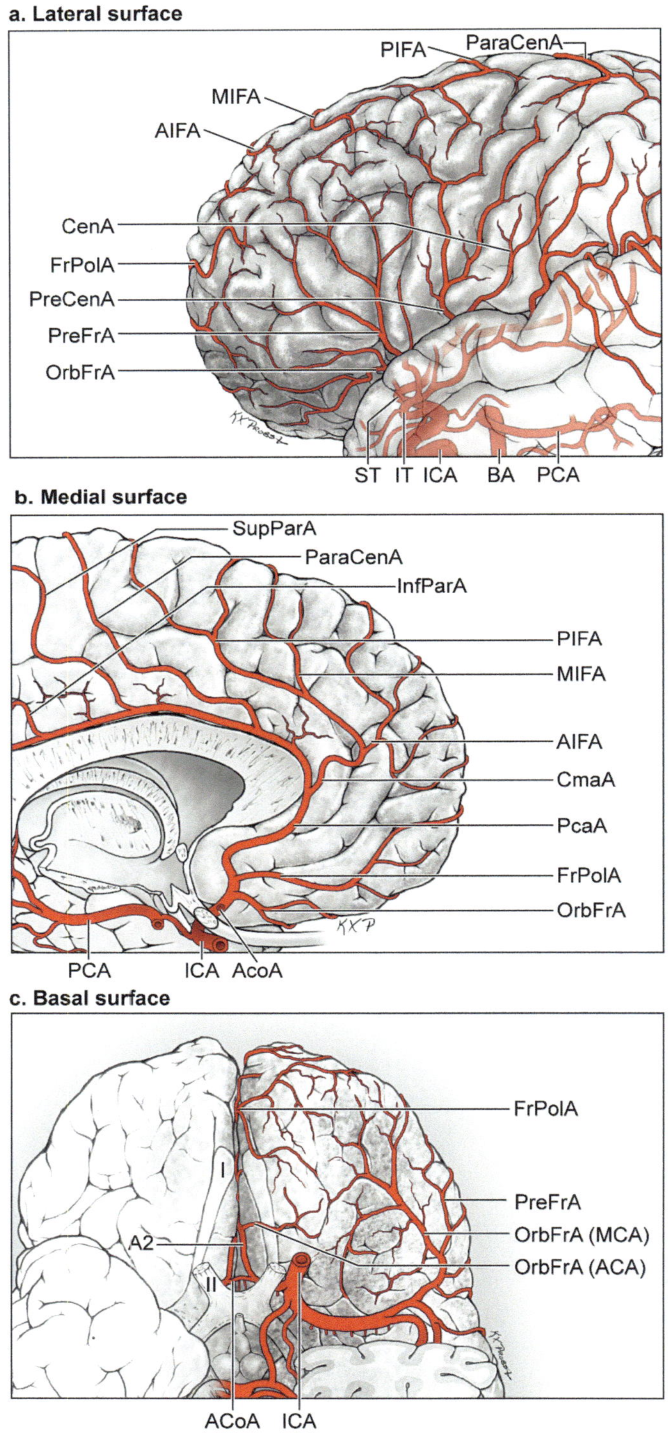

Fig. 11.2 Microsurgical anatomy of frontal lobe arteries. (**a**) The lateral frontal surface is supplied by the superior trunk of the MCA, which divides into stem arteries and terminates in four cortical arteries: OrbFrA, PreFrA, PreCenA, and CenA. Branches from the ACA also extend to the medial part of the lateral frontal surface. (**b**) The medial frontal surface is supplied by eight cortical ACA branches: OrbFrA, FrPolA, CmaA, AIFA, MIFA, PIFA, ParaCenA, and PcaA. (**c**) The basal frontal surface is supplied by orbitofrontal arteries from both the ACA and MCA, as well as FrPolA and PreFrA.

posteriorly. The anterior internal frontal artery (AIFA) originates from the infracallosal A2 segment adjacent to the rostrum; the middle internal frontal artery (MIFA) originates from the precallosal A3 segment adjacent to the genu, or from the callosomarginal artery; and the posterior internal frontal artery (PIFA) originates from the supracallosal A4 segment adjacent to the body of the corpus callosum. The paracentral artery arises from the A4 segment or the callosomarginal artery and supplies the paracentral lobule and its premotor, motor, and somatosensory areas.

Veins

Each frontal surface has its own network of cortical veins, anastomotic veins, and dural sinuses (**Fig. 11.3**). The lateral convexity is drained by the frontal veins that ascend to the superior sagittal sinus (SSS): the frontopolar vein (FrPolV); anterior (AntFrV), middle (MidFrV), and posterior frontal veins (PosFrV); and precentral (PreCenV) and central veins (CenV). The sylvian surface is drained by the frontosylvian veins (FrSylV) that descend to the superficial (SupSylV) and deep sylvian veins (DeepSylV). The medial surface of the frontal lobe is drained by the ascending medial frontal veins (MedFrV; anterior, central, and posterior). These veins course up to the superior margin of the hemisphere where they connect to the SSS or join the terminal ends of the lateral convexity veins before they connect to the SSS. The medial surface below the cingulate sulcus also has descending drainage to the anterior and posterior pericallosal veins (PcaV) that empty into the inferior sagittal sinus (ISS). The basal surface of the frontal lobe is drained by the orbitofrontal veins (OrbFrV, anterior and posterior), frontopolar vein (FrPolV), and olfactory vein (OlfV). The anterior veins (anterior OrbFrV and FrPolV) course forward to the frontal pole and empty in the SSS, whereas the posterior veins (posterior OrbFrV and OlfV) course backward to the DeepSylV in the medial sylvian fissure and continue to the basal vein of Rosenthal (BVR).

Five Frontal AVM Subtypes

Frontal AVM subtypes include the lateral frontal, medial frontal, paramedian frontal, basal frontal, and sylvian frontal. There is a subtype for each of the four frontal lobe surfaces, and an additional subtype for AVMs that have sides on both the medial and lateral surfaces. The surgical exposure of paramedian frontal AVMs requires access to two surfaces and two arterial territories, which alters the surgical strategy

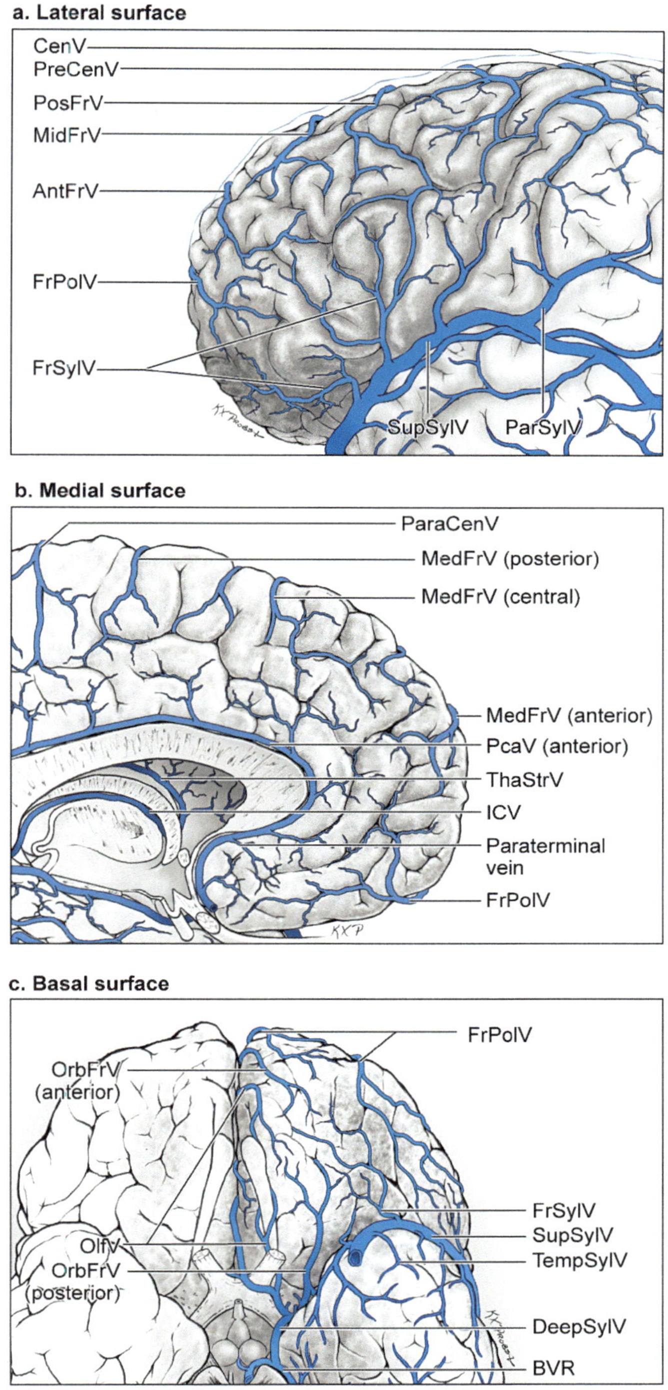

Fig. 11.3 Microsurgical anatomy of frontal lobe veins. (**a**) Veins of the lateral frontal surface (lateral view). (**b**) Veins of the medial frontal surface (medial view). (**c**) Veins of the basal frontal surface (inferior view).

to warrant the additional subtype. Other frontal AVMs that have sides on two surfaces (e.g., lateral + sylvian or lateral + basal) do not require access to an additional arterial territory and can be resected with the strategy defined by its predominant surface.

The Lateral Frontal AVM

Lateral frontal AVMs are the stereotypical cone-shaped convexity AVMs based on the lateral frontal surface with extension toward the ventricle (**Fig. 11.4**). The lateral convexity is such a large surface that this subtype was the most common frontal AVM subtype, accounting for over one third of all frontal AVMs and twice as many as the other frontal subtypes. Lateral frontal AVMs are fed by MCA branches that originate from the superior trunk. More anterior frontal AVMs are fed by OrbFrA and PreFrA; more posterior frontal AVMs are fed by PreCenA and CenA; and larger AVMs are fed by all four frontal arteries. These arteries emerge from the sylvian fissure and ascend on the cortical surface to reach the inferior AVM margin. Contributions from the ACA are absent or minimal. Venous drainage is superficial, ascending

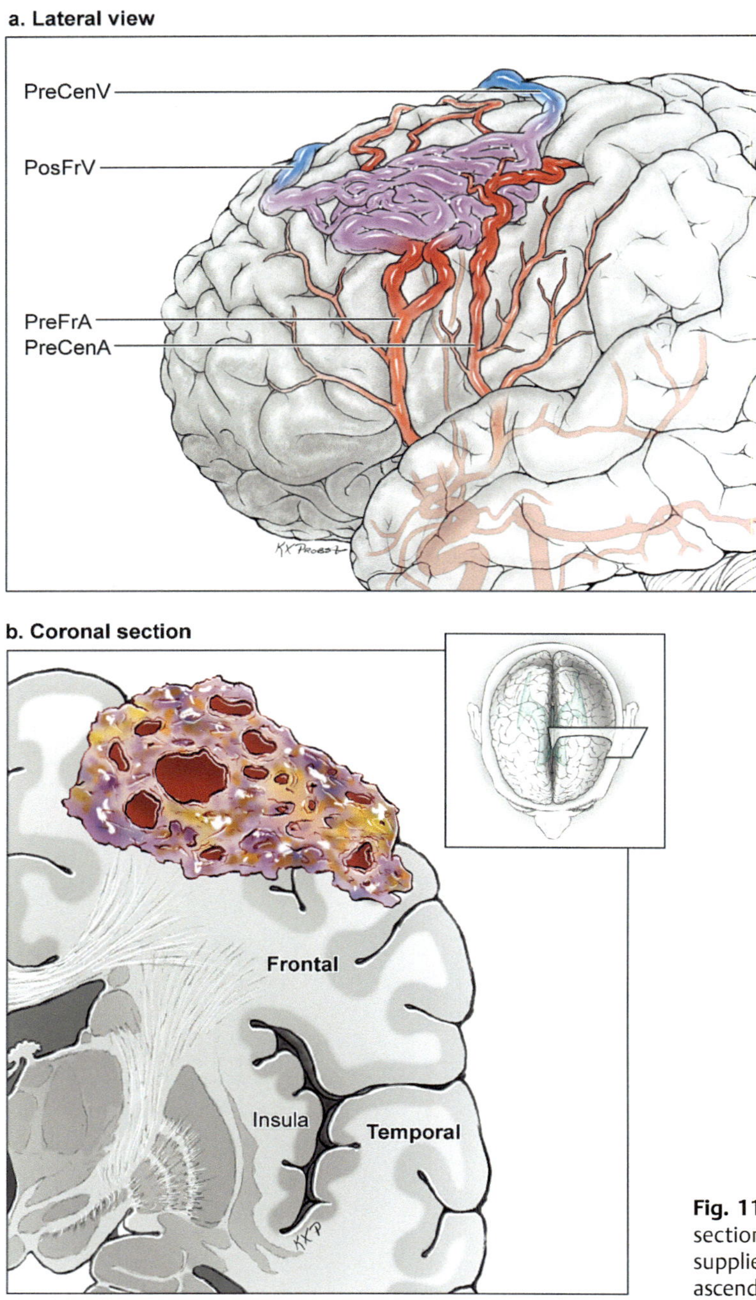

Fig. 11.4 The lateral frontal AVM: (**a**) lateral and (**b**) coronal cross-sectional views. This AVM is located on the lateral frontal surface, supplied by branches from the superior MCA trunk, and drained by ascending veins to the SSS or descending veins to SupSylV.

to the SSS (via FrPolV, AntFrV, MidFrV, PosFrV, PreCenV, and CenV), descending to superficial sylvian veins, or both. Eloquent areas associated with lateral frontal AVMs include the motor areas posteriorly and Broca's area inferiorly in the dominant hemisphere.

The Medial Frontal AVM

Medial frontal AVMs are located on the medial frontal surface (**Fig. 11.5**). Not visible on the lateral surface, they are visible on the medial surface only after opening the interhemispheric fissure. They can be superficially located in the medial aspect of the superior frontal gyrus, or deeply located in the cingulate gyrus. Cingulate AVMs are included in the medial frontal subtype, but not callosal AVMs. In contrast to lateral frontal AVMs fed by MCA branches, medial frontal AVMs are fed by ACA branches. More anterior medial AVMs are fed by OrbFrA and FrPolA; more posterior medial AVMs are fed by the internal frontal arteries and ParaCenA; and deep medial AVMs are fed by the PcaA and CmaA. The

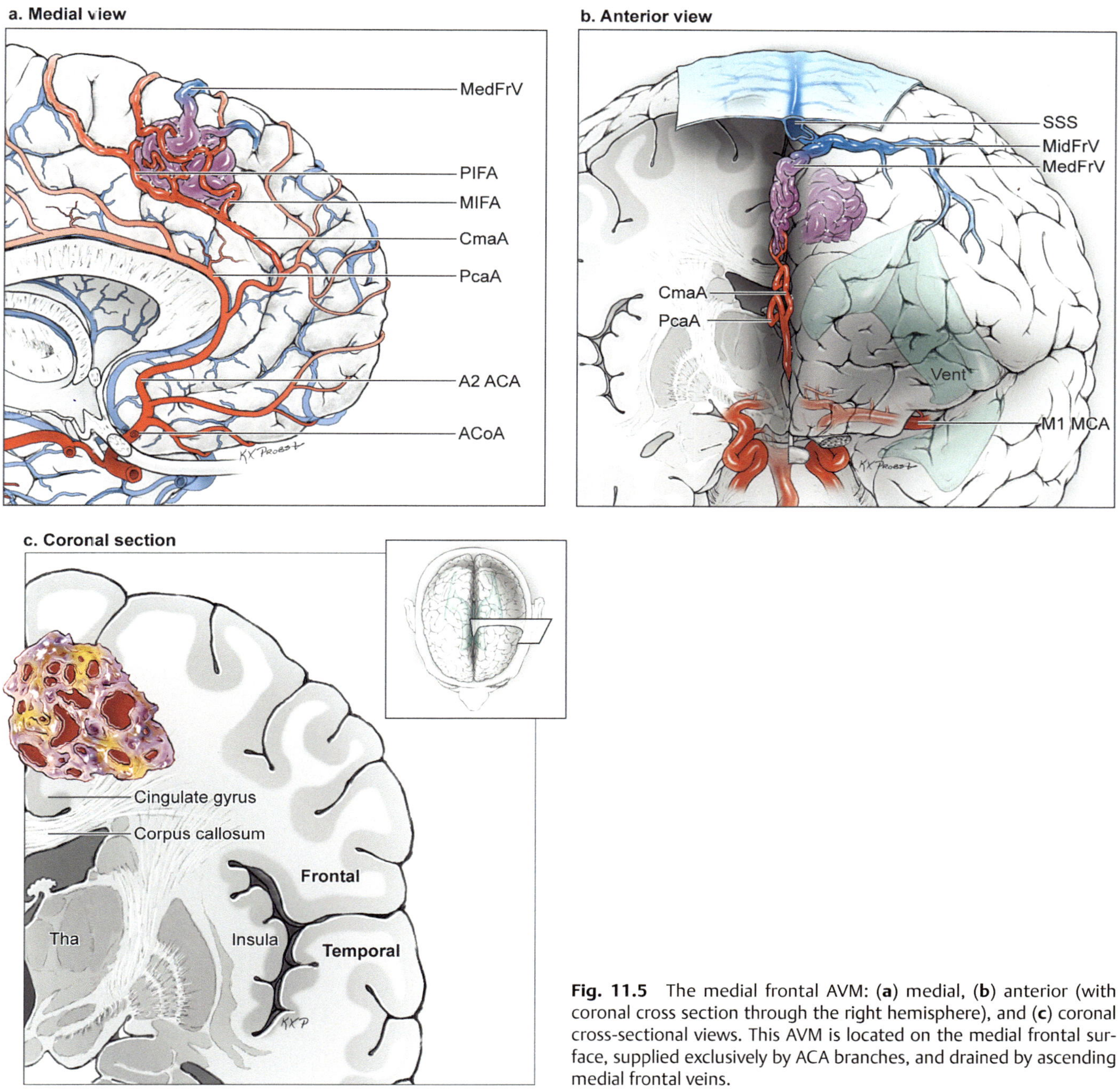

Fig. 11.5 The medial frontal AVM: (**a**) medial, (**b**) anterior (with coronal cross section through the right hemisphere), and (**c**) coronal cross-sectional views. This AVM is located on the medial frontal surface, supplied exclusively by ACA branches, and drained by ascending medial frontal veins.

ACA feeding arteries originate from various points around the corpus callosum and arrive at the nidus along its anteroinferior margins. Cortical branches from the MCA do not contribute to medial frontal AVMs. Drainage ascends to the SSS through the medial frontal veins, which may be the only sign of a medial frontal AVM at initial exposure. Cingulate AVMs and large medial AVMs have descending drainage to the pericallosal veins that empty into the ISS. Medial frontal AVMs are eloquent when they abut the motor strip in the paracentral lobule.

The Paramedian Frontal AVM

The paramedian frontal AVM is a combination of lateral and medial frontal AVMs. The paramedian AVM occupies two surfaces at the medial corner of the frontal lobe, unlike the lateral and medial frontal AVMs that occupy just one (**Fig. 11.6**). The paramedian frontal AVM is visible on the lateral surface *and* on the medial surface after opening the interhemispheric fissure. The difference geographically between the medial and paramedian frontal AVMs is small. In order to transform a medial AVM into a paramedian AVM, one would pull the AVM up out of the interhemispheric fissure to gain additional representation on the lateral surface and enter the watershed between the MCA and ACA territories. In this spot, the paramedian AVM is supplied by two arterial territories, unlike the lateral and medial subtypes that are supplied by just one. Any of the four cortical MCA branches and any of the eight cortical ACA branches can feed the AVM, depending on its size and location in the anteroposterior

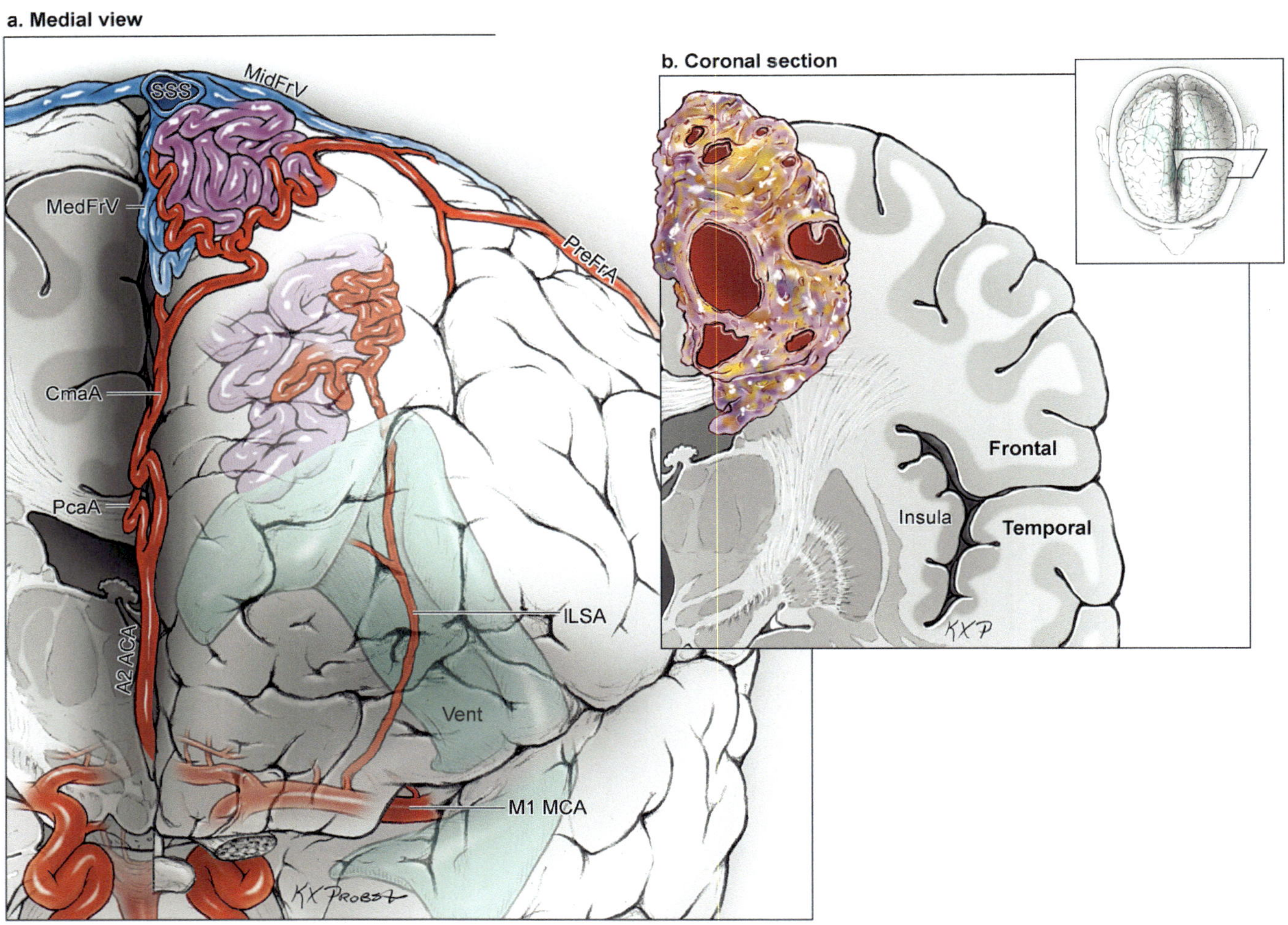

Fig. 11.6 The paramedian frontal AVM: (**a**) anterior (with coronal cross section through the right hemisphere), and (**b**) coronal cross-sectional views. This AVM is located on both lateral and medial surfaces, supplied by both MCA and ACA branches, and drained by both lateral and medial frontal veins.

plane. The paramedian nidus receives robust supply along two separate margins laterally and medially. Similarly, venous drainage is through both lateral and medial frontal veins that course to the SSS. Posteriorly located paramedian frontal AVMs are adjacent to eloquent motor areas.

The Basal Frontal AVM

Basal frontal AVMs are located on the basal frontal surface along the anterior cranial fossa floor (**Fig. 11.7**). They can be medial in the gyrus rectus and olfactory apparatus, or lateral in the orbital gyri. They can be anterior at the frontal pole or posterior adjacent to the anterior perforated substance. Basal frontal AVMs stay out of the interhemispheric and sylvian fissures, differentiating them from medial frontal and sylvian frontal subtypes, respectively. Like the paramedian frontal AVM, the basal frontal AVM receives a dual arterial supply from the MCA and ACA branches. OrbFrA and PreFrA from the MCA exit the sylvian fissure and travel to the AVM's posterolateral border. OrbFrA and FrPolA from the ACA exit the interhemispheric fissure and travel to the AVM's anteromedial border. Basal frontal AVMs also receive arterial input from unnamed A1 segment ACA branches that course over the olfactory tract and along the medial orbital gyrus to supply the AVM's posteromedial border. Venous drainage is usually superficial to the SSS via an anterior OrbFrV or FrPolV, but occasionally may be deep to the BVR via OlfV or posterior OrbFrV. Basal frontal AVMs are located in noneloquent cortex, but preservation of the patient's smell, taste, and appetite requires careful handling of the olfactory apparatus and its blood supply. Although olfaction is not considered eloquent when grading AVMs, postoperative deficits are obvious to patients and impact their satisfaction with surgery.

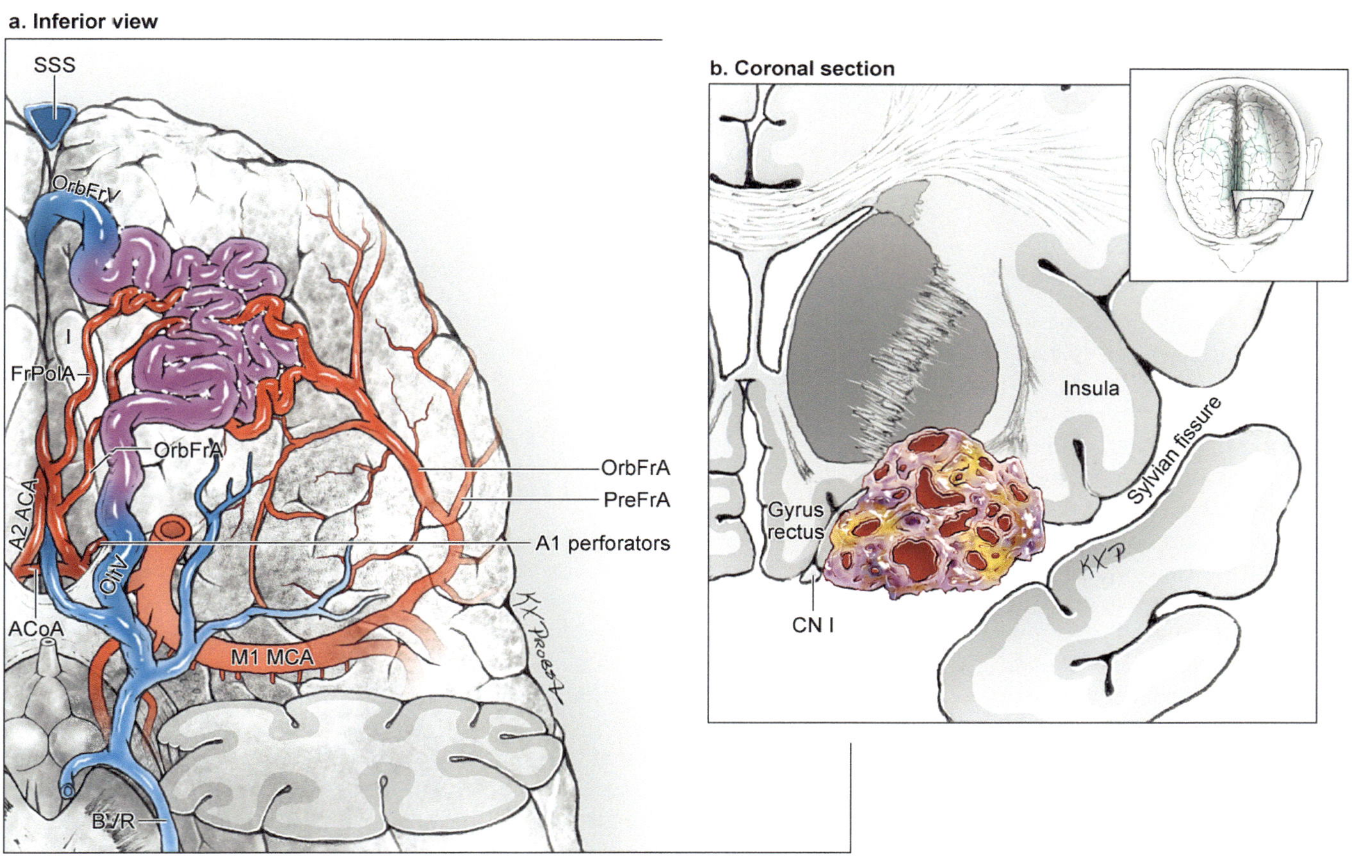

Fig. 11.7 The basal frontal AVM: (**a**) inferior (with left temporal pole removed), and (**b**) coronal cross-sectional views. This AVM is located on the basal frontal surface, supplied by both ACA branches (OrbFrA, FrPolA, and A1 segment perforators) and MCA branches (OrbFrA and PreFrA), and drained both superficially to the SSS and deep to the BVR.

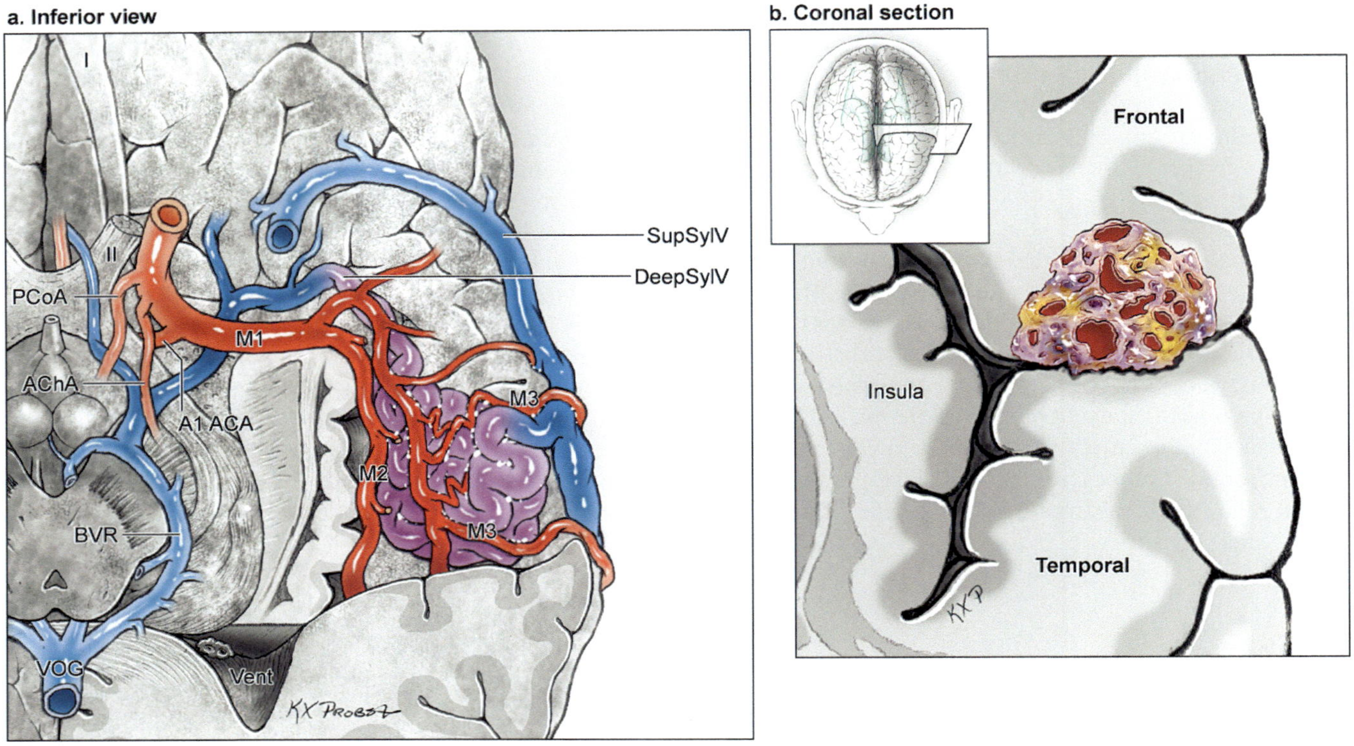

Fig. 11.8 The sylvian frontal AVM: (**a**) inferior (with left temporal pole removed), and (**b**) coronal cross-sectional views. This AVM is located on the sylvian surface of the frontal lobe in the pars orbitalis, pars triangularis, and/or pars opercularis as these gyri fold into the frontal operculum. Sylvian frontal AVMs are fed by M3 opercular branches and drained by sylvian veins, both superficial and deep.

The Sylvian Frontal AVM

Sylvian frontal AVMs are based on the sylvian surface of the frontal lobe, facing the sylvian fissure and temporal lobe on the opposite side of the cistern (**Fig. 11.8**). The inferior frontal gyrus forms an inferior convolution that consists of the pars orbitalis, pars triangularis, and pars opercularis. Sylvian frontal AVMs are located in these gyri as they fold into the opercular surface of the frontal lobe. In contrast, lateral frontal AVMs are located in the inferior frontal gyrus above these convolutions, and basal frontal AVMs are located in the lateral or posterior orbital gyri anterior to pars orbitalis, neither of them with representation on the frontal operculum. Sylvian frontal AVMs are also different from insular AVMs, which lie deeper in insular cortex, medial to M2 segments of MCA. In contrast, sylvian frontal AVMs are deep to the M3 opercular segments that course along the frontal operculum, and are supplied by M3 branches. Cortical M4 arteries do not supply these AVMs unless they enter the nidus as they arrive at the cortical surface or double back to its superolateral margin. The ACA does not supply sylvian frontal AVMs. They drain through SupSylV, DeepSylV, or both. Pars opercularis and pars triangularis in the dominant hemisphere comprise Broca's speech area, making these AVMs highly eloquent.

Frontal AVM Resection Strategies

Lateral Frontal AVM Resection

Lateral frontal AVMs are convexity lesions that are among the easiest to expose (**Fig. 11.9**). A unilateral frontal craniotomy with the patient positioned supine and the head rotated to align the AVM box parallel to the neurosurgeon provides direct access to the cortical surface and circumferential access to the four sides (step 1). Sulcal dissection identifies the nidal margins, feeding arteries, and draining veins (step 2). Lateral frontal AVMs have dual drainage with ascending and descending venous systems. Draining veins are identified at the superior margin if ascending to the SSS, or at the inferior margin if descending to SupSylV or other anastomotic veins, with care devoted to the dominant vein (step 3). Feeding arteries from the superior trunk of the MCA are found along the frontal side of the sylvian fissure

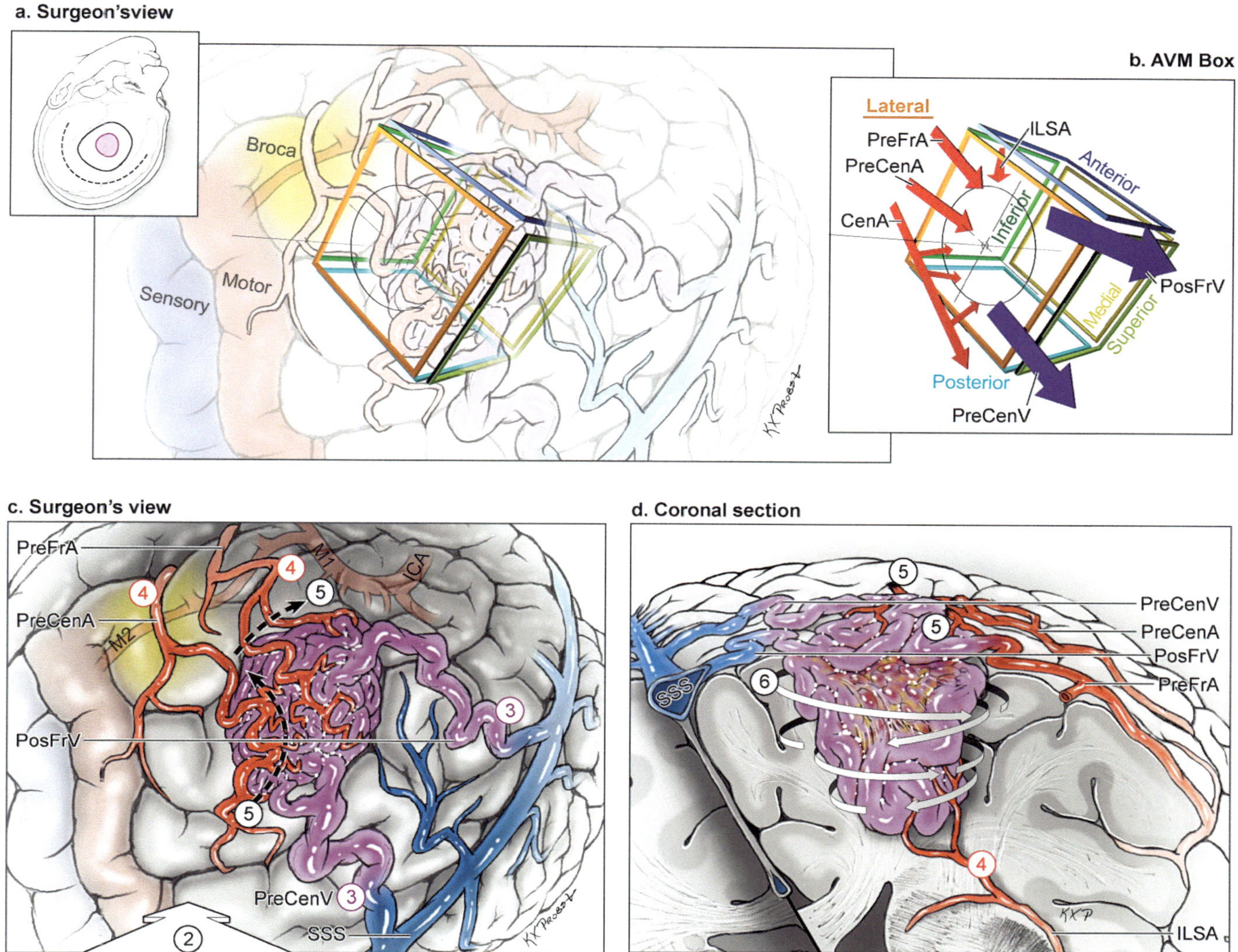

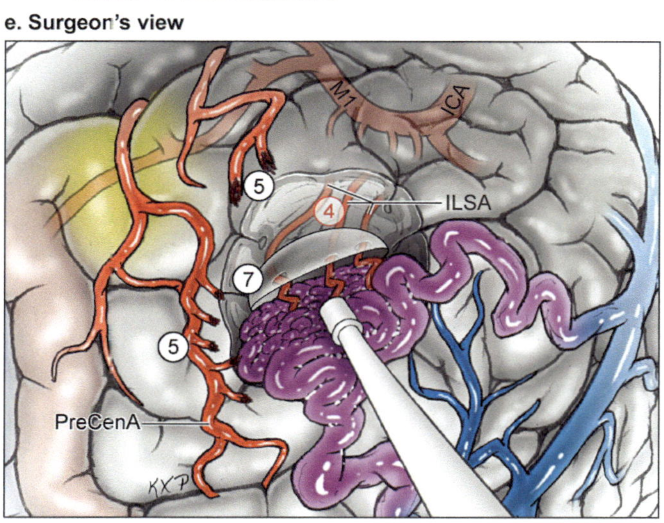

Fig. 11.9 Resection strategy for lateral frontal AVMs. (**a**) Step 1, exposing the AVM with a unilateral frontal craniotomy [surgeon's view, with scalp incision (*dashed line*), craniotomy (*solid line*), and AVM (*purple circle*) shown on inset]. (**b**) AVM box showing arterial inputs from the MCA branches, superficial venous drainage to the SSS, and proximity to Broca's area (yellow) and motor cortex (red). Note that the AVM's cortical surface is depicted with a circle on its base side and that side's label underlined. The AVM's axis is depicted with a line through the box. Arterial and venous anatomy is superimposed on the box with red inflow arrows and blue outflow arrows, respectively. (**c**) Step 2, dissecting margins in the lateral frontal sulci (broad white arrow); step 3, identifying ascending convexity veins; step 4, locating cortical MCA feeders; and step 5, interrupting the inferior front of arteries near the MFG (dashed black line), with care to preserve en passage flow in transit arteries (PreCenA, surgeon's view). (**d**) Step 6, circumdissecting into frontal parenchyma (encircling arrows, coronal cross-sectional view). (**e**) Step 7, mobilizing the AVM (spherical scoop) to expose lenticulostriate artery feeders on inferior side.

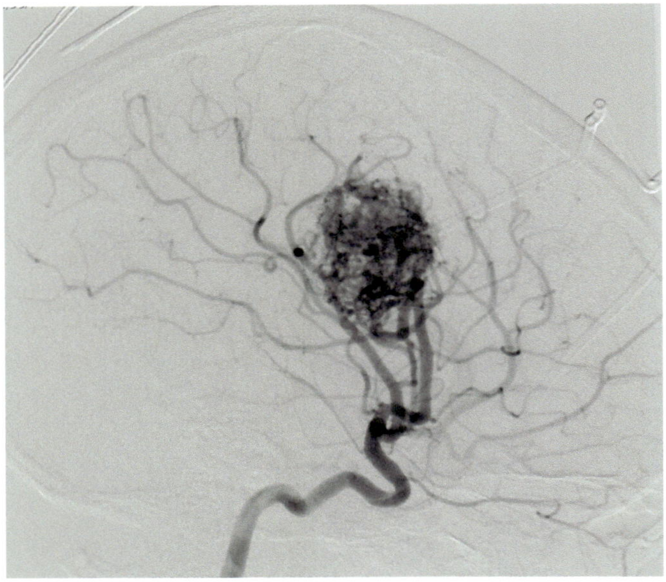
a

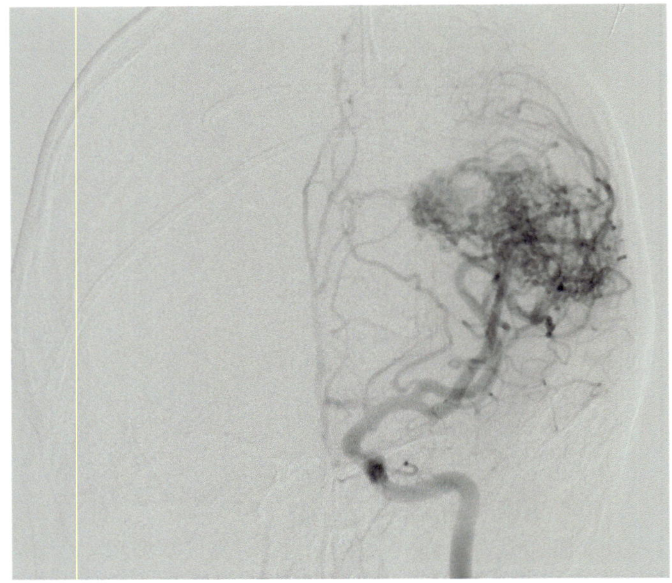
b

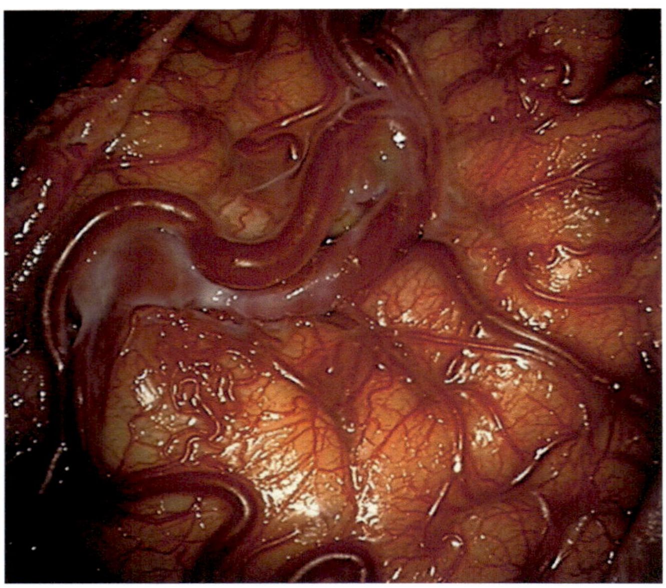
c

Fig. 11.10 This 13-year-old girl presented with a ruptured left frontal AVM (supplemented Spetzler-Martin grade 4: S2V0E1/A1B0C0), fed by PreCenA and CenA from the frontal trunk of the MCA (left ICA angiogram, (**a**) lateral and (**b**) anteroposterior views), and drained inferiorly by FrSylV and SupSylV and superiorly by PreCenV and CenV. (**c**) A left pterional craniotomy exposed these arterialized veins in the sylvian fissure.

as they exit the fissure, making it unnecessary to split the fissure (step 4). These arteries are traced from the sylvian fissure to the nidus where they form an inferior front of cortical arteries (OrbFrA, PreFrA, PreCenA, and/or CenA) that joins the nidus at its inferior margin near the IFG (step 5). Parenchymal dissection preserves Broca's area and motor strip, as well as deep white matter tracts containing corticospinal fibers (step 6). Deep dissection may extend to the frontal horn of the lateral ventricle where there may be an ependymal component of AVM (step 7). The lateral lenticulostriate arteries (lLSA) may also supply the deep plane and arterialize the nidus until the end to the dissection. These perforators are often difficult to visualize and cauterize, requiring AVM retraction and microclips (**Figs. 11.10** and **11.11**).

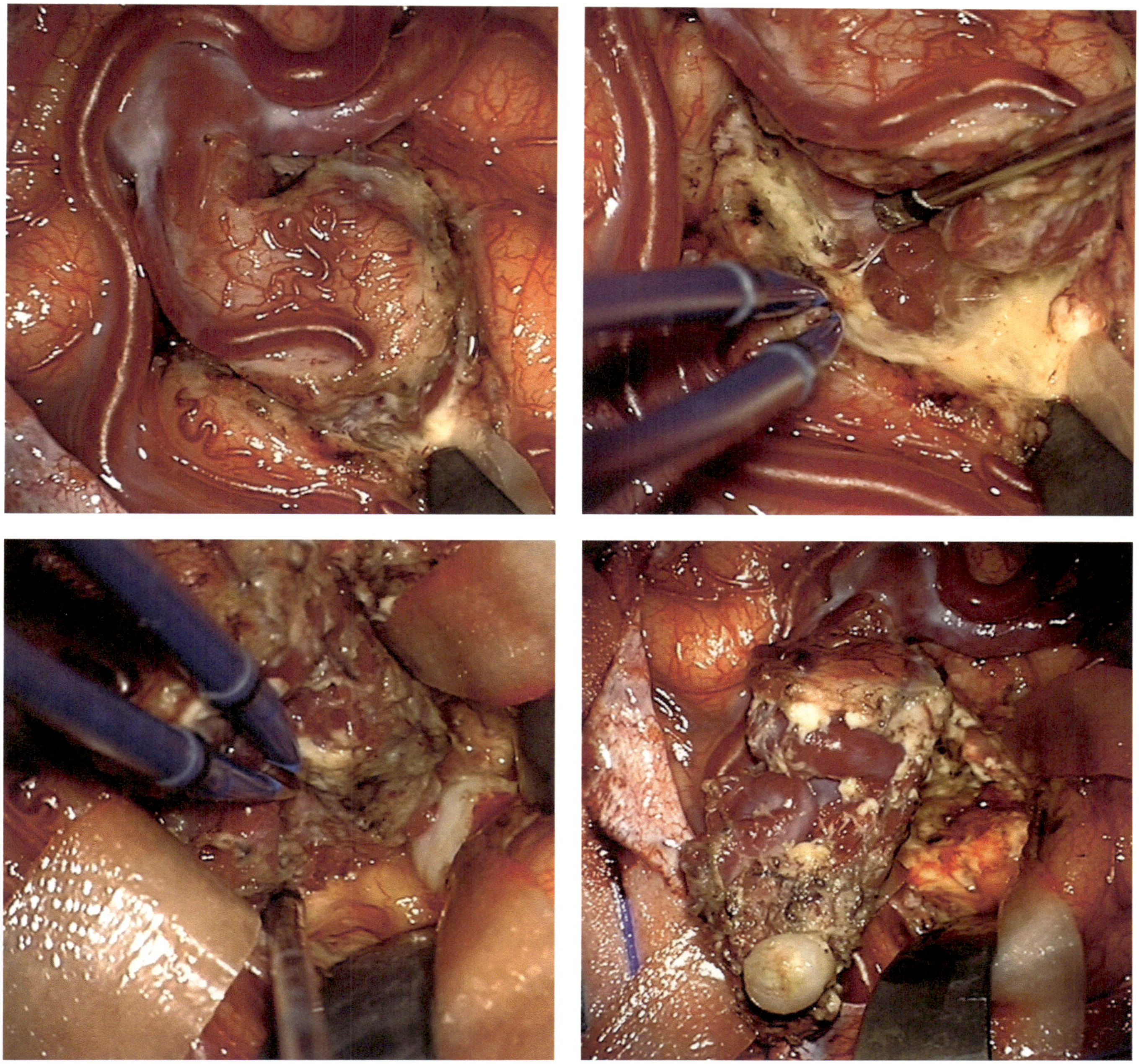

d e f g

Fig. 11.10 (*continued*) (**d**) A circumscribing pial incision revealed a compact nidus, and (**e**) a gliotic plane was followed around the AVM's parenchymal sides. (**f**) The AVM coned down to a venous varix at its tip and an adjacent hematoma that extended to the lateral ventricle (not shown). (**g**) After dissecting the deep side, the AVM was rolled out of the resection cavity based on its blue venous pedicle, indicating complete interruption of arterial input.

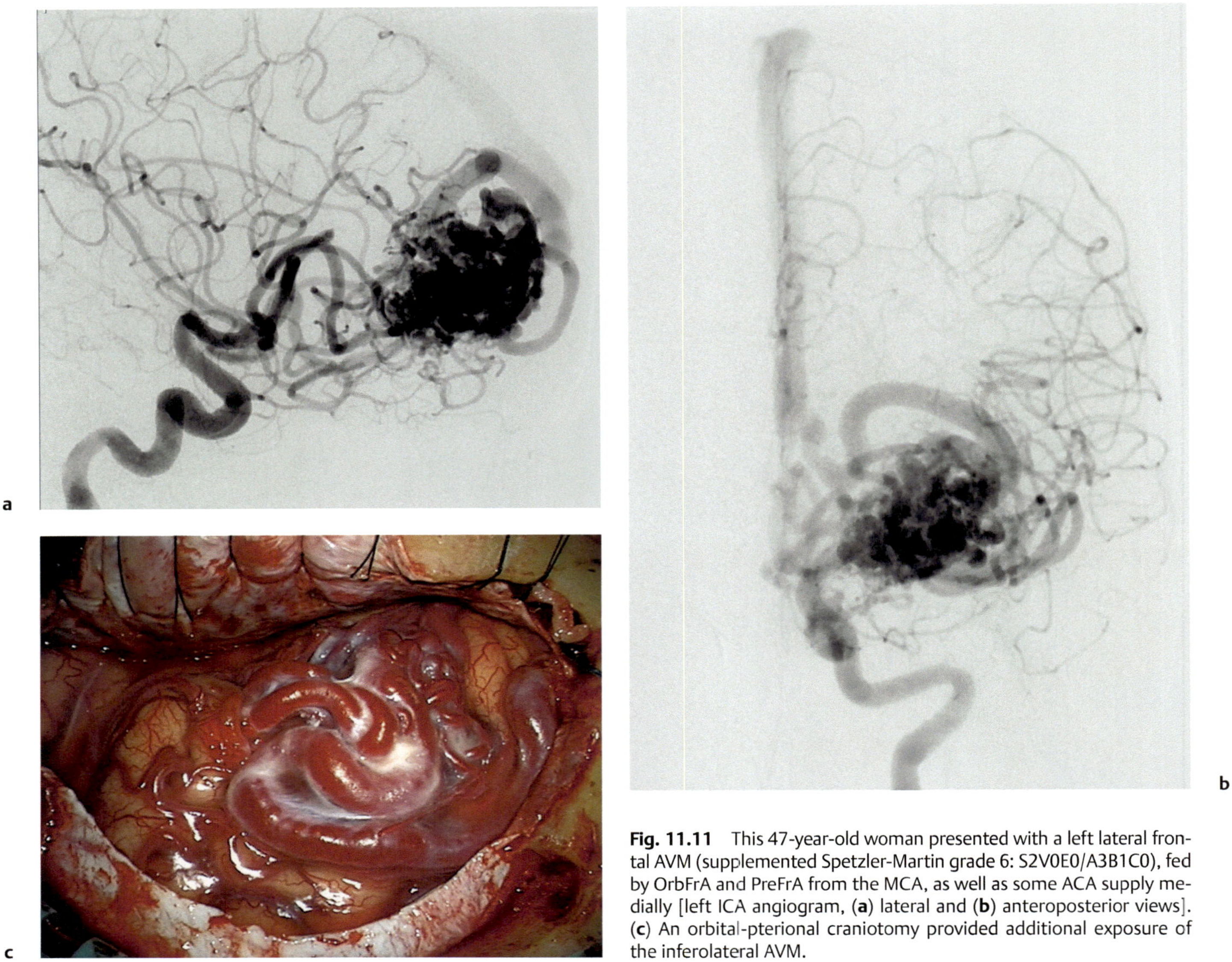

Fig. 11.11 This 47-year-old woman presented with a left lateral frontal AVM (supplemented Spetzler-Martin grade 6: S2V0E0/A3B1C0), fed by OrbFrA and PreFrA from the MCA, as well as some ACA supply medially [left ICA angiogram, (**a**) lateral and (**b**) anteroposterior views]. (**c**) An orbital-pterional craniotomy provided additional exposure of the inferolateral AVM.

d e

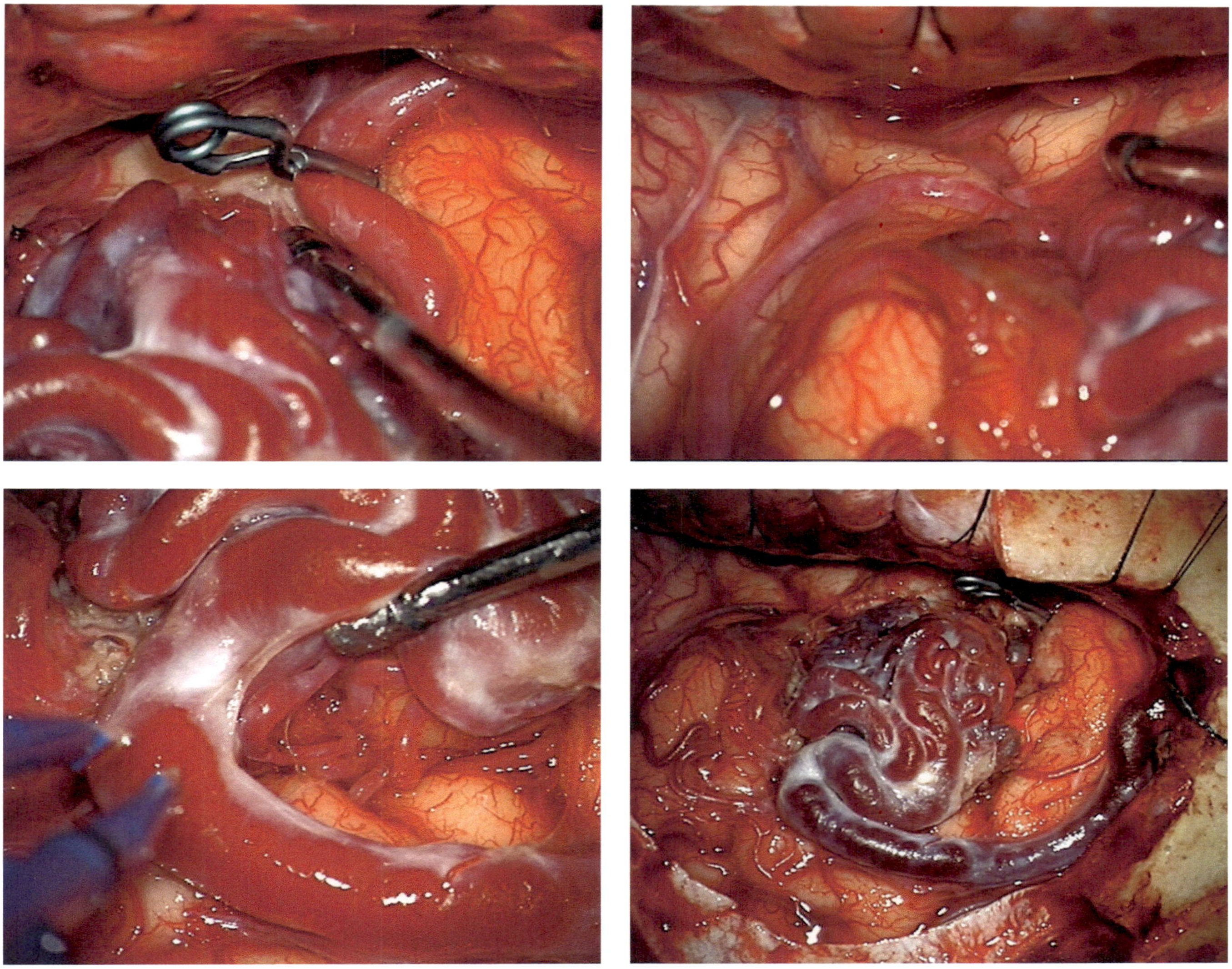

f g

Fig. 11.11 (*continued*) (**d**) A dilated OrbFrA was clip occluded at the AVM's anteroinferior margin, and (**e**) a smaller PreFrA was traced from the sylvian fissure to the posteroinferior margin. (**f**) Additional feeders from MCA were hidden by a turn in the overlying AntFrV. (**g**) After complete circumdissection, the AVM darkened.

Medial Frontal AVM Resection

Medial frontal AVMs are perhaps the most difficult frontal AVMs to expose. They require a complex approach to access their only cortical surface, and the angle of attack is perpendicular (**Fig. 11.12**). The interhemispheric fissure is widened by gravity retraction of the frontal lobe ipsilateral to the AVM. A bifrontal craniotomy is performed with the patient positioned supine, the contralateral shoulder bolstered, and the head turned 90 degrees to align the midline horizontally, with the AVM on the dependent (down) side (step 1). Bilateral craniotomy across the SSS opens an unobstructed view down the falx to the medial frontal surface and the superficial AVM plane. Arachnoidal adhesions between the frontal lobe and overlying dura are released; subdural dissection between the falx and medial frontal lobe reaches the corpus callosum cistern; and subarachnoid dissection between the medial frontal lobes through the cistern exposes the corpus callosum at the bottom of the interhemispheric fissure (step 2). The perspective is deep and perpendicular, with limited access to the sides of the AVM box. Venous drainage ascends to the SSS through MedFrV (step 3), which becomes an obstacle centered in the surgical corridor that must be preserved throughout the operation and cannot be sacrificed out of convenience. The draining vein can also tether the hemisphere and lessen the benefit of gravity retraction. The angle of attack can be redirected anteriorly and posteriorly to work around the vein. Identification of the

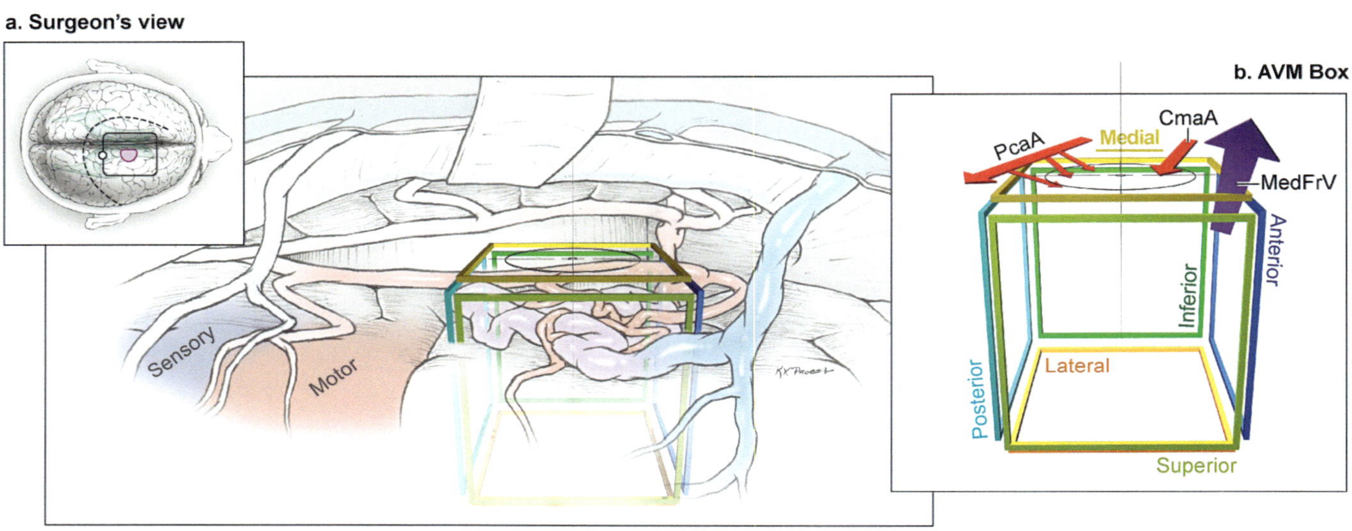

Fig. 11.12 Resection strategy for medial frontal AVMs. (**a**) Step 1, exposing the AVM with a semicircular scalp incision (*inset, dashed line*), bifrontal craniotomy (*inset, solid line*), and an anterior interhemispheric approach with the midline oriented horizontally for gravity retraction of the right hemisphere (surgeon's view). (**b**) AVM box showing arterial supply from ipsilateral ACA branches (CmaA and PcaA), ascending venous drainage through medial frontal veins, and proximity to the motor strip.

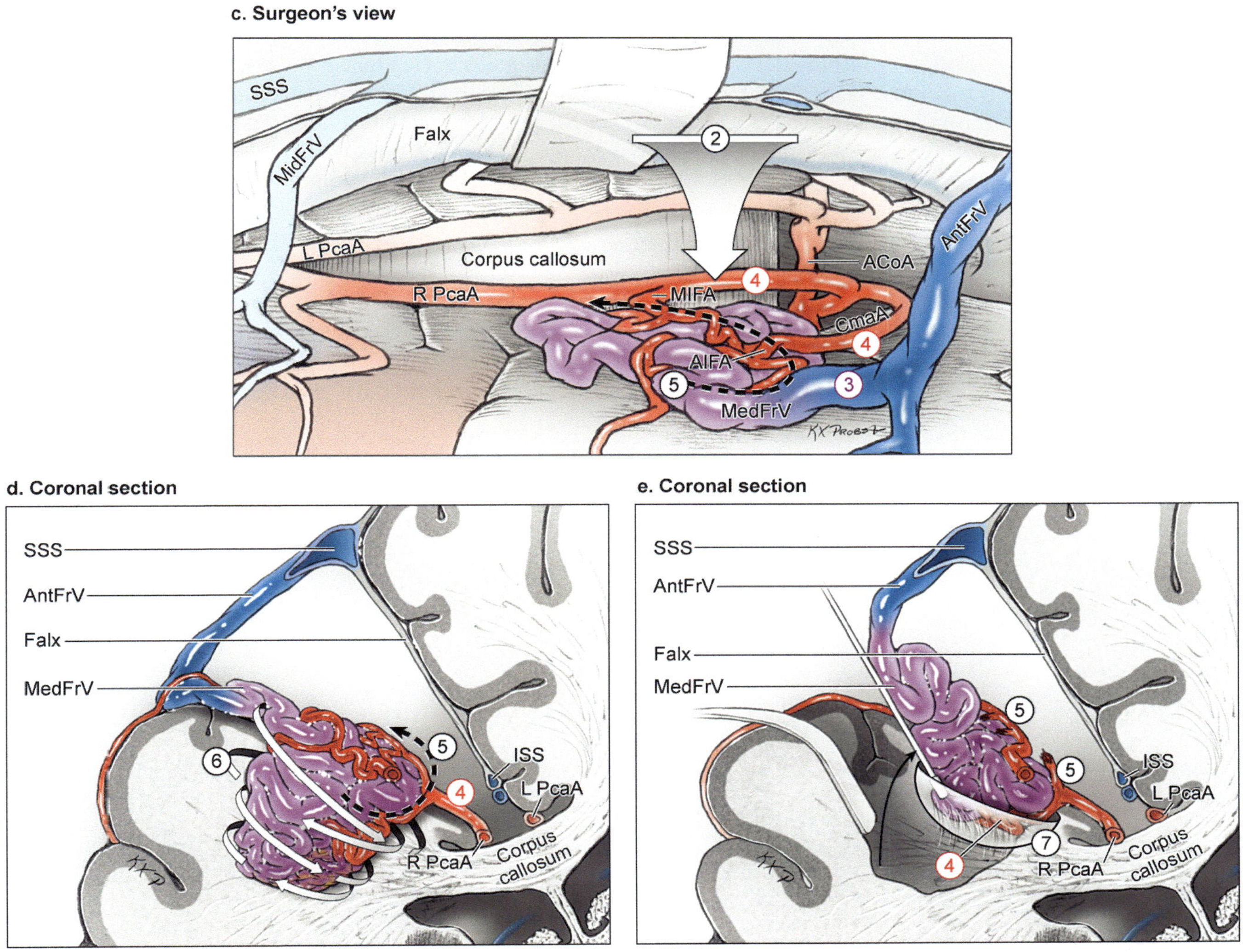

Fig. 11.12 (*continued*) (**c**) Step 2, widely opening the interhemispheric fissure down to the corpus callosum (surgeon's view). Although the dura and a bridging vein have been resected in this illustration to v ew venous connections to the SSS, the dura is elevated medially as a flap that requires release of arachnoidal adhesions, and bridging veins are preserved. Step 3, identifying draining veins on the medial surface; step 4, locating feeding arteries from CmaA and PcaA; and step 5, dividing the anterior front of feeders from ACA along or near cingulate gyrus. (**d**) Step 6, circumdissecting laterally into the frontal lobe (coronal cross-sectional view). (**e**) Step 7, mobilizing the AVM medially into interhemispheric fissure to access the inferolateral feeders.

feeding ACA branches (OrbFrA, FrPolA, internal frontal arteries, CmaA, and PcaA) usually requires interhemispheric dissection down to the corpus callosum anterior to the nidus (step 4). The anterior-to-posterior course of the ACA feeders creates an anterior front of arteries that are occluded along the cingulate gyrus (step 5). Perpendicular exposure requires nidus dissection up from the sagging frontal lobe, drawing the AVM medially as the parenchymal dissection progresses (step 6). Deep dissection may uncover feeding arteries along the inferior AVM margin from the PcaA (step 7). The distal continuation of the PcaA is preserved en passage. Deep dissection may also expose descending drainage to the PcaV and ISS. Medial frontal AVMs exemplify the challenges of perpendicularity. Perpendicular approaches expose the cortical base of the AVM with restricted access to other planes, which compromises visualization of anatomy and demands more nidal mobilization (**Figs. 11.13** and **11.14**).

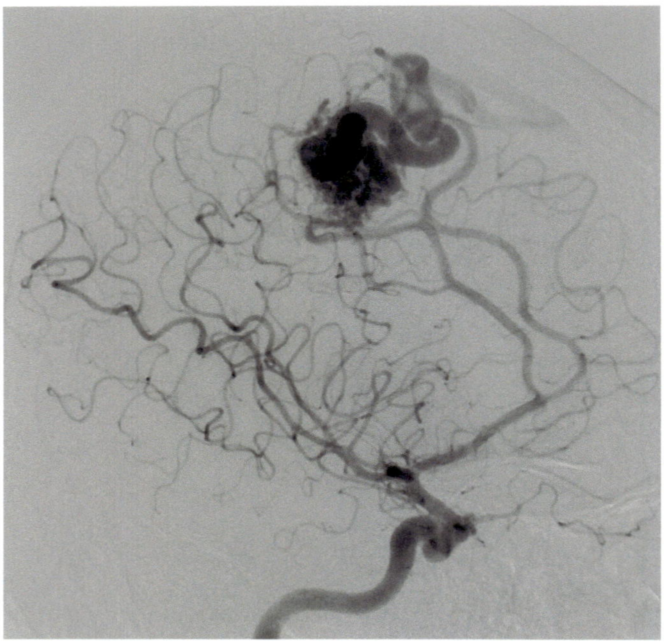
a

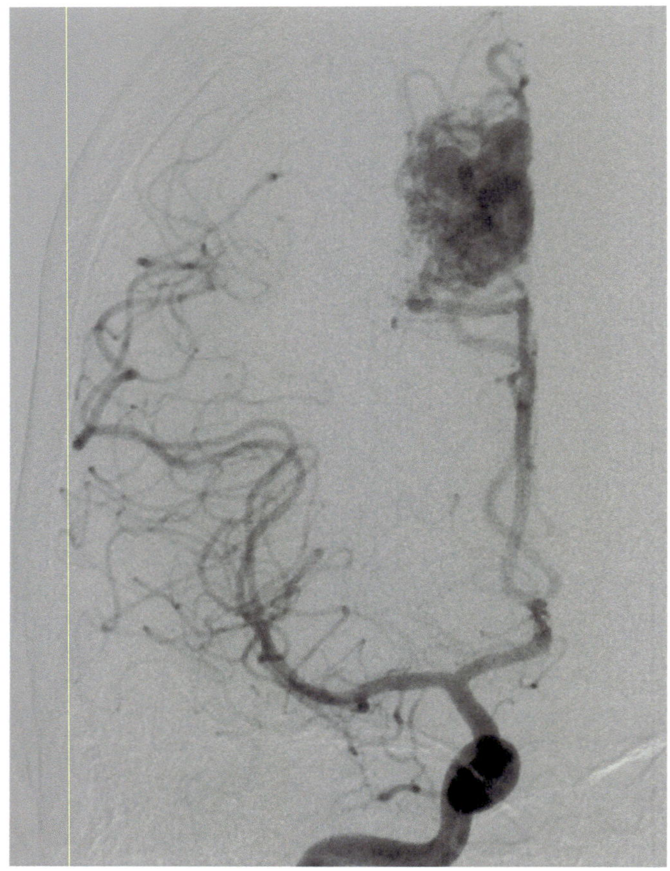
b

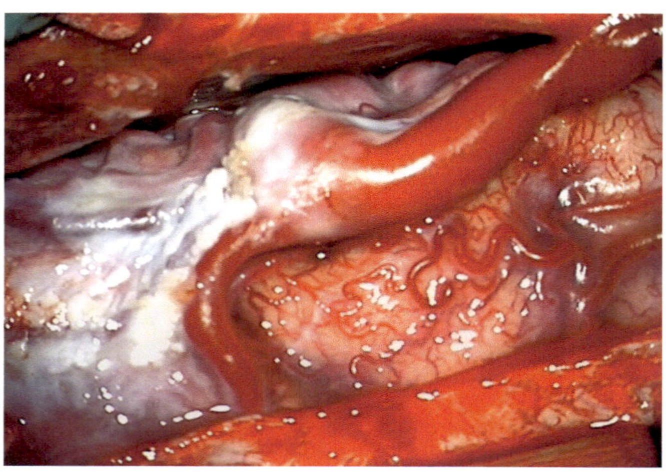
c

Fig. 11.13 This 50-year-old man presented with clumsiness in his left leg related to a right medial frontal AVM (supplemented Spetzler-Martin grade 6: S1V0E1/A3B1C0), fed by the PcaA and CmaA [right ICA angiogram, (**a**) lateral and (**b**) anteroposterior views]. (**c**) With the patient's head turned 90 degrees to the right to align the midline horizontally and the AVM in the dependent hemisphere, a bifrontal craniotomy exposed the interhemispheric fissure and the arterialized central MedFrV. Release of dense adhesions between this vein and the dura allowed gravity to retract the frontal lobe.

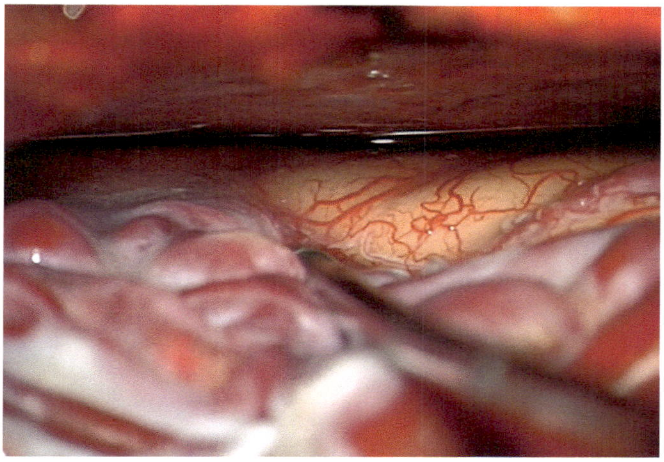

d

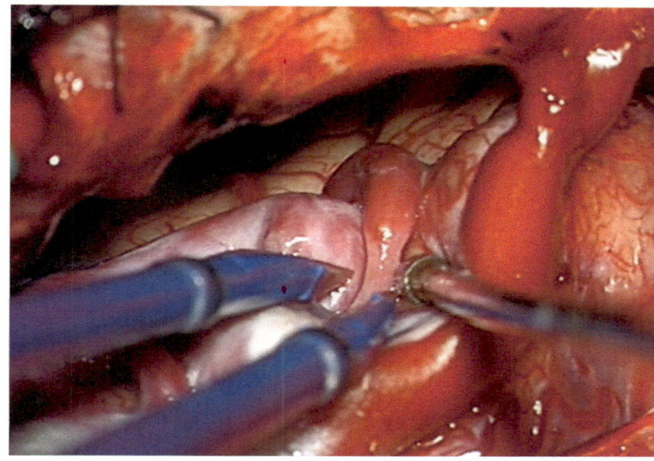

e

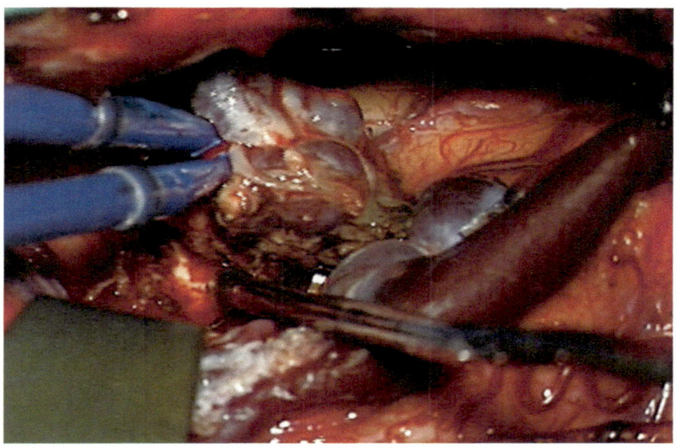

f

Fig. 11.13 (*continued*) (**d**) Bilateral craniotomy and gravity retraction provided a view down the falx to normal cingulate gyrus below the AVM. (**e**) CmaA input along the anterosuperior front was identified and coagulated. (**f**) Occlusion of PcaA input anteroinferiorly darkened MedFrV and the nidus, which was then mobilized upward to dissect the deep plane.

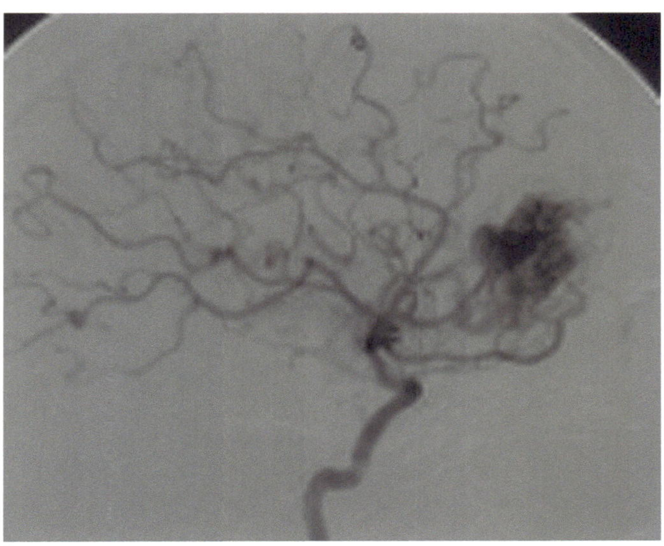

a

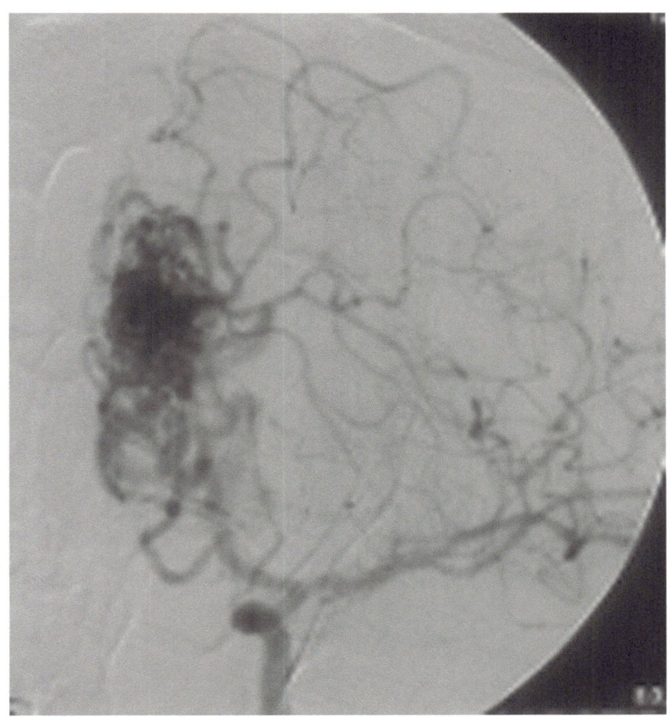

b

Fig. 11.14 This 50-year-old man presented with a left medial frontal AVM (supplemented Spetzler-Martin grade 6: S1V1E0/A3B1C0), fed by OrbFrA and FrPolA (left ICA angiogram, (**a**) lateral and (**b**) anteroposterior views). (*continued on next page*)

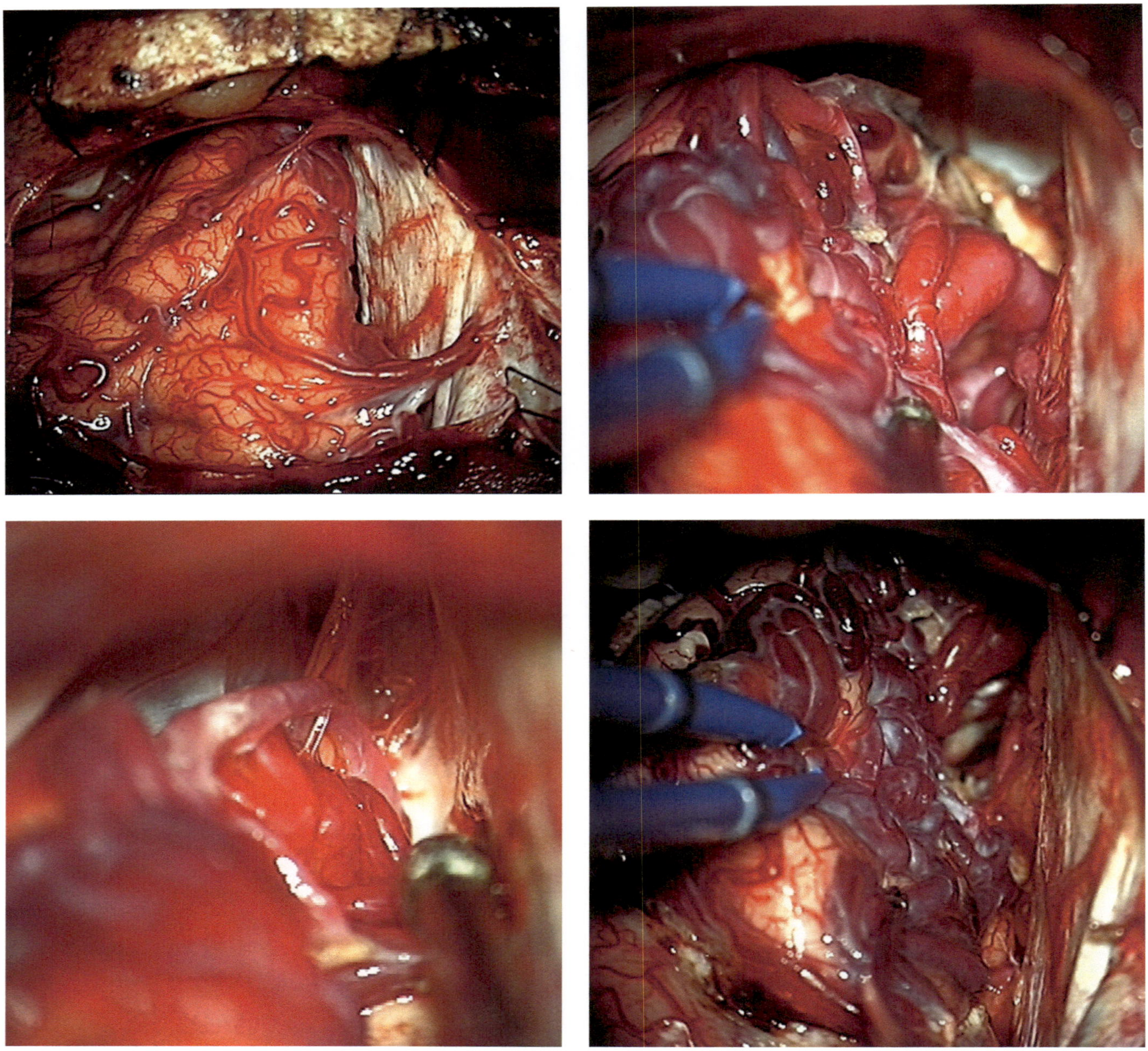

c d e f

Fig. 11.14 (*continued*) (**c**) This anteriorly located medial frontal AVM was exposed with a bifrontal craniotomy to access the interhemispheric fissure, but the midline was aligned vertically ("nose up"). (**d**) Venous drainage from the AVM did not ascend to medial frontal veins, but descended to OrbFrV (deep to the sucker tip) that ultimately drained to VoG. (**e**) OrbFrA coursed above the olfactory tract to supply the anteroinferior front. (**f**) After interrupting OrbFrA, FrPolA, and feeders on the lateral side, the AVM darkened.

Paramedian Frontal AVM Resection

Just as the paramedian frontal AVM is a combination of lateral and medial frontal AVMs, the exposure of the paramedian frontal AVM is a combination of two surgical approaches (**Fig. 11.15**). A bifrontal craniotomy exposes the intersection of the medial and lateral frontal surfaces forming the paramedian corner of the lobe, but gravity retraction is not used (step 1). The patient is positioned supine with the head in a neutral position ("nose up"), with the midline vertical and, with contralateral table rotation, the AVM on the upside. This position accesses the lateral convexity for occlusion of

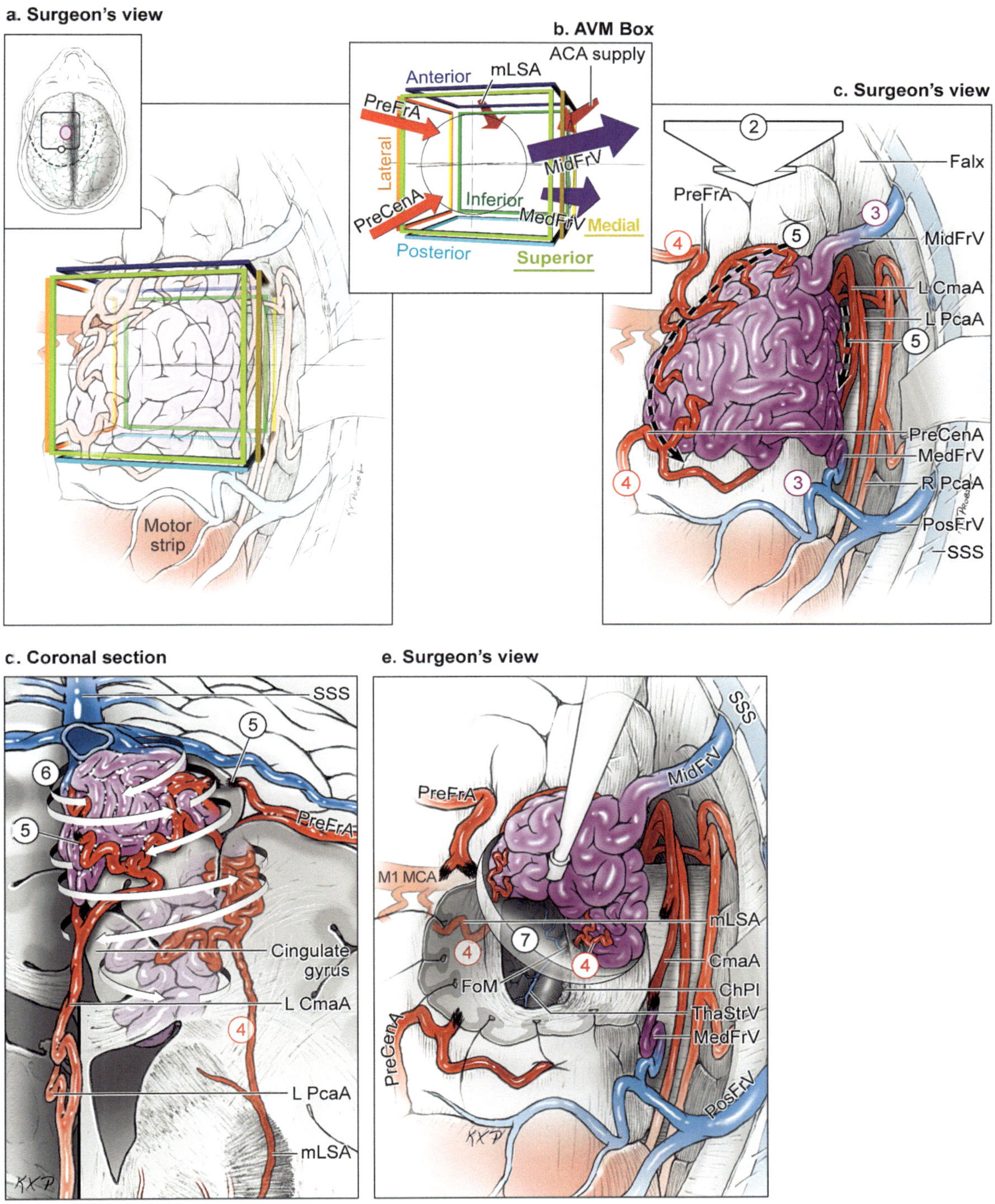

Fig. 11.15 Resection strategy for paramedian frontal AVMs. (**a**) Step 1, exposing the AVM with a semicircular scalp incision (*inset, dashed line*), bifrontal craniotomy (*inset, solid line*), and anterior interhemispheric approach with the midline oriented vertically ("nose up," surgeon's view). (**b**) AVM box showing arterial supply from both the MCA (PreFrA and PreCenA) and ACA branches (CmaA and mLSA). (**c**) Step 2, dissecting the AVM margins in the lateral sulci and opening the interhemispheric fissure. Although the dura has been resected in this illustration to view venous connections to the SSS, it is elevated medially as a flap that requires release of arachnoidal adhesions and preservation of bridging veins. Step 3, identifying draining veins laterally (MidFrV) and medially (MedFrV); step 4, locating feeding arteries laterally (PreFrA and PreCenA) and medially (CmaA); and step 5, dividing the lateral front of the MCA supply at or near the SFG and the anteromedial front of the ACA supply at or near the cingulate gyrus. (**d**) Step 6, circumdissecting into the frontal lobe (coronal cross-sectional view). (**e**) Step 7, mobilizing the AVM upward, dissecting across the deep lenticulostriate feeding arteries, and following the ependymal tip into the lateral ventricle.

the MCA supply and the medial surface for occlusion of the ACA supply. Gravity retraction, with the midline horizontal and the AVM in the dependent position (down), would eliminate access to the lateral convexity. Subarachnoid dissection consists of both an anterior interhemispheric fissure split and lateral sulcal dissection along AVM margins (step 2). Drainage ascends to the SSS via frontal veins and medial frontal veins, which can again be obstacles centered in the surgical corridor (step 3). However, this parallel approach offers greater mobility to work around the vein or veins. The paramedian frontal AVM receives supply from the ACA and MCA, which send their feeders to the AVM from the interhemispheric fissure and sylvian fissure, respectively (step 4). These two arterial supplies are interrupted along the anteromedial (cingulate gyrus) and inferolateral (MFG and SFG) margins (step 5). All four parenchymal sides can be accessed in parallel (step 6), taking care to protect the motor strip posteriorly. The deep plane can receive perforator supply from the medial lenticulostriate artery (mLSA) and lLSA. In addition, paramedian frontal AVMs can extend to the lateral ventricle where the ependymal nidus and draining ventricular veins must be identified (step 7). Their dual arterial supply makes paramedian frontal AVMs more robust than other frontal AVMs (**Figs. 11.16, 11.17, 11.18**)

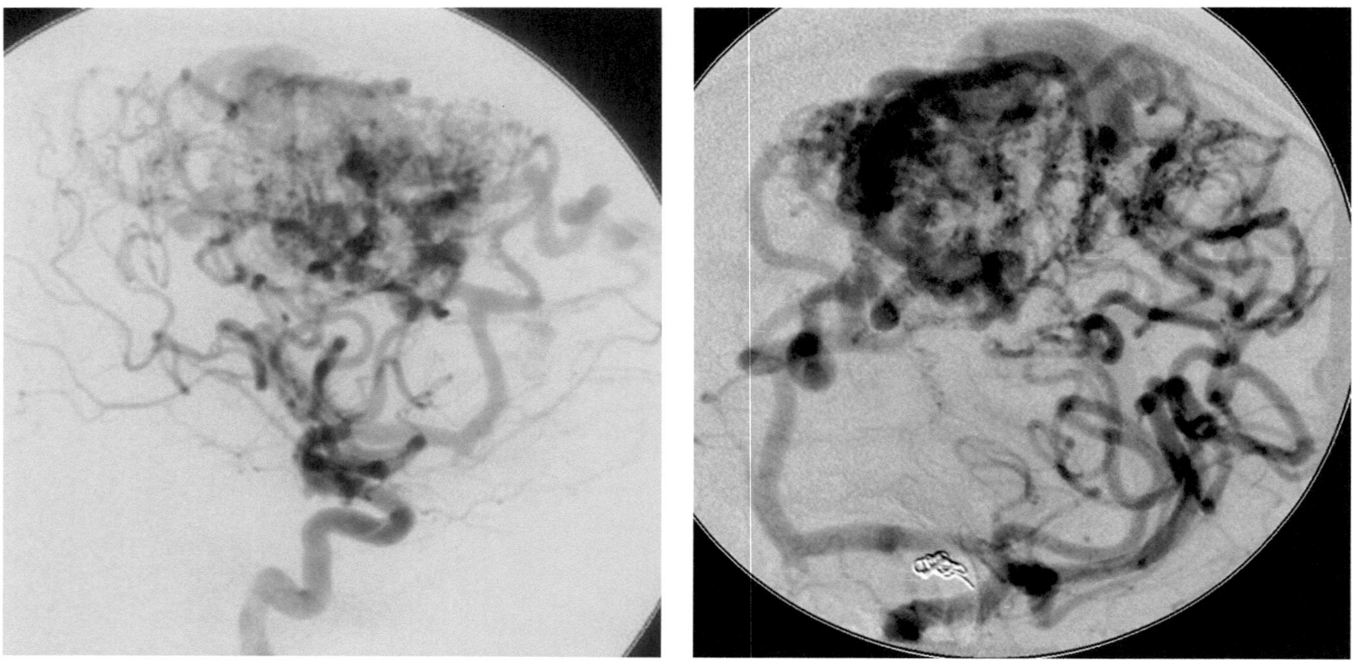

a b

Fig. 11.16 This 62-year-old woman had a left paramedian frontal AVM (supplemented Spetzler-Martin grade 8: S3V0E1/A3B1C0) supplied medially by the ACA branches (MIFA, PIFA, CmaA, and ParaCenA) and laterally by the MCA branches (PreCenA and CenA) (left ICA angiogram, (**a**) lateral and (**b**) anterior oblique views). She was initially treated with volume-staged radiosurgery with significant size reduction, prompting surgical resection.

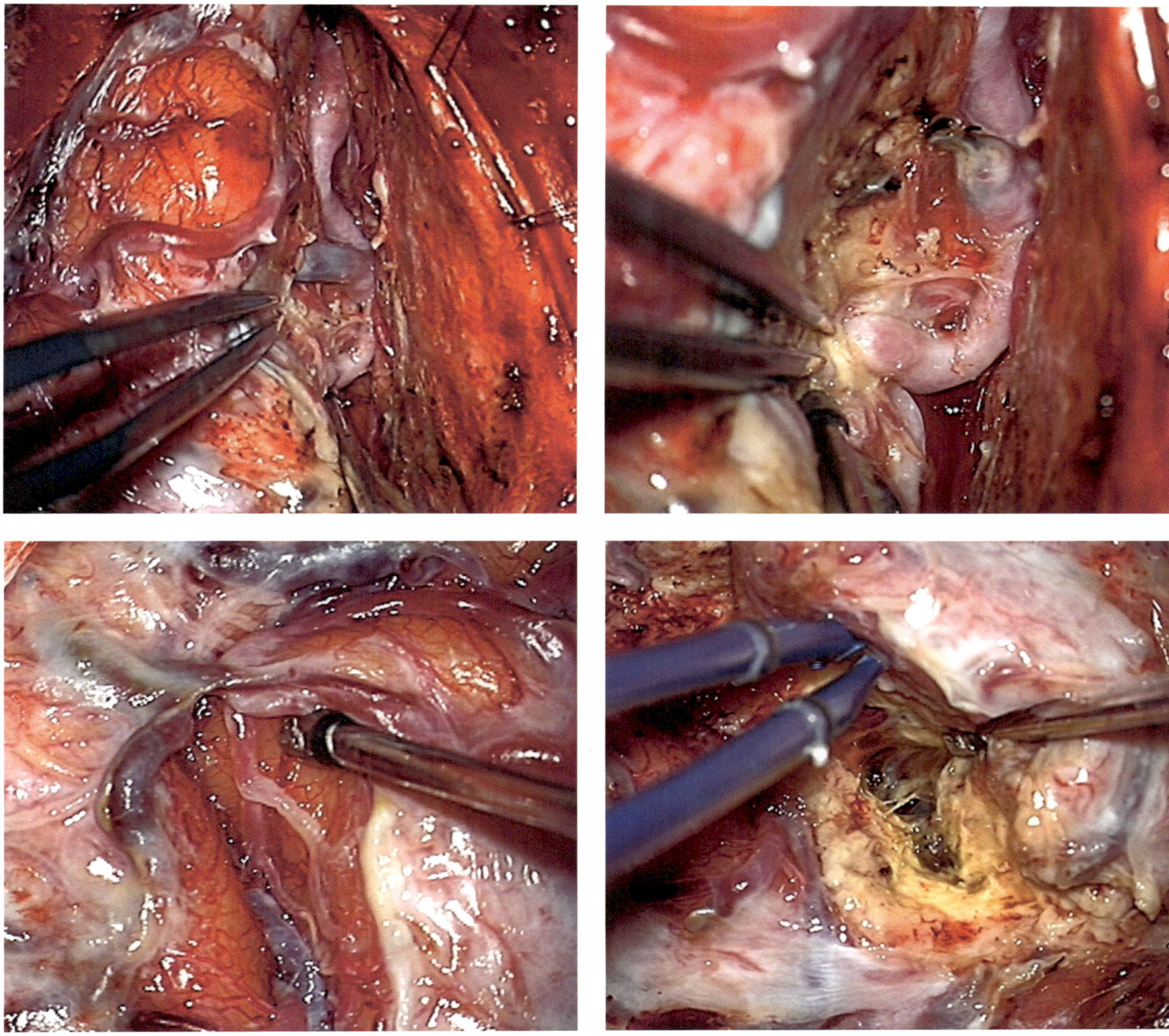

c d e f

Fig. 11.16 (*continued*) (**c**) The AVM was exposed through a bifrontal craniotomy with the midline aligned vertically ("nose up"), accessing a dilated ACA in the interhemispheric fissure that bifurcated into two feeding arteries (**d**) that were cauterized and divided. (**e**) This exposure also provided parallel access to the AVM's lateral border where PreCenA and CenA feeders were interrupted. (**f**) Prior radiosurgery sclerosed the AVM and induced gliosis, creating favorable dissection planes around the parenchymal sides.

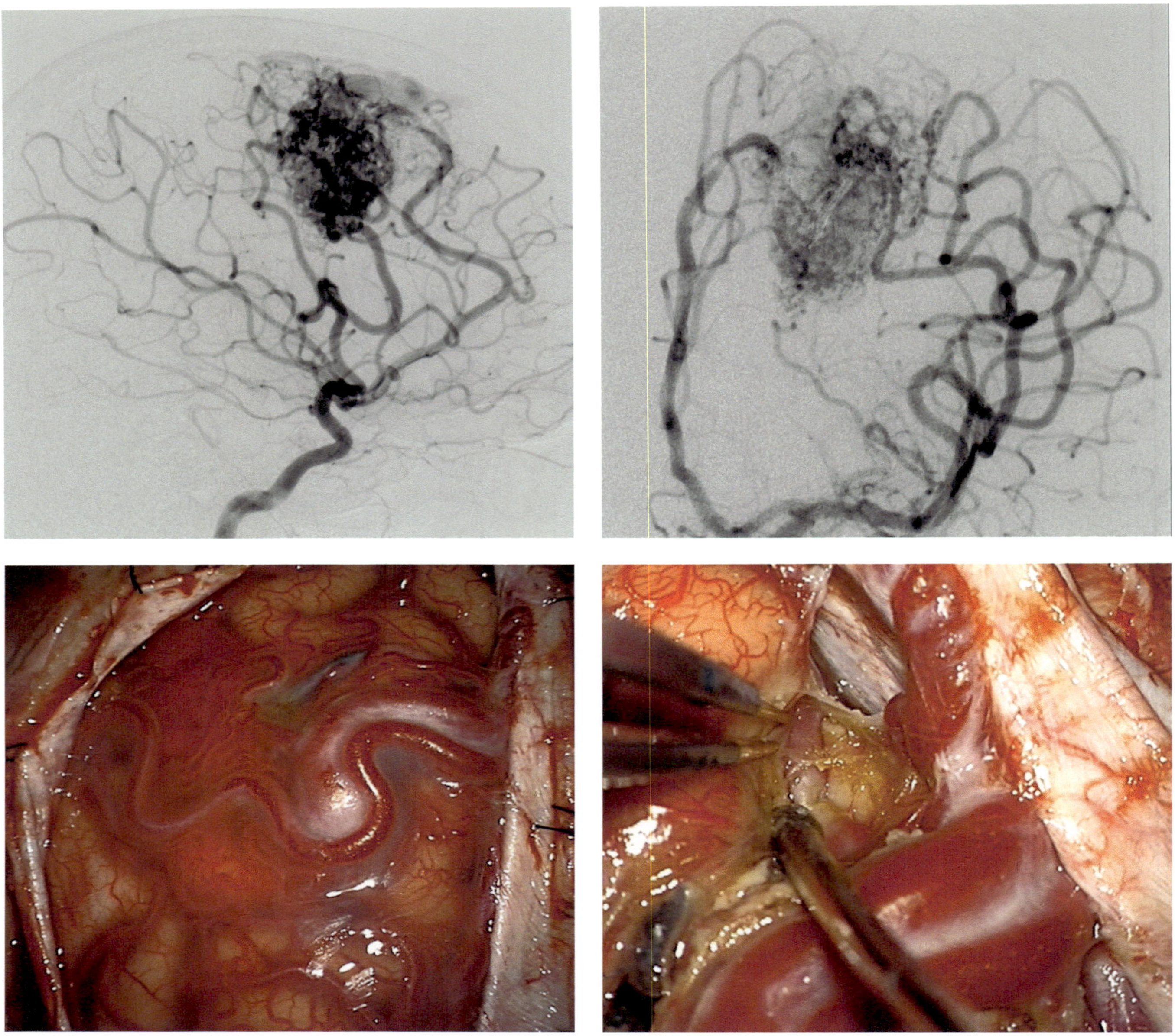

Fig. 11.17 This 21-year-old woman presented with seizures and a left paramedian frontal AVM adjacent to the motor strip (supplemented Spetzler-Martin grade 6: S2V0E1/A2B1C0). Angiography demonstrated the dual supply from the ACA medially (MIFA and PIFA) and the MCA laterally (PreCenA, CenA, and lLSA) [left ICA angiogram, (**a**) lateral and (**b**) anteroposterior views]. (**c**) Bifrontal craniotomy with the nose up exposed an arterialized PreCenV coursing to the SSS and an embolized PreCenA. (**d**) Dissection along the falx into the interhemispheric fissure, anterior to the draining vein, led to the PIFA along the anterior front.

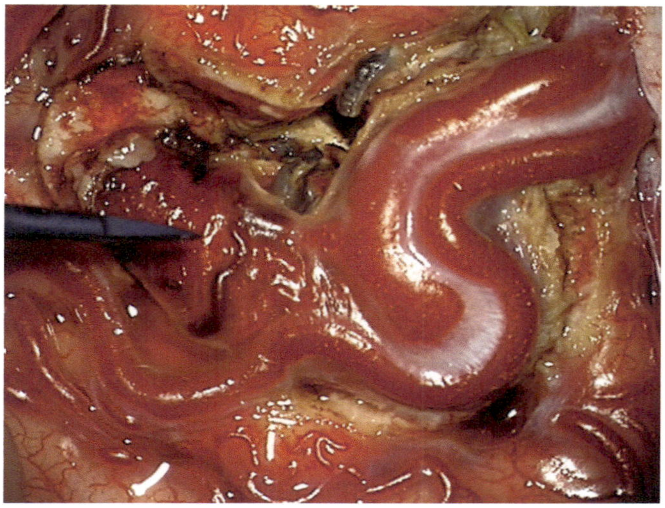

e

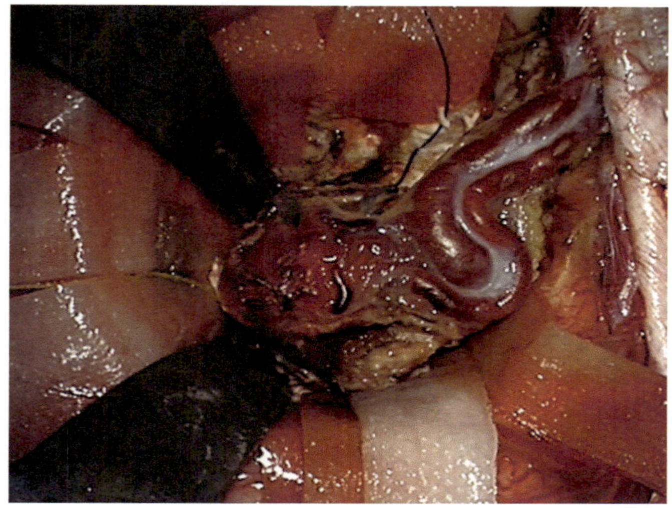

f

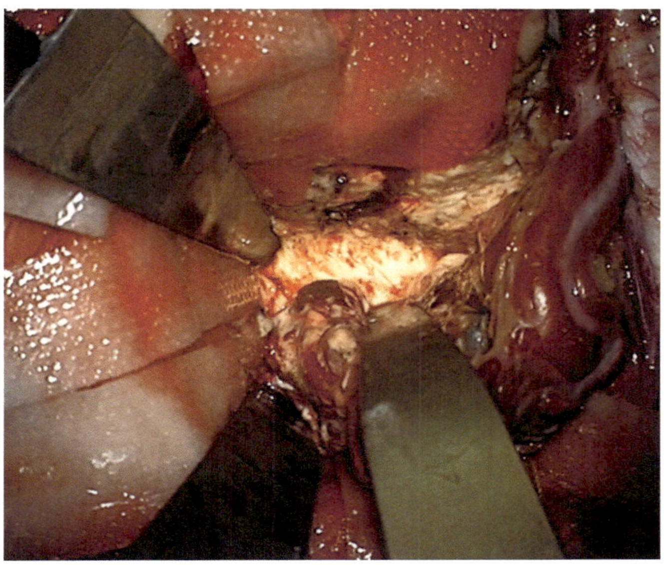

g

Fig. 11.17 (*continued*) (**e**) Lateral pial and parenchymal dissection interrupted inputs from the MCA. (**f**) Before attacking the lLSA feeder on the ependymal plane, the cavity was lined with Telfa strips and retractors were inserted. (**g**) Retraction on the AVM exposed the deep side where the lLSA was occluded with microclips.

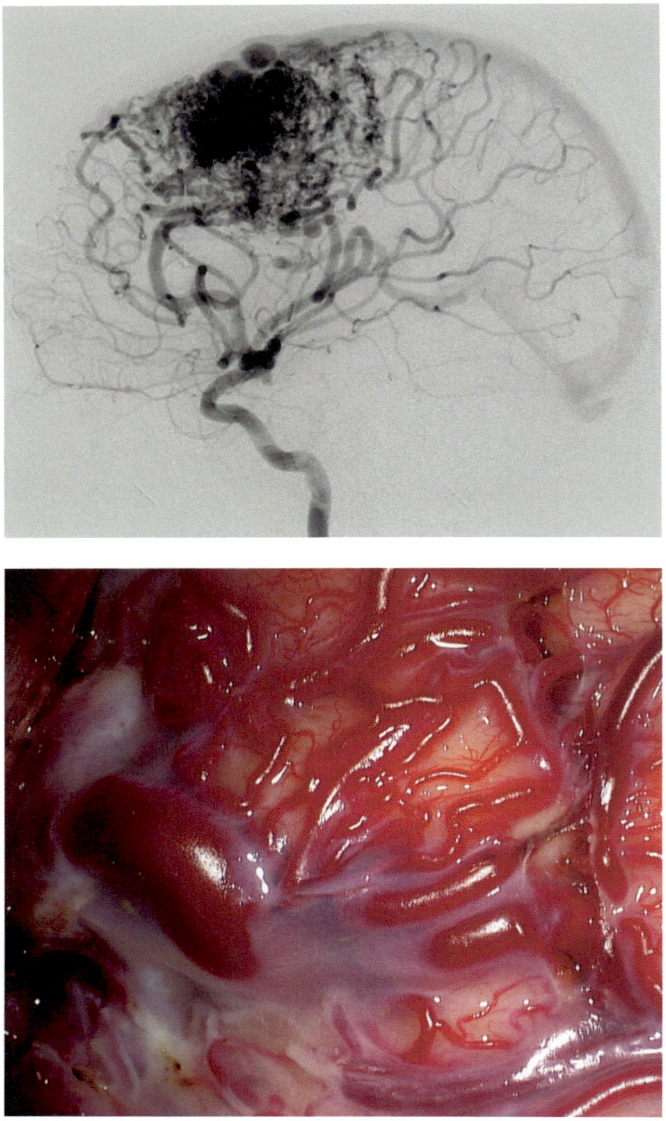

a

c

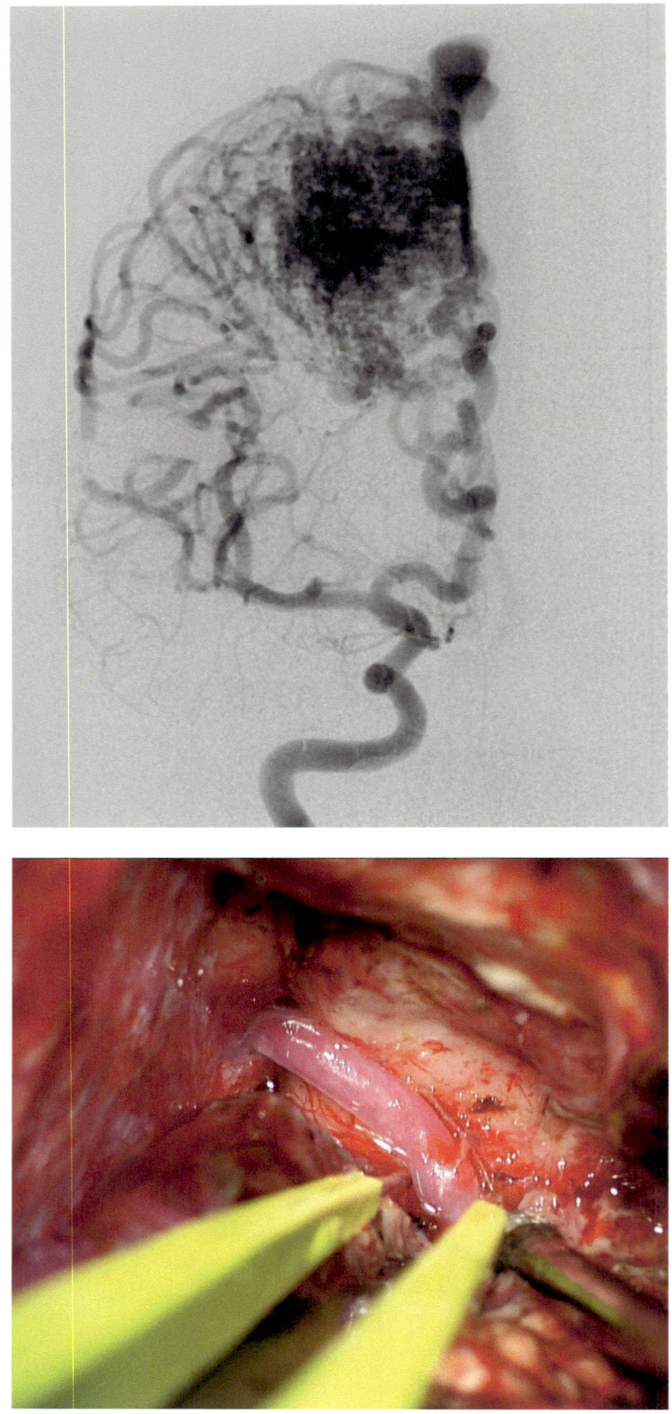

b

d

Fig. 11.18 This 16-year-old girl presented with a right paramedian frontal AVM (supplemented Spetzler-Martin grade 8: S3V1E1/A1B1C1), fed by dilated internal frontal arteries from the ACA, smaller cortical MCA branches, and a deep ILSA [right ICA angiogram, (**a**) lateral and (**b**) anteroposterior views]. The AVM was considered too high-risk for surgery. She underwent volume-staged radiosurgery with significant size reduction and decided on surgical resection. (**c**) A bifrontal craniotomy with the nose up exposed the arterialized PreCenV, and (**d**) dissection into the interhemispheric fissure along the falx exposed feeding arteries from the ACA.

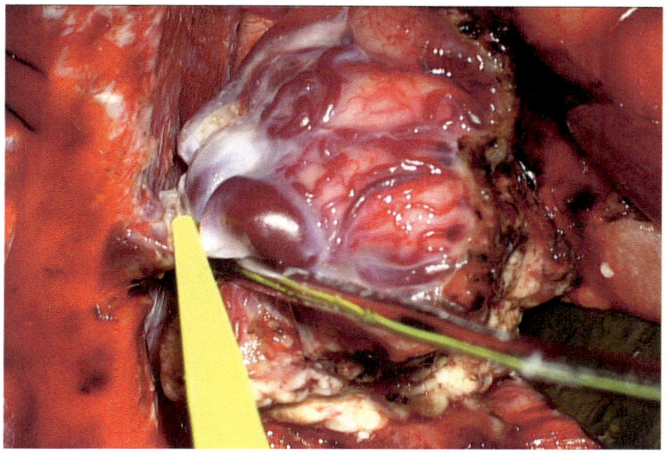

e

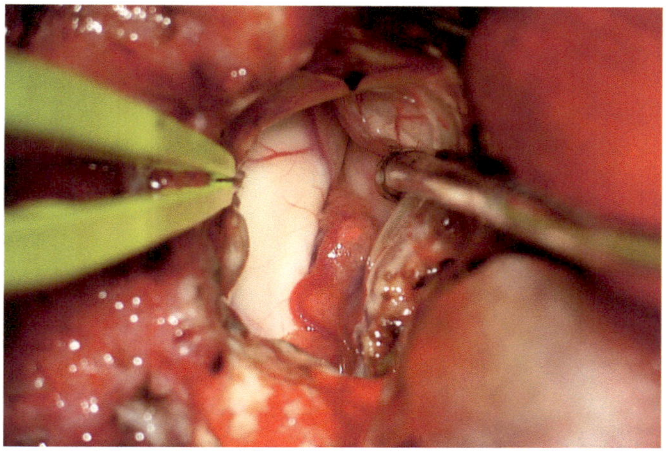

f

Fig. 11.18 (*continued*) (**e**) The draining vein was coagulated and divided. (**f**) After removing the AVM and dissecting into the lateral ventricle, an arterialized ependymal vein was found, traced back to a small portion of residual AVM in the lateral wall of the cavity fed by the lLSA, and resected. The postoperative angiogram confirmed complete resection.

Basal Frontal AVM Resection

Basal frontal AVMs are exposed with an orbital-pterional craniotomy, with the patient positioned supine and the head turned 30 degrees contralaterally, as for an anterior communicating artery aneurysm (step 1, **Fig. 11.19**). An orbitotomy opens the subfrontal plane and widens exposure of the basal surface. An orbitozygomatic craniotomy adds nothing, and a simple pterional craniotomy may be sufficient for smaller AVMs. The important anatomy on the basal surface is found after a subfrontal approach and sulcal dissection (step 2). Ascending drainage to the SSS via anterior OrbFrV or FrPolV is identified at the anterior margin (step 3), but deep drainage via the posterior OrbFrV or OlfV may not be appreciated until later. Basal frontal AVMs have three arterial fronts: MCA feeders from the sylvian fissure (OrbFrA and PreFrA); A2 ACA feeders from the interhemispheric fissure (OrbFrA and FrPolA); and A1 ACA feeders from the

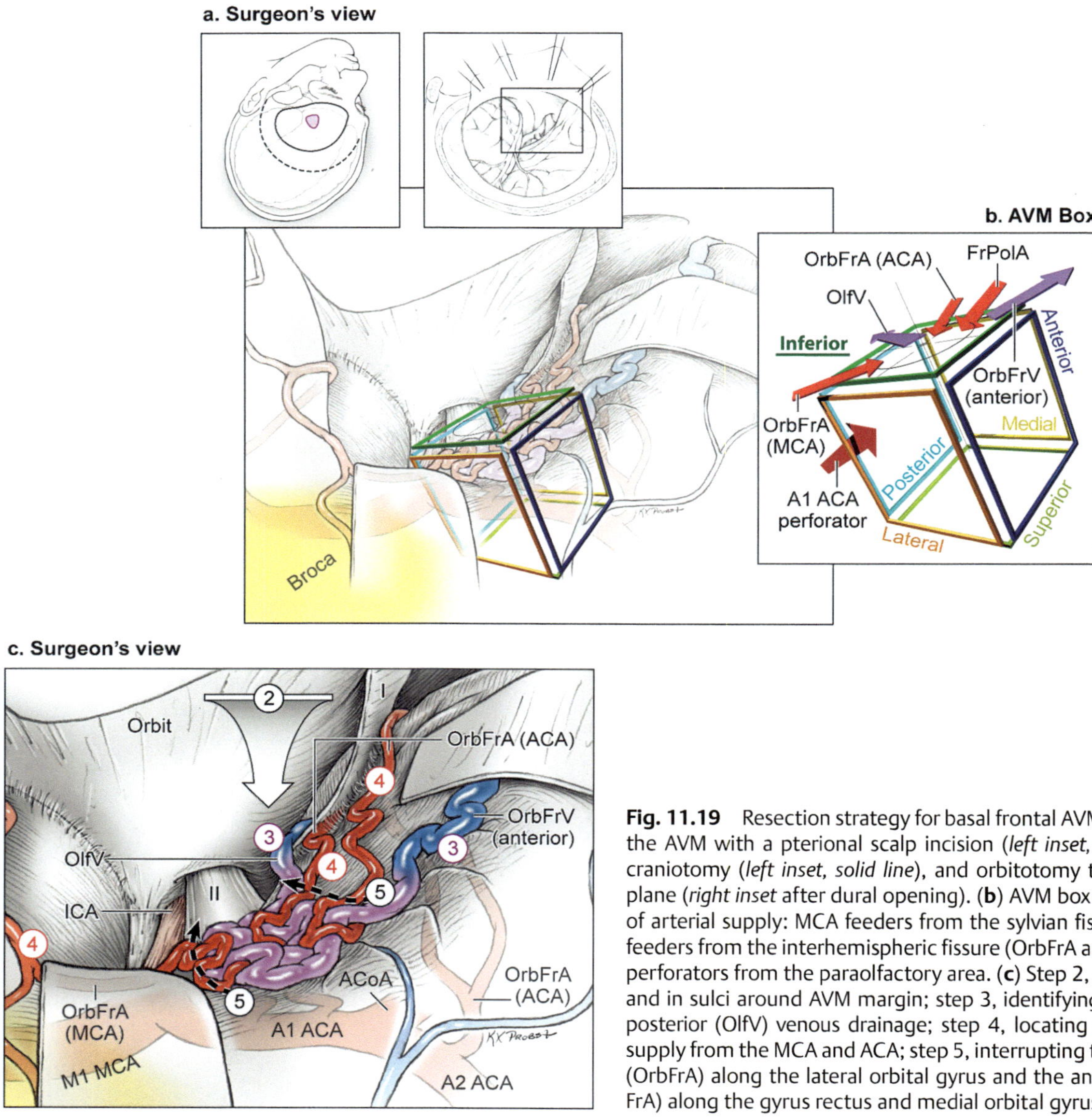

Fig. 11.19 Resection strategy for basal frontal AVMs. (**a**) Step 1, exposing the AVM with a pterional scalp incision (*left inset, dashed line*), pterional craniotomy (*left inset, solid line*), and orbitotomy to open the subfrontal plane (*right inset* after dural opening). (**b**) AVM box showing three sources of arterial supply: MCA feeders from the sylvian fissure (OrbFrA); A2 ACA feeders from the interhemispheric fissure (OrbFrA and FrPolA); and A1 ACA perforators from the paraolfactory area. (**c**) Step 2, dissecting subfrontally and in sulci around AVM margin; step 3, identifying anterior (OrbFrV) and posterior (OlfV) venous drainage; step 4, locating the superficial arterial supply from the MCA and ACA; step 5, interrupting the posterolateral front (OrbFrA) along the lateral orbital gyrus and the anteromedial front (OrbFrA) along the gyrus rectus and medial orbital gyrus (surgeon's view).

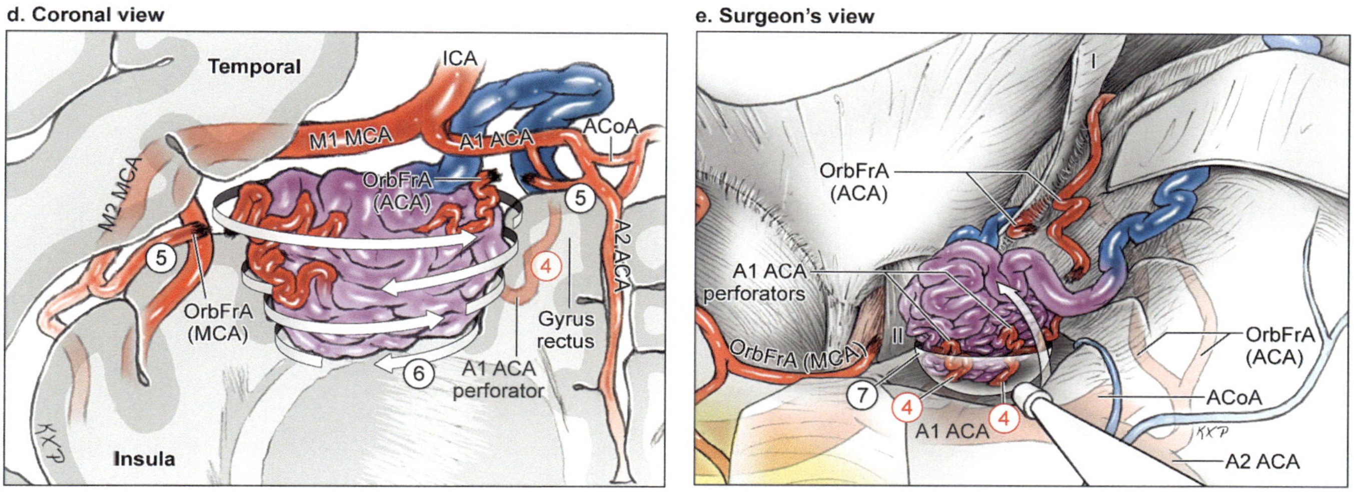

Fig. 11.19 *(continued)* (**d**) Step 6, circumdissecting superiorly into frontal lobe (coronal cross-sectional view). (**e**) Step 7, mobilizing the AVM inferiorly to interrupt the posteromedial front (A1 ACA perforators) along the posterior orbital gyrus (surgeon's view).

paraolfactory area (step 4). Two of these three fronts are superficial and can be interrupted in the pia of the posterolateral (M4 MCA and LOG) and anteromedial (A2 ACA and gyrus rectus) margins (step 5). The third posteromedial front lies along the deep medial margin and may not be visualized until after the nidus has been mobilized (step 6). Through this perpendicular exposure, the AVM is mobilized down from the frontal lobe into the subfrontal corridor to dissect the A1 ACA feeders coursing across the posterior orbital gyrus and olfactory tract, interrupting them just lateral to the olfactory tract along the AVM's posteromedial border (step 7). There are no eloquent structures along the paraolfactory plane, but olfactory nerve rootlets can be avulsed from the olfactory bulb and perforating arteries supplying the olfactory tract can be damaged during this dissection (**Figs. 11.20** and **Fig. 11.21**).

a

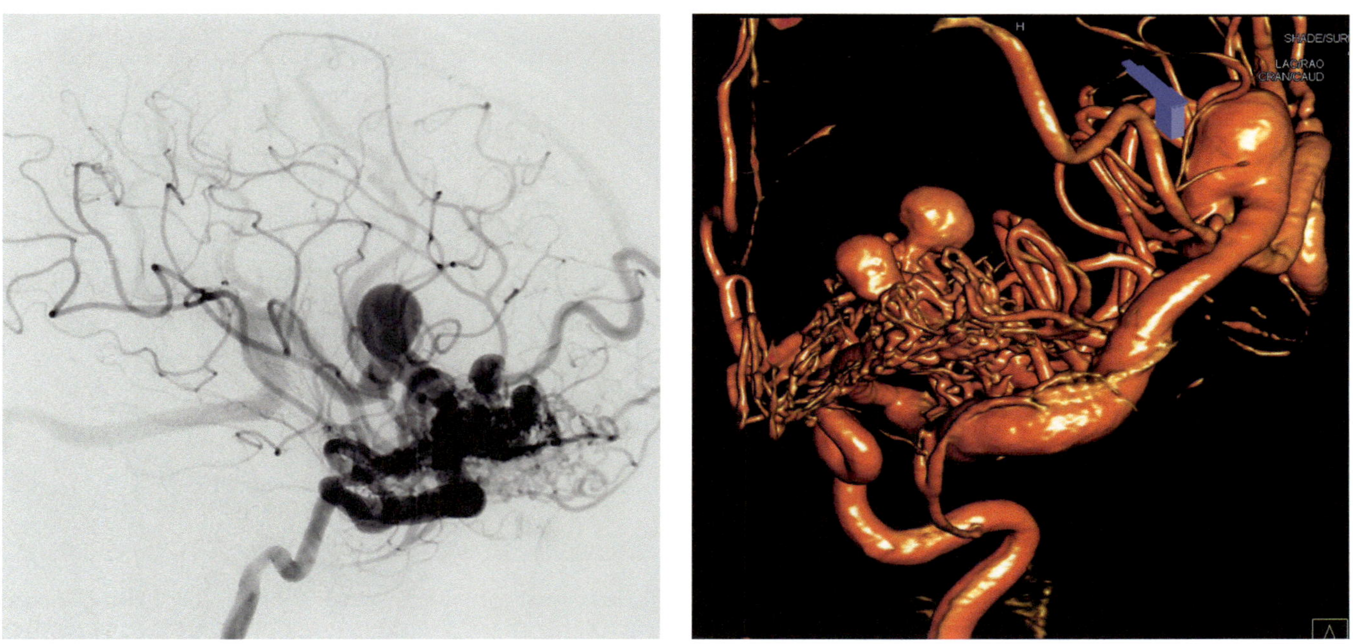

b

Fig. 11.20 This 21-year-old woman presented with a ruptured left basal frontal AVM (supplemented Spetzler-Martin grade 3: S1V0E0/A2B0C0), fed by the M4 MCA (OrbFrA), A1 ACA branches, and A2 ACA (OrbFrA and FrPolA), as seen on left ICA angiography [(**a**) lateral and (**b**) anterior 3D reconstructed views]. *(continued on next page)*

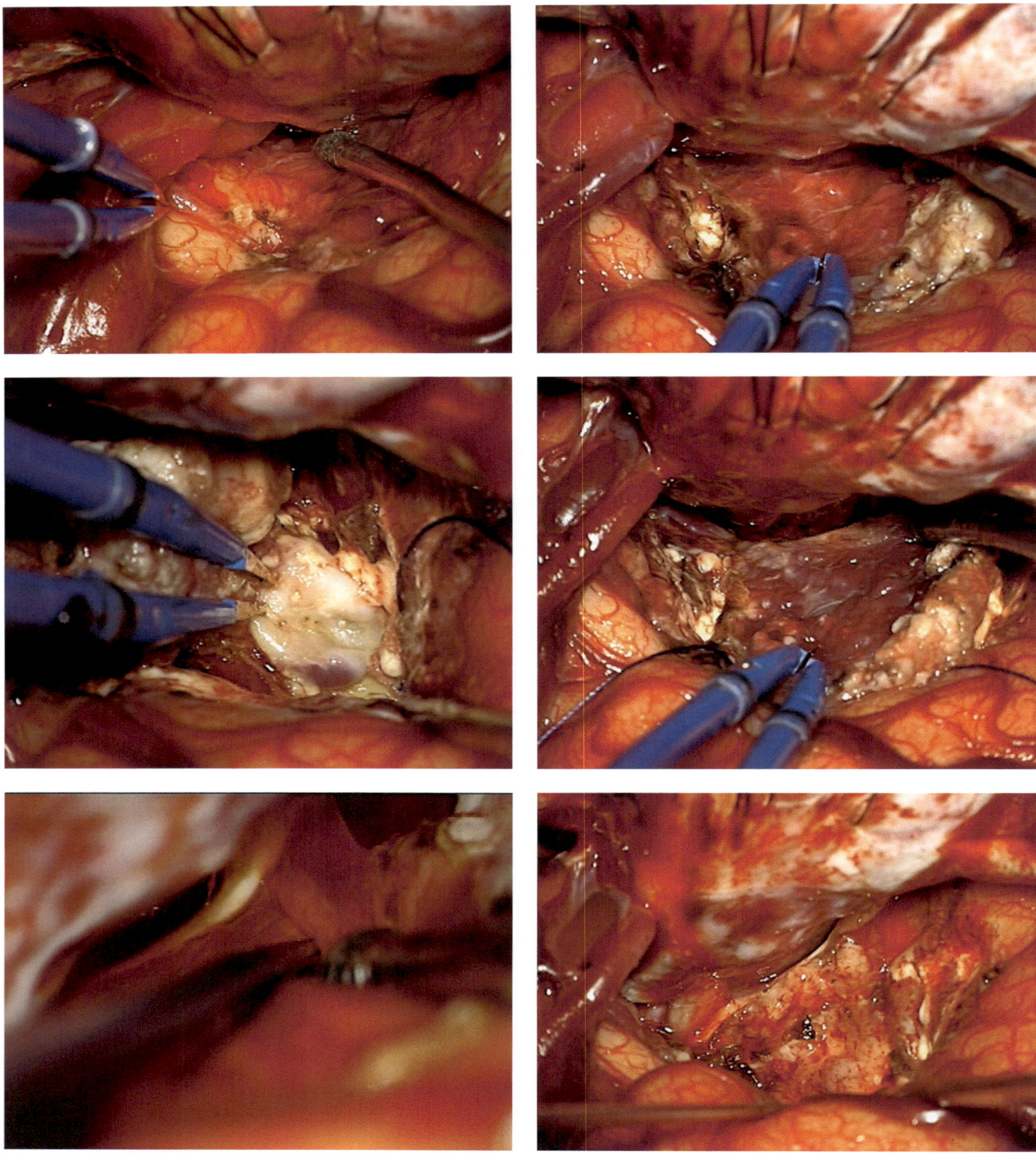

Fig. 11.20 (*continued*) (**c**) An orbital-pterional craniotomy optimized exposure of the basal frontal surface, and OrbFrA emerged from the sylvian fissure to supply the AVM's posterolateral front. (**d**) A circumscribing pial incision interrupted FrPolA feeders from the ACA anteriorly. (**e**) The AVM was mobilized inferiorly to dissect around the venous varix superiorly. (**f**) The AVM darkened, (**g**) leaving just the deep posteromedial front of arterial feeders (OrbFrA and A1 ACA branches) which intersected the AVM lateral to gyrus rectus and above olfactory tract. (**h**) This posteromedial border of the resection parallels the olfactory tract (seen above optic nerve and anterior cranial fossa floor) after AVM removal.

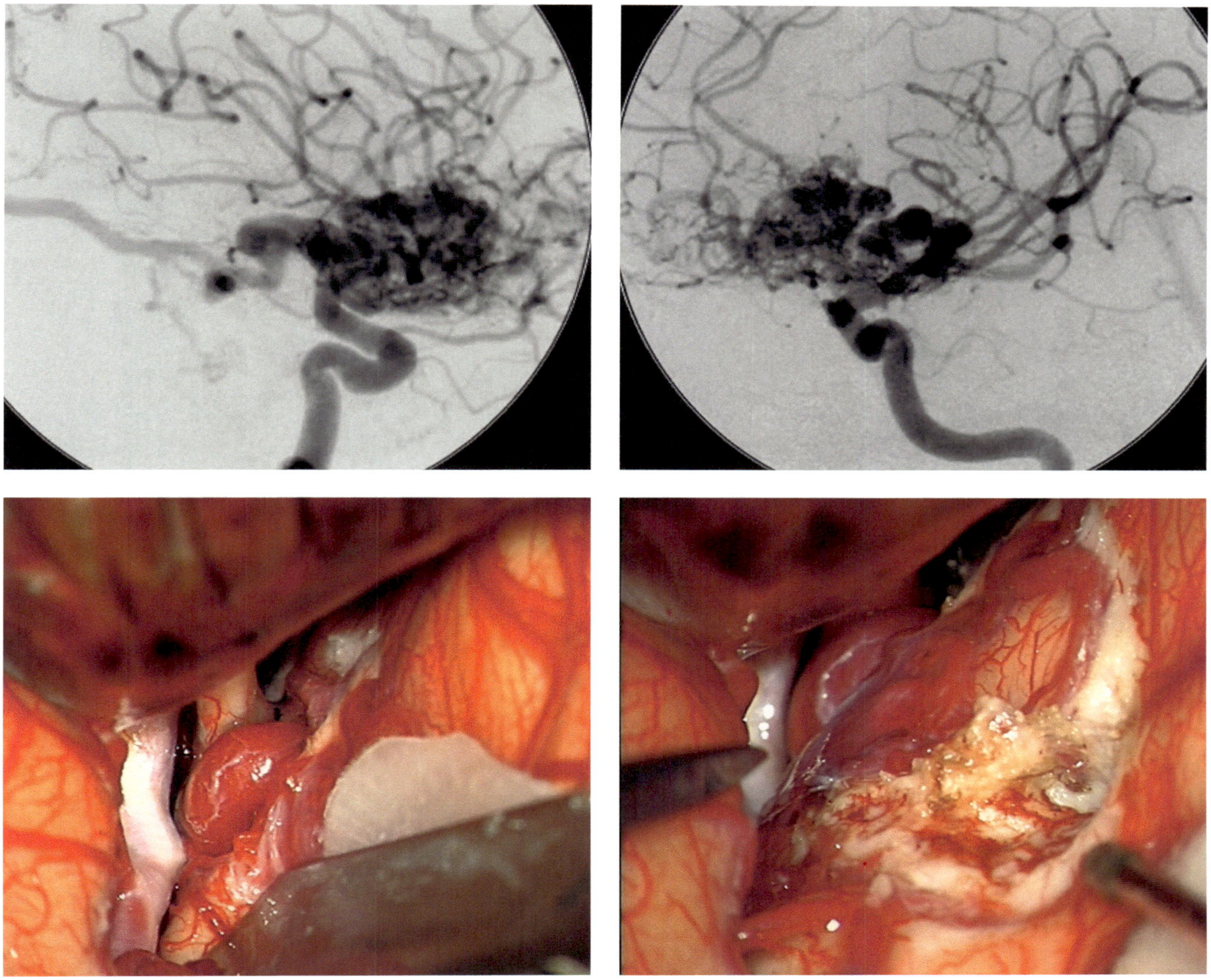

a b c d

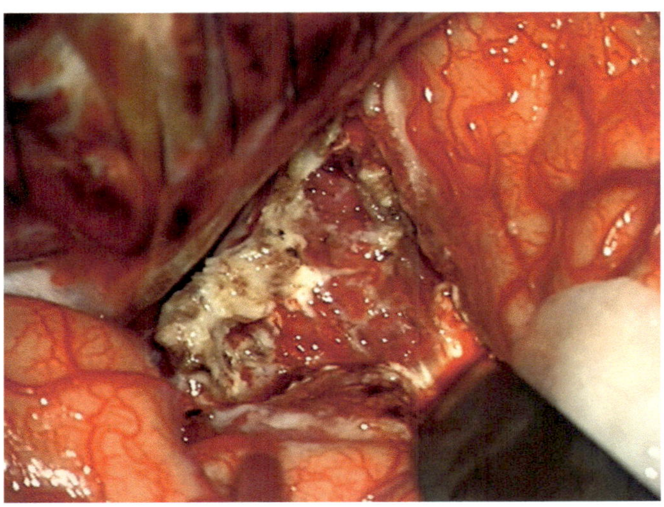

e

Fig. 11.21 This 53-year-old woman presented with a left basal frontal AVM (supplemented Spetzler-Martin grade 6: S1V1E0/A3B1C0), supplied by OrbFrA from the ACA, OrbFrA from the MCA, and A1 ACA branches [left ICA angiogram, (**a**) lateral and (**b**) anterior oblique views]. Note the deep drainage to the OlfV and BVR. (**c**) The AVM sat on the basal frontal surface, anterior to the ICA terminus and lateral to the olfactory tract, as exposed through an orbital-pterional craniotomy. The arterialized OlfV coursed between the olfactory tract and optic nerve to join the BVR. (**d**) A pial incision in the lateral orbital gyrus interrupted the small MCA feeders that formed the posterolateral front, and (**e**) some frontal lobe retraction exposed the AVMs lateral border. (*continued on next page*)

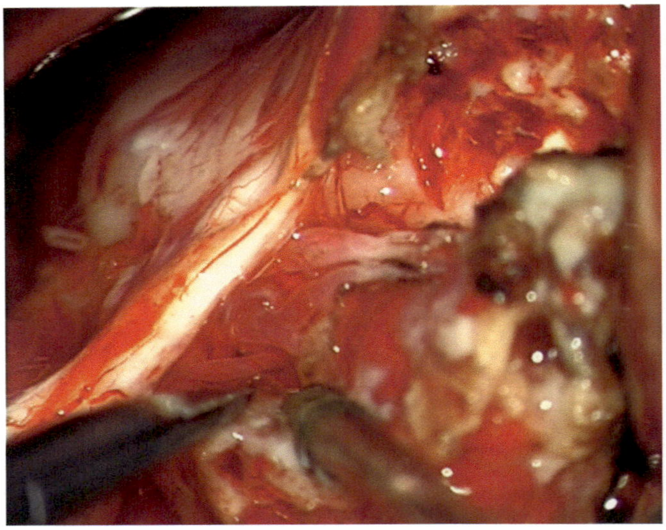

f

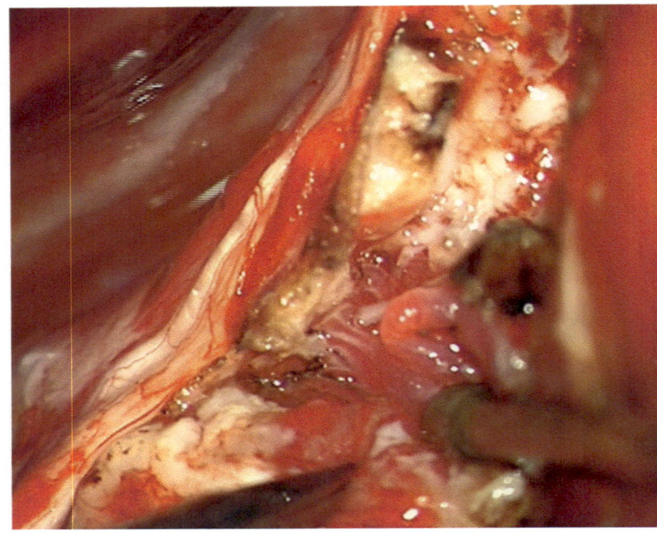

g

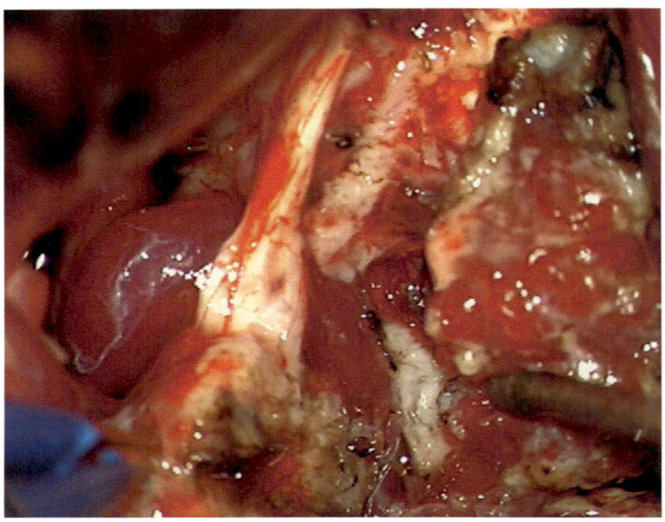

h

Fig. 11.21 (*continued*) (**f**) Arterial feeders along the lateral edge of olfactory tract and medial orbital gyrus formed the AVM's anteromedial front of supply from the A2 ACA (OrbFrA). (**g**) More posteriorly, arterial feeders along the olfactory tract and posterior orbital gyrus formed the AVM's posteromedial front of supply from A1 ACA. (**h**) Deep dissection exposed the OlfV coursing medial to olfactory tract.

Sylvian Frontal AVM Resection

Sylvian frontal AVMs are exposed like MCA aneurysms through a standard pterional craniotomy (step 1, **Fig. 11.22**). The sylvian fissure is split widely to separate the frontal and temporal lobes and lay out the stem arteries and branches from the superior trunk, from the insular M2 segments to the cortical M4 segments (step 2). Drainage is via the sylvian veins that are also exposed with the sylvian split (step 3). An arterialized DeepSylV at the bottom of the surgical field is out of the way, but an arterialized SupSylV can post a venous obstacle in the center of the field. Sylvian frontal AVMs are deep to and fed by M3 opercular arteries that may terminate in the AVM or send branches to the AVM before continuing en passage (step 4). Arteries are established as terminal feeders, transit arteries, or bystanders, and each is managed differently: terminal feeders are occluded at the AVM margin; transit arteries are skeletonized; and bystanders are separated.

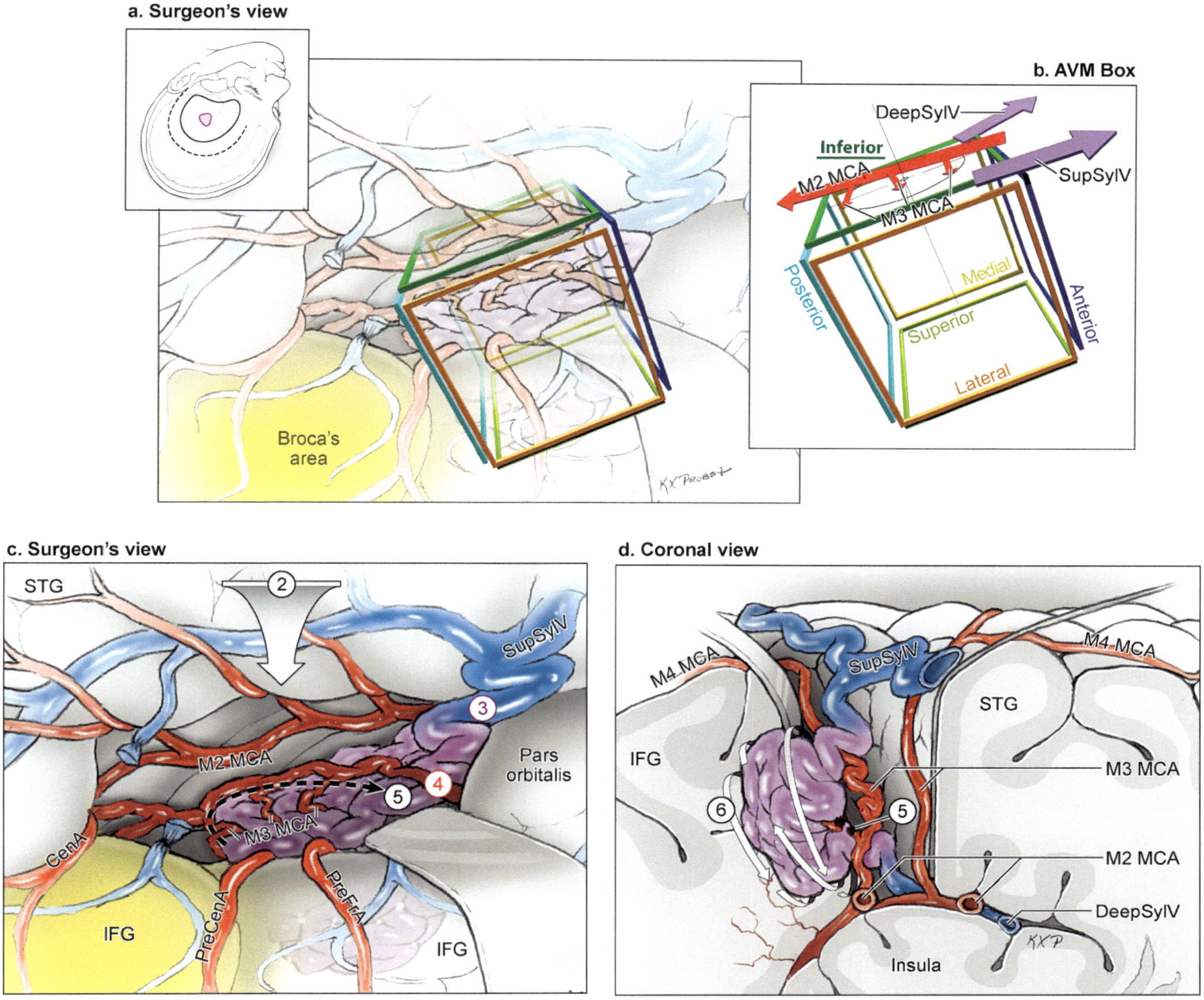

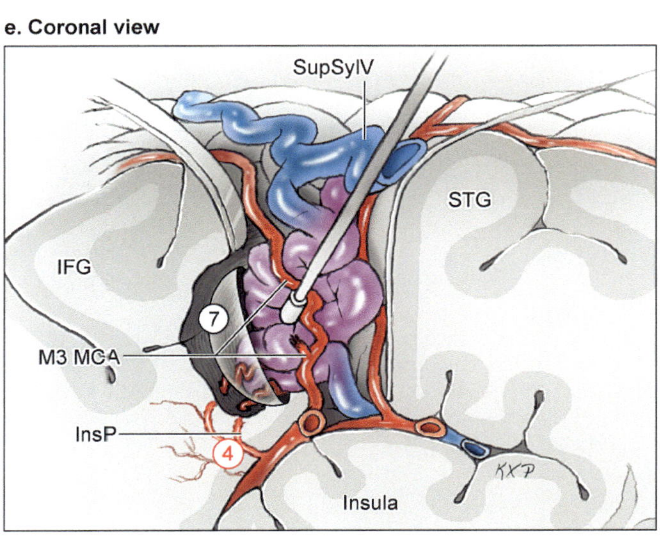

Fig. 11.22 Resection strategy for sylvian frontal AVMs. (**a**) Step 1, exposing the AVM with a hairline scalp incision (*inset, dashed line*), pterional craniotomy (*left inset, solid line*), and a transsylvian approach (surgeon's view). (**b**) AVM box showing arterial supply from the M3 MCA branches, drainage to the superficial and deep sylvian veins, and proximity to Broca's area. (**c**) Step 2, splitting the sylvian fissure to expose the frontal operculum; step 3, mobilizing the superficial sylvian veins temporally; step 4, laying out the superior trunk and its M2 and M3 branches feeding the AVM; and step 5, interrupting the inferomedial front on or near the pars orbitalis by skeletonizing the M2 stem arteries in a distal-to-proximal direction. (**d**) Step 6, dividing the terminal feeding arteries, skeletonizing the transit arteries, and separating the bystander arteries (coronal cross-sectional view). (**e**) Step 7, mobilizing the AVM into the sylvian fissure to interrupt the deep supply from the insular perforators.

The sheer number of arteries coursing through the sylvian fissure and their variable nature makes this dissection challenging. The insular-to-opercular course of the MCA creates an inferomedial front of arteries on the sylvian frontal surface, but some feeders can be found on the lateral surface of the inferior frontal gyrus (step 5). Despite rolling into the sylvian fissure, these AVMs are still superficial, and circumdissection in the IFG is parallel to and respectful of Broca's area in the dominant hemisphere (step 6). The deep plane may be fed by insular perforators and the lLSA (step 7) (**Figs. 11.23, 11.24, 11.25**).

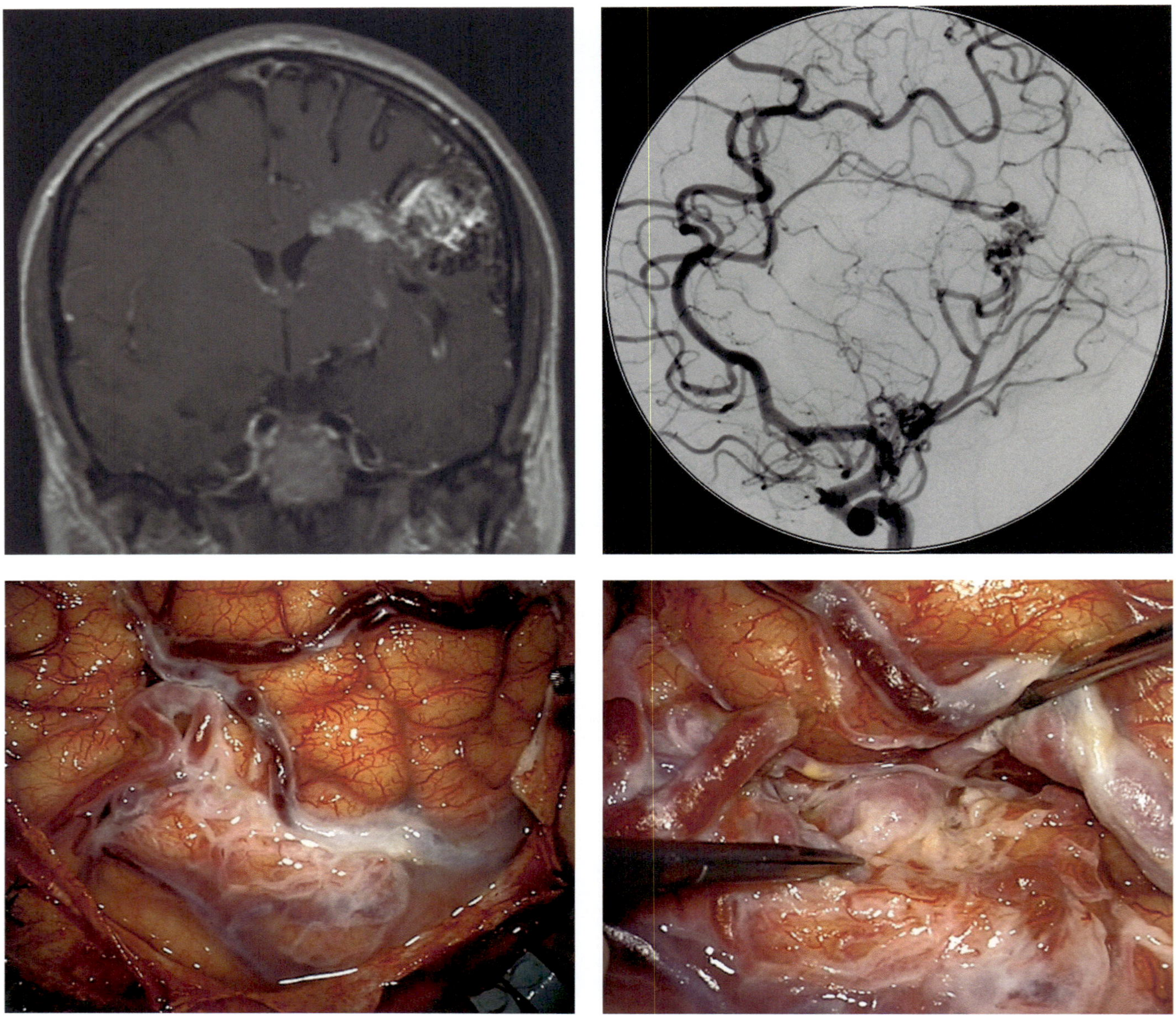

a b c d

Fig. 11.23 This 43-year-old woman presented with a left sylvian frontal AVM (supplemented Spetzler-Martin grade 7: S2V0E1/A3B1C0), (**a**) seen on T1-weighted MRI with gadolinium enhancement (coronal view). She was treated with Gamma Knife radiosurgery, and the AVM shrank to a small remnant on the sylvian surface of the frontal lobe, fed by M3 MCA branches [(**b**) left ICA angiogram, anterior oblique view]. (**c**) Cortical feeding arteries were sclerotic, arachnoid was thickened, and an arterialized FrSylV emerged from the distal sylvian fissure. (**d**) The anterior border of the AVM was dissected on this opercular surface.

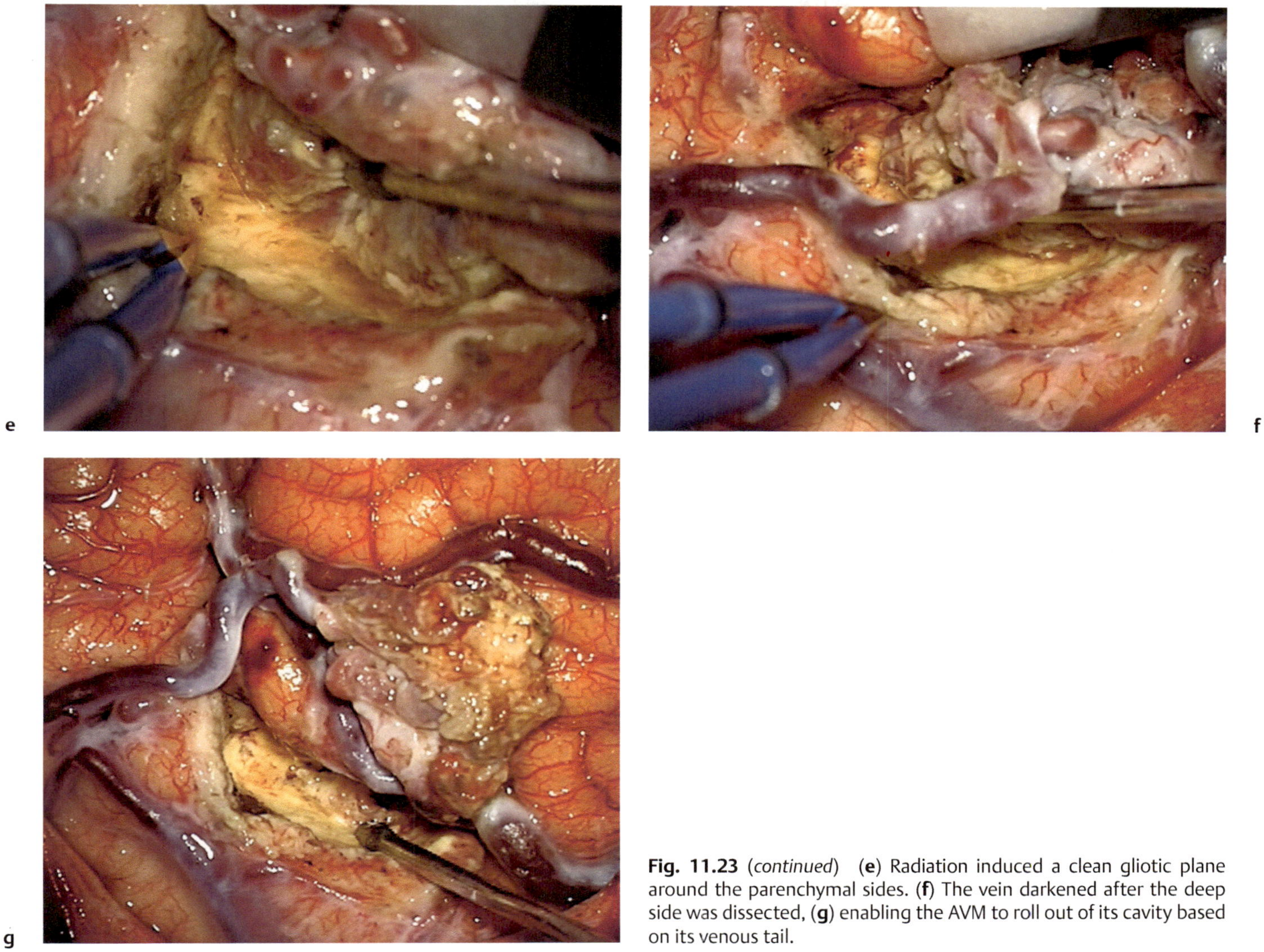

Fig. 11.23 (*continued*) (**e**) Radiation induced a clean gliotic plane around the parenchymal sides. (**f**) The vein darkened after the deep side was dissected, (**g**) enabling the AVM to roll out of its cavity based on its venous tail.

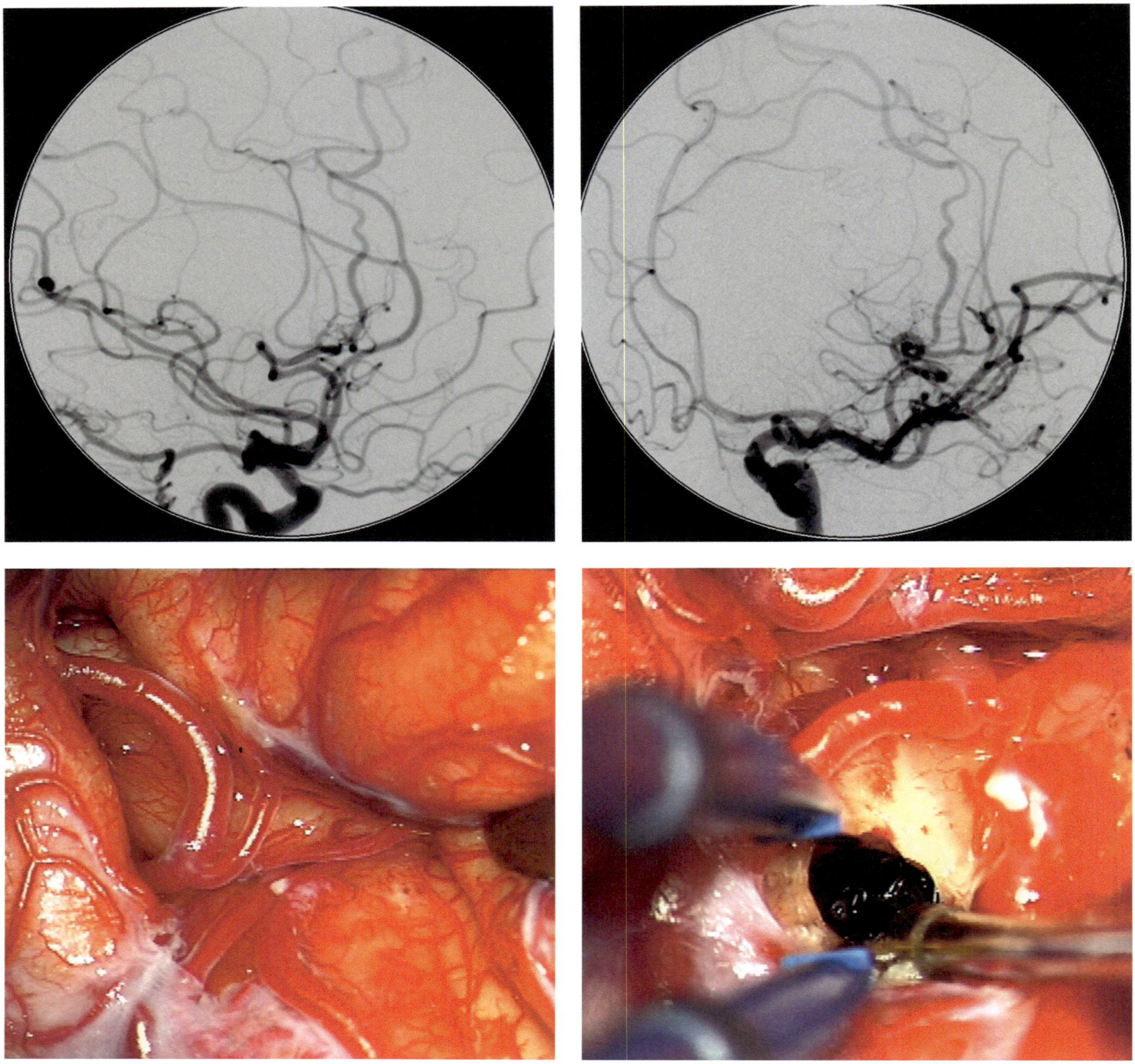

a b c d

Fig. 11.24 This 61-year-old man presented with a large intracerebral hemorrhage from this tiny left sylvian frontal AVM (supplemented Spetzler-Martin grade 5: S1V0E1/A3B0C0), fed by M3 MCA branches [left ICA angiogram, (**a**) lateral and (**b**) anterior oblique views]. The nidus was difficult to appreciate angiographically, but the early draining vein ascending to the SSS was unmistakable. (**c**) Sylvian fissure dissection exposed the opercular MCA segments and the arterialized vein on the pars triangularis. (**d**) A small pial incision through hemosiderin-stained cortex alongside the draining vein entered the hematoma cavity.

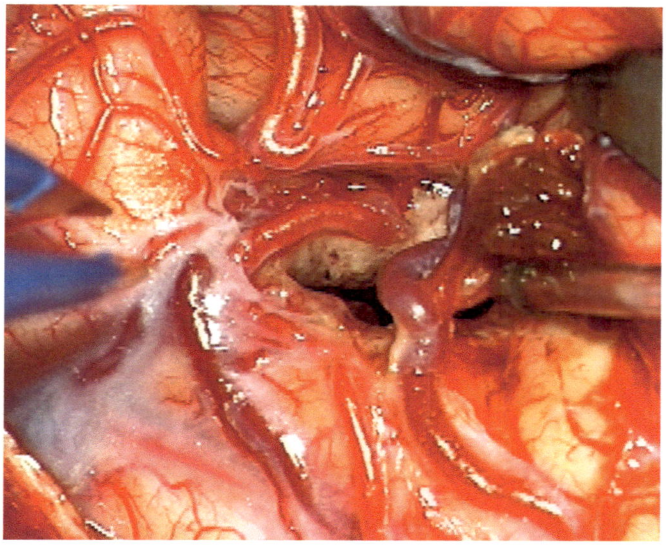

e

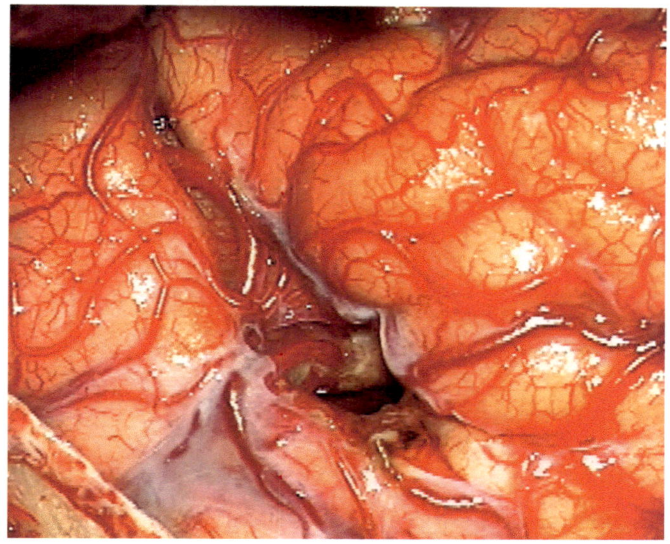

f

Fig. 11.24 (*continued*) (**e**) After evacuating hematoma and identifying AVM in the wall of the hematoma cavity, it was circumdissected and rolled out of the cavity on a darkened venous tail. (**f**) Extensive subarachnoid dissection of the sylvian fissure exposed this opercular region in the dominant hemisphere with no adverse effect on his speech function.

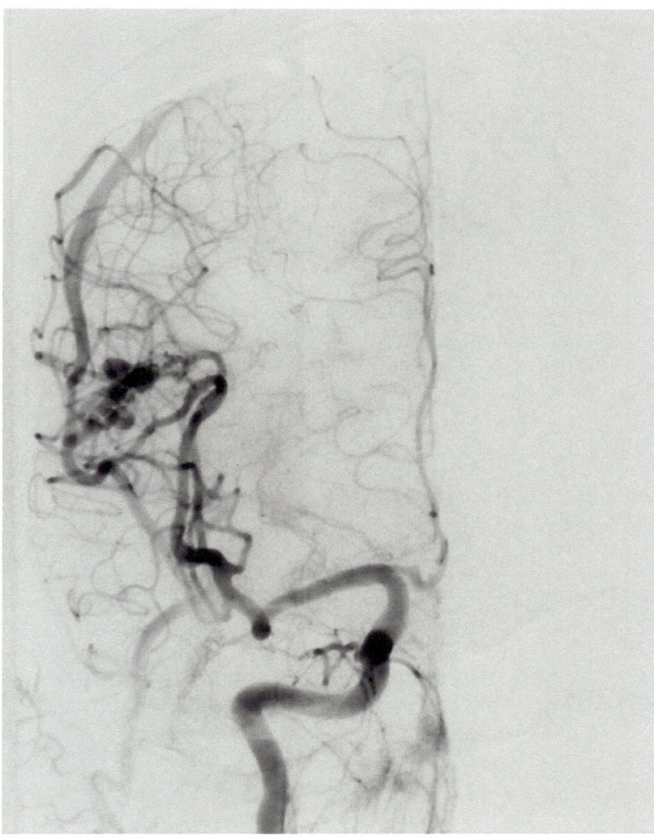

a

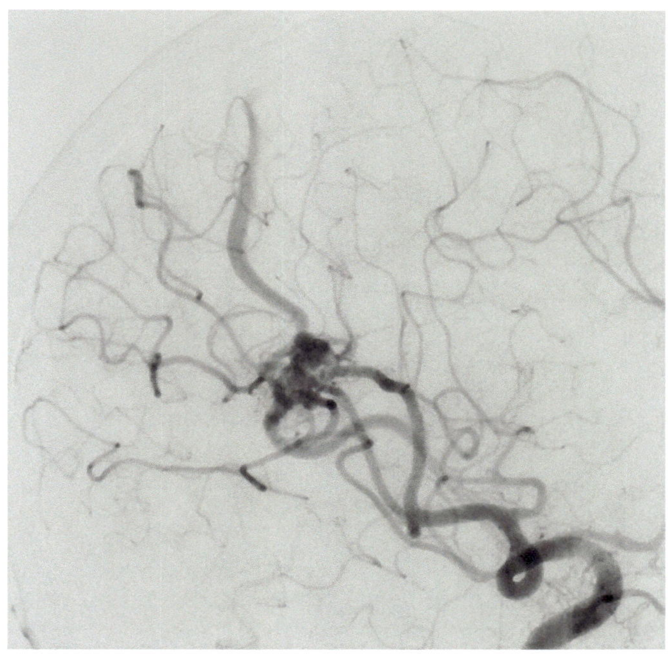

b

Fig. 11.25 This 52-year-old woman presented with an intracerebral hemorrhage and a right sylvian frontal AVM (supplemented Spetzler-Martin grade 5: S1V0E1/A3B0C0), fed by opercular MCA branches and drained superiorly by the CenV/vein of Trolard and inferiorly by SupSylV [right ICA angiogram, (**a**) anteroposterior and (**b**) lateral oblique views]. (*continued on next page*)

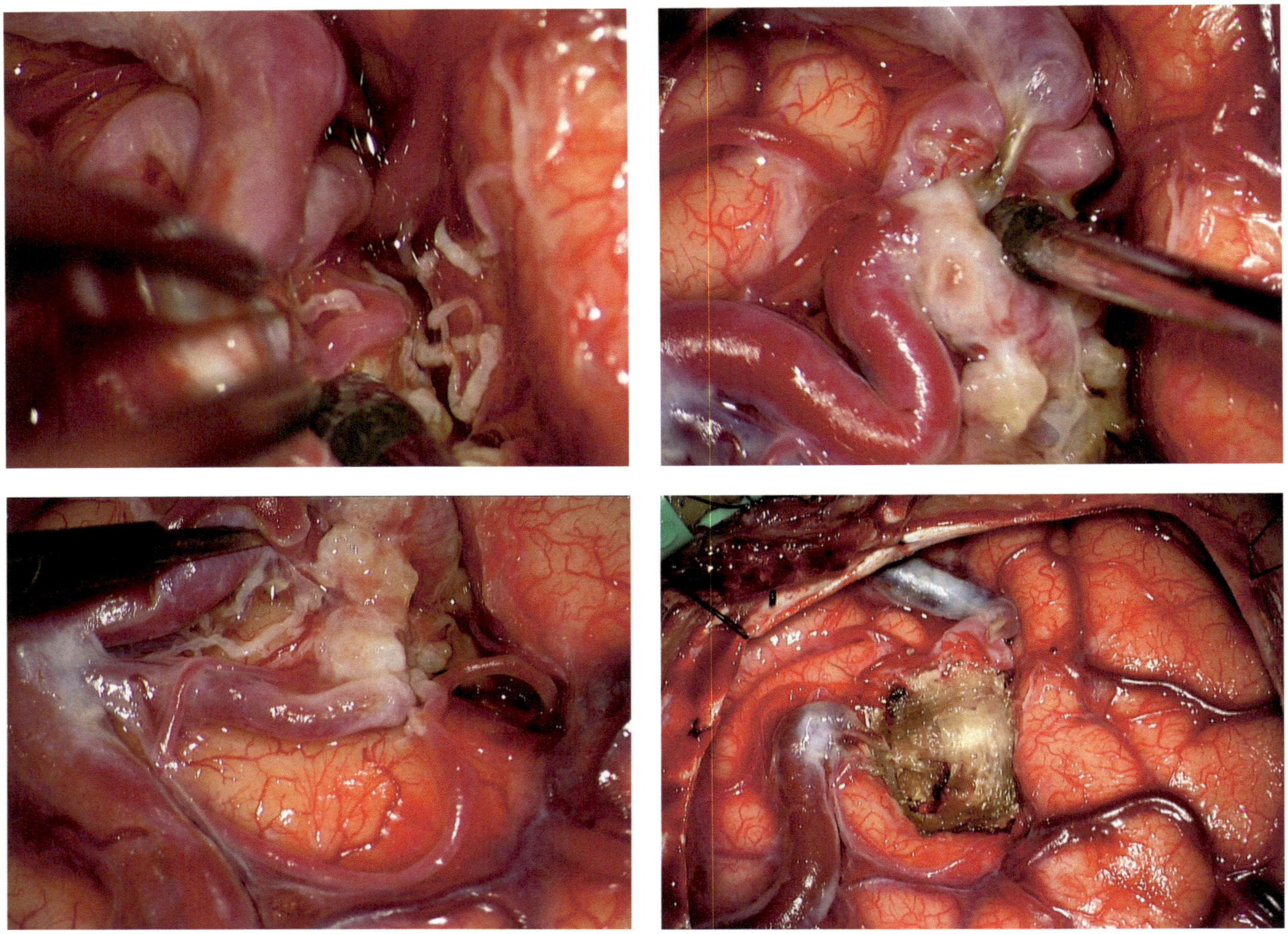

c d e f

Fig. 11.25 (*continued*) (**c**) Opercular feeding arteries traversed the frontal side of the operculum (*left*) to reach the AVM and did not involve the temporal side of the operculum (*right*). (**d**) Cauterizing the SupSylV anteriorly exposed a large MCA feeding artery underneath. (**e**) Another feeding artery emerged from the posterior end of the sylvian fissure, beyond which a normal CenA was seen on the cortical surface. (**f**) The large CenV posteriorly allowed the SupSylV anteriorly to be divided early. The resection cavity, here lined with Nu-Knit, was in the pars opercularis of the frontal lobe and the superior temporal gyrus was uninvolved.

Conclusion

The frontal lobe is the brain's largest lobe, and consequently frontal AVMs are the most common of the seven AVMs. Nearly one quarter of AVMs (22.5%) in this surgical experience were frontal AVMs, and all five frontal subtypes were among the most frequently operated AVMs (**Table 11.1**). Therefore, it is necessary to master the anatomic subtleties of these five frontal AVM subtypes and the surgical strategies for resecting them.

Table 11.1 Summary of the Most Common AVM Subtypes in 600 Surgical Patients in the Author's 16-Year Experience

Frequency	AVM Subtype	*n*	%
1	Lateral temporal AVM	76	13%
2	Lateral parieto-occipital AVM	52	9%
3	Lateral frontal AVM	48	8%
4	Paramedian parieto-occipital AVM	29	5%
5	Insular AVM	25	4%
	Vermian cerebellar AVM	25	4%
7	Paramedian frontal AVM	24	4%
8	Callosal AVM	23	4%
9	Medial frontal AVM	21	4%
	Basal frontal AVM	21	4%
	Sylvian frontal AVM	21	4%

12 Temporal Arteriovenous Malformations

Microsurgical Anatomy

Brain

The temporal lobe has four surfaces: lateral, basal, sylvian, and medial (**Fig. 12.1**). The lateral temporal surface consists of three horizontal gyri that lie below and run parallel to the sylvian fissure: superior, middle, and inferior temporal gyri (STG, MTG, and ITG). Superior and inferior temporal sulci separate the three gyri and lie above and below the MTG, respectively. The basal surface also consists of three longitudinal gyri: the lower portion of the ITG, the occipitotemporal (fusiform) gyrus (OTG), and the lower portion of the parahippocampal gyrus. The basal surface is traversed longitudinally by the occipitotemporal sulcus, which separates the fusiform gyrus from the ITG. The collateral sulcus lies between the fusiform and parahippocampal gyri and parallels the occipitotemporal sulcus. The medial temporal surface consists of the parahippocampal gyrus, uncus, and hippocampus (which is composed of the dentate gyrus, Ammon's horn, and the subiculum). The hippocampal sulcus separates the parahippocampal and dentate gyri. The fimbriodentate sulcus separates the dentate gyrus and the fimbria of the hippocampus, which collects hippocampal efferents as a bundle at the edge of the choroid plexus before leaving the hippocampus to form the crus of the fornix. The amygdala and hippocampal formation lie beneath the medial temporal surface. The sylvian surface forms the superior boundary of the temporal lobe and the lower lip of the opercular cleft. The anterior sylvian surface consists of the planum polare, formed by the upper edge of the STG. The posterior sylvian surface consists of the planum temporale, formed by Heschl's gyrus and the transverse temporal gyri. The temporal lobe houses important neurologic functions: memory and learning in the hippocampus and parahippocampus; language reception in Wernicke's area in the dominant STG; auditory reception in Heschl's gyrus; and transmission of visual signals in the optic radiations.

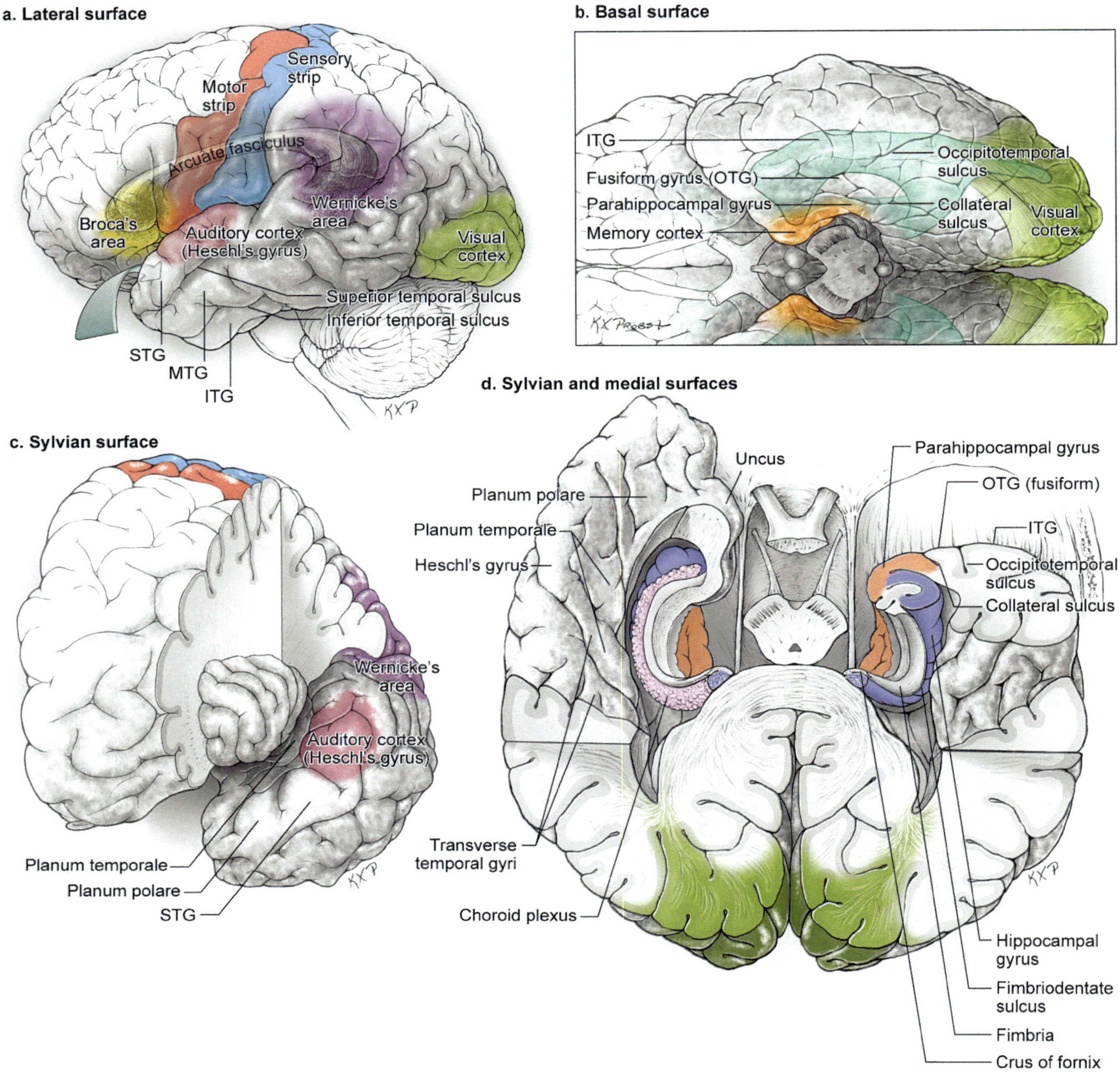

Fig. 12.1 Microsurgical anatomy of the temporal lobe. (**a**) Lateral temporal surface (lateral view). (**b**) Basal temporal surface (inferior view). (**c**) Sylvian surface (anterior view with frontal and parietal lobes partially removed). (**d**) Sylvian and medial surfaces (superior view with axial sections through the temporal horns and partial removal of the occipital lobes, and on the right side, a coronal section through the temporal pole with choroid plexus removed).

Arteries

The temporal lobe has an intimate relationship with the middle cerebral artery (MCA) coursing through the sylvian fissure, with the posterior cerebral artery (PCA) coursing through the crural and ambient cisterns, and with the anterior choroidal artery (AChA) supplying the choroid plexus of the temporal horn of the lateral ventricle (**Fig. 12.2**). In contrast to frontal arteriovenous malformations (AVMs) that are supplied by branches from the superior trunk of the MCA, temporal AVMs are supplied by branches from the inferior trunk. The inferior trunk divides into approximately four unnamed stem arteries devoted to the temporal lobe and comprising the M2 insular and M3 opercular segments. These arteries emerge from the sylvian fissure distally to become M4 cortical arteries: middle temporal (MidTempA), poste-

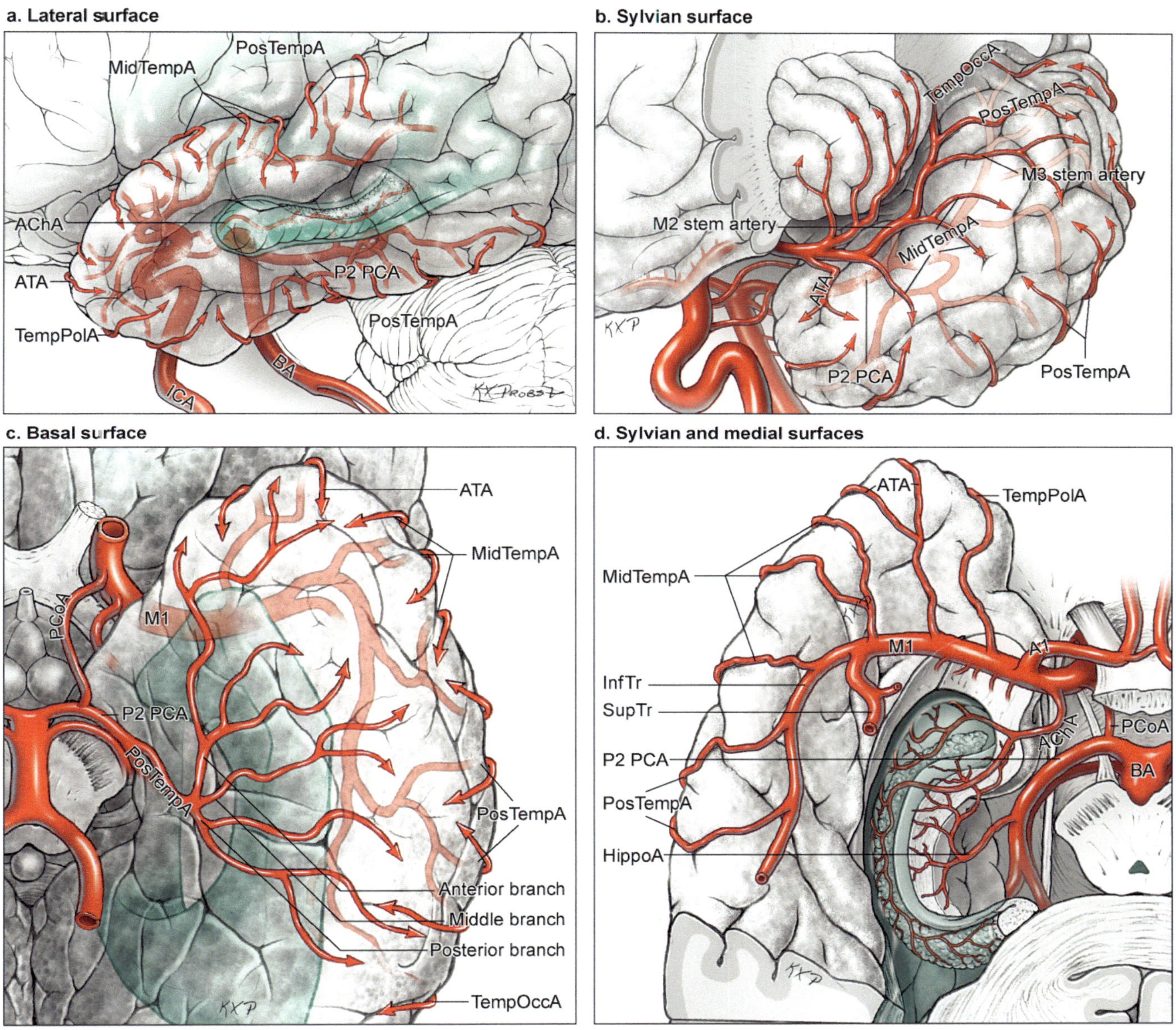

Fig. 12.2 Microsurgical anatomy of temporal lobe arteries. (**a**) The lateral surface is supplied by "early branches" arising from the M1 MCA (TempPolA and ATA), "superior temporal arteries" from the inferior trunk of the MCA (MidTempA, PosTempA, TempOccA, and AngA), and "inferior temporal arteries" from the PCA (HippoA and PosTempA) (lateral view). (**b**) The sylvian surface is supplied by M2 and M3 segments of MCA stem arteries (anterior view frontal and parietal lobes partially removed). (**c**) The basal surface is supplied by posterior temporal artery, shown here as a common trunk that divides into anterior, middle, and posterior branches. (**d**) Arteries of the sylvian and medial surfaces (superior view with axial section through the left temporal horn and partial removal of the occipital lobe). (*continued on next page*)

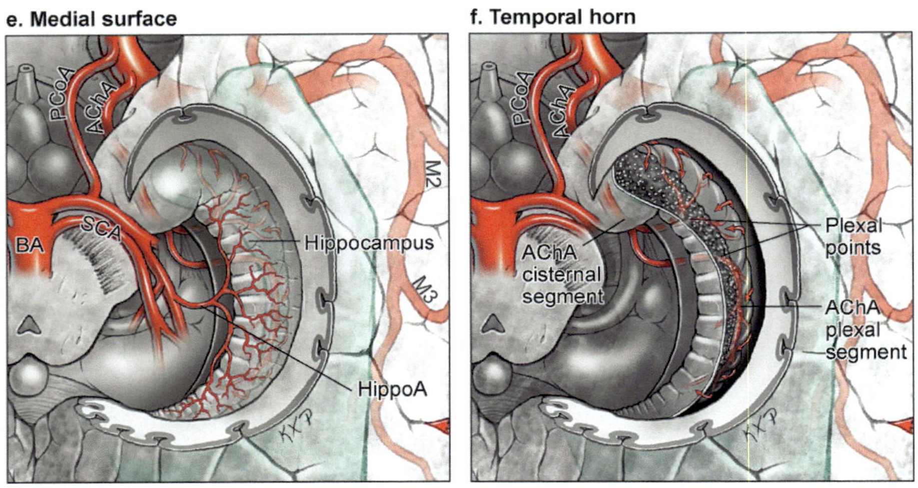

Fig. 12.2 (*continued*) (**e**) The medial surface is supplied by HippoA (inferior view with parahippocampus removed). (**f**) The temporal horn is supplied by anterior choroidal artery (inferior view with parahippocampus removed).

rior temporal (PosTempA), temporo-occipital (TempOccA), and angular artery (AngA). They course downward from the sylvian fissure in an inferior direction and supply the lateral temporal surface. Collectively, they are referred to as "superior temporal arteries" because of this superior relationship to their territories. Temporopolar (TempPolA) and anterior temporal arteries (ATAs) are "early branches" that do not arise from the inferior trunk or travel the long course of the sylvian fissure, but instead arise from the M1 segment proximal to the MCA bifurcation. TempPolA is a small branch distal to the internal carotid artery (ICA) bifurcation and proximal to the ATA, but it enlarges in the presence of an AVM. Both of these arteries originate from the inferior surface of the M1 segment, course inferiorly, and supply the temporal pole.

The posterior cerebral artery (PCA) supplies the basal surface of the temporal lobe with branches originating from the P2 segment: hippocampal (HippoA) and posterior temporal arteries (PosTempA). The HippoA is the first PCA cortical branch, arising in the crural or ambient cistern and supplying the uncus, anterior parahippocampal gyrus, hippocampus, and dentate gyrus. The PosTempA can arise as a common trunk that branches into anterior, middle, and posterior branches, or it can originate as individual anterior, middle, and posterior branches. Collectively, these hippocampal and posterior temporal arteries are referred to as "inferior temporal arteries." They originate from the inferolateral PCA surface and course over the tentorial incisura in the subtemporal plane. They continue past the lateral margin of the basal surface to reach the lateral surface (ITG) and can ascend to the MTG.

Veins

Venous anatomy of the temporal lobe is a complex collateral network with drainage anteriorly to temporopolar veins and the sphenoparietal sinus, posteriorly to the vein of Labbé and transverse sinus, medially to the basal vein of Rosenthal (BVR) and Galenic system, and superiorly to the sylvian veins and the superior sagittal sinus (SSS) (**Fig. 12.3**). The lateral temporal convexity is drained by descending veins (AntTempV, MidTempV, and PosTempV) that collect in the vein of Labbé and transverse sinus (TrvS) proximal to the transverse–sigmoid junction. The basal surface is drained by temporobasal veins (TempBasV; anterior, middle, and posterior) that collect laterally in tentorial sinuses and rarely in sphenobasal and sphenopetrosal sinuses, or medially in the BVR. The medial surface of the temporal lobe is drained by the uncal (UncV), anterior hippocampal (HippoV), and medial temporal vein (MedTempV), which collect in the BVR en route to the vein of Galen (VoG). The sylvian surface of the temporal lobe, as well as some of the STG along the sylvian fissure, drain into the temporosylvian veins (TempSylV) that ascend to SupSylV. Anastomotic veins can direct this venous flow anteriorly to SphParS and the cavernous sinus, superiorly to the frontoparietal veins, or deep to DeepSylV and the BVR.

Fig. 12.3 (*opposite*) Microsurgical anatomy of the temporal lobe veins. (**a**) Veins of the lateral surface (lateral view). (**b**) Veins of the sylvian surface (anterior view with frontal and parietal lobes partially removed). (**c**) Veins of the medial surface (anterior view with frontal and parietal lobes partially removed). (**d**) Veins of the temporal horn (anterior view with frontal and parietal lobes partially removed). (**e**) Veins of the basal surface (inferior view). (**f**) Veins of the sylvian and medial surfaces (superior view with axial section through the left temporal horn and partial removal of the occipital lobe).

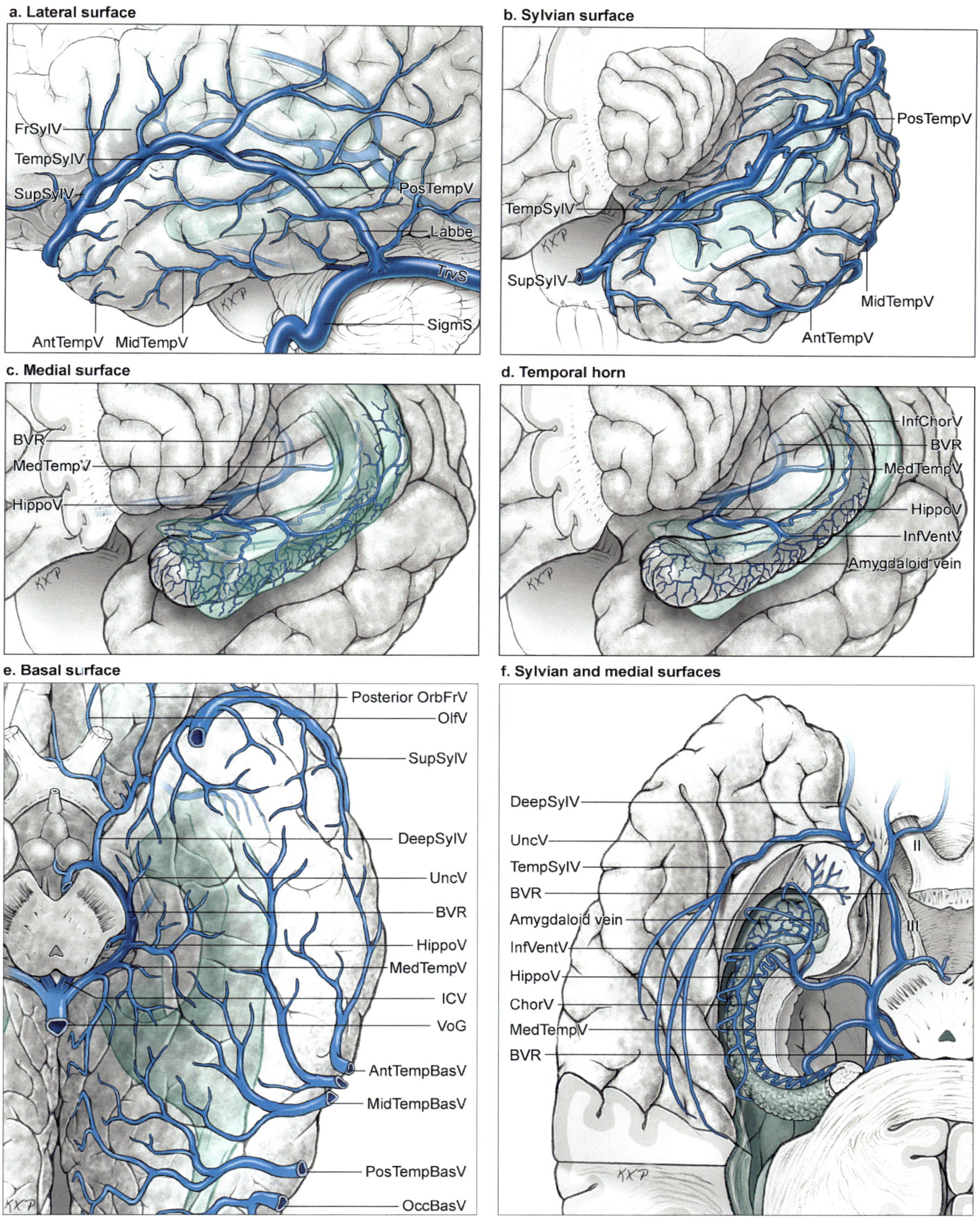
a. Lateral surface
FrSylV
TempSylV
SupSylV
PosTempV
Labbe
TrvS
SigmS
AntTempV
MidTempV
KXP
b. Sylvian surface
PosTempV
TempSylV
SupSylV
MidTempV
AntTempV
KXP
c. Medial surface
BVR
MedTempV
HippoV
KXP
d. Temporal horn
InfChorV
BVR
MedTempV
HippoV
InfVentV
Amygdaloid vein
KXP
e. Basal surface
Posterior OrbFrV
OlfV
SupSylV
DeepSylV
UncV
BVR
HippoV
MedTempV
ICV
VoG
AntTempBasV
MidTempBasV
PosTempBasV
OccBasV
KXP
f. Sylvian and medial surfaces
DeepSylV
UncV
TempSylV
BVR
Amygdaloid vein
InfVentV
HippoV
ChorV
MedTempV
BVR
II
III
KXP

Four Temporal AVM Subtypes

The Lateral Temporal AVM

Temporal AVM subtypes include one for each surface: lateral temporal, basal temporal, sylvian temporal, and medial temporal. Lateral temporal lobe AVMs are based on or immediately beneath the lateral convexity (**Fig. 12.4**). These are the most common of all subtypes, and by far the most common temporal subtype, accounting for over two thirds of temporal AVMs. Superior temporal arteries from the inferior trunk of the MCA are the feeders to these lateral AVMs. The dominant feeding artery varies with the nidus location in the lateral temporal lobe, with the ATA and MidTempA feeding anterior temporal AVMs and PosTempA and TempOccA feeding posterior temporal AVMs. The MCA feeding arteries emanate from the sylvian fissure and intersect the nidus along its superior border. The ATA and TempPolA wrap around the temporal pole and intersect anteriorly. The PosTempA from the P2 PCA contributes to AVMs that are inferiorly located in the ITG. The AChA is involved with larger AVMs with an ependymal plane in the temporal horn. Venous drainage is superficial, with minor deep drainage only with larger AVMs. Drainage usually descends posteriorly through AntTempV, MidTempV, and PosTempV to the vein of Labbé and the TrvS, but may also ascend to TempSylV, SupSylV, and SphParS. Wernicke's speech area is associated with lateral temporal AVMs in the STG beyond 5 cm from the temporal pole.

The Basal Temporal AVM

Arteriovenous malformations on the basal temporal surface reside in the ITG, fusiform, and/or parahippocampal gyri (**Fig. 12.5**). They are not visible on the lateral temporal surface and become apparent only after subtemporal dissection. Basal temporal AVMs are fed by MCA and PCA branches, but PCA dominates. PosTempA emanates from the crural or ambient cisterns, courses over the tentorial incisura, and supplies the medial AVM border. These feeders are deep to the AVM and may not be accessible until after circumferential dissection around the anterior and posterior sides of the nidus. The MCA branches (AntTempA, MidTempA, and PosTempA) wrap around the ITG to supply the lateral margin. The basal surface is intimate with the dura of the middle fossa and has meningeal feeders in nearly one quarter of patients. The AChA is not involved with these lesions. The TempBasVs (anterior, middle, and posterior) drain basal temporal AVMs and typically remain superficial, but one third will have deep connections to the BVR.

The Sylvian Temporal AVM

Sylvian AVMs in the temporal lobe are based on its superior surface, which is oriented vertically down the fissure (**Fig. 12.6**). The nidus may be apparent on this cortical surface or it may lie just beneath, in which case an arterialized vein can offer a landmark. Sylvian temporal AVMs respect insular and

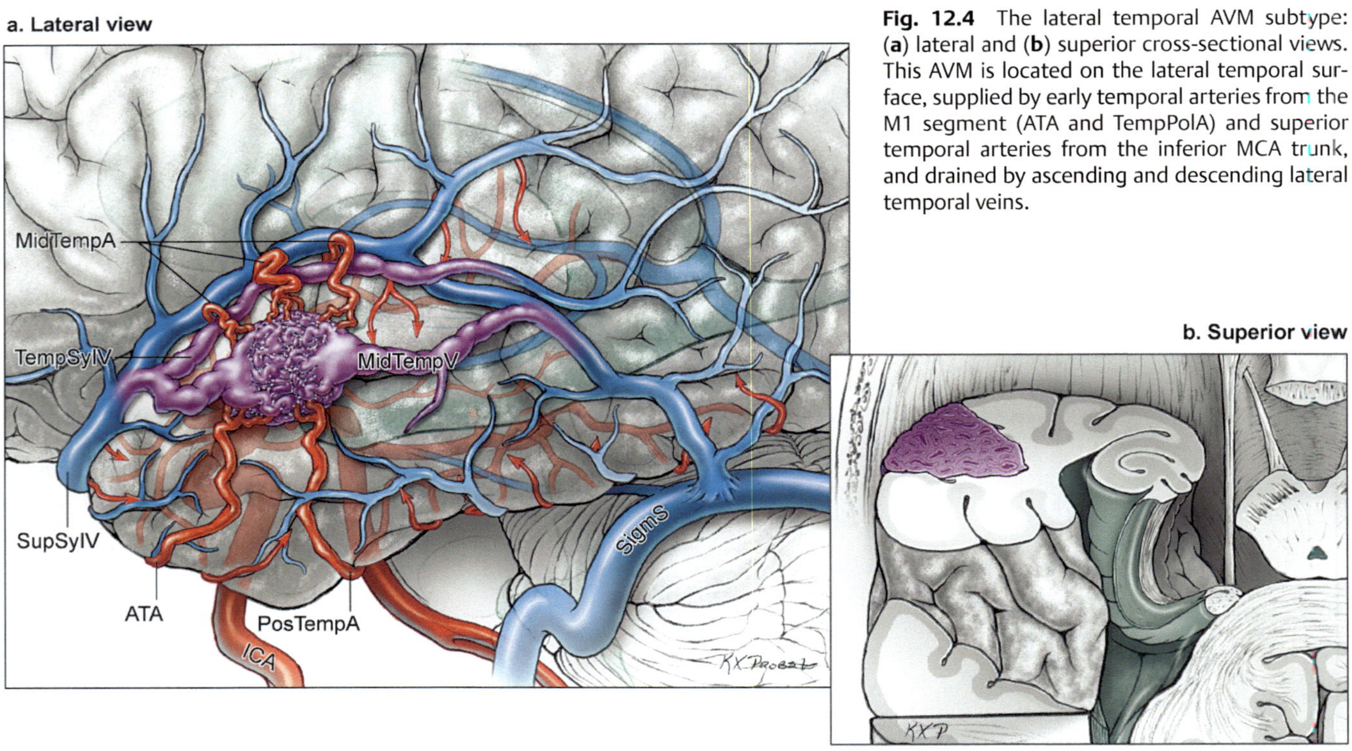

Fig. 12.4 The lateral temporal AVM subtype: (**a**) lateral and (**b**) superior cross-sectional views. This AVM is located on the lateral temporal surface, supplied by early temporal arteries from the M1 segment (ATA and TempPolA) and superior temporal arteries from the inferior MCA trunk, and drained by ascending and descending lateral temporal veins.

a. Inferior view

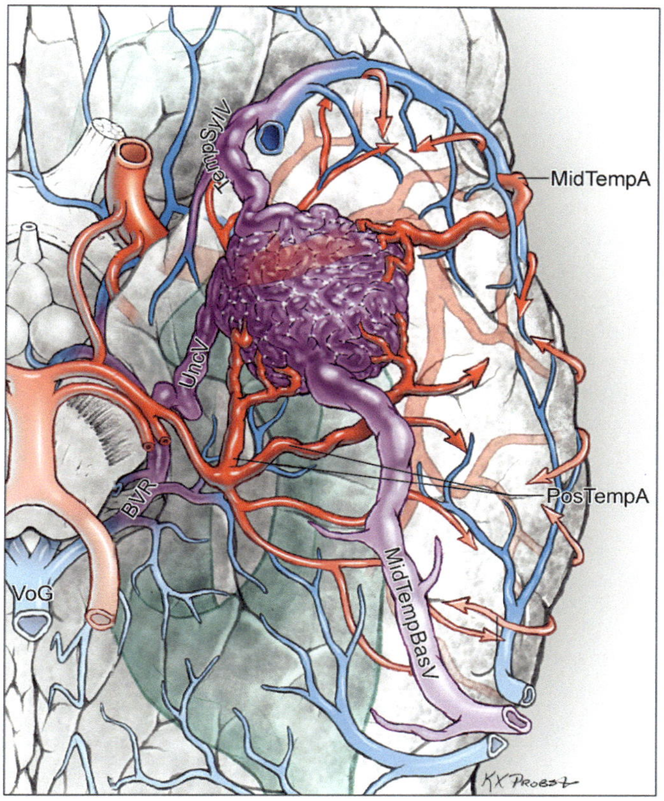

b. Superior view

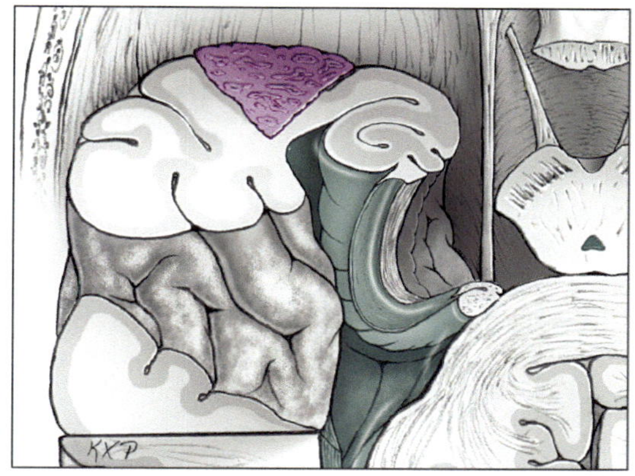

Fig. 12.5 The basal temporal AVM subtype: (**a**) inferior and (**b**) superior cross-sectional views. This AVM is located on the basal temporal surface, supplied by inferior temporal arteries from the PCA (PosTempA), with minor contributions from MCA branches, and drained by temporal basal veins.

a. Lateral view

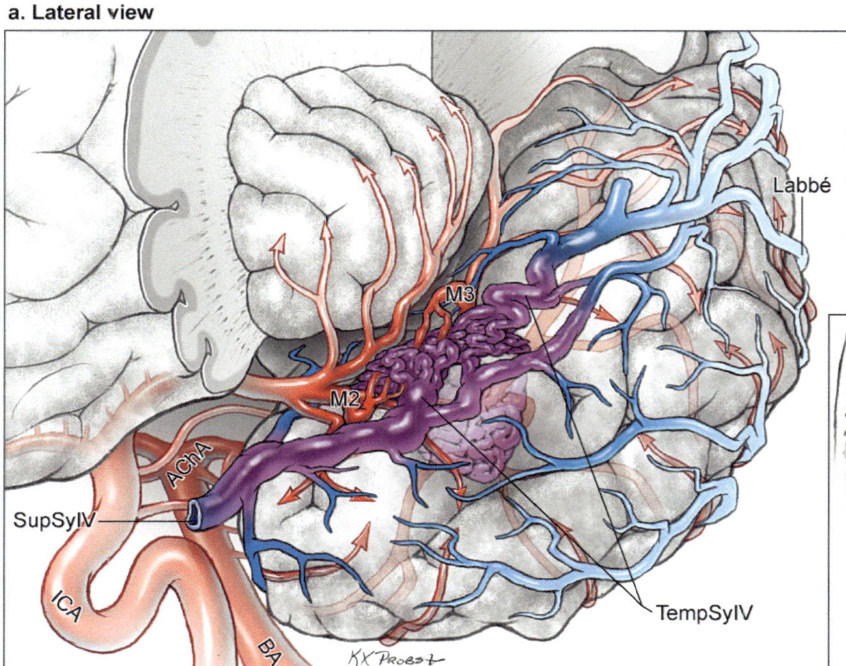

b. Superior view

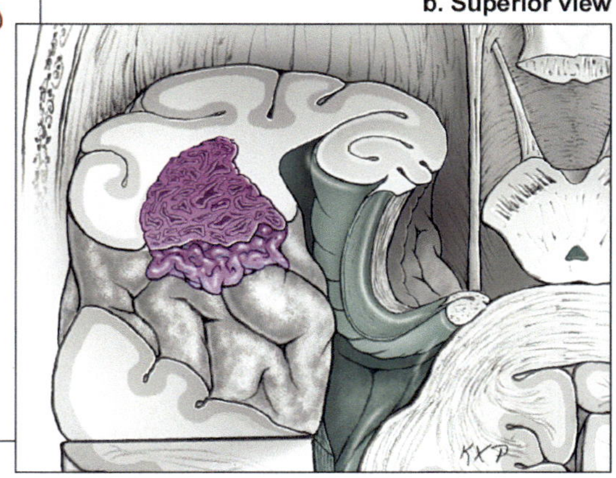

Fig. 12.6 The sylvian temporal AVM subtype: (**a**) anterior view with frontal and parietal lobes partially removed, and (**b**) superior cross-sectional view. This AVM is located on the sylvian temporal surface, supplied by M3 opercular stem arteries, and drained by sylvian veins (TempSylV, SupSylV, and DeepSylV).

frontal cortex, and separate from them completely. Sylvian temporal AVMs are deep to and supplied by M3 opercular segments. These stem arteries supply the AVM as feeding trunks or insular branches before they exit the sylvian fissure to become cortical M4 arteries (MidTempA, PosTempA, TempOccA). These arteries supply the medial and superior margins of the AVM. The AChA may supply the medial margin when it extends to the temporal horn. The PCA does not typically feed these AVMs. Venous drainage is superficial via TempSylV, SupSylV, and DeepSylV. These AVMs are only eloquent when they are in Heschl's gyrus or posterior enough to involve Wernicke's area in the dominant hemisphere.

The Medial Temporal AVM

The medial temporal AVM resides in the block of tissue medial to the temporal horn in the uncus, parahippocampal gyrus, and/or hippocampus (**Fig. 12.7**). This cortical surface is the inside edge of the temporal lobe. A deep transsylvian dissection that follows the AChA, mobilizes the temporal lobe away from the frontal lobe, opens the crural and ambient cisterns, and traces the tentorial incisura around the midbrain affords the only surgical view of this region, and it is limited at best. Inaccessibility makes medial temporal AVMs challenging. Transsylvian dissection leads to feeders from the AChA and the P2 PCA running along the medial and inferior aspect of the nidus, respectively. The cisternal segment of the AChA is always a transit artery that continues to supply the optic tract and internal capsule. HippoA and PosTempA supply these AVMs, with the parent P2 PCA also continuing to supply the occipital lobe while transmitting normal branches like the peduncular (PedP), circumflex (CirP), and thalamogeniculate perforators (ThGenP). The arterial supply may also come from the anterior thalamoperforators

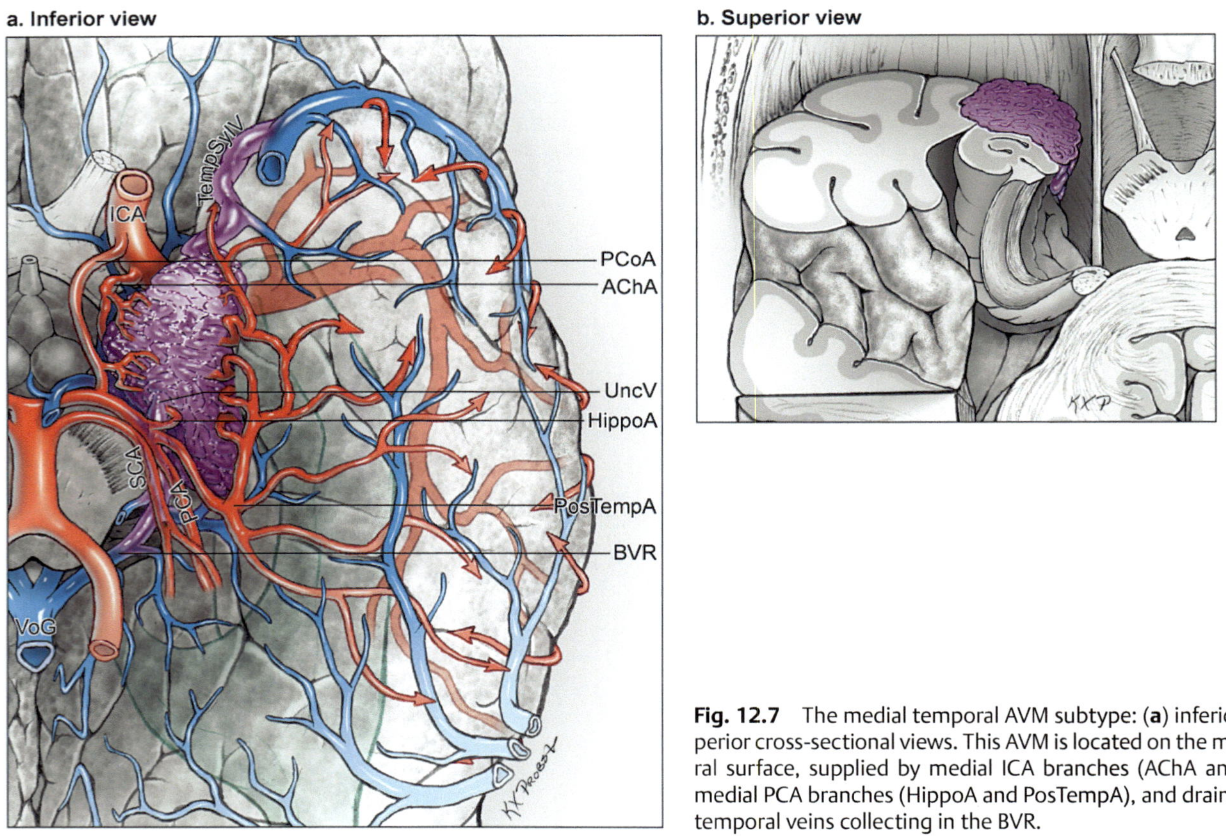

Fig. 12.7 The medial temporal AVM subtype: (**a**) inferior and (**b**) superior cross-sectional views. This AVM is located on the medial temporal surface, supplied by medial ICA branches (AChA and PCoA) and medial PCA branches (HippoA and PosTempA), and drained by medial temporal veins collecting in the BVR.

(ThaP) from the posterior communicating artery (PCoA), TempPolA, and ATA, particularly with more anteriorly located (i.e., uncus) medial temporal AVMs. Medial temporal AVMs that are more posteriorly located (i.e., behind the lateral edge of the cerebral peduncle, or parahippocampal gyrus) have increasing supply from PCA branches, including PosTempA and lPChA. Medial temporal AVMs drain deep to the BVR, and may have minor venous drainage posterolaterally through the basal temporal veins or anterolaterally through deep sylvian veins. Involvement of the hippocampus in memory function makes these AVMs eloquent, particularly in the dominant hemisphere.

Temporal AVM Resection Strategies

Lateral Temporal AVM Resection

Lateral temporal AVMs are convexity lesions that are the easiest temporal AVMs to expose. A pterional craniotomy is used for AVMs in front of the external auditory canal (one fourth of lateral AVMs), and a temporal craniotomy is used for AVMs behind the external auditory canal (EAC) (three fourths of lateral AVMs) (**Fig. 12.8**). Patients are positioned supine with 45 degrees of lateral head rotation for antero-

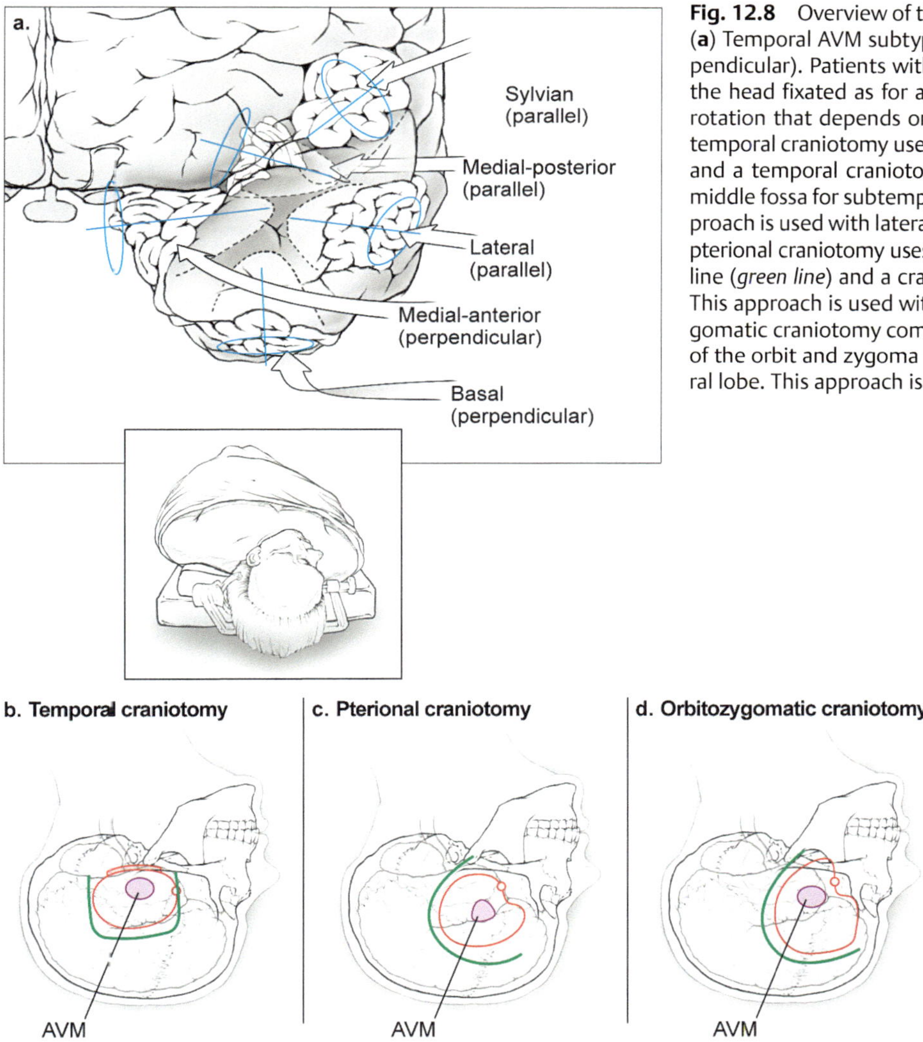

Fig. 12.8 Overview of temporal AVMs and their surgical approaches. (**a**) Temporal AVM subtypes and their angle of attack (parallel or perpendicular). Patients with temporal AVMs are positioned supine with the head fixated as for an MCA aneurysm (*inset*), with variable head rotation that depends on the craniotomy and AVM subtype. (**b**) The temporal craniotomy uses horseshoe-shaped scalp incision (*green line*) and a temporal craniotomy (*red circle*) extending to the floor of the middle fossa for subtemporal exposure (*red-shaded rectangle*). This approach is used with lateral, basal, and medial (posterior) AVMs. (**c**) The pterional craniotomy uses a semicircular scalp incision behind the hairline (*green line*) and a craniotomy centered on the pterion (*red circle*). This approach is used with lateral and sylvian AVMs. (**d**) The orbitozygomatic craniotomy combines the pterional craniotomy with removal of the orbit and zygoma for increased exposure of the medial temporal lobe. This approach is used with medial (anterior) AVMs.

lateral AVMs and 90 degrees of lateral head rotation for posterolateral AVMs. A "horse shoe" or "question mark" incision is used for temporal craniotomies, and a semicircular hairline incision is used for pterional craniotomies. Temporal craniotomies are centered over the EAC and typically extended inferiorly to the middle fossa floor. The dural opening is based on the pterion with pterional craniotomies, and inferiorly with temporal craniotomies (**Fig. 12.9,** step 1). Only sulcal dissection is needed to identify margins, cortical feeding arteries, and draining veins (step 2); sylvian fissure dissection is rarely or minimally needed. Drainage to the vein of Labbé is identified at the posterior margin, and drainage to the sylvian veins is identified superiorly (step 3). Superior feeding arteries are found along the temporal side of the sylvian fissure and traced to the AVM margin (step 4). Lateral temporal AVMs can have three arterial fronts: one superiorly from the MCA inferior trunk branches (MidTempA, PosTempA, and TempOccA) that are interrupted along the AVM's superior margin near the STG; one anteriorly from the M1 MCA branches (TempPolA and ATA) that are interrupted pially along the anterior margin near the pole; and one inferiorly from the P2 PCA branches (PosTempA) that are

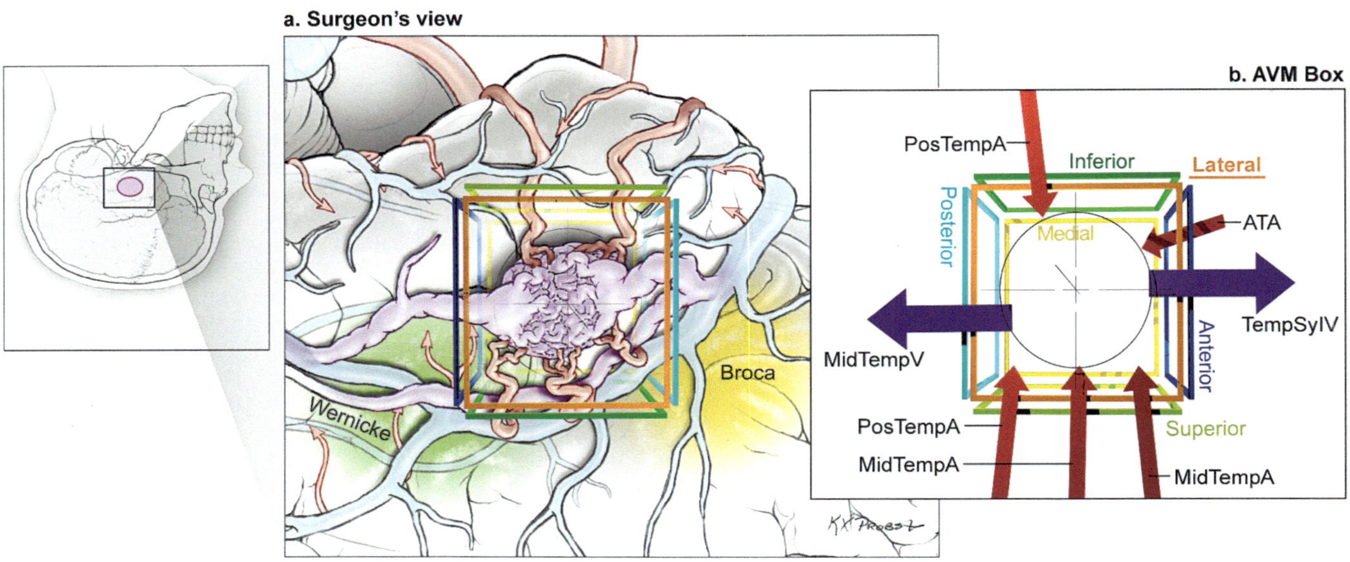

Fig. 12.9 Resection strategy for lateral temporal AVMs. (**a**) Step 1, exposing the AVM with a temporal craniotomy (surgeon's view). (**b**) AVM box showing arterial inputs superiorly from MCA branches off the inferior trunk and inferiorly from PCA branches, with eloquence posteriorly (Wernicke's area).

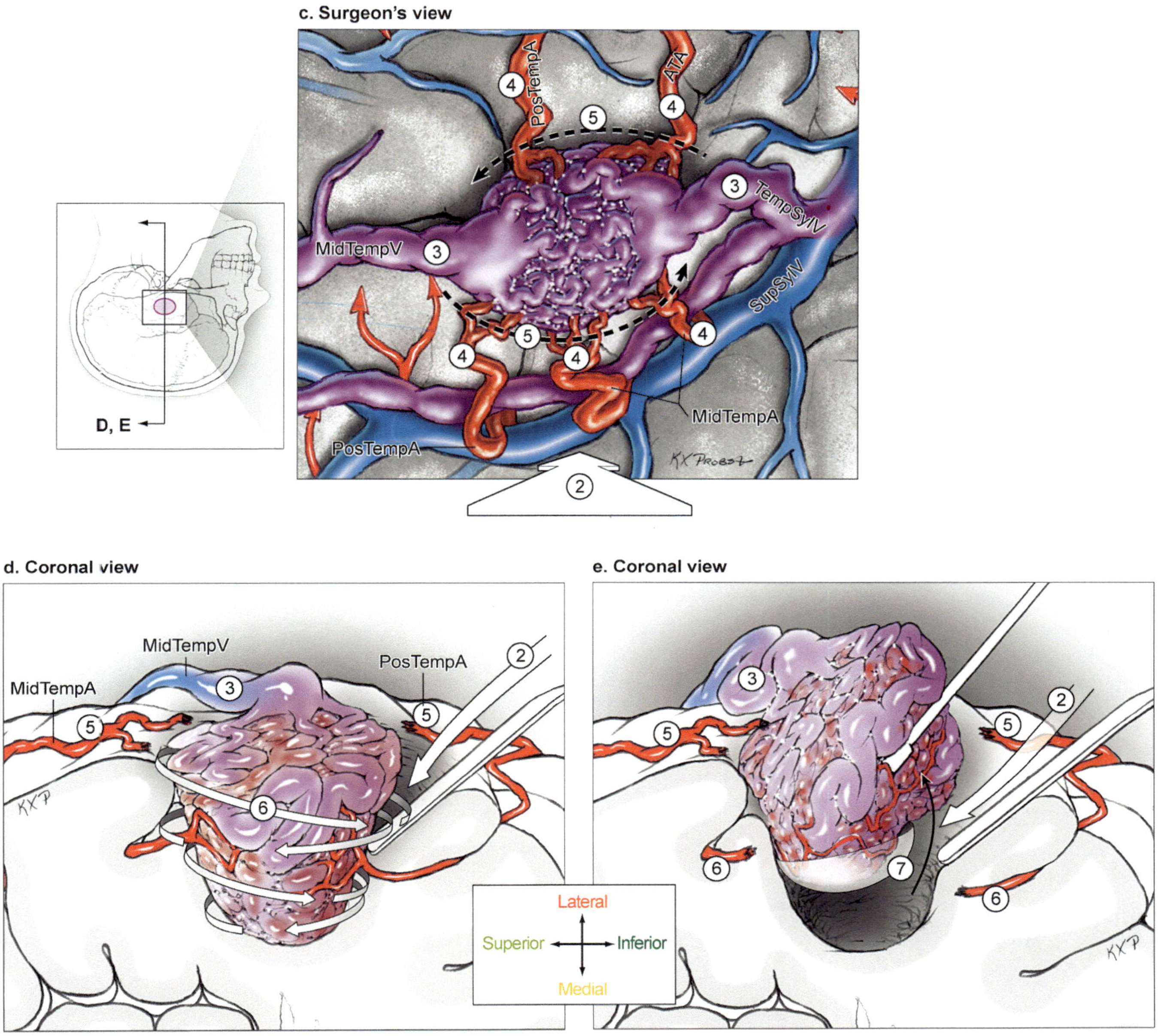

Fig. 12.9 (*continued*) (**c**) Step 2, dissecting surface margins on the lateral temporal lobe; step 3, identifying draining convexity veins; step 4, identifying cortical MCA and PCA feeders; and step 5, interrupting the superior front along the STG and the inferior front along the ITG (surgeon's view). (**d**) Step 6, circumdissecting into temporal parenchyma (coronal cross-sectional view). (**e**) Step 7, delivering the AVM from the temporal lobe.

interrupted along the inferior margin near the ITG (step 5). Parenchymal dissection proceeds with a circumferential and parallel attack (step 6). Awake anesthesia and intraoperative stimulation mapping may be indicated at this point in selected patients to localize speech function (a total of five patients in my experience). Deep dissection may extend to ependymal AVM in the temporal horn with AChA supply (step 7). The choroidal fissure can be opened in the horn medially and the AChA can be interrupted proximally (**Figs. 12.10** and **12.11**).

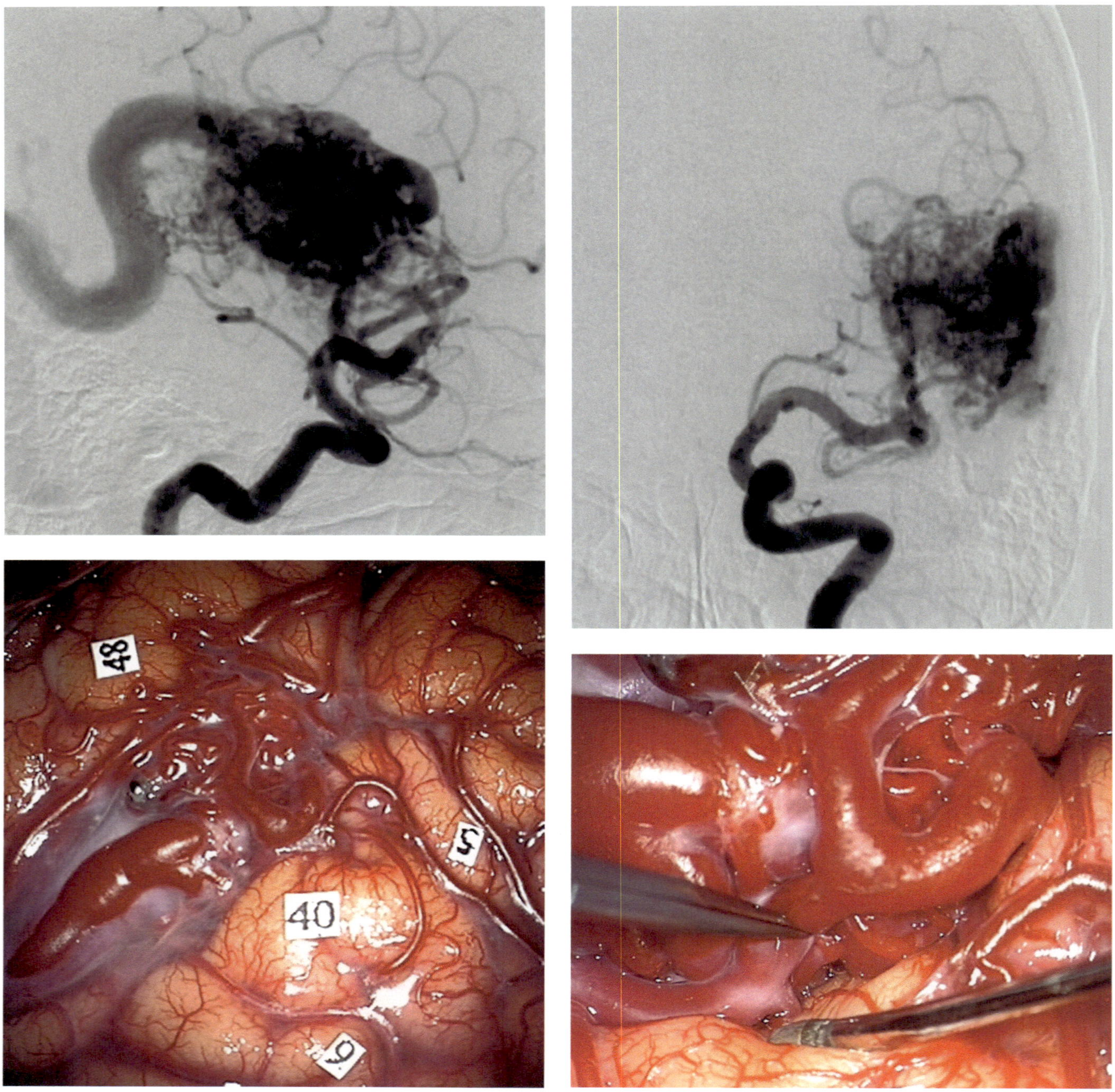

a b c d

Fig. 12.10 This 30-year-old woman presented with a left lateral temporal AVM (supplemented Spetzler-Martin grade 6: S2V0E1/A2B1C0), fed by MidTempA and PosTempA, and drained by a large PosTempV, as seen on left ICA angiography [(**a**) lateral and (**b**) anteroposterior views]. (**c**) The lateral temporal surface was exposed through a large temporal craniotomy and speech areas were mapped with awake anesthesia (48 = Wernicke's area, and 40 = Broca's area). (**d**) By splitting the distal sylvian fissure, this compact AVM was separated from the frontal operculum.

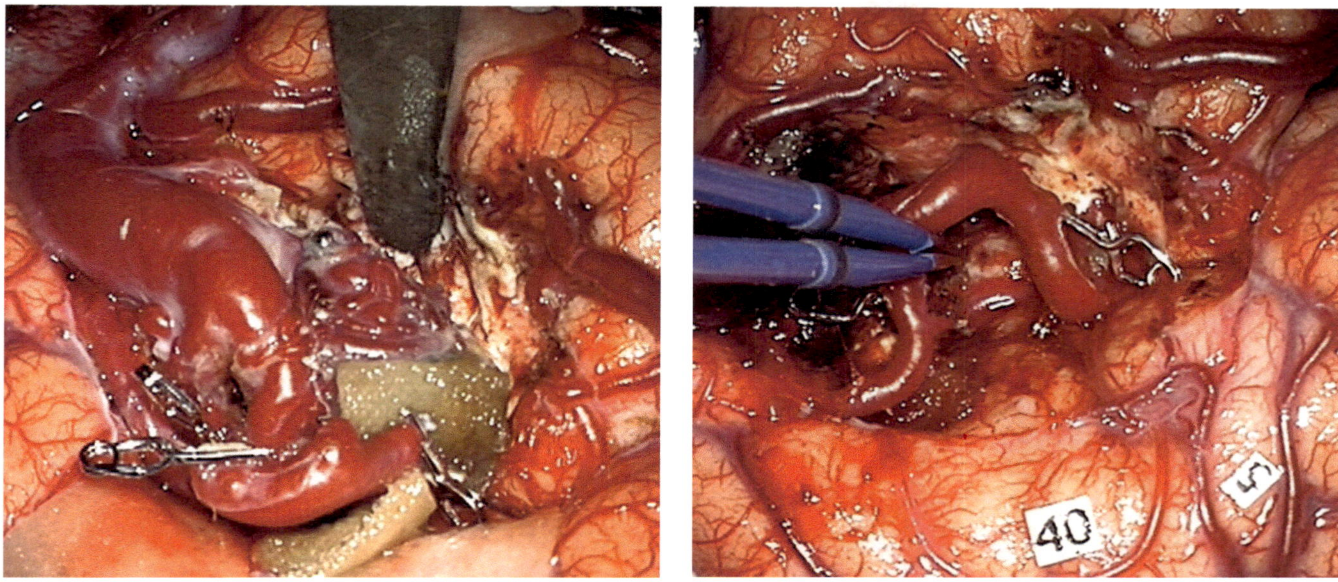

e f

Fig. 12.10 (*continued*) (**e**) Telfa strips and careful dissection protected speech areas, and MidTempA was skeletonized to occlude feeding arteries and preserve en passage arteries. (**f**) After AVM resection, the skeletonized MidTempA courses to distal territories supplying speech conduction pathways. The patient had no postoperative speech deficits.

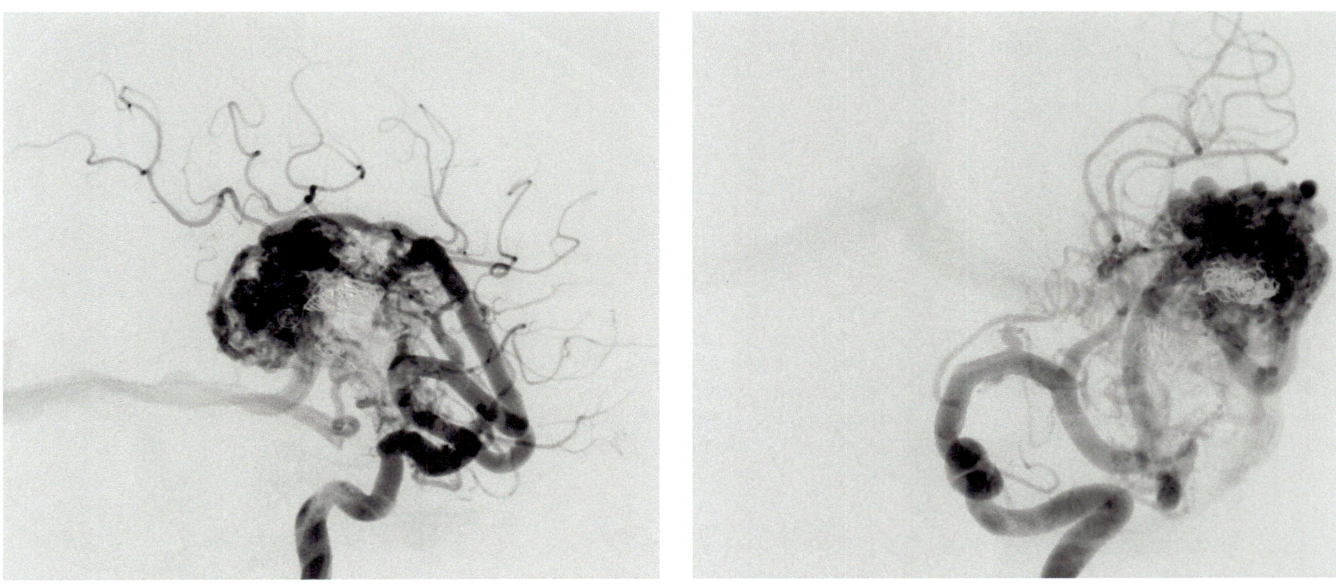

a b

Fig. 12.11 This 20-year-old man presented with a left lateral temporal AVM (supplemented Spetzler-Martin grade 7: S3V0E1/A2B1C0) occupying most of the lateral surface, fed by the ATA, all branches of the inferior MCA trunk, the AChA, and PosTempA from the PCA, and drained by MidTempV. It was embolized preoperatively in three stages, with coils occluding large intranidal shunts (left ICA angiography [(**a**) lateral and (**b**) anteroposterior views]). (*continued on next page*)

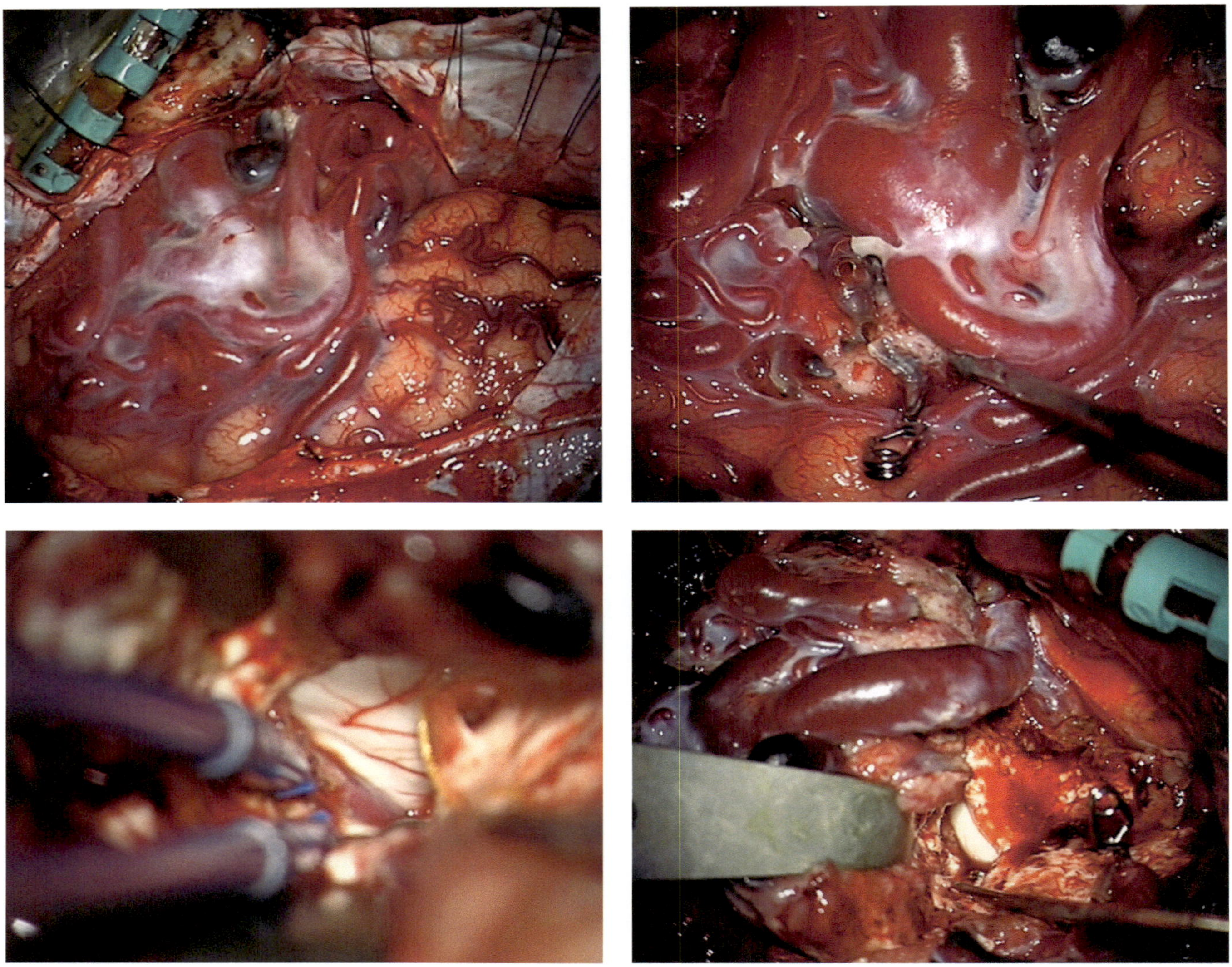

c d e f

Fig. 12.11 (*continued*) (**c**) A combined orbitozygomatic-temporal craniotomy exposed the entire AVM, including the temporal pole. (**d**) MidTempA was clipped proximal to the intraluminal coils and divided. (**e**) Temporal horn of lateral ventricle was entered through the superior temporal gyrus and the AChA identified in the choroidal fissure, where it was clipped, coagulated, and divided. (**f**) The anterior AVM margin was retracted posteriorly to dissect the ependymal surface of the temporal horn. The primary draining MidTempV coursing to the middle fossa floor was preserved throughout the dissection.

Basal Temporal AVM Resection

Basal temporal AVMs are exposed with a temporal craniotomy and a subtemporal approach (**Fig. 12.12**, step 1). The patient is positioned supine and the head is rotated 90 degrees, with the midline horizontal and the neck flexed laterally to drop the vertex downward toward the floor, allowing the temporal lobe to fall away from the middle fossa floor. The inferior extent of the craniotomy is drilled flat to remove the lip of the temporal squamosal bone and widen exposure to the floor. Entrance into mastoid air cells is closed with wax. Subtemporal dissection exposes the basal surface (step 2). Release of tentorial adhesions and arachnoid granulations frees the temporal lobe, and cerebrospinal fluid (CSF) drainage from the carotid and ambient cisterns slackens the brain. These maneuvers facilitate subtemporal retraction and bring the basal temporal surface into view, but in contrast to lateral temporal AVMs, it is a perpendicular rather than a parallel view. Arteriovenous malformation drainage is through the TempBasV (anterior, middle, and posterior), and an arterialized vein is often the first and only sign of the AVM (step 3). The draining vein is a landmark to follow into the collateral or occipitotemporal sulci or into a basal gyrus when the AVM is subcortical. Subtemporal retraction must

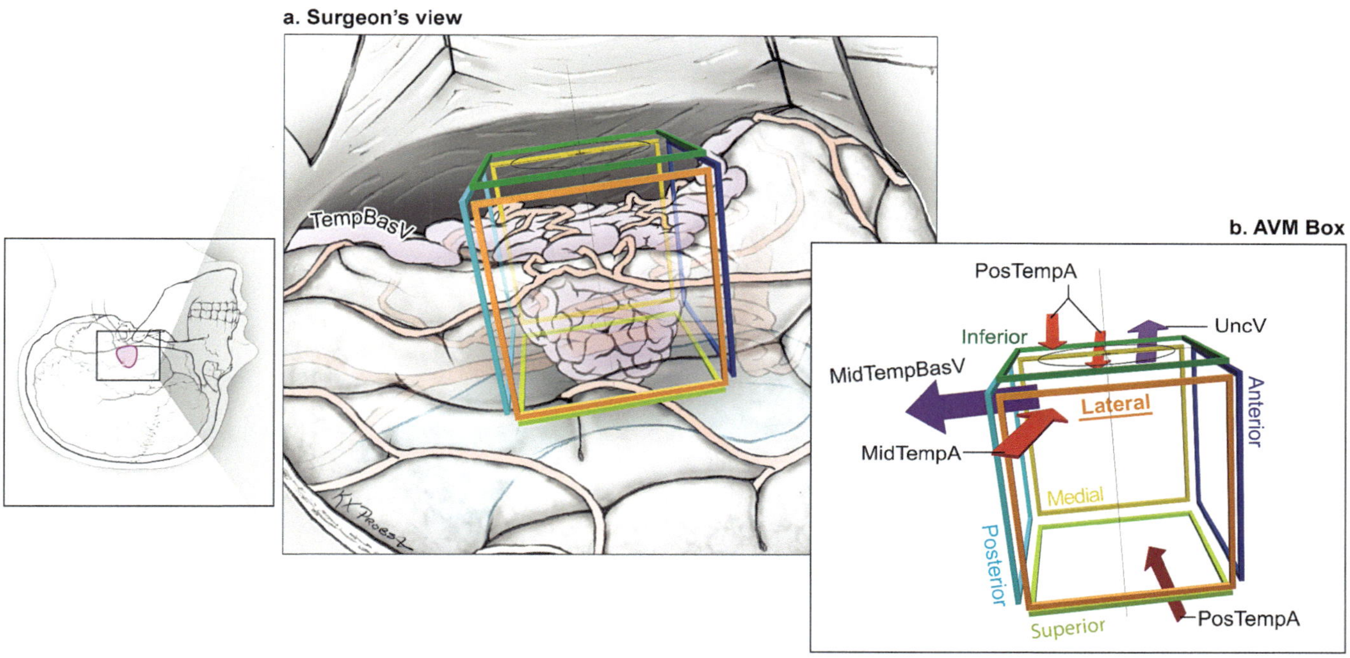

Fig. 12.12 Resection strategy for basal temporal AVMs. (**a**) Step 1, exposing the lateral temporal lobe through a temporal craniotomy (surgeon's view). (**b**) AVM box showing arterial inputs from the PosTempA on medial, inferior, and superior sides. (*continued on next page*)

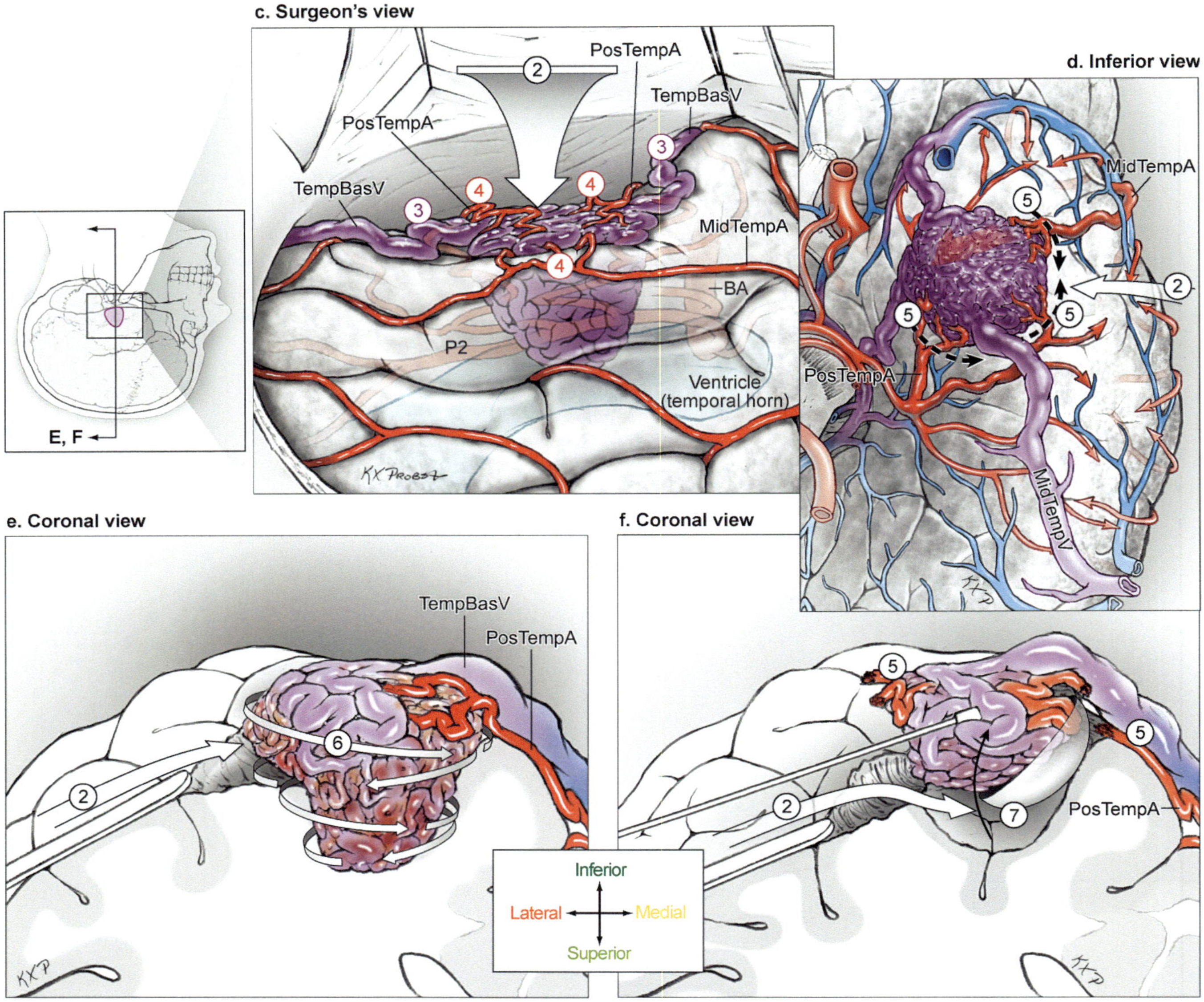

Fig. 12.12 (*continued*) (**c**) Step 2, approaching the AVM subtemporally; step 3, locating the draining vein on the basal surface; and step 4, identifying feeding arteries from the PCA medially and the MCA laterally (surgeon's view). The AVM blocks access to feeders from PCA. (**d**) Step 5, dividing the medial front along parahippocampal gyrus and the lateral front along the ITG (inferior view). (**e**) Step 6, circumdissection upward into the temporal lobe with some subtemporal retraction and resection of the ITG (coronal cross-sectional view). (**f**) Step 7, mobilizing AVM inferiorly into the subtemporal corridor and interrupting final medial feeders from the PCA.

avoid avulsing the draining vein or the vein of Labbé. The PosTempA and its branches are the major supply to basal temporal AVMs, with minor supply from the MCA's superior temporal arteries (step 4). Superior temporal arteries are interrupted early as a lateral front on the basal surface along the ITG (step 5), but the posterior temporal arteries are interrupted much later as a medial front near the parahippocampus after circumdissection. Perpendicular exposure of basal temporal AVMs requires that the AVM be drawn downward toward the middle fossa floor and into the subtemporal corridor (step 6). As the nidus mobilizes, the deep medial plane becomes accessible and PosTempA feeders are interrupted at the tentorial incisura (step 7). There are no eloquent areas on the basal temporal surface (**Figs. 12.13** and **12.14**).

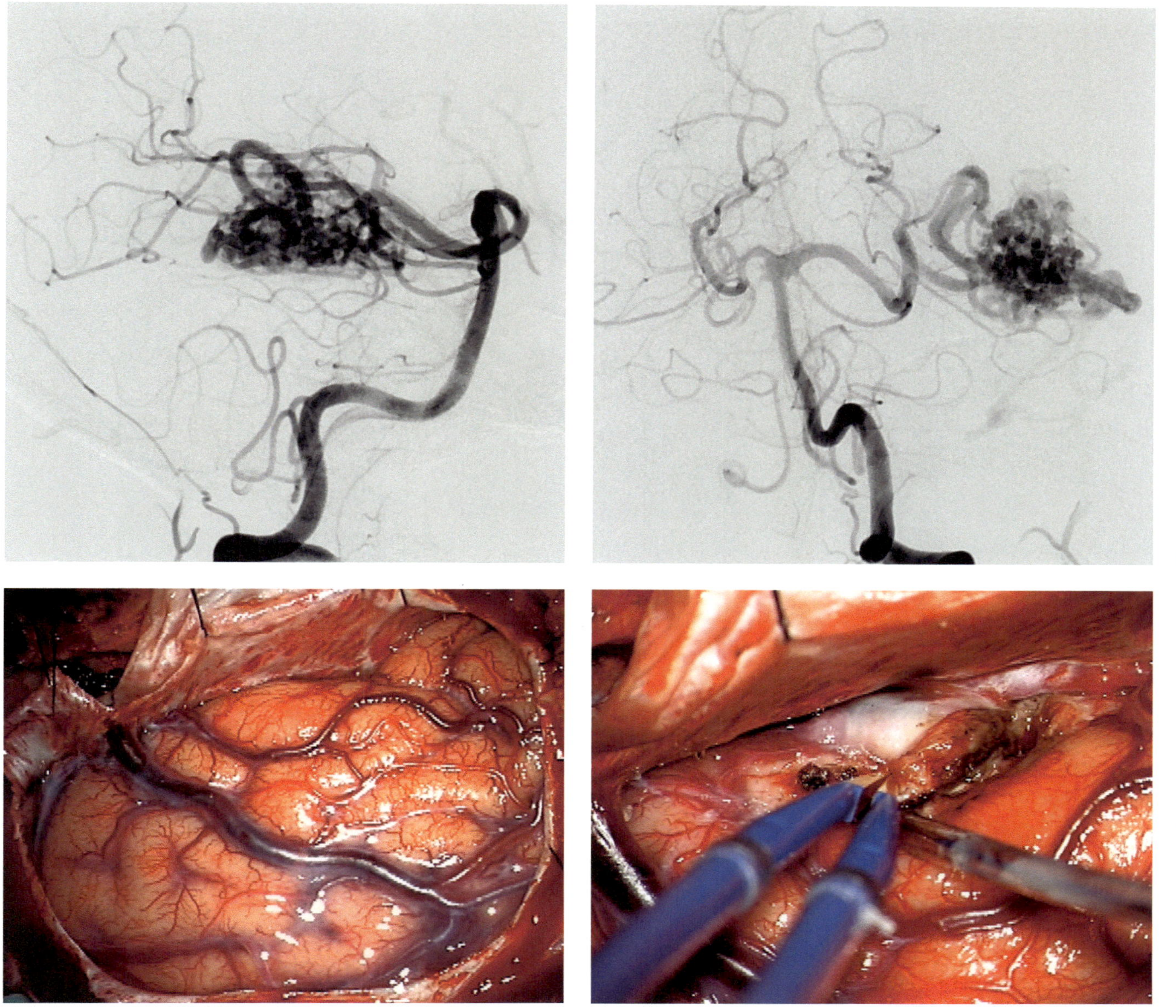

Fig. 12.13 This 50-year-old woman presented with a left basal temporal AVM (supplemented Spetzler-Martin grade 6: S1V1E0/A3B1C0), fed by PosTempA branches from the P2 PCA [left vertebral artery angiogram, (**a**) lateral and (**b**) anteroposterior views] and drained by anterior and posterior TempBasV and the BVR. (**c**) A temporal craniotomy extending inferiorly to the middle fossa floor facilitated the subtemporal approach and AVM exposure. (**d**) After identifying the arterialized TempBasV, the pia of the inferior temporal gyrus was cauterized and incised circumferentially. (*continued on next page*)

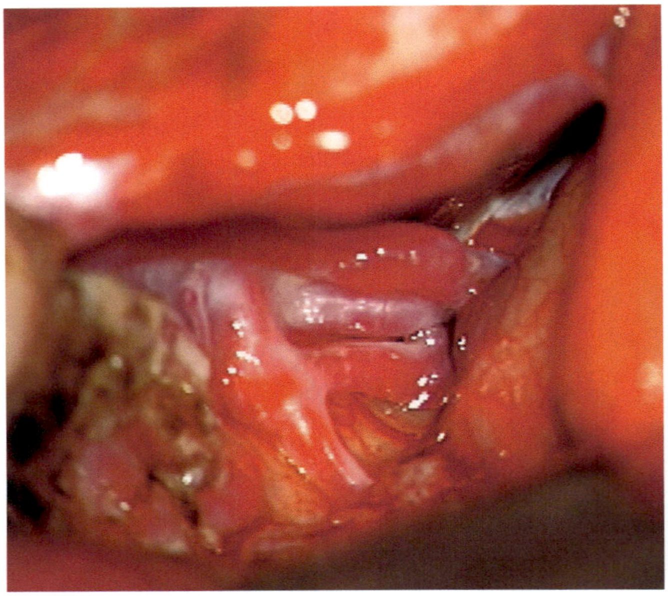

e

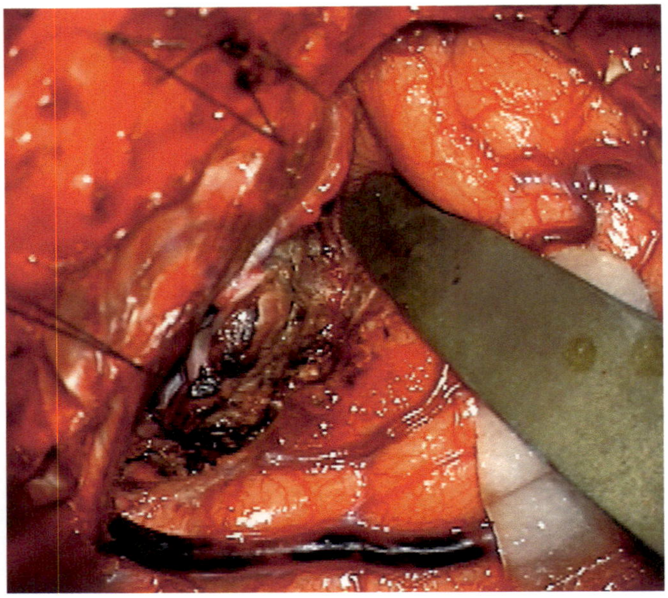

f

Fig. 12.13 (*continued*) (**e**) PosTempA branches supplying the medial margin of the AVM were encountered along the tentorium later in the dissection. (**f**) The AVM was mobilized down toward the tentorium, with some retraction of the inferior temporal gyrus, to dissect across the superior surface.

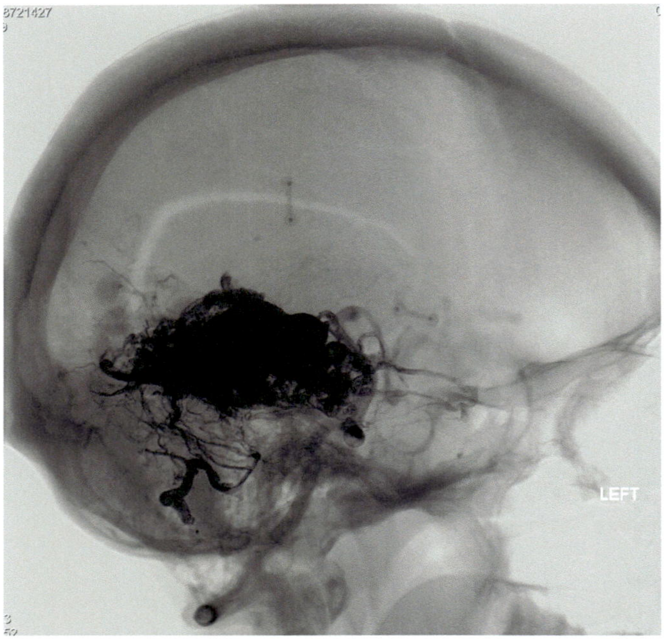

a

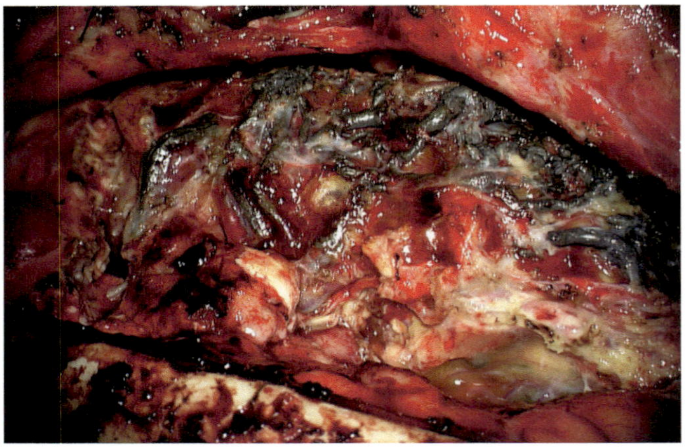

b

Fig. 12.14 This 32-year-old man was referred for surgery after undergoing multiple sessions AVM embolization with Onyx and attempted surgical resection at an outside hospital. He had a large right basal temporal AVM (supplemented Spetzler-Martin grade 8: S3V1E1/A2B1C0). (**a**) He needed no further embolization (right carotid angiogram, lateral view). (**b**) The AVM was centered on the basal surface, but extended to the lateral temporal surface and to the floor of the temporal horn, and was heavily injected with Onyx (black cast).

c d e f

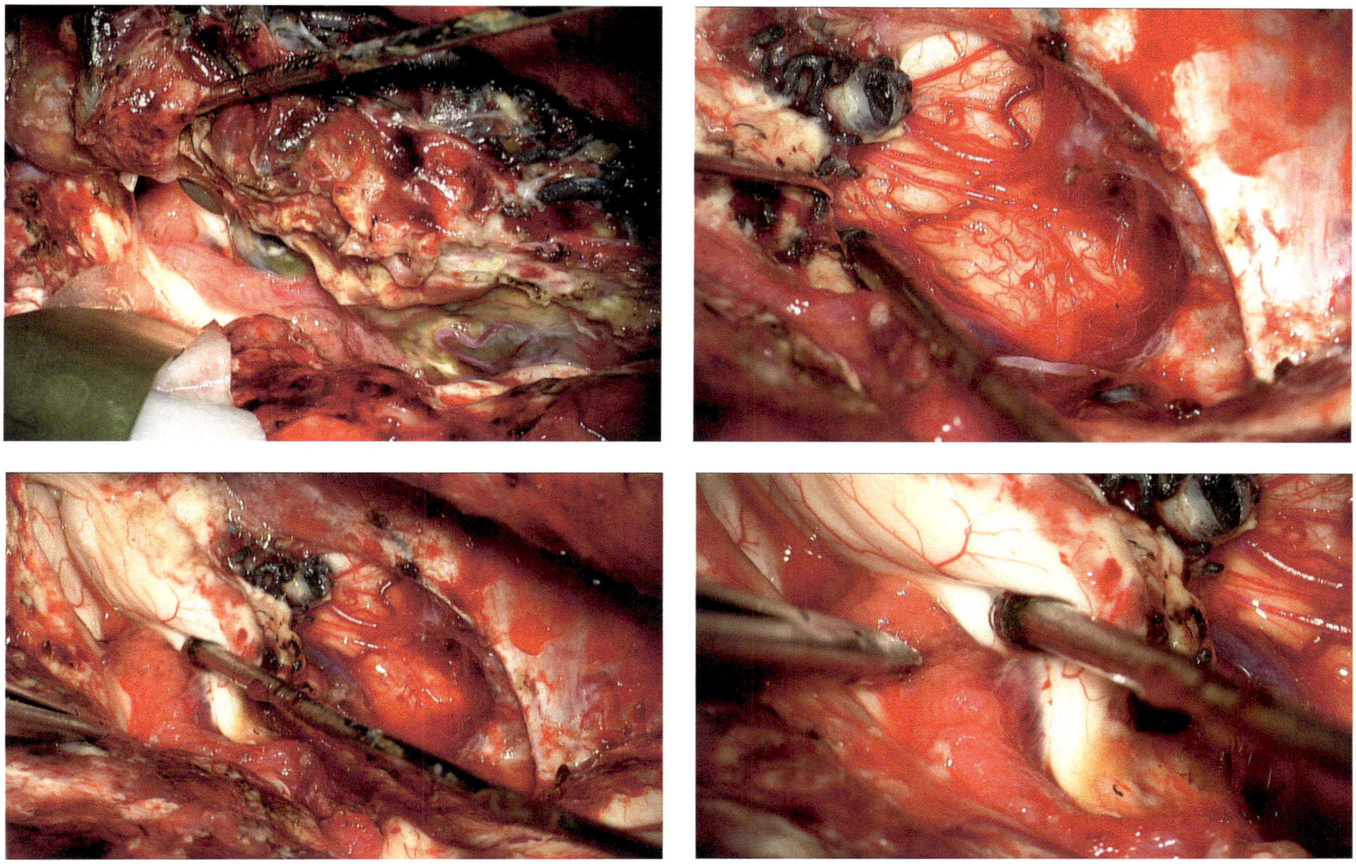

Fig. 12.14 (*continued*) (**c**) Choroid plexus coursed along the superomedial border of the AVM, as seen through the temporal horn that was opened widely. (**d**) PosTempA was transected above the tentorial incisura, seen after resection of the AVM. (**e**) Temporal lobe medial to the temporal horn (hippocampus, parahippocampus, and uncus) was not involved with the AVM. (**f**) The choroidal fissure, choroid plexus, and fimbria of fornix were visualized through the resection cavity.

Sylvian Temporal AVM Resection

Sylvian temporal AVMs are resected similarly to sylvian frontal AVMs, except on the opposite side of the sylvian fissure (**Fig. 12.15**). They are exposed through a standard pterional craniotomy (step 1). Transsylvian dissection widely separates the frontal and temporal lobes and lays out the inferior trunk's stem arteries from insular M2 segments to cortical M4 segments (step 2). Draining sylvian veins are also exposed with the sylvian split, and the SupSylV is mobilized temporally to preserve its connection to the SphParS, which can position an arterialized vein directly over the nidus (step 3). Sylvian temporal AVMs are deep to and fed by unnamed M3 opercular arteries that may terminate in the AVM or send branches to the AVM before continuing en passage (step 4). Arteries are established as terminal feeders, transit arteries, or bystanders, and each is managed differently: terminal feeders are occluded at the AVM margin; transit arteries are skeletonized; and bystanders are separated away from the nidus. Skeletonization in a distal-to-

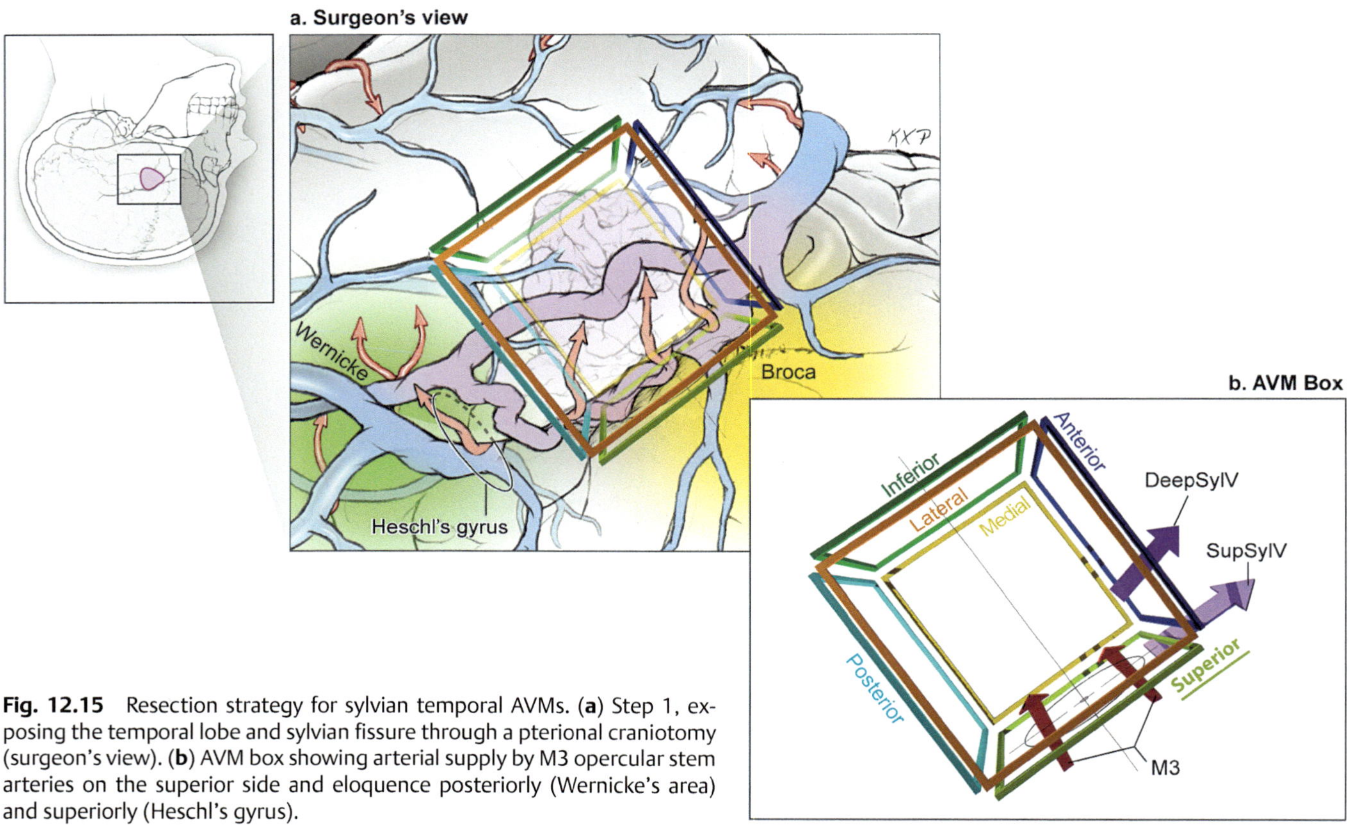

Fig. 12.15 Resection strategy for sylvian temporal AVMs. (**a**) Step 1, exposing the temporal lobe and sylvian fissure through a pterional craniotomy (surgeon's view). (**b**) AVM box showing arterial supply by M3 opercular stem arteries on the superior side and eloquence posteriorly (Wernicke's area) and superiorly (Heschl's gyrus).

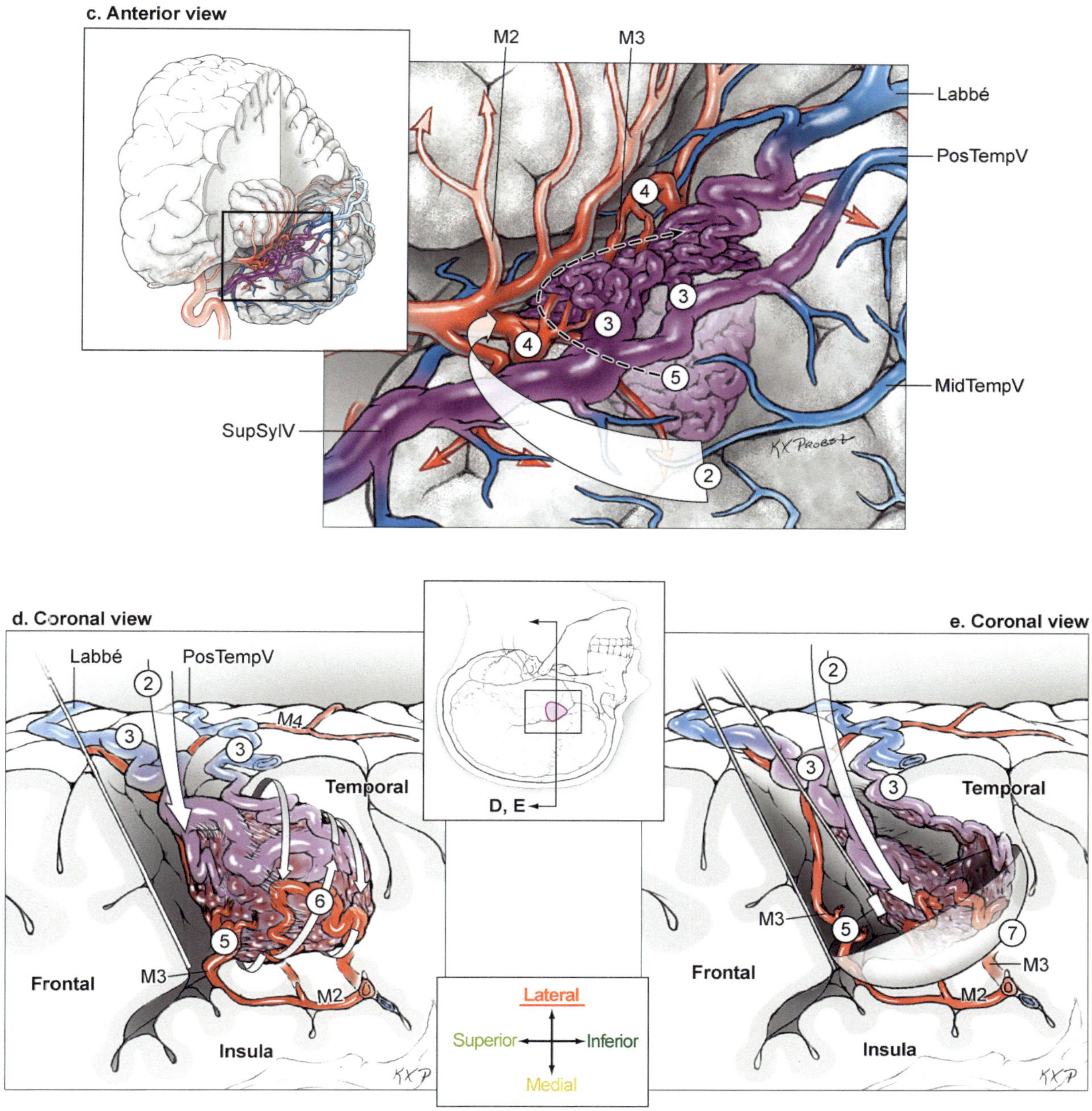

Fig. 12.15 *(continued)* (**c**) Step 2, splitting the sylvian fissure and exposing the sylvian surface; step 3, mobilizing draining sylvian veins temporally; step 4, exposing insular and opercular MCA segments from the inferior trunk; and step 5, dividing terminal feeders on the superomedial frontal along planum polare/planum temporale (anterior view). (**d**) Step 6, circumdissecting downward into temporal lobe and skeletonizing transit arteries in a distal-to-proximal direction (coronal cross-sectional view). (**e**) Step 7, interrupting deep proximal M3 feeders and identifying any extensions to temporal horn.

proximal direction helps preserve the transit artery. Opercular feeders create a superomedial front of arteries on the sylvian temporal surface (planum polare and temporale), and additional feeders can be found on the lateral surface of the superior temporal gyrus (step 5). The sylvian temporal AVMs are accessible superficially in the sylvian fissure and through the STG, facilitating parallel circumdissection that protects Heschl's gyrus and Wernicke's area (step 6). The dissection is often conducted between M3 and M4 segments and between sylvian veins. The deep plane may extend to the temporal horn and receive AChA supply (step 7) (**Figs. 12.16** and **12.17**).

a

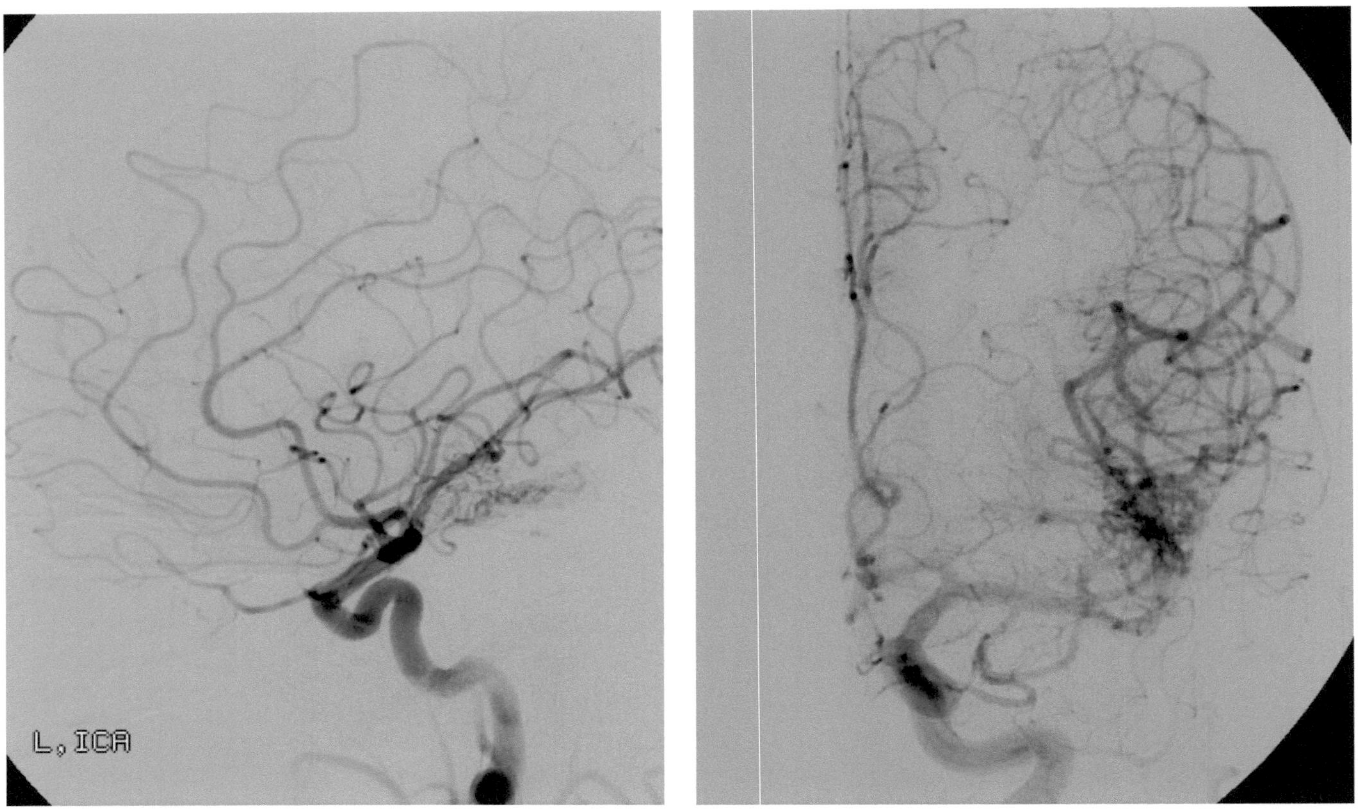

b

Fig. 12.16 This 47-year-old man presented with a hemorrhage from this left sylvian temporal AVM (supplemented Spetzler-Martin grade 6: S1V1E1/A3B0C0), fed by branches from the M2 (insular) and M3 (opercular) MCA [left ICA angiogram, (**a**) lateral and (**b**) anteroposterior views].

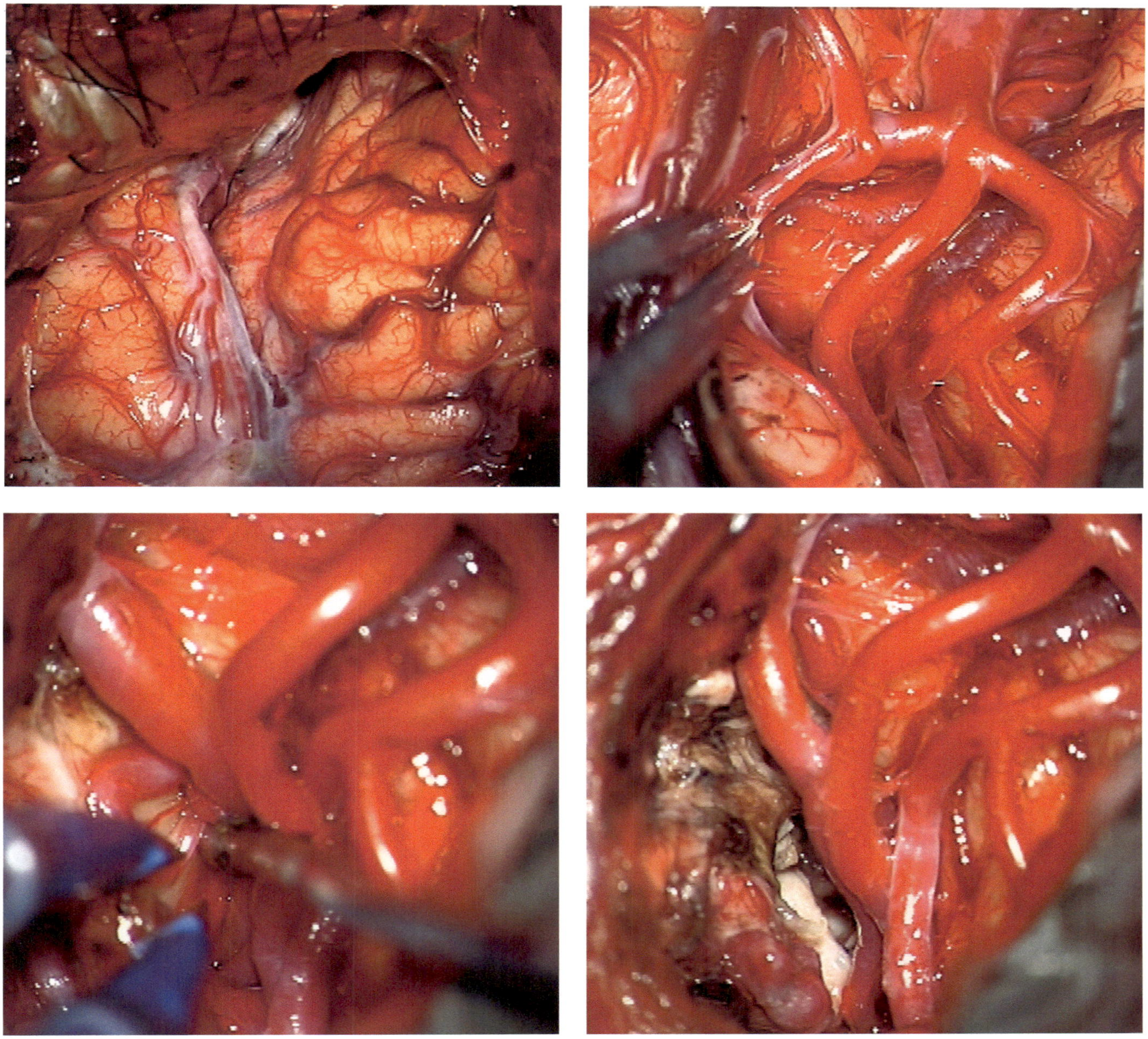

c d e f

Fig. 12.16 (*continued*) (**c**) Left pterional craniotomy revealed arterialized SupSylVs draining to SphParS. (**d**) After splitting the sylvian fissure, an arterialized DeepSylV was identified deep to the MCA trifurcation and followed to the AVM in the planum polare of the sylvian surface. (**e**) The nidus was supplied by small branches from the inferior trunk and MCA stem arteries, (**f**) which were skeletonized and separated from the AVM. The AVM was resected completely.

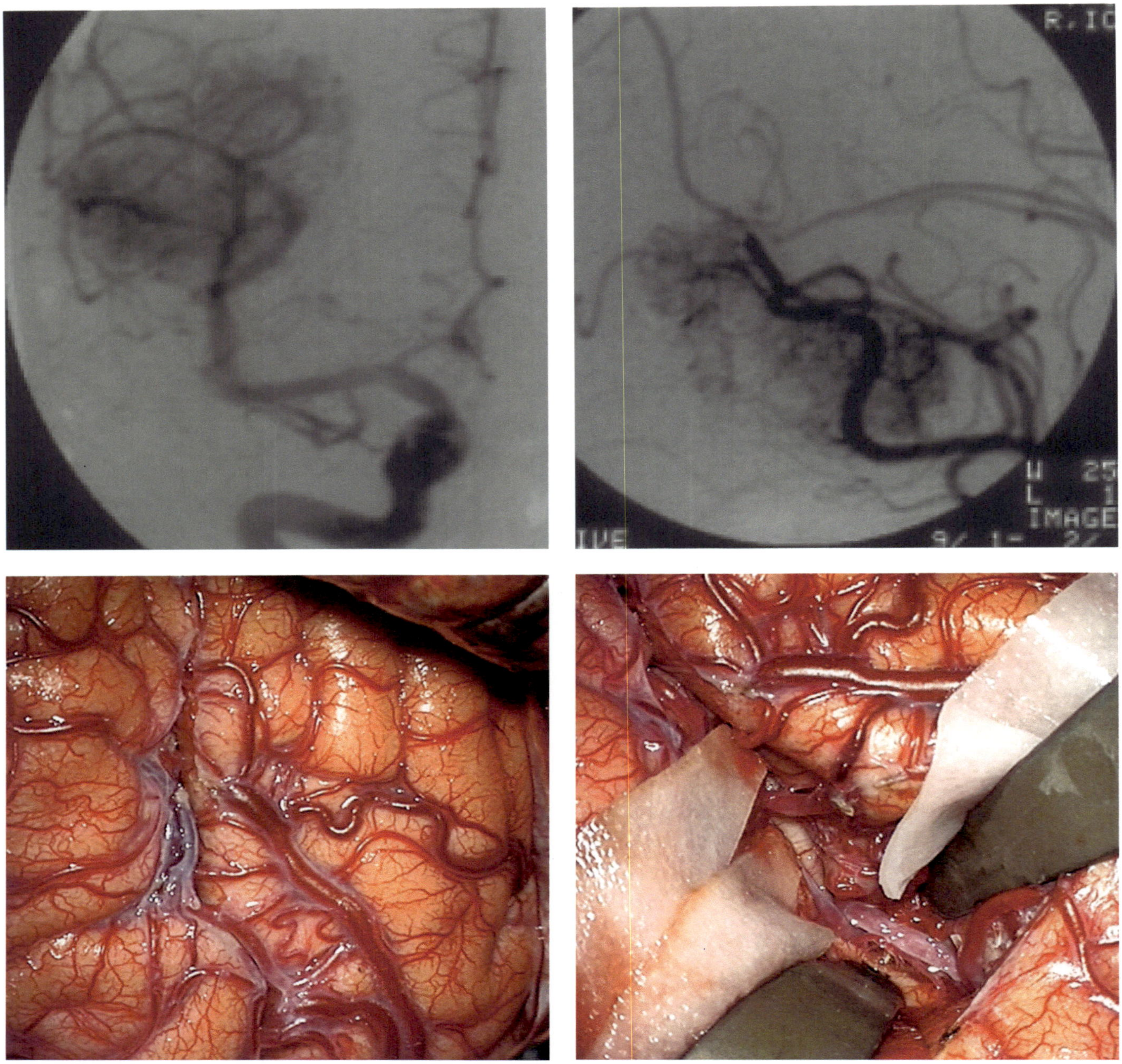

a b c d

Fig. 12.17 This 42-year-old man presented with a right sylvian temporal AVM (supplemented Spetzler-Martin grade 6: S2V0E0/A3B1C0), fed by small branches from the M2 and M3 MCA segments [right ICA angiogram, (**a**) anteroposterior and (**b**) anterior oblique views]. (**c**) Normal transit arteries emerged from the distal sylvian fissure, together with two arterialized TempSylVs. (**d**) Splitting the distal sylvian fissure exposed the AVM on the planum temporale and M2 and M3 segments of MCA.

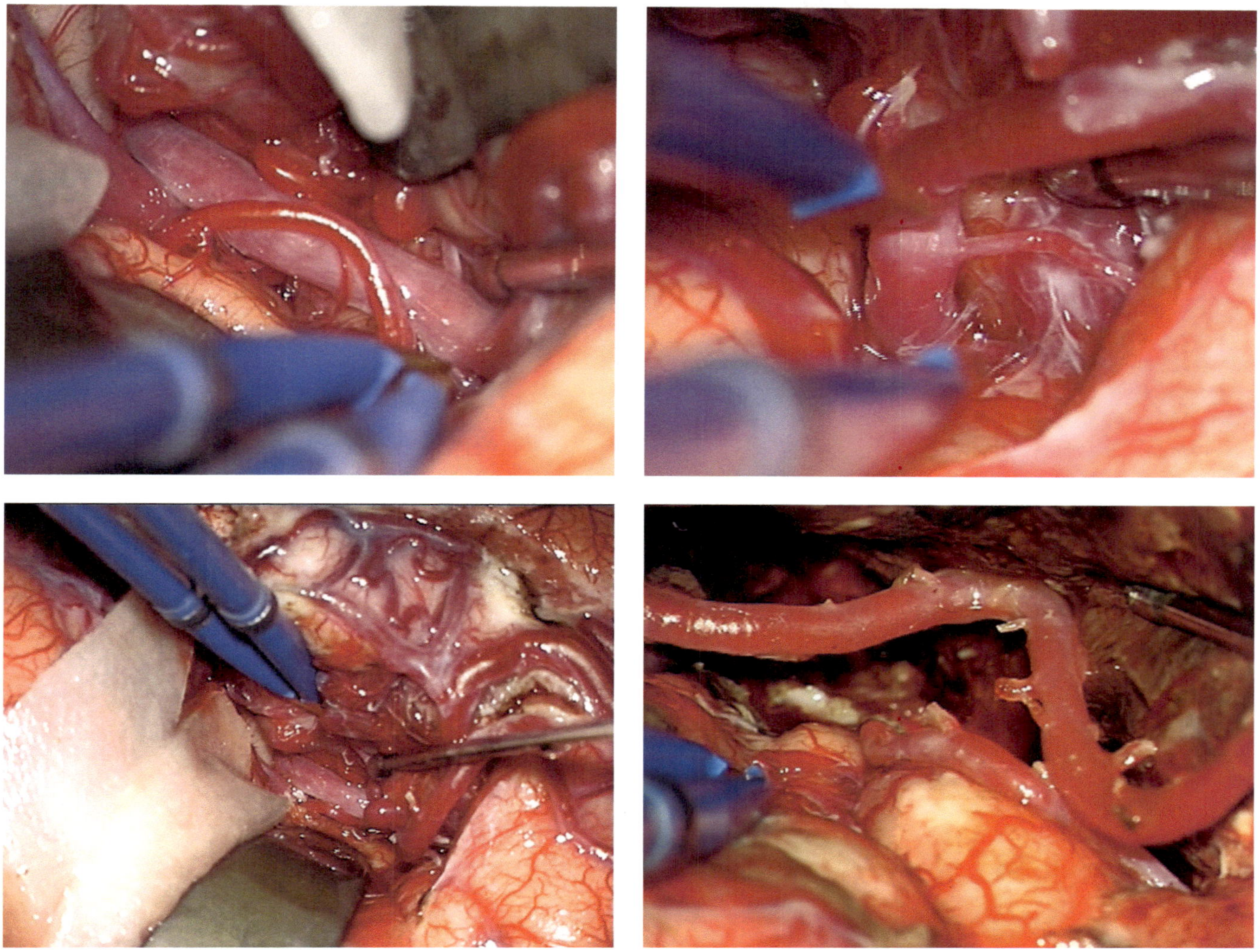

e f g h

Fig. 12.17 (*continued*) (**e**) Small feeding arteries from MCA's insular segment and (**f**) opercular segment supplied the AVM. (**g**) Their cauterization and division interrupted AVM supply on the sylvian surface, and a circumscribing incision in the superior temporal gyrus accessed the parenchymal sides. (**h**) After AVM resection, a skeletonized MCA emerged from the distal sylvian fissure, with perfusion to its distal territories preserved.

Medial Temporal AVM Resection

The surgical approach to medial temporal AVMs is an extreme variation of the approach to sylvian temporal AVMs (**Fig. 12.18**). Medial AVMs are exposed perpendicularly with an orbitozygomatic craniotomy and transsylvian dissection, as with an approach to a basilar bifurcation aneurysm (step 1). Orbital removal opens a trajectory that is more anterior than with a pterional approach, creating a view along the medial temporal surface. Zygoma removal facilitates temporal lobe retraction in a posterolateral direction that opens this view further. Posterolateral retraction exposes the medial temporal surface and makes this more of a convexity approach. Overall, the orbitozygomatic craniotomy shortens the working distance to the AVM and widens the exposure. The medial temporal lobe is separated from its adhesions to the frontal lobe by splitting the sylvian fissure, opening the carotid cistern and crural cisterns, and dissecting the AChA along its course around the uncus (step 2). Further dissection leads to the PCA along the medial and inferior aspects of the nidus. Medial temporal AVMs drain deep to the BVR (step 3), which enables the temporal pole to be retracted without sacrificing a critical draining vein. The orbitozygomatic-transsylvian exposure of the medial AVM base gives early access to feeders from the AChA and P2 PCA, as well as from the PCoA (AntThaP), TempPolA, and ATA (step 4). These feeders join the nidus along the medial pial border (uncus) to form a medial front (step 5). The AChA and P2 PCA are skeletonized; terminal feeders from the PCA, including HippoA, PosTempA, and lPChA, are occluded; and medial midbrain perforators (PosThaP, PedP, CirP, ThGenP, and mPChA) are protected by moving them medially. Circumdissection through the uncus and amygdala defines the AVM's lateral border and has no detectable effect on

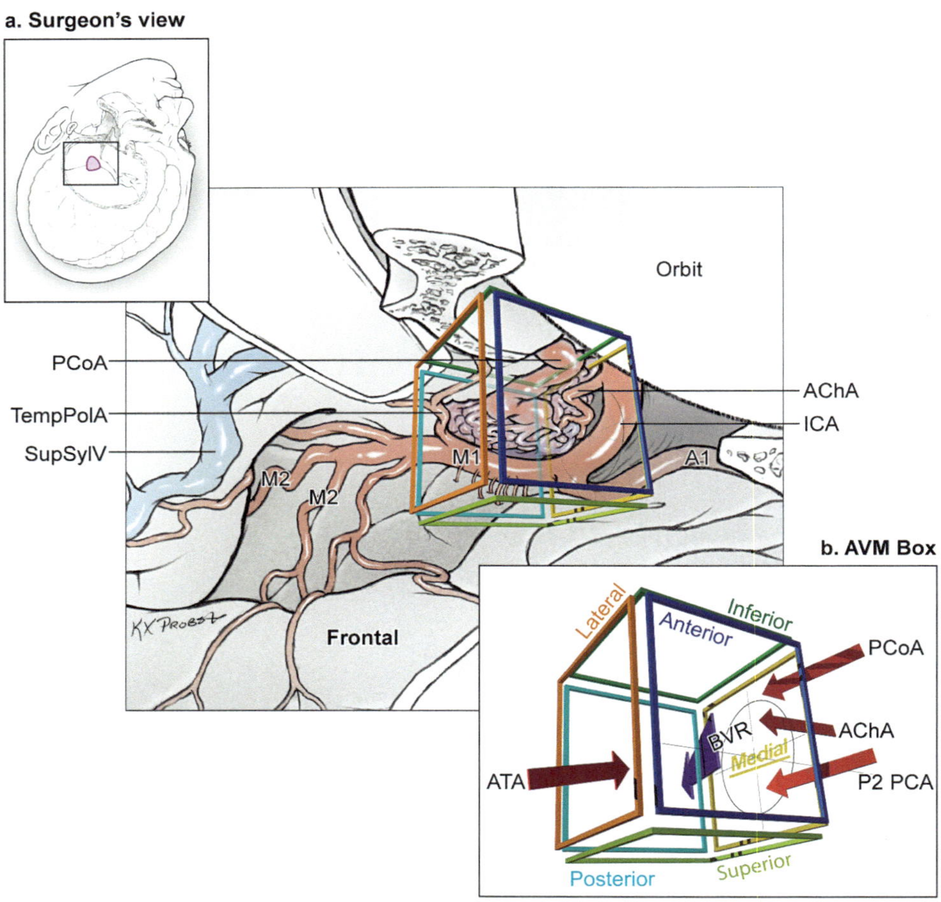

Fig. 12.18 Resection strategy for medial temporal AVMs (anterior to the crus of cerebral peduncle). (**a**) Step 1, exposing the sylvian fissure through an orbitozygomatic-pterional craniotomy (surgeon's view). (**b**) AVM box showing arterial supply medially from the AChA, PCoA, and P2 PCA, and venous drainage posteriorly through the BVR.

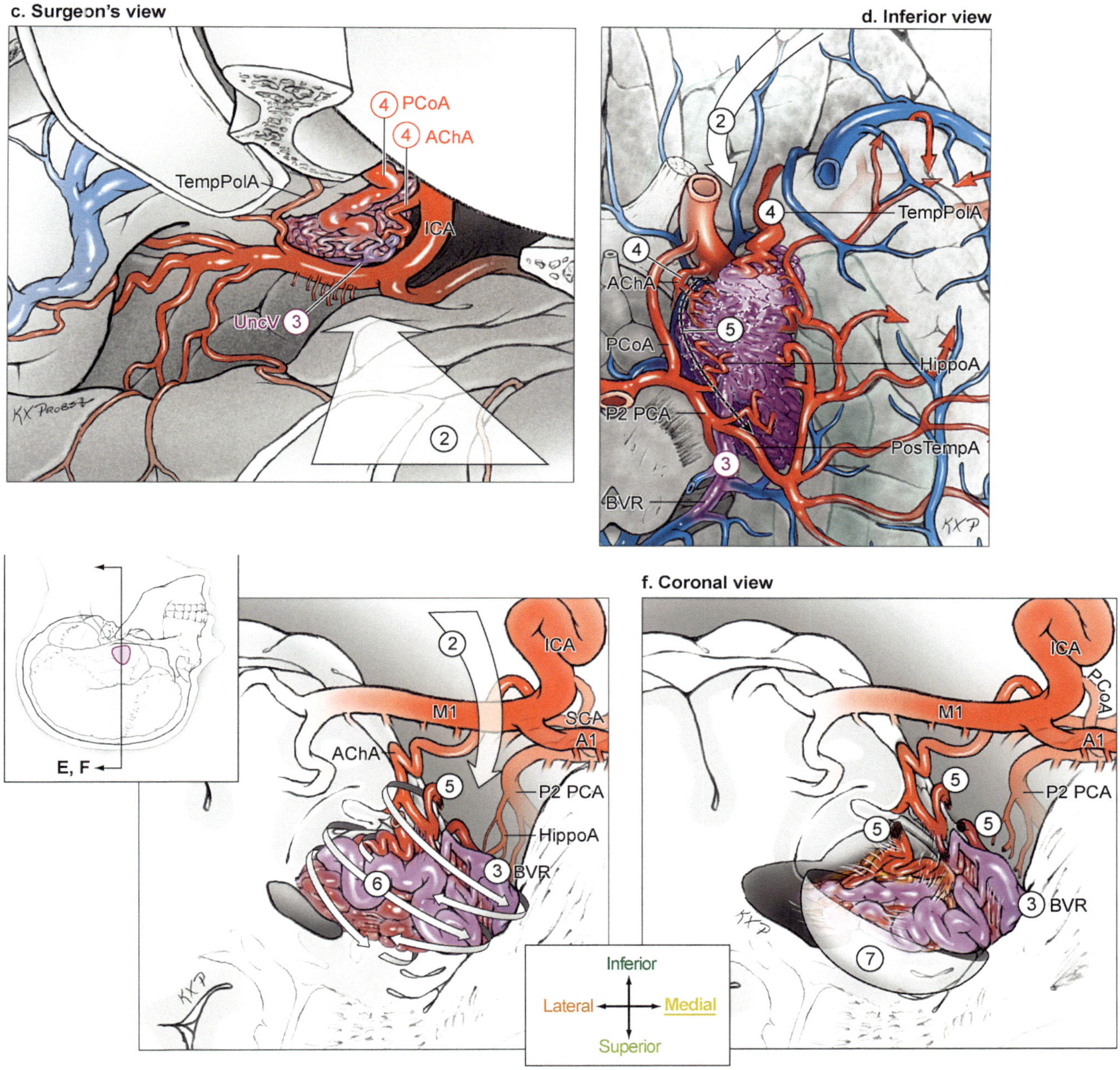

Fig. 12.18 (*continued*) (**c**) Step 2, splitting the sylvian fissure, opening carotid and crural cisterns, dissecting the AChA around the uncus, and mobilizing the temporal pole posterolaterally; step 3, defining medial venous drainage, which may not be visible until later; and step 4, identifying medial feeders from the ICA (AChA and PCoA), MCA (TempPolA and ATA), and PCA (HippoA and PosTempA). (**d**) Step 5, interrupting the medial front along the uncus (inferior view). (**e**) Step 6, circumdissecting laterally into the uncus and amygdala, and skeletonizing the AChA and P2 PCA (coronal cross-sectional view). (**f**) Step 7, mobilizing AVM inferomedially and dividing drainage to the BVR.

memory function (step 6). Larger AVMs may extend to the temporal horn, in which case definition of the lateral margin may require opening into the ventricle. Posterior hippocampal circuitry that is more critical for memory is easier to preserve. The perpendicularity of this approach obscures the posterosuperior margins of the AVM and it must be drawn inferomedially into the surgical corridor. The deep side of the AVM box connects to the BVR, which is often dark by the time it is visualized at the end of the dissection (step 7) (**Figs. 12.19** and **12.20**).

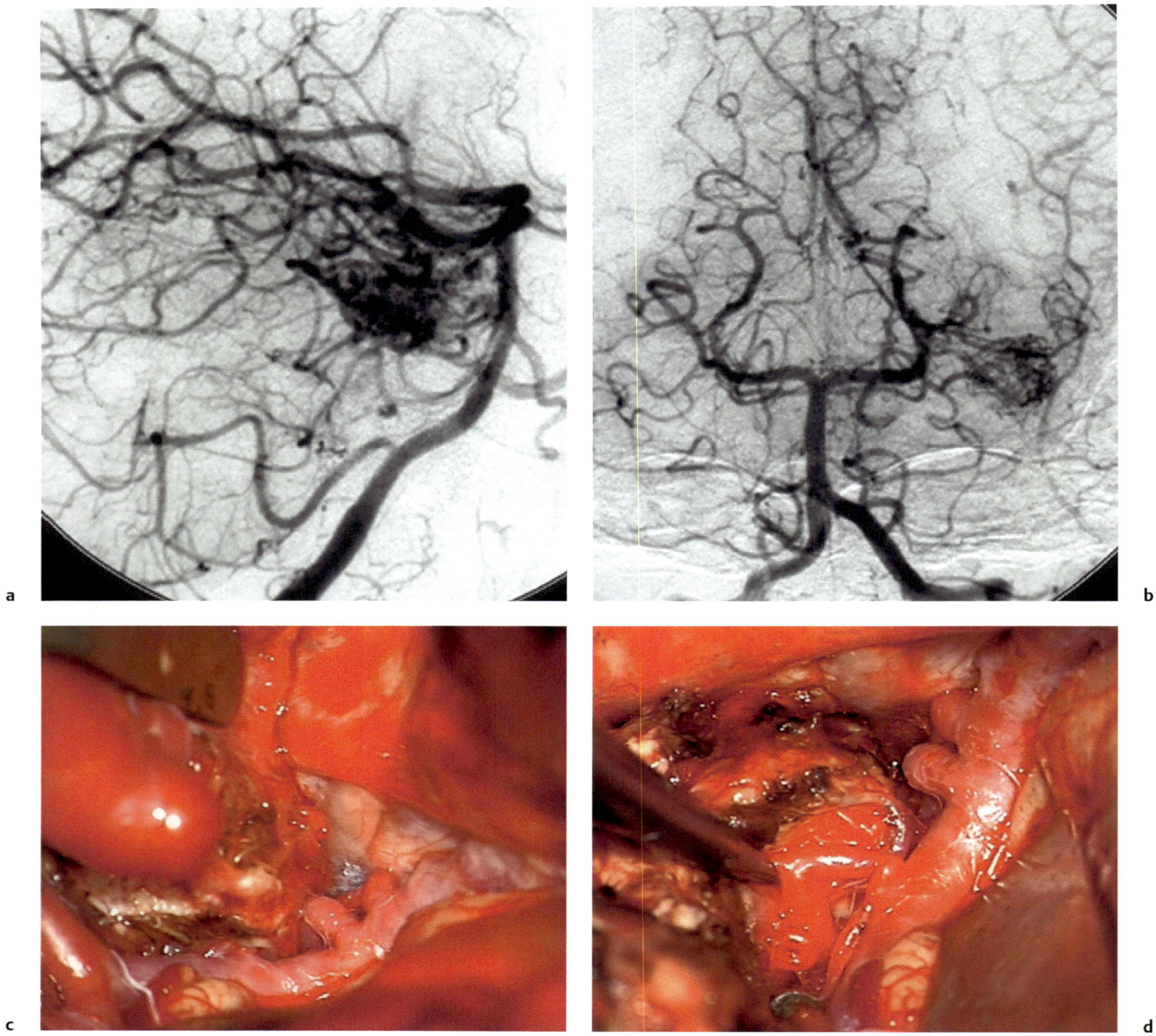

Fig. 12.19 This 31-year-old man presented with a left medial temporal AVM (supplemented Spetzler-Martin grade 6: S1V1E1/A2B1C0), fed by the PCoA, AChA, TempPolA, and PosTempA, which all lie along the tentorial edge at the AVM's medial margin. PosTempA feeders [left vertebral artery angiogram, (**a**) lateral and (**b**) anteroposterior views] were embolized preoperatively. Left orbitozygomatic craniotomy and sylvian fissure split exposed an AVM in the uncus. (**c**) An enlarged PCoA and AChA originated from the supraclinoidal ICA above the oculomotor nerve, and (**d**) an enlarged TempPolA originated from the proximal M1 MCA.

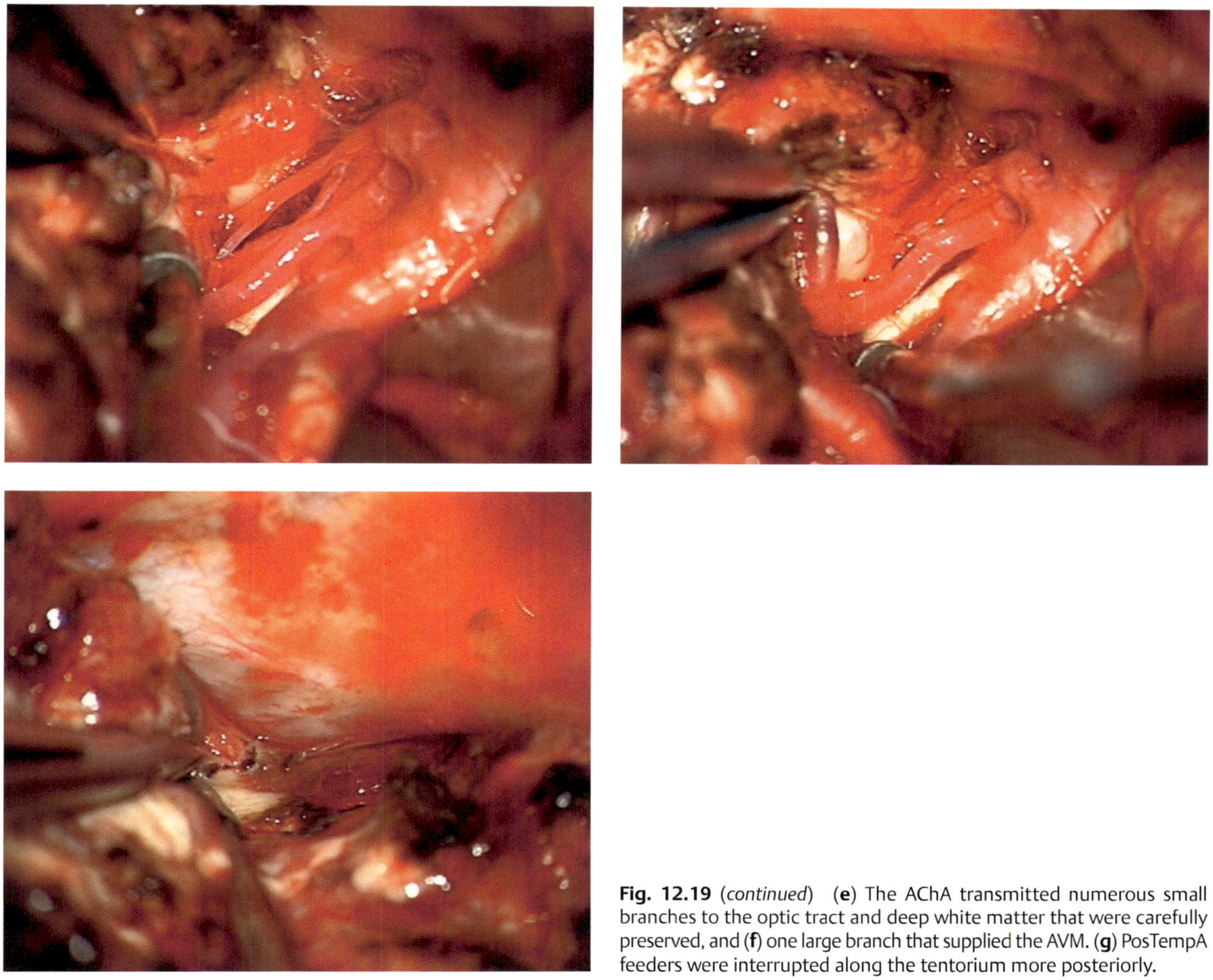

e f g

Fig. 12.19 (*continued*) (**e**) The AChA transmitted numerous small branches to the optic tract and deep white matter that were carefully preserved, and (**f**) one large branch that supplied the AVM. (**g**) PosTempA feeders were interrupted along the tentorium more posteriorly.

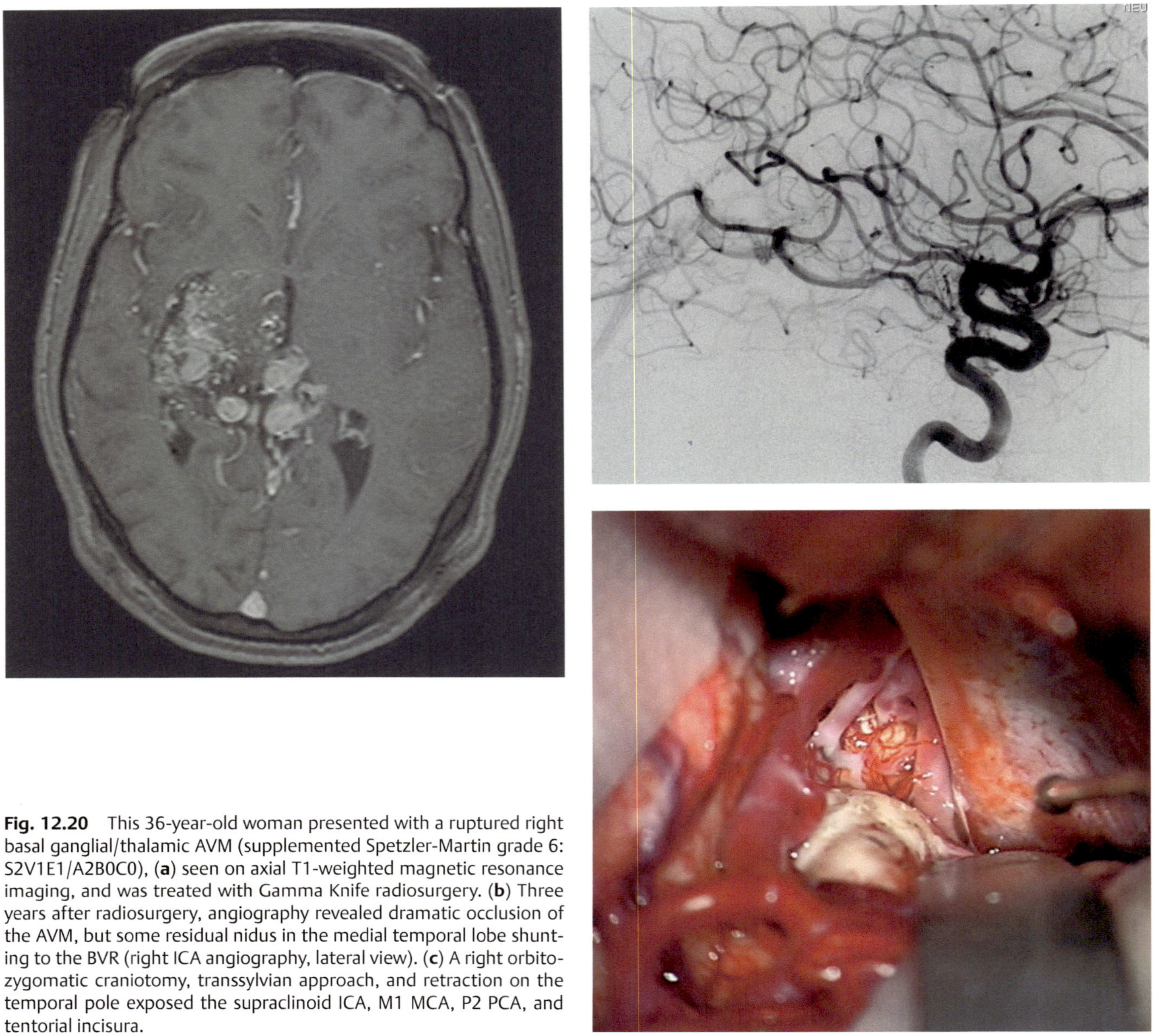

Fig. 12.20 This 36-year-old woman presented with a ruptured right basal ganglial/thalamic AVM (supplemented Spetzler-Martin grade 6: S2V1E1/A2B0C0), (**a**) seen on axial T1-weighted magnetic resonance imaging, and was treated with Gamma Knife radiosurgery. (**b**) Three years after radiosurgery, angiography revealed dramatic occlusion of the AVM, but some residual nidus in the medial temporal lobe shunting to the BVR (right ICA angiography, lateral view). (**c**) A right orbitozygomatic craniotomy, transsylvian approach, and retraction on the temporal pole exposed the supraclinoid ICA, M1 MCA, P2 PCA, and tentorial incisura.

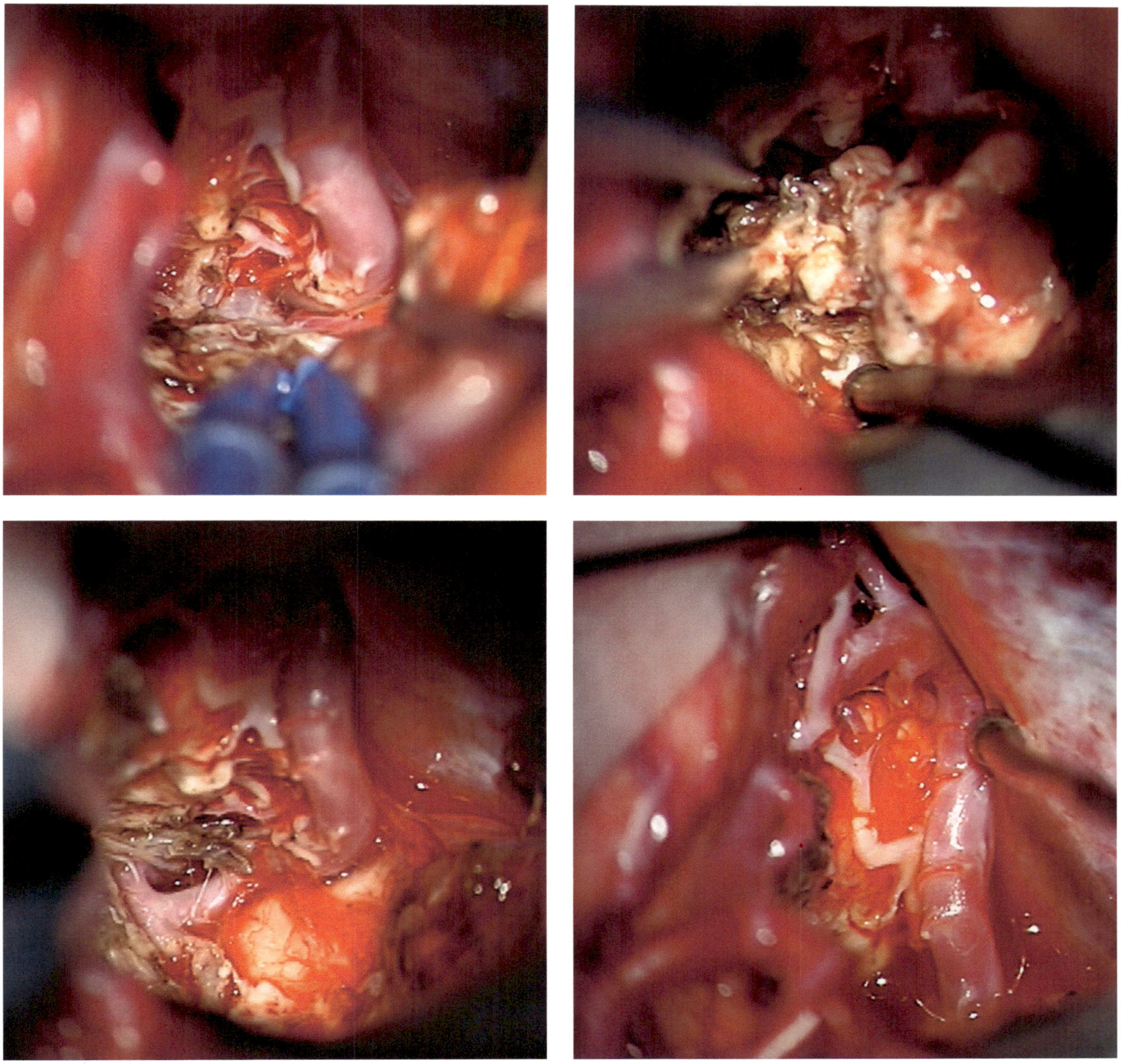

d e f g

Fig. 12.20 (*continued*) (**d**) Branches from the P2 PCA supplying this medial temporal lobe AVM were coagulated to de-arterialize the nidus. (**e**) The AVM was removed, (**f**) exposing the ambient segment of the PCA to its bifurcation into ParOccA and CalcA (P2P). (**g**) The crural segment of the PCA (P2A) and its sclerosed feeders were seen along the tentorial incisura.

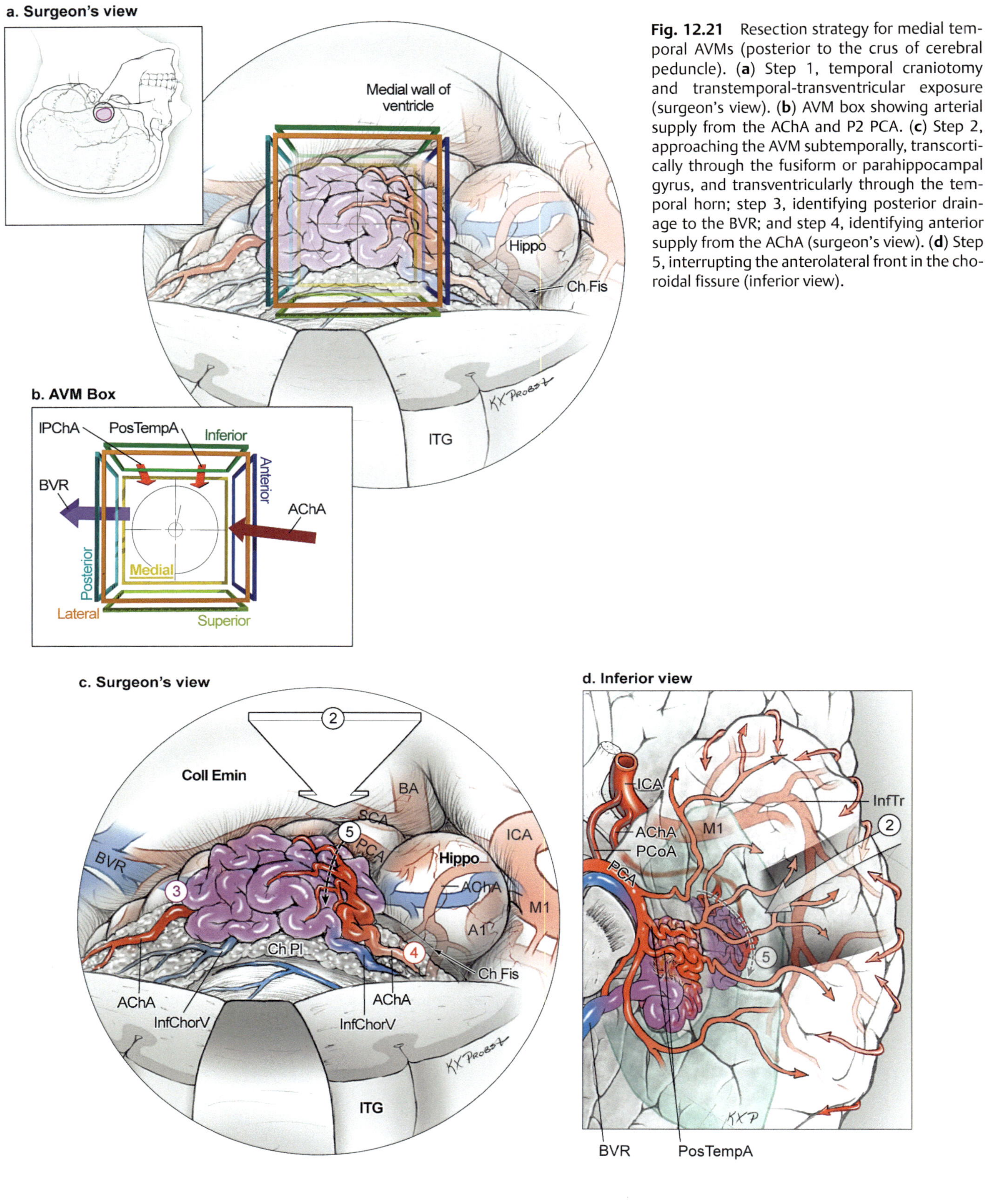

Fig. 12.21 Resection strategy for medial temporal AVMs (posterior to the crus of cerebral peduncle). (**a**) Step 1, temporal craniotomy and transtemporal-transventricular exposure (surgeon's view). (**b**) AVM box showing arterial supply from the AChA and P2 PCA. (**c**) Step 2, approaching the AVM subtemporally, transcortically through the fusiform or parahippocampal gyrus, and transventricularly through the temporal horn; step 3, identifying posterior drainage to the BVR; and step 4, identifying anterior supply from the AChA (surgeon's view). (**d**) Step 5, interrupting the anterolateral front in the choroidal fissure (inferior view).

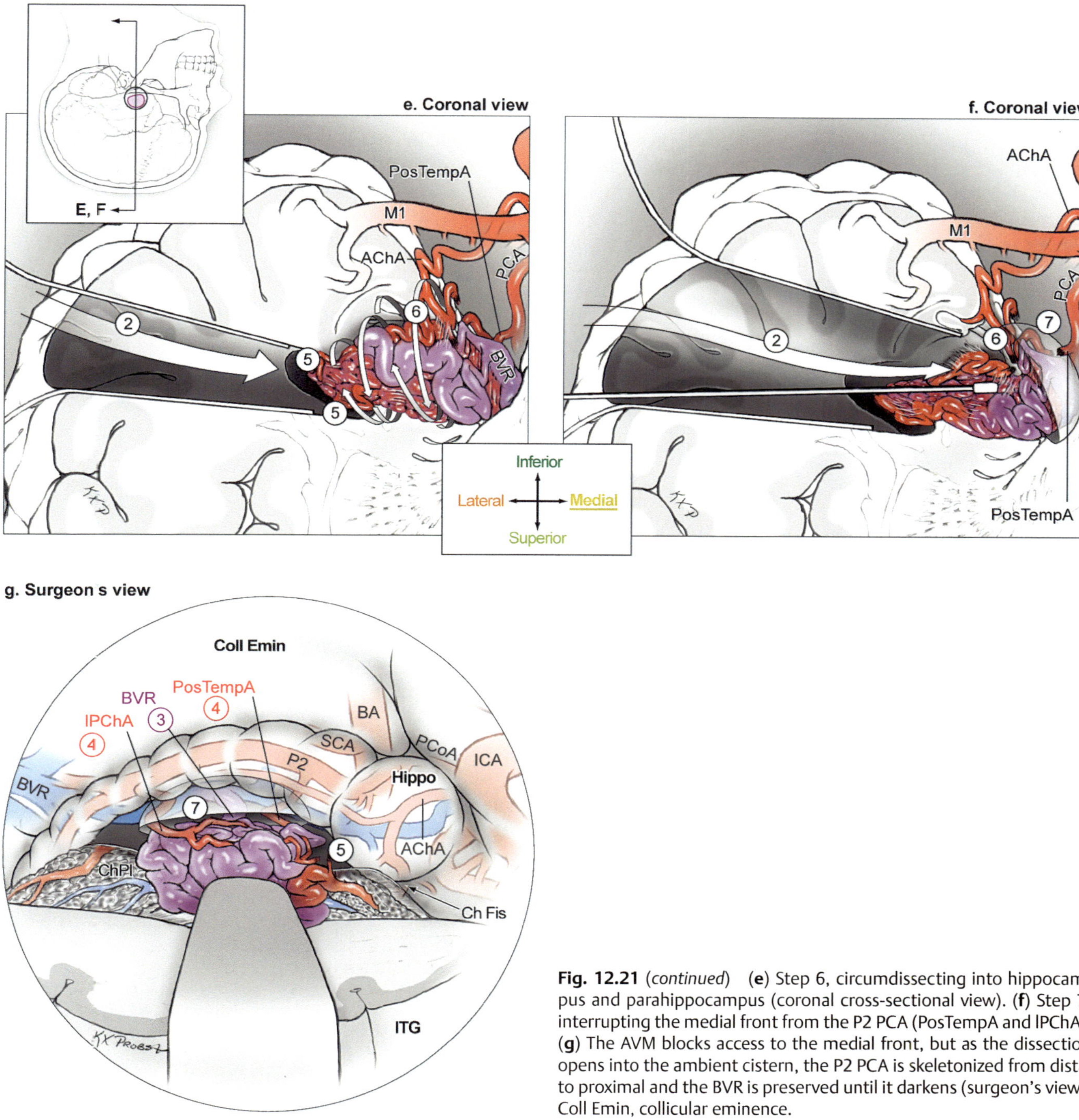

Fig. 12.21 (*continued*) (**e**) Step 6, circumdissecting into hippocampus and parahippocampus (coronal cross-sectional view). (**f**) Step 7, interrupting the medial front from the P2 PCA (PosTempA and lPChA). (**g**) The AVM blocks access to the medial front, but as the dissection opens into the ambient cistern, the P2 PCA is skeletonized from distal to proximal and the BVR is preserved until it darkens (surgeon's view). Coll Emin, collicular eminence.

Medial temporal AVMs that are posterior to the crus of the cerebral peduncle and wrap around the posterolateral midbrain require a transtemporal-transventricular approach rather than an orbitozygomatic-transsylvian approach (**Fig. 12.21**). The transsylvian view becomes inadequate, whereas the transcortical approach offers wider views and a parallel attack angle. The approach is like that described for basal temporal AVMs, with a temporal craniotomy (step 1) and a subtemporal approach (step 2), but the transcortical dissection is more medial, working through fusiform or parahippocampal gyrus rather than the ITG. Transcortical corridors are limiting and should be widened to encompass the entire nidus. Opening the ventricle accesses the lateral border of medial temporal AVMs. Unlike with the transsylvian exposure of these AVMs, drainage to the BVR is identified posteriorly early in the dissection (step 3). However, arterial supply from the AChA and PCA is on the deep plane and not well visualized until late in the dissection (step 4). Anterior supply from the AChA can be occluded anteriorly in the choroidal fissure of the temporal horn and PCA feeders are occluded in the ambient cistern (step 5). Transcortical dissection through the posterior hippocampus and parahippocampus is associated with increased risk to memory (step 6). When present, hematomas open these corridors of exposure without additional morbidity. This transbasal approach avoids SupSyV and DeepSylV that might be compromised with a transsylvian approach. However, this transbasal approach requires some superior retraction on the temporal lobe, which can injure or avulse the vein of Labbé. Tributaries to the vein of Labbé that cross the path of the cortical incision can be spared with separate incisions that straddle the veins. The BVR is followed into the ambient cistern to ensure that the entire nidus has been circumscribed and that the feeding arteries (PosTempA and lPChA) on the posterior margin have been interrupted (step 7). The distal PCA is protected to continue its posterior course (**Fig. 12.22**).

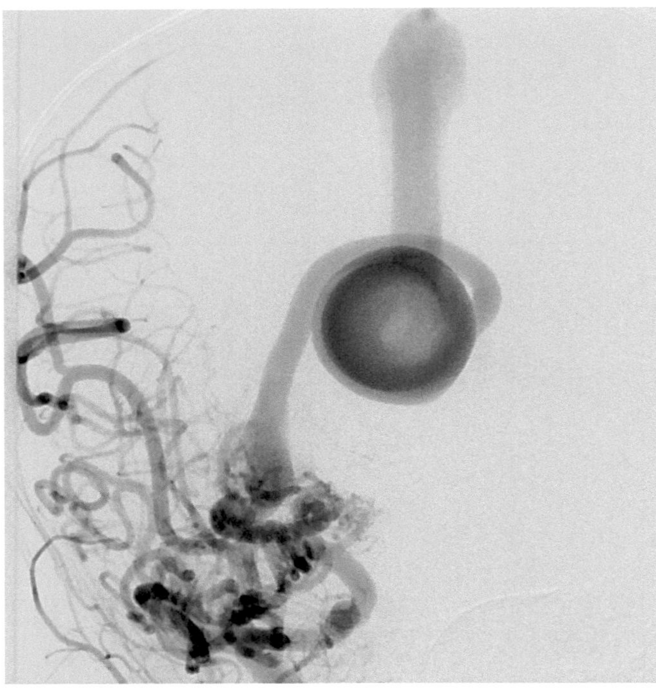

a

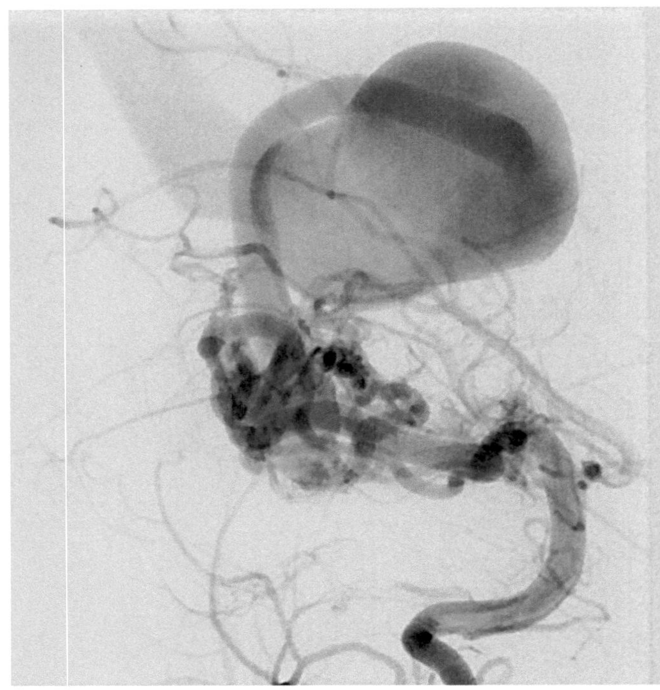

b

Fig. 12.22 This 3-year-old girl presented with a right medial temporal AVM (supplemented Spetzler-Martin grade 4: S2V1E0/A1B0C0), fed by the PCoA, AChA, TempPolA, and ATA [(**a**) right ICA angiogram, anteroposterior view] and by PosTempA, HippoA, and PChA [(**b**) right vertebral artery angiogram, anterior oblique view]. The AVM drained to the BVR, a variceal VoG, and a falcine sinus (prosencephalic vein of Markowski). She was incompletely treated with coil embolization of PosTempA feeding arteries, and later thrombosed her distal SSS and torcula, leading to venous hypertension, neurologic deterioration, and retrograde drainage in the SSS to convexity veins and cavernous sinus.

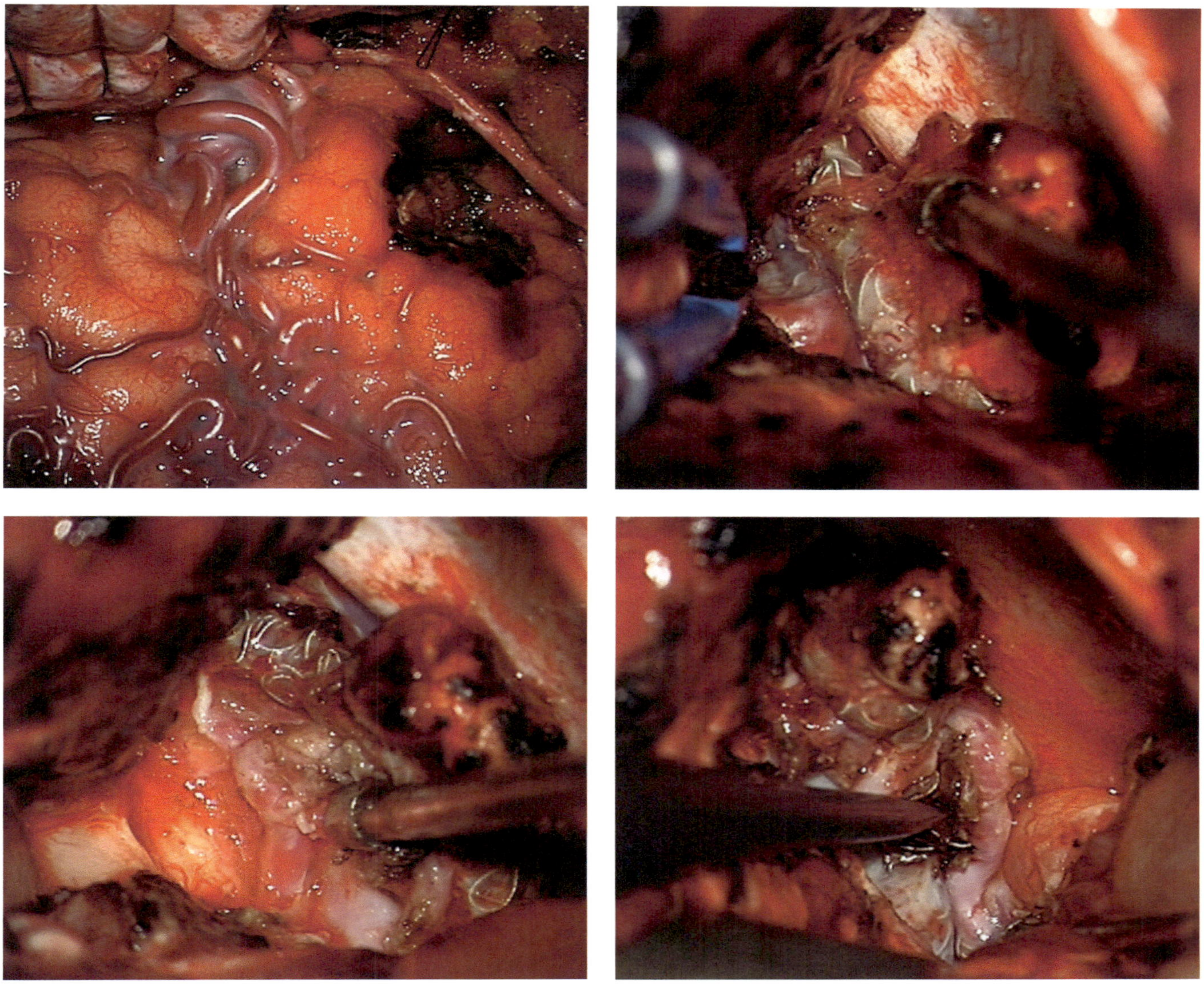

Fig. 12.22 (*continued*) (**c**) Pterional-temporal craniotomy exposed the lateral temporal lobe and engorged sylvian veins. (**d**) The AVM was approached transcortically through the OTG, transventricularly through the temporal horn, and finally through the choroidal fissure, arriving medially to the PosTempA that had been packed with coils. (**e**) Feeders from the AChA and PChA were occluded in the choroidal fissure superiorly, and (**f**) feeders from the PCA were occluded in the ambient cistern inferiorly, darkening the BVR (medial to microscissors). (*continued on next page*)

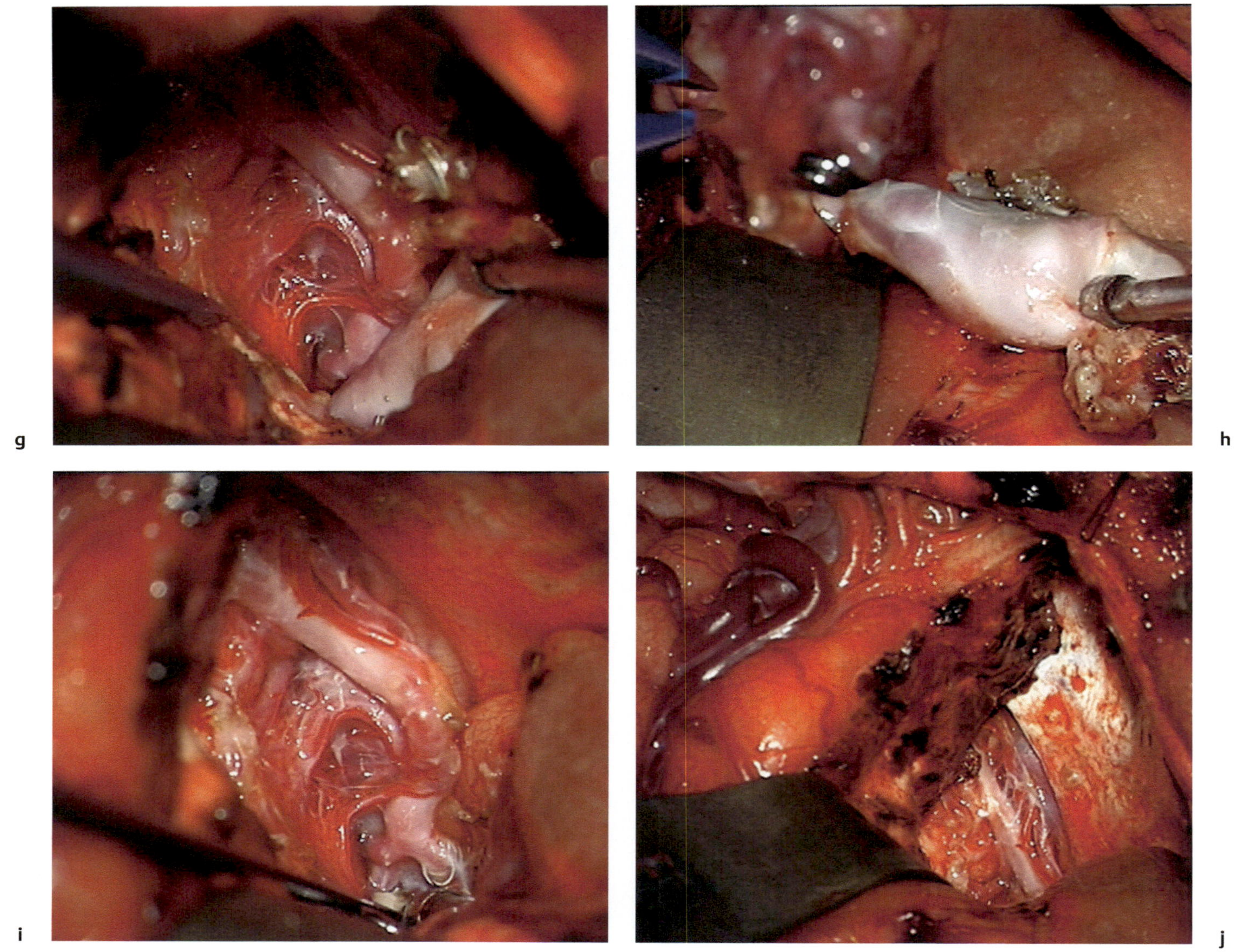

Fig. 12.22 *(continued)* (**g**) Normal perforators from the PCA, visualized after pulling the BVR laterally with the sucker, coursed medially and were protected. (**h**) The BVR was clip occluded distally after it had darkened completely, and the AVM was resected. (**i**) The skeletonized P2 PCA segment and its thalamic and midbrain perforators were preserved throughout its crural and ambient course. (**j**) This transcortical-transventricular approach through the OTG and temporal horn exposed the tentorial ring and preserved the sylvian veins, which darkened after AVM resection.

Conclusion

The temporal lobe is hospitable territory for AVM surgery. Craniotomies provide good exposures; approaches are familiar because of their similarity to aneurysm approaches; microsurgical techniques for opening subarachnoid planes and fissures are well practiced; the vasculature is accessible; and much of the lobe is non-eloquent. Surgical results with temporal AVMs are generally excellent in terms of curative resection and seizure control. Therefore, as a group, temporal lobe AVMs are gratifying to treat and treated often, second only to frontal AVMs in their frequency and having the most common subtype (the lateral temporal AVM).

13 Parieto-Occipital Arteriovenous Malformations

■ Microsurgical Anatomy

Brain

Divisions between the parietal and occipital lobes are somewhat arbitrary. Although they are divided by the parieto-occipital sulcus on the medial hemisphere, there is no such separating sulcus on the lateral hemisphere. Instead, the extended sylvian line drawn along the long axis of the sylvian fissure divides these two lobes arbitrarily. The parietal and occipital lobes have defined boundaries, but they are anatomically contiguous and continuous. They are considered as a unit in this book because their vascular anatomy is interrelated and arteriovenous malformations (AVMs) in parietal and occipital lobes are managed so similarly. Even combining two lobes, the parieto-occipital unit still has only three anatomic surfaces (lateral, medial, and basal) and lacks the anatomic complexity of a major fissure or convolution (**Fig. 13.1**). Technically, the parietal lobe has a sylvian surface between the central sulcus and supramarginal gyrus, but it is short and an AVM here would be handled just like a sylvian frontal AVM.

The lateral parietal surface is made up of three parts: the postcentral gyrus, which is vertically oriented and parallels the central and postcentral sulci; the superior parietal lobule (SPL), which extends from the superior border of the hemisphere to the horizontally oriented intraparietal sulcus; and the inferior parietal lobule (IPL), the larger of the two lobules that contains the supramarginal and angular gyri. The lateral occipital surface is composed of the superior occipital (SOG) and inferior occipital gyri (IOG), which are divided by the lateral occipital sulcus. The medial parietal surface is made up of the posterior paracentral lobule (medial extension of postcentral gyrus), the posterior cingulate gyrus, and the precuneus (medial extension of SPL). The parieto-occipital sulcus defines the medial boundary between the parietal and occipital lobes. The calcarine fissure extends forward from the occipital pole and joins the parieto-occipital sulcus behind the isthmus of the cingulate gyrus, dividing the medial occipital surface into the cuneus (above) and lingula (below). The basal occipital surface is composed of the lower part of the lingula, the posterior continuation of occipitotemporal gyrus (OTG, or fusiform gyrus), and the medial continuation of the IOG, divided by posterior extensions of the collateral and occipitotemporal sulci.

Arteries

The parieto-occipital lobe is supplied by all three of the major cerebral arteries, unlike the other cerebral lobes that

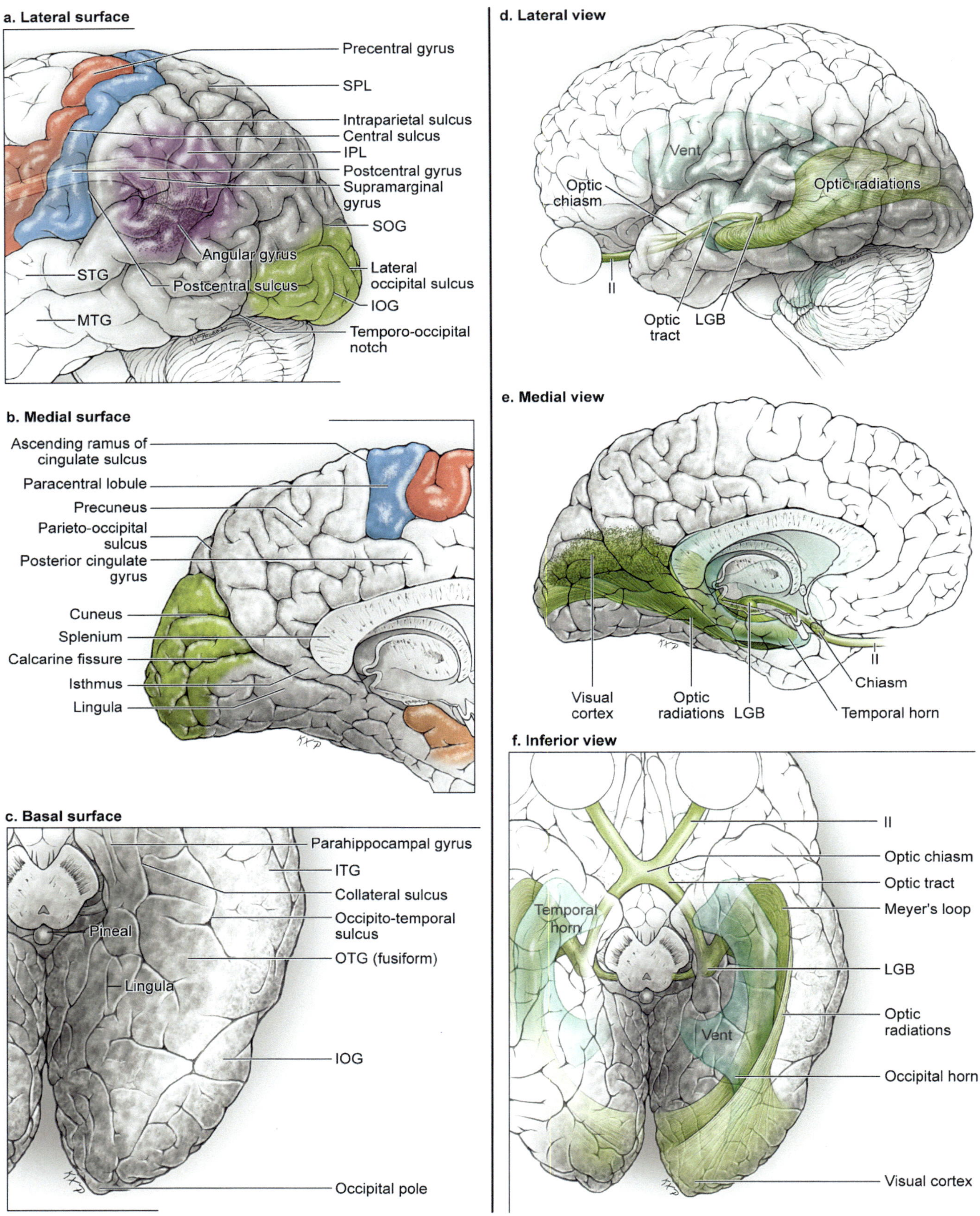
a. Lateral surface
Precentral gyrus
SPL
Intraparietal sulcus
Central sulcus
IPL
Postcentral gyrus
Supramarginal gyrus
SOG
Angular gyrus
Lateral occipital sulcus
STG
Postcentral sulcus
IOG
MTG
Temporo-occipital notch
b. Medial surface
Ascending ramus of cingulate sulcus
Paracentral lobule
Precuneus
Parieto-occipital sulcus
Posterior cingulate gyrus
Cuneus
Splenium
Calcarine fissure
Isthmus
Lingula
c. Basal surface
Parahippocampal gyrus
ITG
Collateral sulcus
Occipito-temporal sulcus
Pineal
OTG (fusiform)
Lingula
IOG
Occipital pole
d. Lateral view
Vent
Optic chiasm
Optic radiations
II
Optic tract
LGB
e. Medial view
II
Chiasm
Visual cortex
Optic radiations
LGB
Temporal horn
f. Inferior view
II
Optic chiasm
Optic tract
Temporal horn
Meyer's loop
LGB
Optic radiations
Vent
Occipital horn
Visual cortex

Fig. 13.1 (*opposite*) Microsurgical anatomy of the parietal and occipital lobes. (**a**) Lateral parieto-occipital surface (lateral view), with eloquent areas shown in color: motor strip (red), somatosensory strip (blue), visual cortex (green), and language conduction area (angular gyrus, supramarginal gyrus, and underlying arcuate fasciculus, purple). (**b**) Medial parieto-occipital surface (medial view). (**c**) Basal parieto-occipital surface (inferior view). (**d**) Visual system consists of the eyes and retina, optic nerves, optic chiasm, optic tracts, lateral geniculate body or nucleus, optic radiations, and visual cortex, shown in lateral, (**e**) medial, and (**f**) inferior views. Note that the optic radiations pass laterally around the temporal horn of lateral ventricle, including Meyer's loop anteriorly in the temporal lobe, and traverse occipital white matter lateral to the occipital horn.

are supplied by only two (**Fig. 13.2**). Distal middle cerebral artery (MCA) cortical arteries supply the lateral parieto-occipital surfaces and originate from both the superior and inferior MCA trunks of bifurcations, from the middle trunk of MCA trifurcations, or from the dominant trunk in unequal bifurcations. These cortical M4 arteries emerge from the distal sylvian fissure and fan out as central (CenA), anterior parietal (AntParA), posterior parietal (PosParA), angular (AngA), and temporo-occipital arteries (TempOccA). Terminal A5 anterior cerebral artery (ACA) cortical arteries supply the medial parietal lobe as the superior (SupParA) and inferior parietal arteries (InfParA). The lateral parietal arteries from the MCA are named "anterior" and "posterior," whereas the medial parietal arteries from the ACA are named "superior" and "inferior." SupParA supplies the precuneus and InfParA supplies the cuneus and precuneus (inferior part).

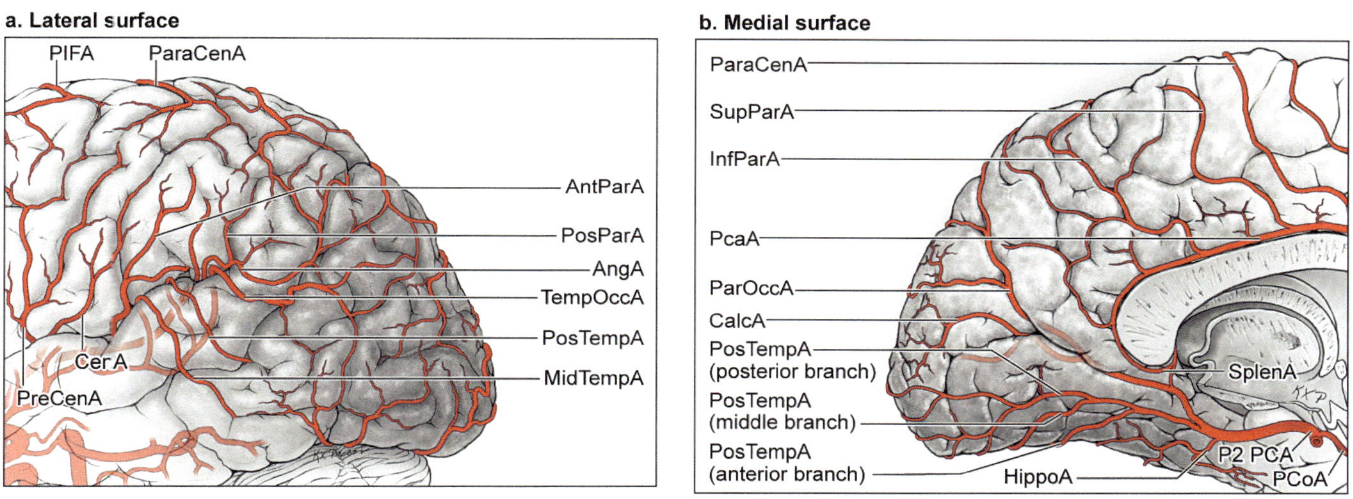

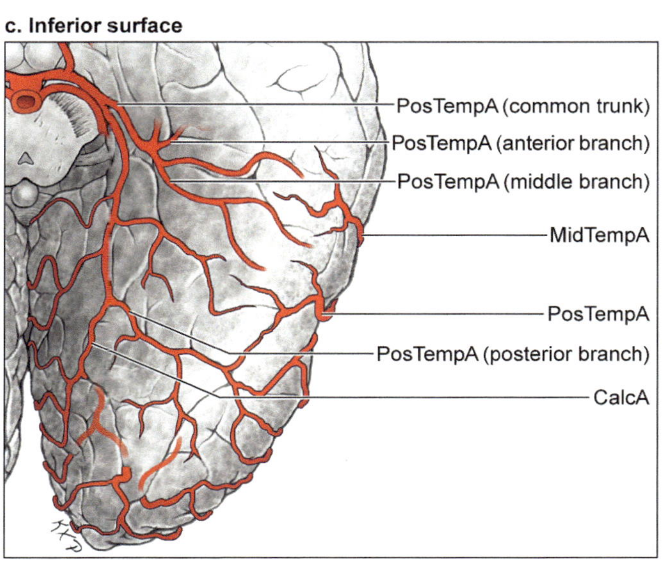

Fig. 13.2 Microsurgical anatomy of parieto-occipital arteries. (**a**) The lateral parieto-occipital surface is supplied by distal MCA cortical branches from both the superior and inferior trunks of an MCA bifurcation, or the middle trunk of an MCA trifurcation (CenA, AntParA, PosParA, AngA, and TempOccA). Branches from the ACA also extend to the medial part of the lateral parieto-occipital surface, and branches from the PCA extend to the inferior part of the lateral surface. (**b**) The medial parieto-occipital surface is supplied by terminal ACA branches (ParaCenA, SupParA, and InfParA) and PCA branches (CalcA and ParOccA). (**c**) The basal occipital surface is supplied by PosTempA, which originates from the P2 PCA as multiple branches (anterior, middle, and posterior) or as a common trunk shown here.

The posterior cerebral artery (PCA) is the major source of blood flow to the parieto-occipital lobe, and it supplies the remaining territories on the medial and basal surfaces. PosTempA, already discussed with temporal AVMs, originates from the P2 PCA in the ambient or sometimes quadrigeminal cistern, runs obliquely in a posterolateral direction to the occipital pole, and supplies the basal temporal and occipital surfaces. PosTempA arises as a common trunk (common temporal artery), as four separate arteries (hippocampal artery, anterior, middle, and posterior temporal arteries), or in various combinations. The PCA divides into the calcarine (CalcA) and parieto-occipital arteries (ParOccA) along its P3 or quadrigeminal segment, which begins lateral to the posterior margin of the midbrain, climbs over the free edge of the tentorium, courses through quadrigeminal cistern, and ends at the anterior limit of the calcarine fissure. CalcA becomes the P4 segment after it enters the calcarine fissure and courses to the cortical surface of occipital lobe. Its branches fan out over the lingula and inferior cuneus, supply the visual cortex in the banks and depths of the calcarine fissure, and continue to the occipital pole. ParOccA runs in the parieto-occipital fissure and supplies the cuneus and precuneus. This artery travels beyond the medial surface to the convexity to supply the SPL and SOG. The splenial artery (SplenA) arises proximally from ParOccA and can anastomose with the pericallosal artery as part of a "limbic loop" that supplies corpus callosum AVMs from a posterior-to-anterior direction.

Veins

The parieto-occipital lobe is drained by cortical veins on the lateral, medial, and basal surfaces (**Fig. 13.3**). Ascending veins to the superior sagittal sinus (SSS) predominate and include the postcentral (PostCenV), anterior (AntParV) and posterior parietal (PostParV), and occipital veins (OccV), with the largest vein designated as the vein of Trolard. Lateral occipital veins course forward to reach the medial parietal lobe and clear an area of 4 to 5 cm along the distal SSS where no large veins bridge to the sinus; this anatomy is exploited for the posterior interhemispheric approaches. Inferolaterally, there are parietosylvian veins that descend to the sylvian fissure. Occipital veins descend laterally to the transverse sinus (TrvS) and vein of Labbé. The medial parieto-occipital veins drain superficially and deep. Ascending veins to the SSS include the paracentral (ParaCenV), medial parietal (MedParV; anterior and posterior), and posterior calcarine veins (PosCalcV); and descending veins to the vein of Galen (VoG) include the posterior pericallosal vein (PcaV) and anterior CalcV (AntCalcV, a.k.a., internal occipital vein). Occipitobasal veins (OccBasV) drain the basal surface under the occipital pole and course to the tentorial sinus (TentS), posterior TempBasV, or anterolaterally to the TrvS.

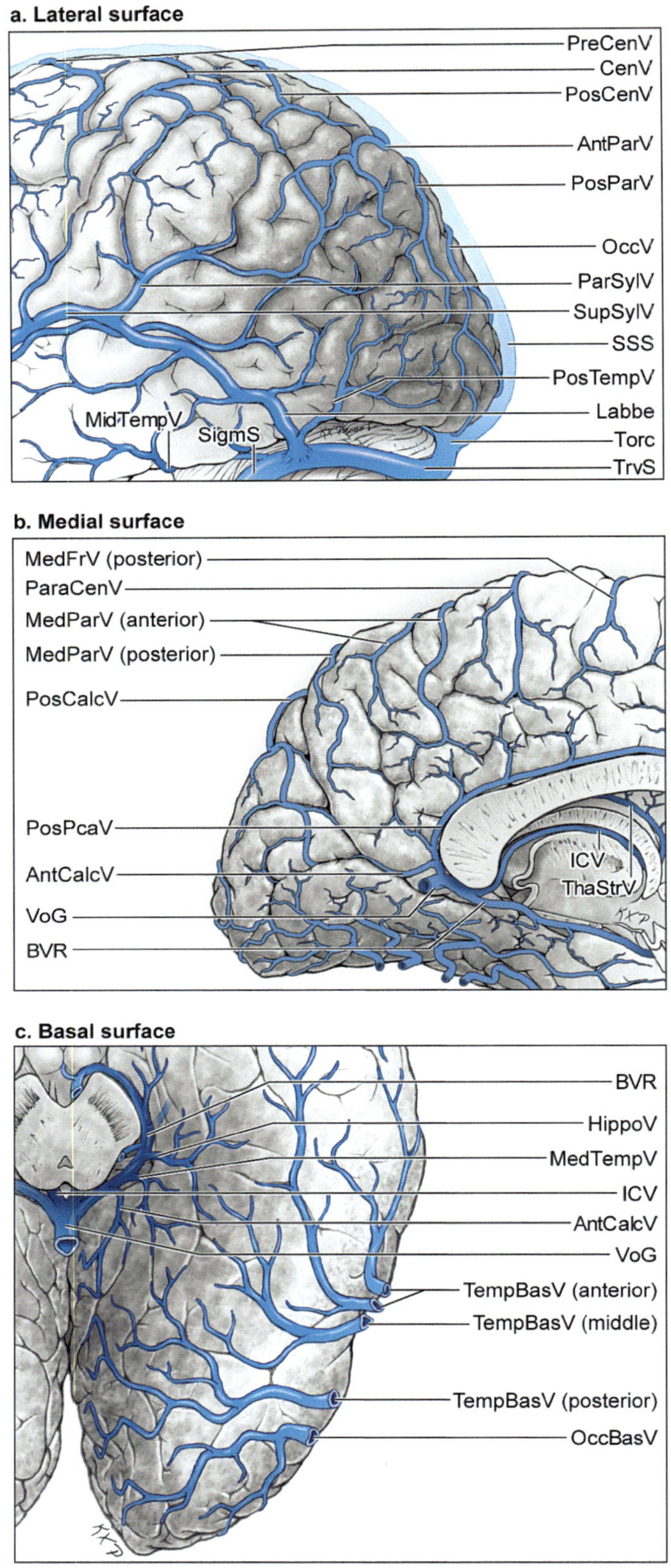

Fig. 13.3 Microsurgical anatomy of parieto-occipital lobe veins. (**a**) Veins of the lateral parieto-occipital surface (lateral view). (**b**) Veins of the medial parieto-occipital surface (medial view). (**c**) Veins of the basal occipital surface (inferior view).

Four Parieto-Occipital AVM Subtypes

Parieto-occipital AVM subtypes include the lateral parieto-occipital, medial parieto-occipital, paramedian parieto-occipital, and basal occipital. As with frontal AVMs, there is a subtype for each surface and an extra one for paramedian AVMs with sides on both the medial and lateral surfaces that require additional access to two surfaces and three arterial territories.

The Lateral Parieto-Occipital AVM

The lateral parieto-occipital AVM is the stereotypical convexity AVM with a cortical base and tapered extension toward the ventricle (**Fig. 13.4**). It is the second most common subtype overall and accounts for half of all parieto-occipital AVMs and more than twice as many as most other parieto-occipital subtypes. It involves only the lateral surface (involvement of the medial surface would make it a paramedian AVM). Most lateral parieto-occipital AVMs have a free side, although some are deep to the cortical surface without a free side. These AVMs are supplied mainly by MCA cortical arteries: CenA, AntParA, PosParA, AngA, and TempOccA. Input depends on the convexity location, with superior AVMs supplied by AntParA and PosParA and inferior AVMs supplied by AngA and TempOccA. Contributions from ACA and PCA are minimal except with AVMs near the MCA–PCA watershed. Lateral parieto-occipital AVMs drain superficially, ascending to the SSS (PosCenV, AntParV, PostParV, and/or OccV) or descending to the sylvian veins (ParSylV and SupSylV). Parietal AVMs are eloquent when located in the postcentral gyrus, and occipital AVMs are eloquent when located near the pole in the visual cortex. A perisylvian AVM in the angular and supramarginal gyrus can involve speech conduction tracts in the arcuate fasciculus connecting Wernicke's and Broca's areas.

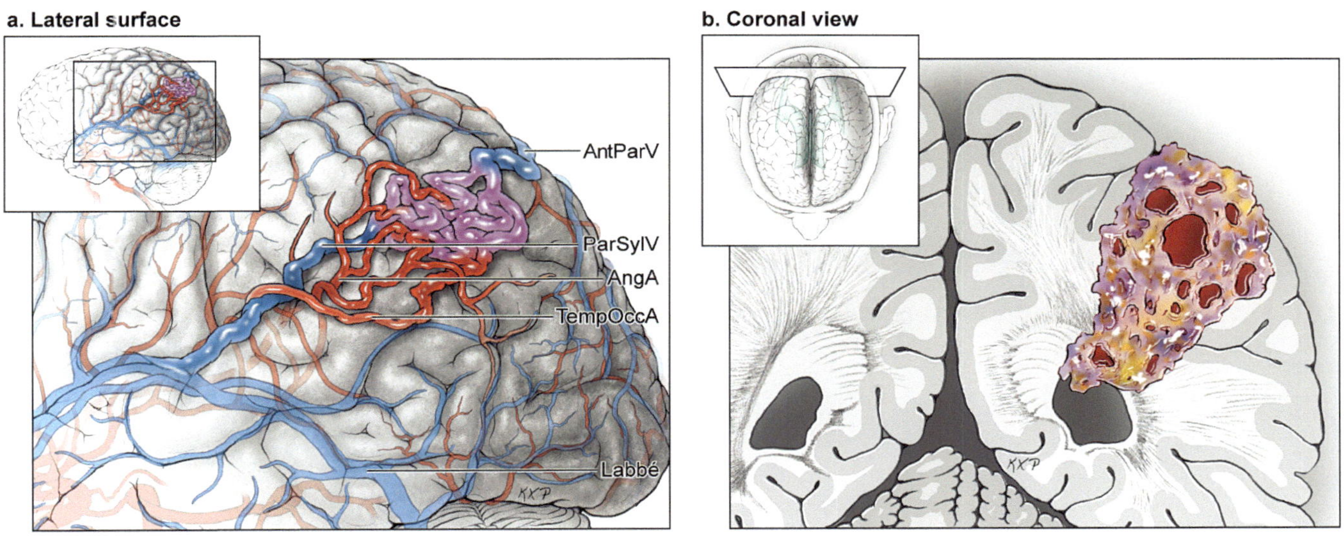

Fig. 13.4 The lateral parieto-occipital AVM: (**a**) lateral and (**b**) coronal cross-sectional views. This AVM is located on the lateral parieto-occipital surface, supplied by branches from the superior and inferior MCA trunks, and drained by ascending veins to the SSS and/or descending veins to SupSylV.

The Medial Parieto-Occipital AVM

The medial parieto-occipital AVM is based on the medial hemisphere with its base in the posterior interhemispheric fissure without extension to the lateral convexity (**Fig. 13.5**). It resides anywhere beyond the central sulcus, and may be superficial below the medial corner of the hemisphere or deep near, but not in, the splenium. These AVMs are fed by cortical PCA branches and, to a lesser degree, the ACA, but not the MCA. Parietal AVMs receive contributions from ParaCenA, SupParA, InfParA, and ParOccA (ACA and PCA), whereas occipital AVMs receive contributions from ParOccA and CalcA (just the PCA). Medial parieto-occipital AVMs drain superficially or deep, ascending to the SSS via ParaCenV, MedParV, and posterior CalcV, or descending to the VoG via the posterior pericallosal vein (PcaV) and anterior CalcV. Medial parietal AVMs in the paracentral lobule are eloquent (somatosensory cortex for leg sensation), as are medial occipital AVMs in the cuneus and lingula around the calcarine fissure (visual cortex). A swath of non-eloquent territory lies between these two eloquent areas.

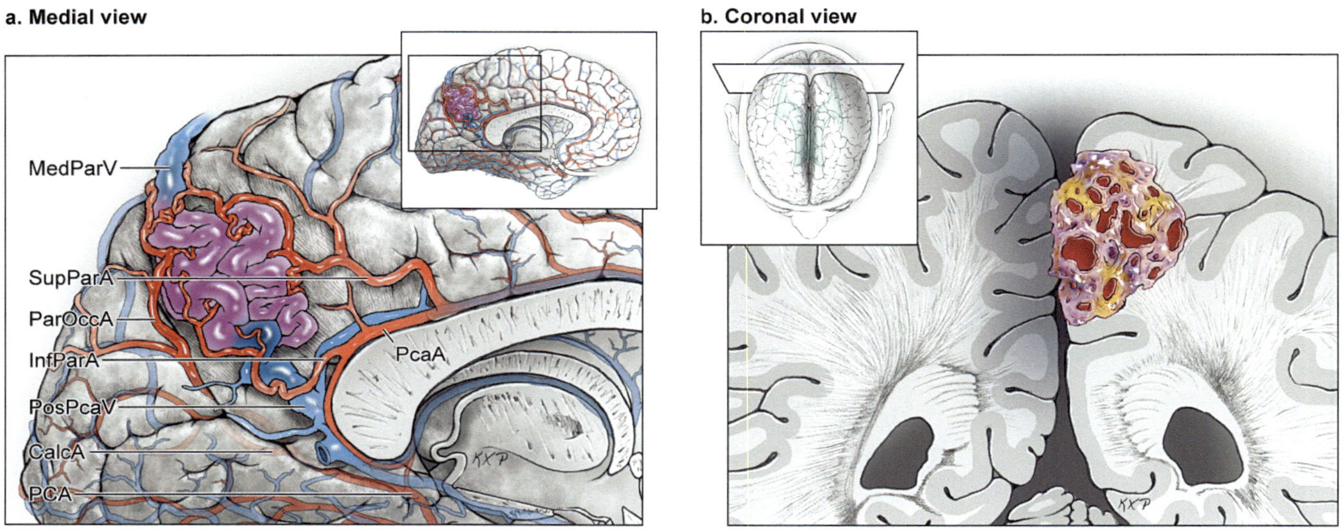

Fig. 13.5 The medial parieto-occipital AVM: (**a**) medial and (**b**) coronal cross-sectional views. This AVM is located on the medial parieto-occipital surface, supplied by cortical PCA branches (ParOccA and CalcA) and ACA branches (ParaCenA, SupParA, and InfParA), and is drained by superficial veins to the SSS (ParaCenV, MedParV, and PosCalcV) and deep veins to the VoG (PosPcaV and AntCalcV).

The Paramedian Parieto-Occipital AVM

The paramedian parieto-occipital AVM is a combination of the medial and lateral subtypes residing on both medial and lateral surfaces and centered at their orthogonal intersection at the medial corner of the hemisphere (**Fig. 13.6**). This AVM has two free surfaces that can expedite resection when exposed properly. Paramedian parieto-occipital AVMs lie at the watershed between the MCA, PCA, and ACA territories, making them the only parieto-occipital subtype and the only cerebral subtype to be fed by all three cerebral arteries. Arterial supply varies with size and location in the parieto-occipital range, with paramedian parietal AVMs having a mix of ACA and PCA supply, and occipital AVMs having mostly PCA supply. Similarly, the more a paramedian AVM extends laterally, the more it will be supplied by the MCA. Venous drainage is predominantly superficial to the SSS. Paramedian AVMs have eloquence when based on the postcentral gyrus/paracentral lobule or the IOG/cuneus. Small AVMs can be resected with good somatosensory and visual outcomes, as can those based in the area between the somatosensory strip and the visual cortex.

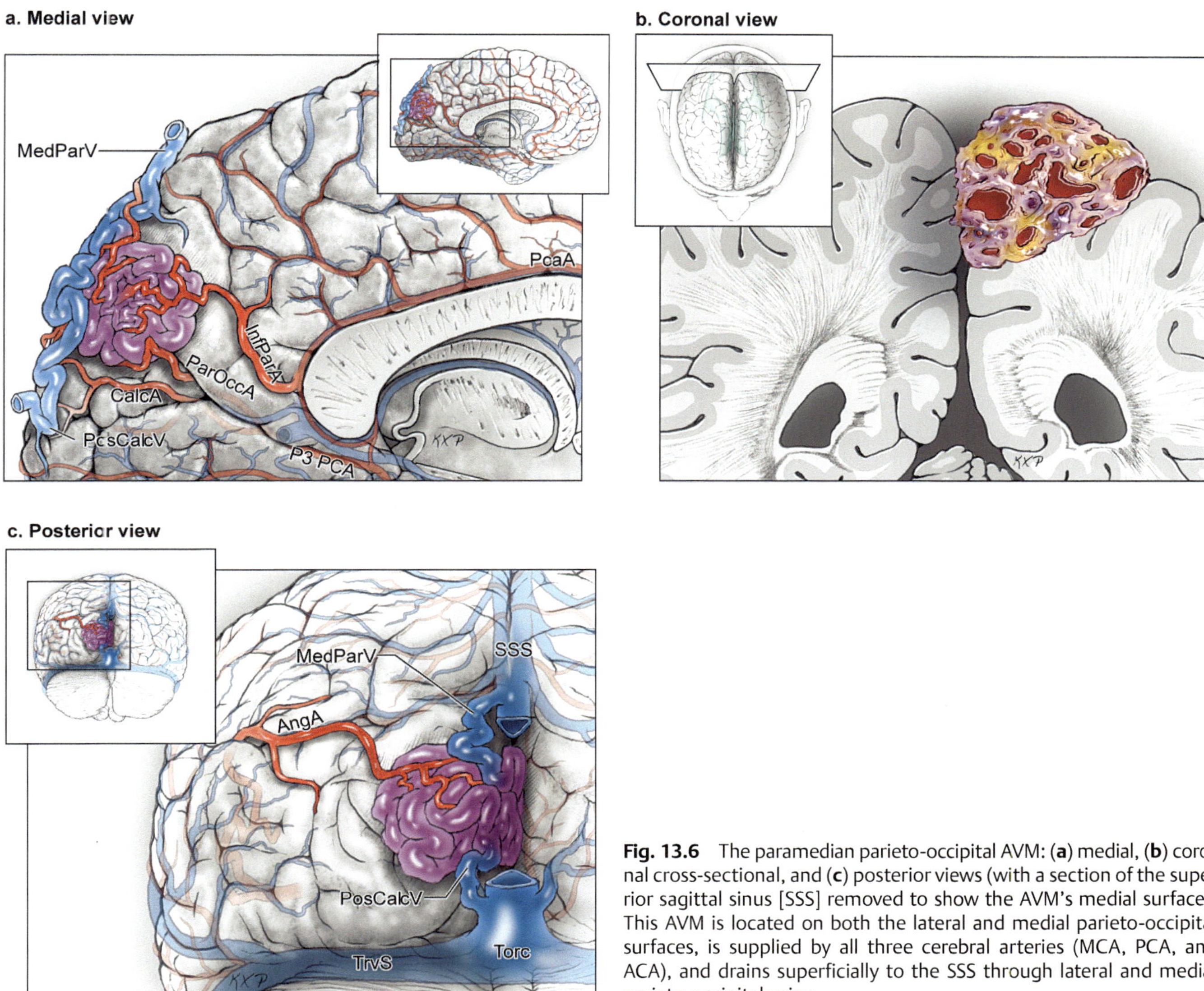

Fig. 13.6 The paramedian parieto-occipital AVM: (**a**) medial, (**b**) coronal cross-sectional, and (**c**) posterior views (with a section of the superior sagittal sinus [SSS] removed to show the AVM's medial surface). This AVM is located on both the lateral and medial parieto-occipital surfaces, is supplied by all three cerebral arteries (MCA, PCA, and ACA), and drains superficially to the SSS through lateral and medial parieto-occipital veins.

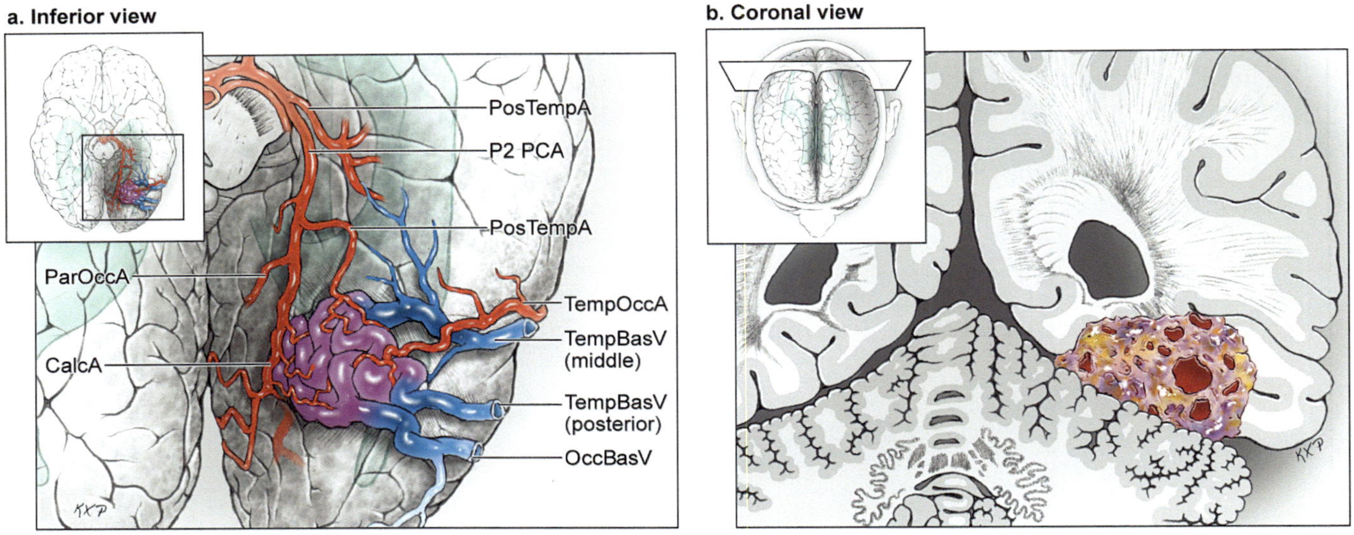

Fig. 13.7 The basal occipital AVM: (**a**) inferior and (**b**) coronal cross-sectional views. This AVM is located on the basal occipital surface and is supplied by PosTempA branches from the PCA, with minor contributions from calcarine artery medially (PCA) and temporo-occipital artery laterally (MCA). This AVM drains to basal veins (TempBasV and OccBasV) that collect in the tentorial or transverse sinuses.

The Basal Occipital AVM

The basal occipital AVMs are the least common of the parieto-occipital AVMs (around 10%). They are located on the basal undersurface of the occipital lobe along the tentorium anywhere from the falcotentorial junction medially to TrvS laterally (**Fig. 13.7**). They also vary in their depth from the occipital pole posteriorly to the tentorial incisura anteriorly. The PCA supplies basal AVMs almost exclusively with PosTempA and inferior branches from CalcA. The ACA is uninvolved, but TempOccA from the MCA may supply basal AVMs adjacent to the TrvS. Venous drainage is typically superficial to the posterior TempBasV and OccBasV, which then collect in the TrvS or TentS. The visual pathways, including optic radiations en route to the occipital pole as well as visual cortex, are intimately associated with basal AVMs, and tight dissection planes are needed to spare the visual fields.

Parieto-Occipital AVM Resection Strategies

Lateral Parieto-Occipital AVM Resection

The lateral parieto-occipital AVM is exposed with a simple convexity craniotomy that does not expose the interhemispheric or infraoccipital planes and therefore does not cross venous sinuses (**Fig. 13.8,** step 1). The patient is positioned laterally with the degree of head rotation depending on the AVM location: neutral (midline horizontal) for parietal lesions and "nose down" for occipital lesions. A horseshoe skin incision is used. These AVMs are based on the lateral surface, and subarachnoid dissection is limited to opening the overlying arachnoid and surrounding sulci (step 2). This base offers a free side, although some lateral parieto-occipital AVMs

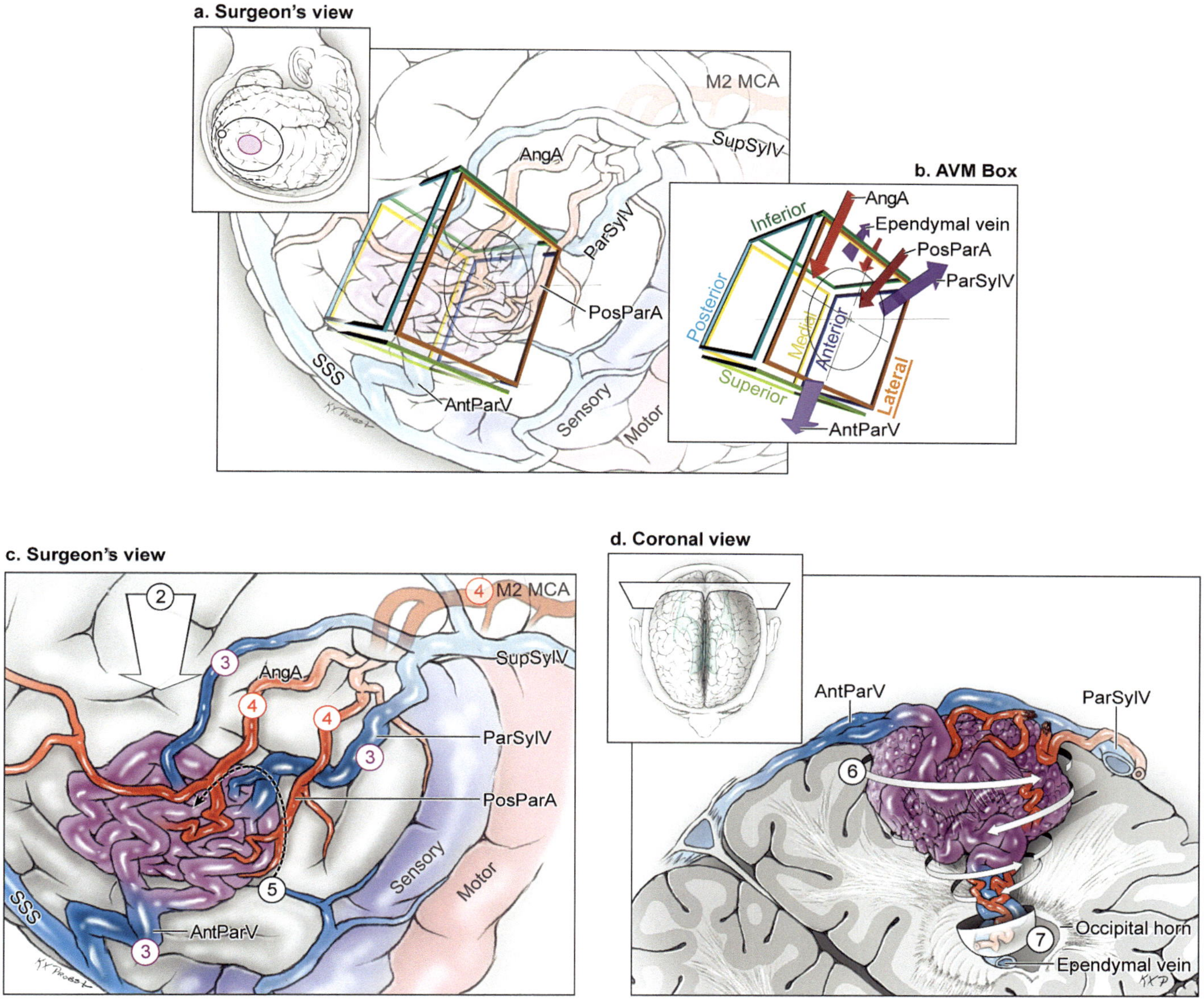

Fig. 13.8 Resection strategy for lateral parieto-occipital AVMs. (**a**) Step 1, exposing the AVM with a unilateral parieto-occipital craniotomy (surgeon's view, with the patient in the lateral position and the head rotated "nose down"; scalp incision (*dashed line*), craniotomy (*solid line*), and AVM (*purple circle*) shown on inset). (**b**) AVM box showing arterial inputs from MCA branches, venous drainage to both the SSS and the sylvian veins, and proximity to the sensory cortex. Note that the AVM's cortical surface is depicted with a circle on its base side and that side's label is underlined. The AVM's axis is depicted with a line through the box. Arterial and venous anatomy is superimposed on the box with red inflow arrows and blue outflow arrows, respectively. (**c**) Step 2, dissecting margins in the lateral sulci (broad white arrow); step 3, identifying ascending convexity veins and descending sylvian veins; step 4, locating cortical MCA feeders; and step 5, interrupting the anteroinferior front of arteries near the supramarginal gyrus (*dashed black line,* surgeon's view). (**d**) Step 6, circumdissecting into parieto-occipital parenchyma (encircling arrows); and step 7, mobilizing the AVM (spherical scoop) to expose deep feeding arteries from white matter or ventricle, as well as ependymal draining veins (coronal cross-sectional view).

are subcortical and are localized by following the arterialized vein. Ascending venous drainage (PosCenV, AntParV, PostParV, and/or OccV) is localized to the AVM's superior margin (step 3). The arterial supply is superficial and travels from the distal sylvian fissure (CenA, AntParA, PosParA, AngA, and/or TempOccA) (step 4). These arterial feeders are found anteroinferiorly, either on pial surfaces or in sulci along the AVMs margin near the supramarginal and angular gyri (step 5). Parenchymal dissection is parallel, with hot sides located anteriorly and inferiorly and eloquent sides associated with the somatosensory strip, visual cortex, optic radiations, and speech conduction tracts (step 6). Deep dissection may extend conically to an ependymal AVM in the atrium or occipital horn, supplied by choroidal arteries (lPChA) or deep MCA branches and drained by ependymal veins (step 7) (**Figs. 13.9, 13.10, 13.11**).

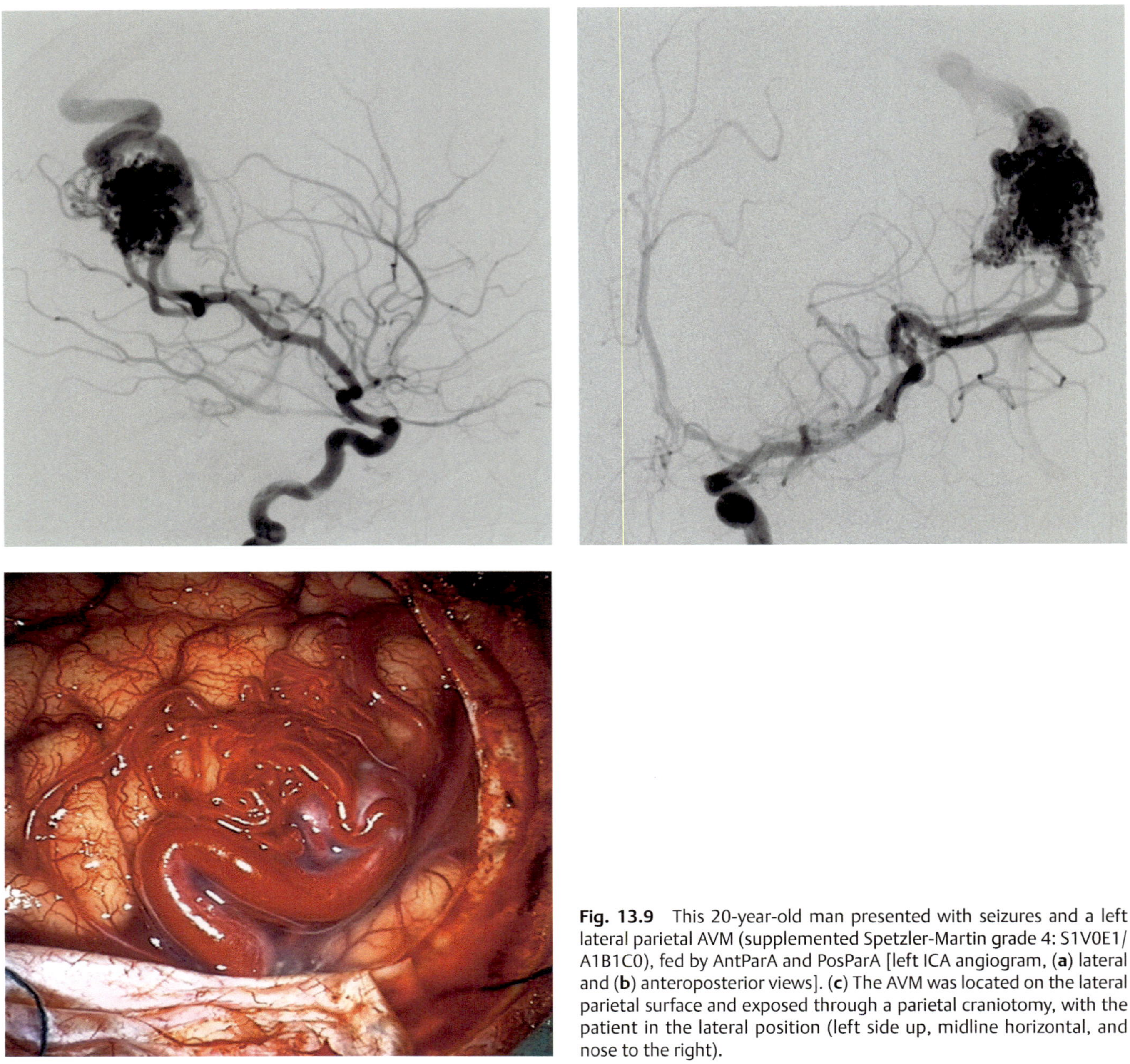

a b c

Fig. 13.9 This 20-year-old man presented with seizures and a left lateral parietal AVM (supplemented Spetzler-Martin grade 4: S1V0E1/A1B1C0), fed by AntParA and PosParA [left ICA angiogram, (**a**) lateral and (**b**) anteroposterior views]. (**c**) The AVM was located on the lateral parietal surface and exposed through a parietal craniotomy, with the patient in the lateral position (left side up, midline horizontal, and nose to the right).

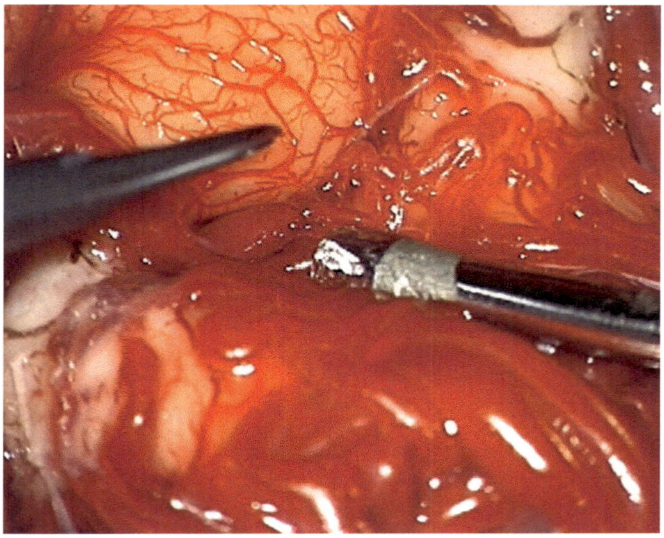
d

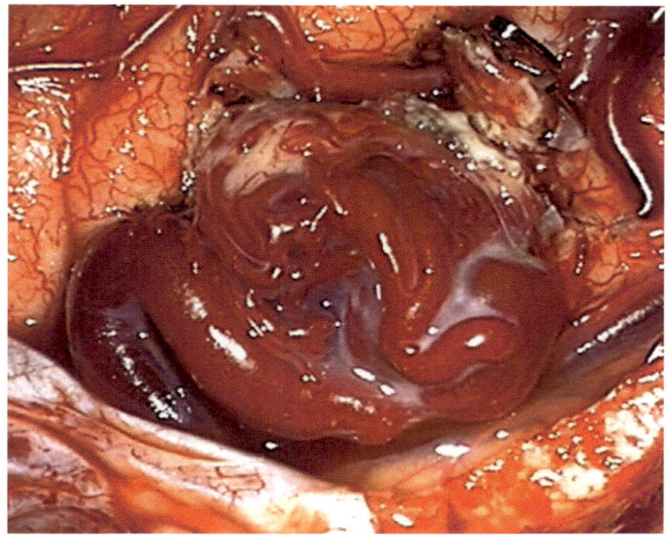
e

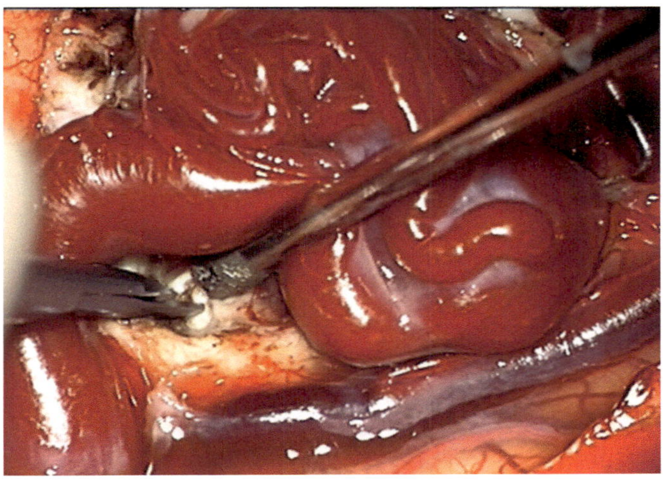
f

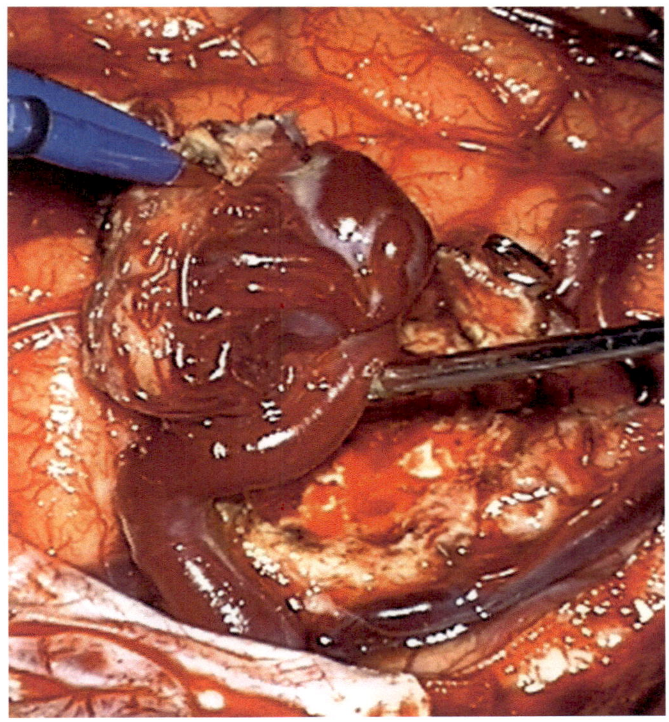
g

Fig. 13.9 (*continued*) (**d**) The two parietal feeding arteries were identified in the sulci along the anteroinferior front and (**e**) occluded with a clip (AntParA) or coagulated (PosParA). (**f**) Smaller feeding arteries were divided along the posterosuperior margin under the draining vein (PostParV). (**g**) The darkened AVM was lifted out of its resection bed before dividing the draining vein.

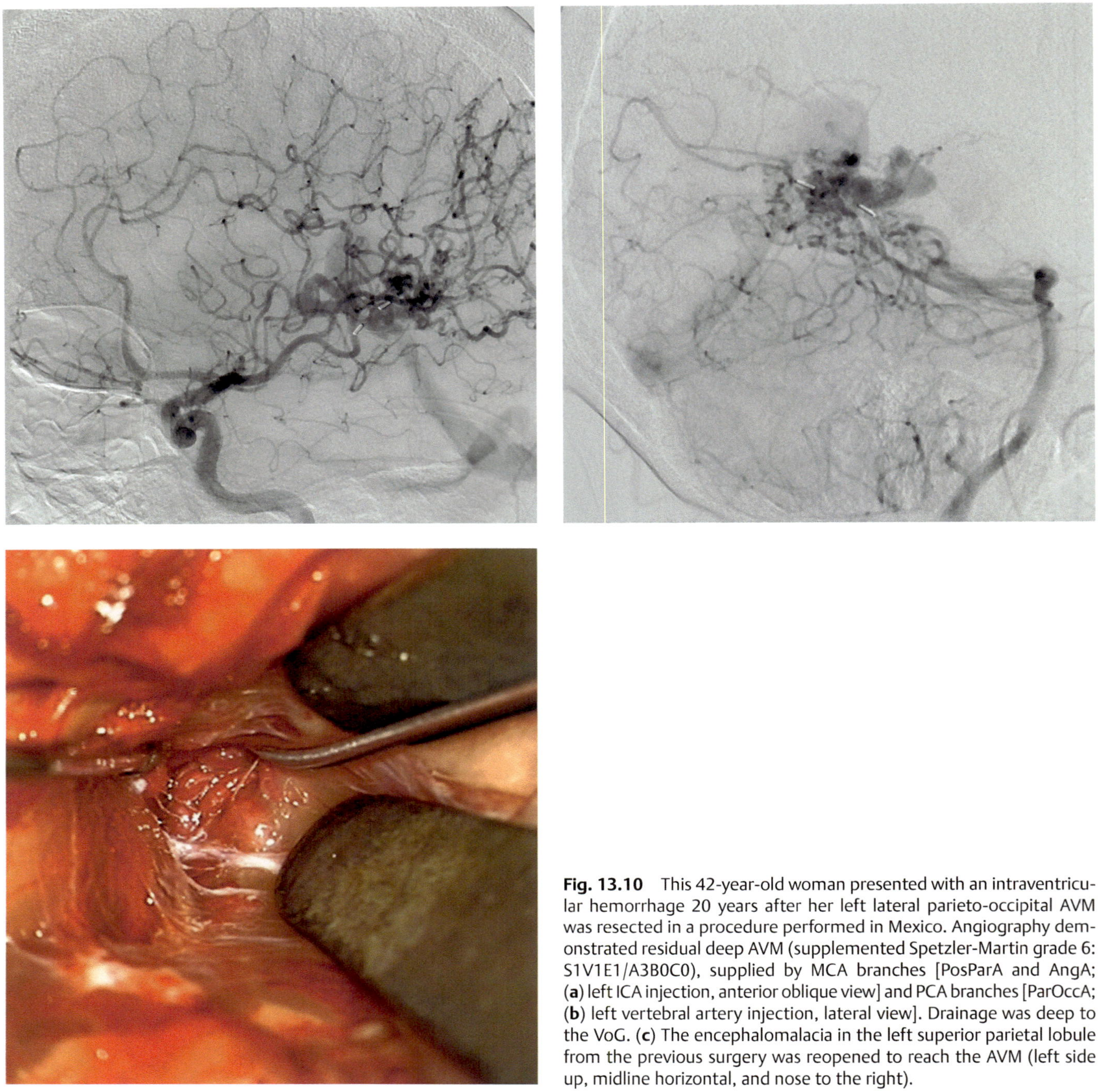

a b c

Fig. 13.10 This 42-year-old woman presented with an intraventricular hemorrhage 20 years after her left lateral parieto-occipital AVM was resected in a procedure performed in Mexico. Angiography demonstrated residual deep AVM (supplemented Spetzler-Martin grade 6: S1V1E1/A3B0C0), supplied by MCA branches [PosParA and AngA; (**a**) left ICA injection, anterior oblique view] and PCA branches [ParOccA; (**b**) left vertebral artery injection, lateral view]. Drainage was deep to the VoG. (**c**) The encephalomalacia in the left superior parietal lobule from the previous surgery was reopened to reach the AVM (left side up, midline horizontal, and nose to the right).

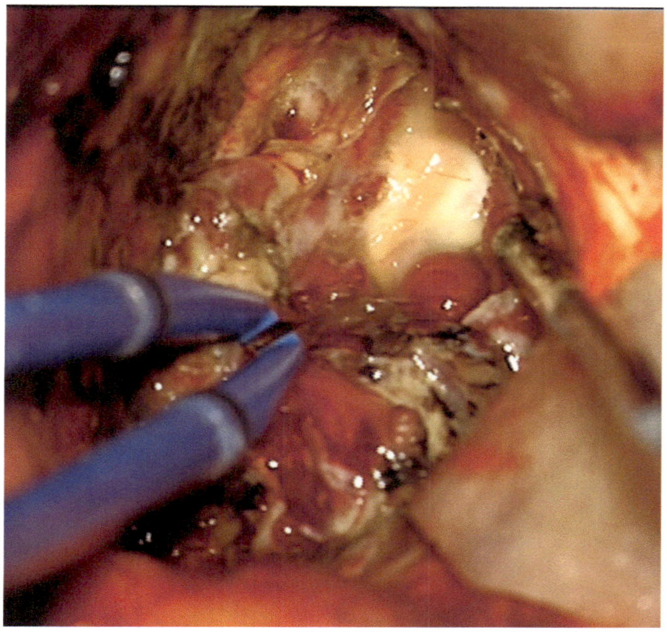

d

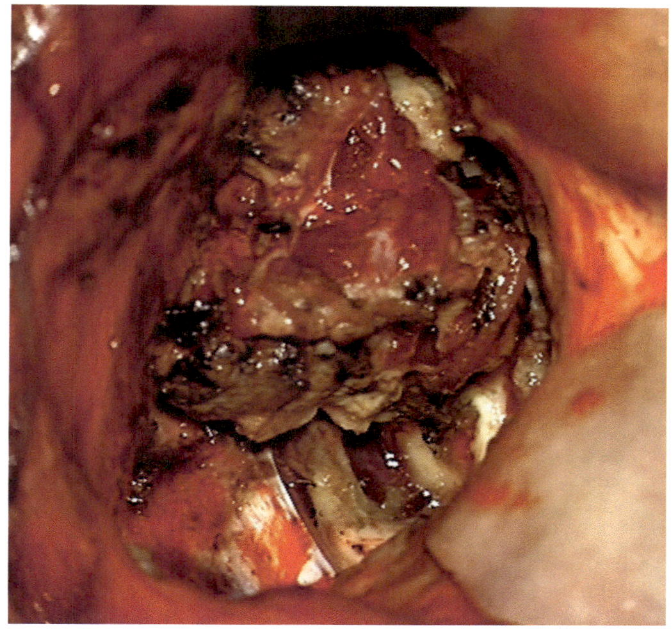

e

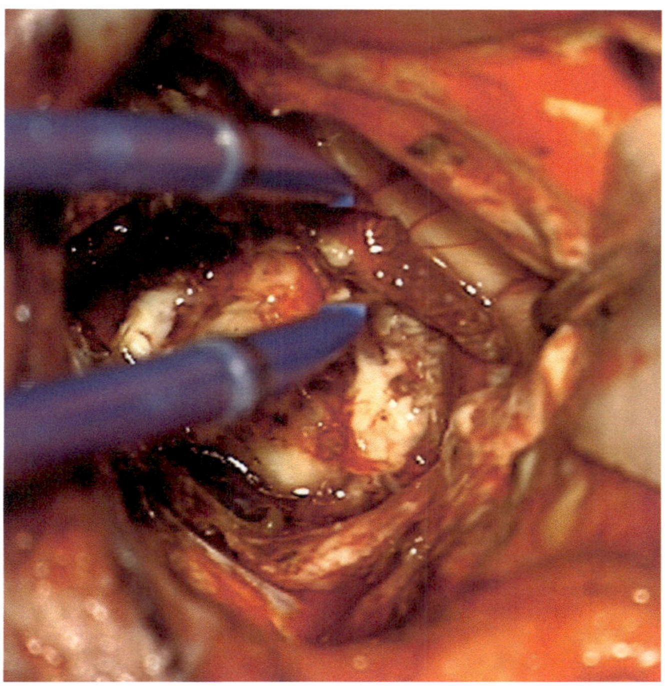

f

Fig. 13.10 (*continued*) (**d**) Surrounding gliosis created a clear parenchymal dissection plane that (**e**) was followed down to the tentorial incisura and (**f**) into the occipital horn. The AVM was resected completely and confirmed with postoperative angiography.

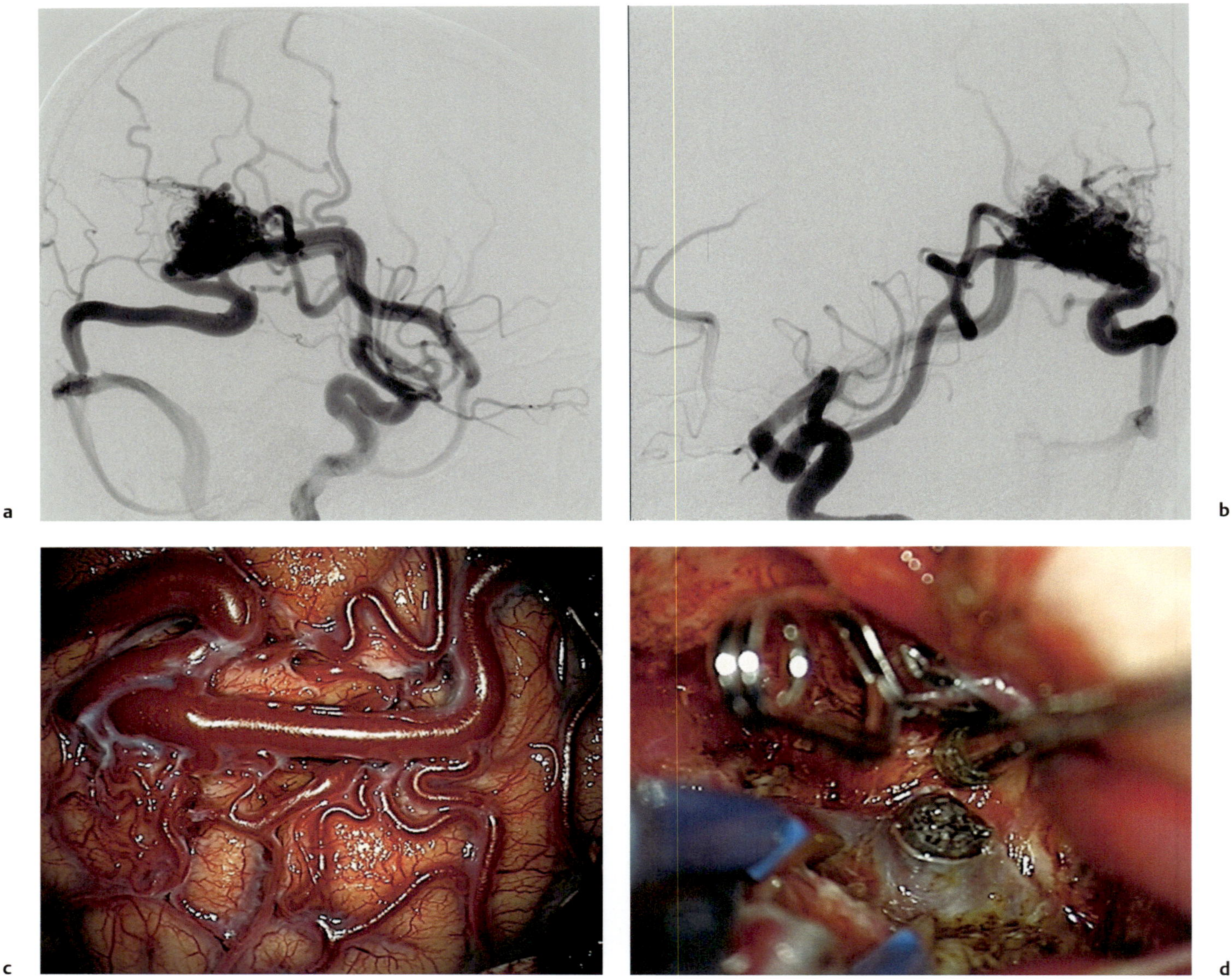

Fig. 13.11 This 46-year-old man presented with a left lateral parieto-occipital AVM in the angular gyrus (supplemented Spetzler-Martin grade 7: S2V0E1/A3B1C0). The AVM was fed by the AngA and drained by SupSylV, PosTempV, and several small parietal veins [left ICA angiogram, (**a**) lateral and (**b**) anterior oblique views]. Note the difference in caliber of the AngA and the normal frontal branches of the MCA, and drainage to a midline occipital sinus posteriorly and a sphenopetrosal sinus anteriorly. (**c**) The AVM's dilated draining veins (SupSylV center and PosTempV top left) were seen at the end of the sylvian fissure, with the patient supine, midline horizontal, and nose to the right. (**d**) The large AngA that had been embolized with Onyx was clipped proximally and transected.

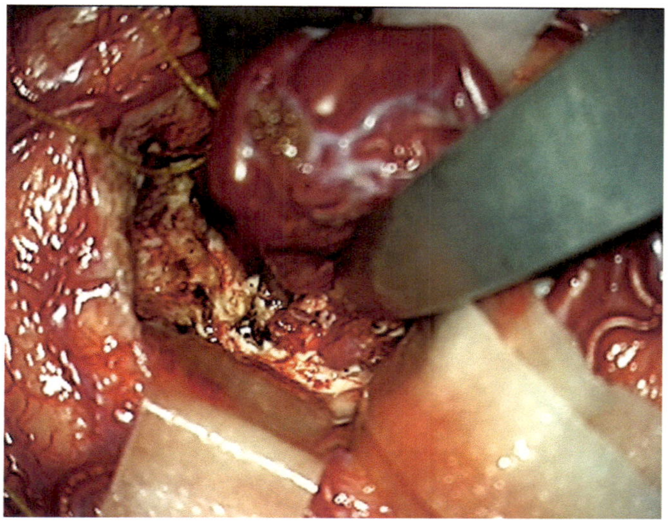

e

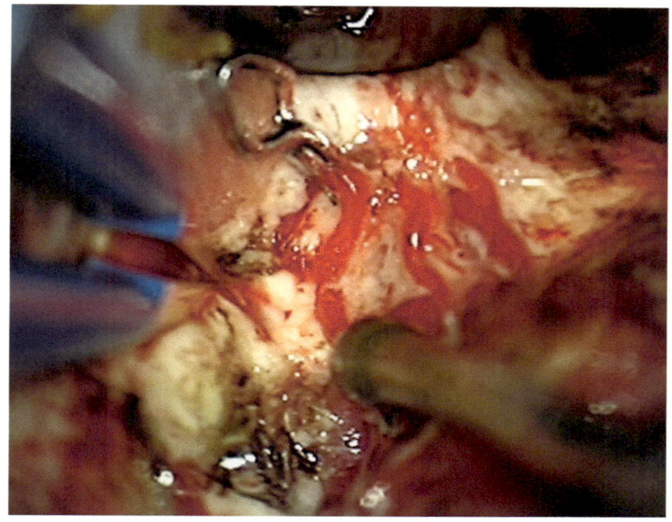

f

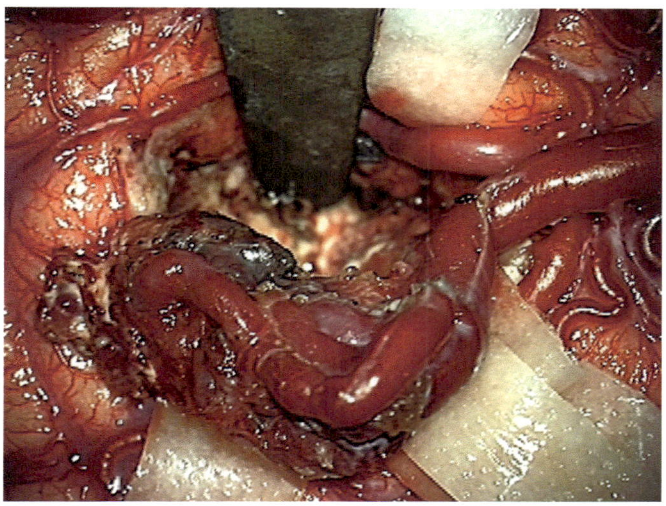

g

Fig. 13.11 (*continued*) (**e**) Small perforating arteries ("red devils") were encountered at the apex of the nidus, requiring retraction on the AVM to expose them and (**f**) microclips to occlude them. (**g**) The dearterialized AVM was rolled out of the resection cavity before dividing the draining SupSylV.

Medial Parieto-Occipital AVM Resection

Medial parieto-occipital AVMs are exposed through a generous torcular craniotomy over the SSS, torcula (Torc), and TrvS, with gravity retraction opening the posterior interhemispheric fissure (**Fig. 13.12,** step 1). The patient is positioned laterally with the AVM in the dependent position (down), and the head is turned "nose down" about 60 degrees from horizontal, with slight neck flexion. With this position and craniotomy, the occipital pole falls away from the falx and splays the interhemispheric fissure. Separate dural flaps based on the SSS medially and TrvS inferiorly remove dural barriers to this occipital migration, and release of arachnoidal granulations and adhesions untethers the brain (step 2). Bridging lateral veins course anteriorly, and the interhemispheric approach is centered behind them. Subarachnoid dissection deepens down the falcotentorial junction to the incisura to open the corpus callosum and/or quadrigeminal cisterns, drain cerebrospinal fluid (CSF), and slacken the brain, which further drops the occipital pole and widens the surgical corridor. This posterior interhemispheric approach accesses the AVM's medial surface with early exposure of its draining veins. Descending veins to VoG (posterior PcaV and anterior CalcV) are out of the way, but ascending veins to the SSS (ParaCenV, MedParV, and posterior CalcV) may not be (step 3). This approach also exposes superficial feeding arteries (ParaCenA, SupParA, InfParA, ParOccA, and CalcA) early in the dissection (step 4). The ACA feeders are exposed in the pia on the anteriorly margin at the cingulate gyrus, and PCA feeders are exposed on the inferior margin at the precuneus, cuneus, and lingula (step 5). The ACA feeders are usually terminal arteries that can be taken, but PCA feeders may be transit arteries that require skeletonization to preserve normal arteries to the occipital pole.

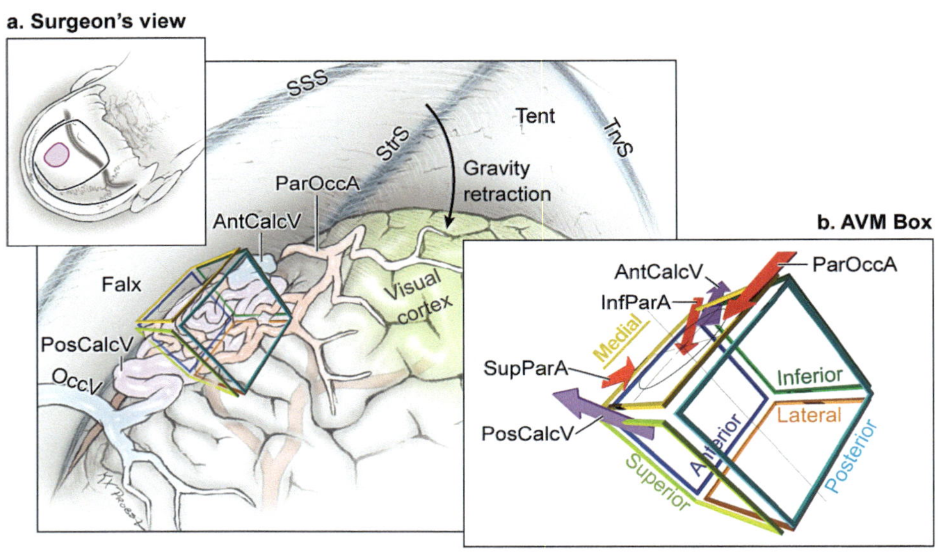

Fig. 13.12 Resection strategy for medial parieto-occipital AVMs. (**a**) Step 1, exposing the AVM with a torcular craniotomy eccentric to the left and a posterior interhemispheric approach [surgeon's view, with the patient in the lateral position, the head rotated "nose down," and the left-sided AVM in the dependent position (down); scalp incision (*dashed line*), craniotomy (*solid line*), and AVM (*purple circle*) are shown on *inset*]. (**b**) AVM box showing arterial supply from the ACA (SupParA and InfParA) and PCA (ParOccA), drainage superficially to PosCalcV and deep to AntCalV, and proximity to the visual cortex.

c. Surgeon's view

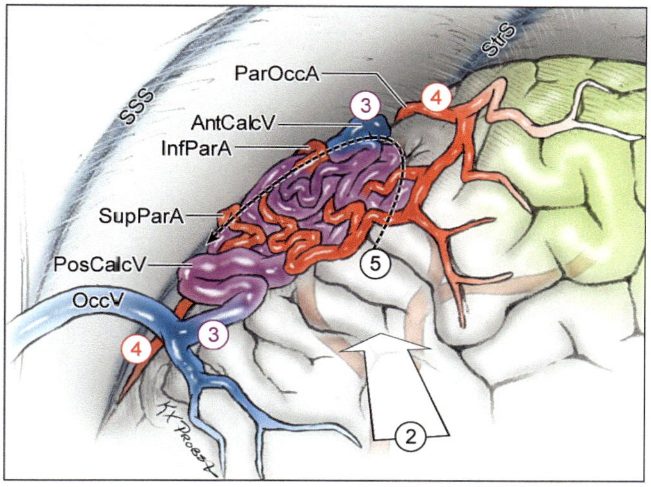

d. Coronal view

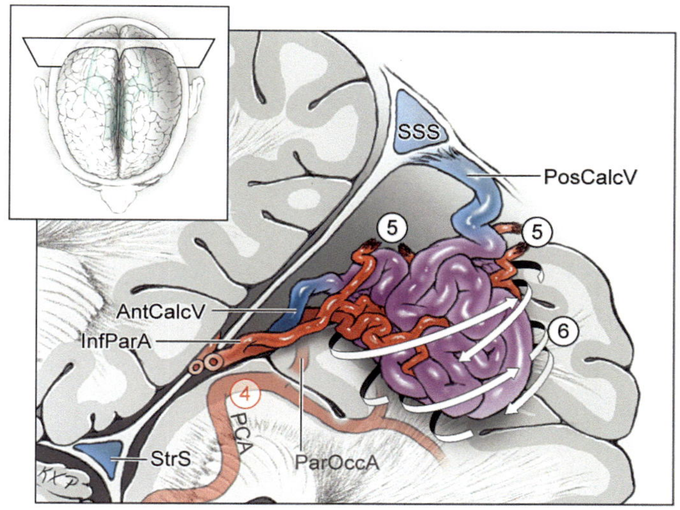

e. Surgeon's view

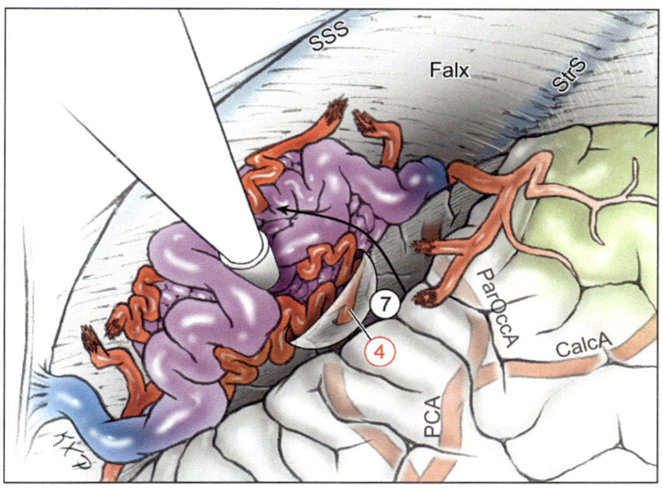

Fig. 13.12 (*continued*) (**c**) Step 2, widely opening the posterior interhemispheric fissure down to the falcotentorial junction; step 3, identifying draining veins on the medial surface; step 4, locating feeding arteries from the ACA and PCA; and step 5, interrupting the anterior and inferior fronts near the cingulate gyrus and precuneus/cuneus, respectively (surgeon's view). (**d**) Step 6, circumdissecting laterally into the parieto-occipital lobe (coronal cross-sectional view). (**e**) Step 7, mobilizing the AVM medially into the interhemispheric fissure to access inferolateral feeders from the PCA and any ependymal draining veins (surgeon's view).

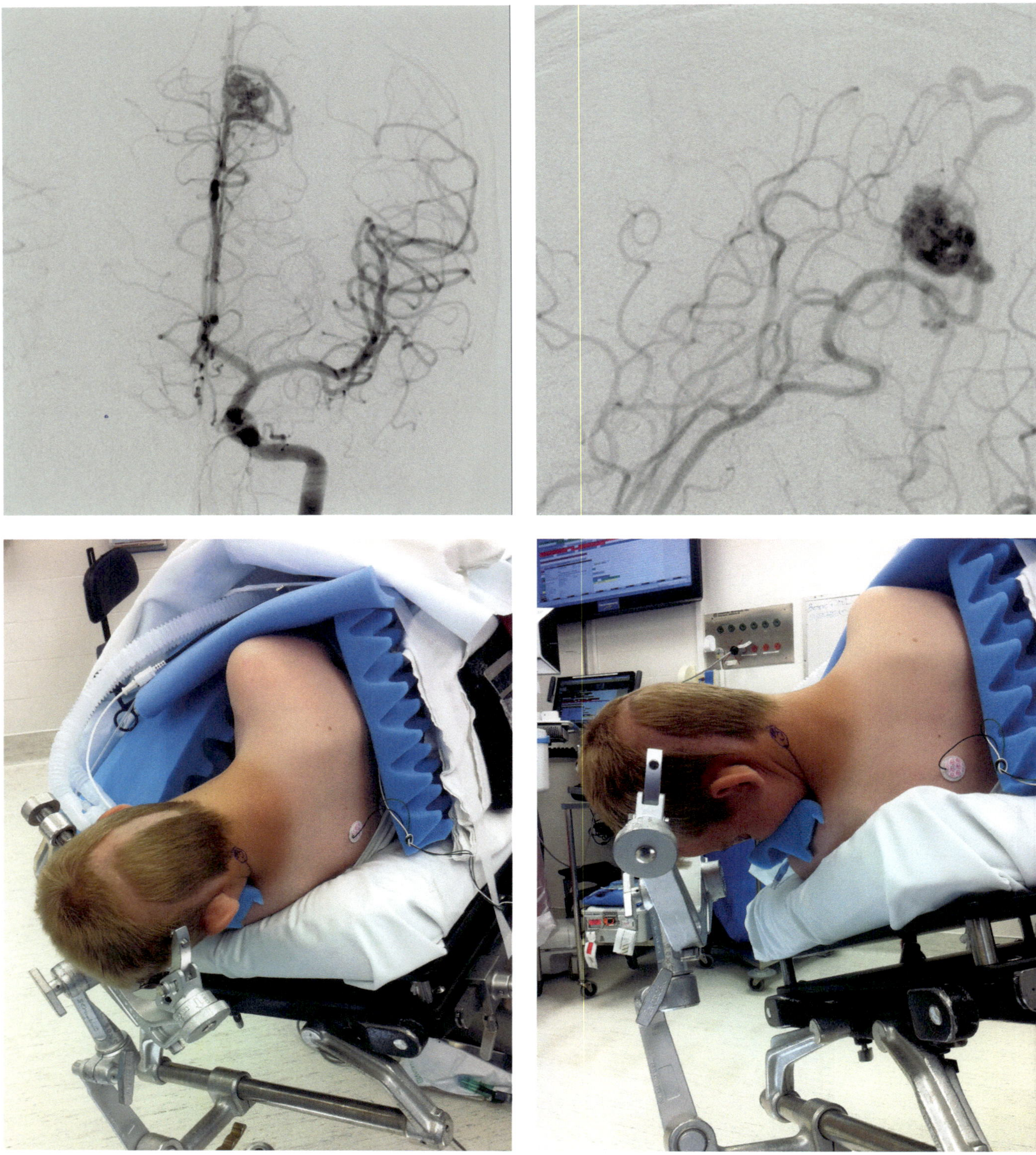
a b c d

Fig. 13.13 This 17-year-old boy presented with a left medial parieto-occipital AVM (supplemented Spetzler-Martin grade 4: S1V1E0/A1B1C0), supplied primarily by the ACA [InfParA; left ICA angiogram, (**a**) anteroposterior and (**b**) anterior oblique magnified views] and small branches from the PCA (ParOccA, not shown). The AVM drained superiorly to PosParV and inferiorly to AntCalcV and VoG. (**c**) The medial parieto-occipital lobe was exposed through a torcular craniotomy, eccentric to the left, with the patient in the lateral position (right side up, midline horizontal, and (**d**) nose turned 45 degrees down toward the floor). Table rotation to the patient's left brought the occiput up for the craniotomy, and table rotation to the patient's right allowed gravity to retract the occipital pole.

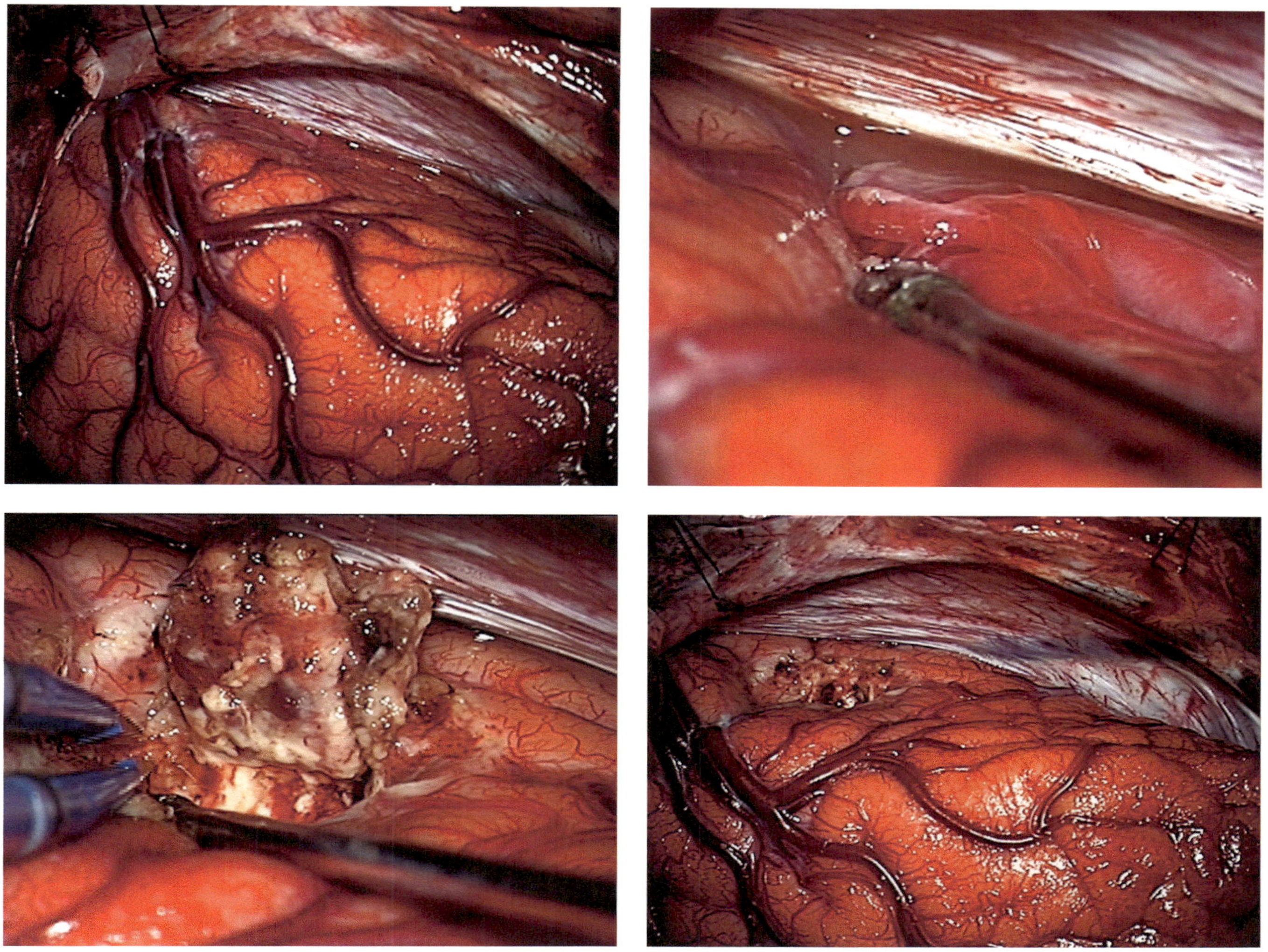

e f g h

Fig. 13.13 (*continued*) (**e**) Torcular craniotomy and wide dural opening with one flap base on the SSS and another based on the left TrvS exposed the interhemispheric fissure. (**f**) InfParA intersected the AVM along its anterior front. (**g**) Parenchymal dissection mobilized the nidus into the interhemispheric fissure and exposed the inferior front of the PCA supply. (**h**) Overview demonstrated the exposure of the posteromedial hemisphere, falcotentorial junction, the StrS, and the absence of bridging veins to the SSS posterior to the OccV, all with gravity retraction and without fixed retraction.

Parenchymal dissection is perpendicular and requires that the nidus be drawn up from the sagging parieto-occipital lobe into the interhemispheric fissure (step 6). The AVMs beneath the medial surface are identified by tracing feeding arteries or draining veins transcortically and sometimes resecting an overlying lobule to reach the lateral AVM border. The more lateral the reach, the more the SSS limits the surgical corridor and the more the nidus must be mobilized medially into view. The hot sides are anterior and inferior. Deep dissection surrounds deep feeders from the PCA, any ventricular extension, and ependymal draining veins (step 7) (**Figs. 13.13, 13.14, 13.15**).

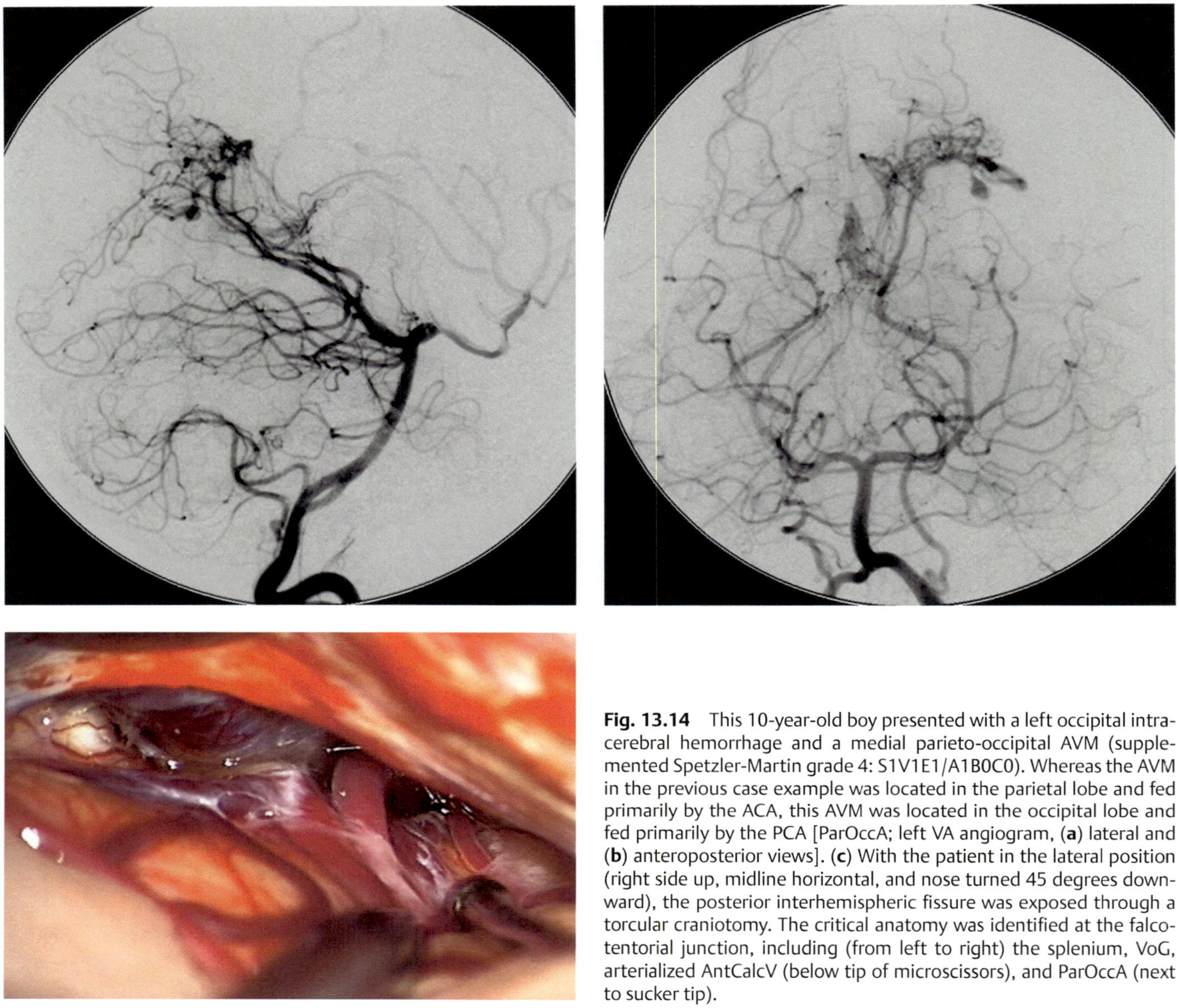

a b c

Fig. 13.14 This 10-year-old boy presented with a left occipital intracerebral hemorrhage and a medial parieto-occipital AVM (supplemented Spetzler-Martin grade 4: S1V1E1/A1B0C0). Whereas the AVM in the previous case example was located in the parietal lobe and fed primarily by the ACA, this AVM was located in the occipital lobe and fed primarily by the PCA [ParOccA; left VA angiogram, (**a**) lateral and (**b**) anteroposterior views]. (**c**) With the patient in the lateral position (right side up, midline horizontal, and nose turned 45 degrees downward), the posterior interhemispheric fissure was exposed through a torcular craniotomy. The critical anatomy was identified at the falcotentorial junction, including (from left to right) the splenium, VoG, arterialized AntCalcV (below tip of microscissors), and ParOccA (next to sucker tip).

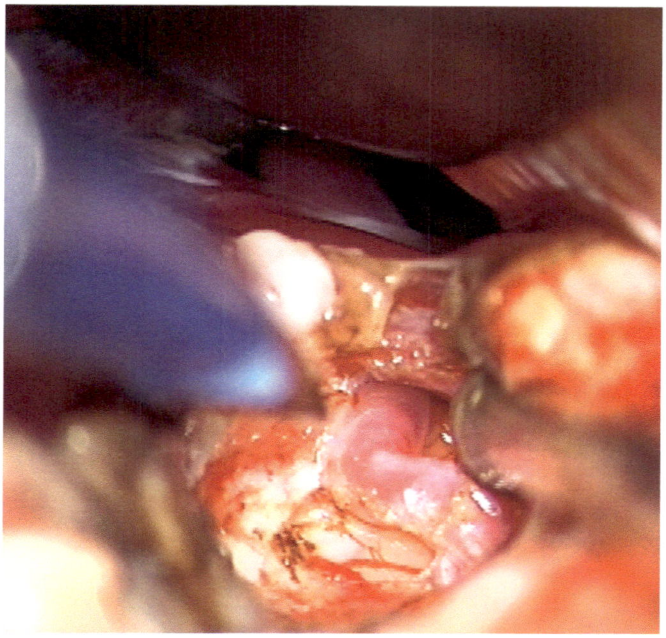
d

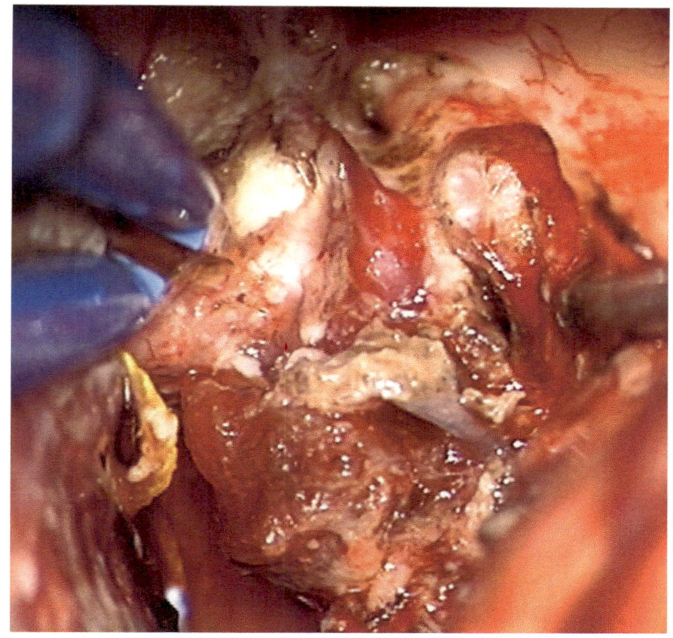
e

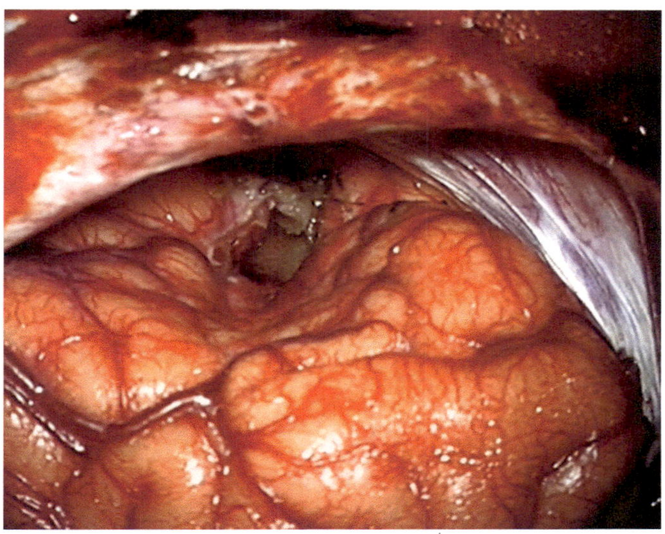
f

Fig. 13.14 (*continued*) (**d**) ParOccA was followed into a sulcus and laterally to the AVM. (**e**) After evacuating the hematoma laterally, circumferential dissection based on the medial draining AntCalcV freed the nidus. (**f**) Gravity retraction, hematoma evacuation, and release of CSF from the deep cisterns slackened the left hemisphere and opened interhemispheric and infraoccipital fissures without fixed retraction.

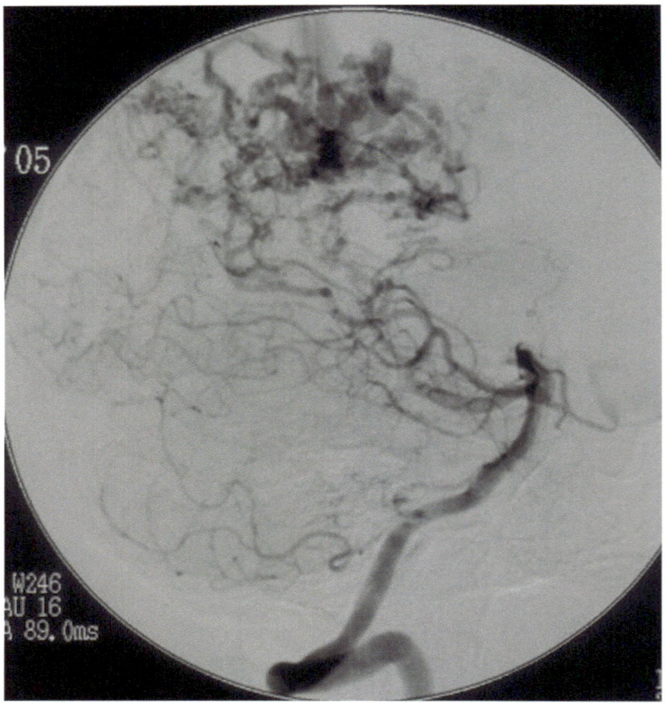

a

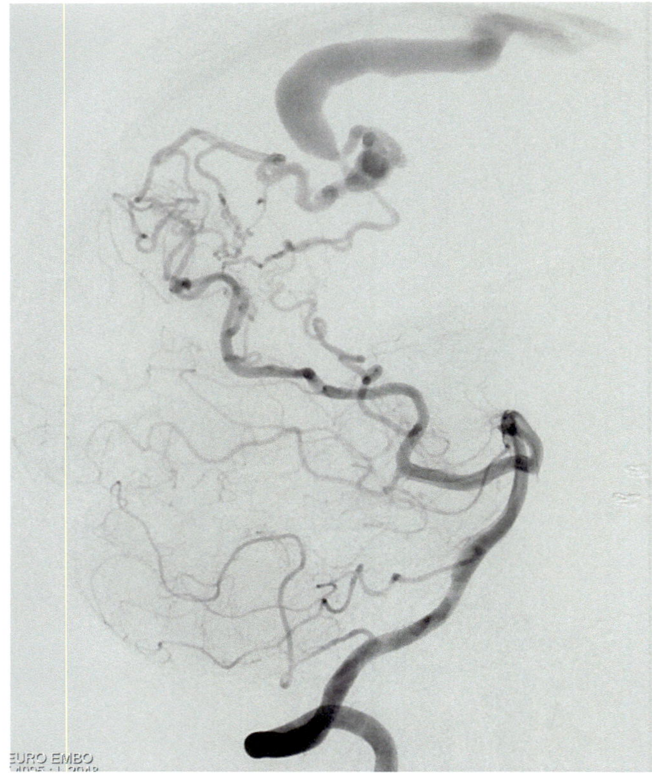

b

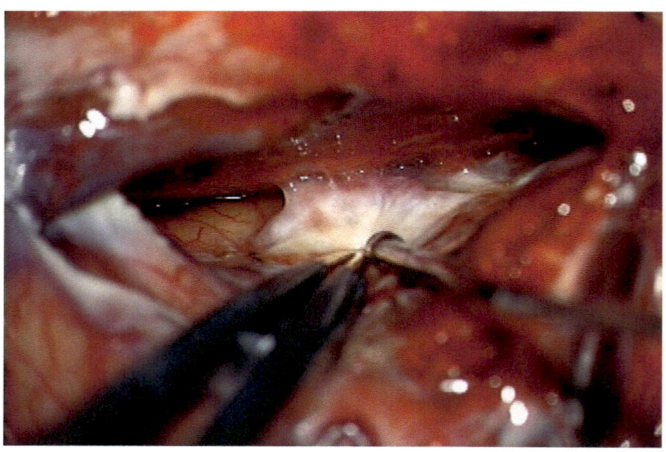

c

Fig. 13.15 This 43-year-old man presented with right medial parieto-occipital AVM (supplemented Spetzler-Martin grade 9: S2V1E1/A3B1C1) that was deemed inoperable because of its size, diffuseness, and benign presentation. It was supplied by ParOccA from the PCA [(**a**) right VA angiogram, lateral view], the parietal arteries from the ACA (InfParA and SupParA), and the parietal arteries from the MCA (AntParA and PosParA). He was treated with Gamma Knife radiosurgery in three stages, with reduction in nidal volume over 5 years [(**b**) right VA angiogram, lateral view]. (**c**) With the patient in the lateral position (left side up, midline horizontal, and nose to the right), the posterior interhemispheric fissure was exposed through a torcular craniotomy, working between normal bridging veins to the SSS.

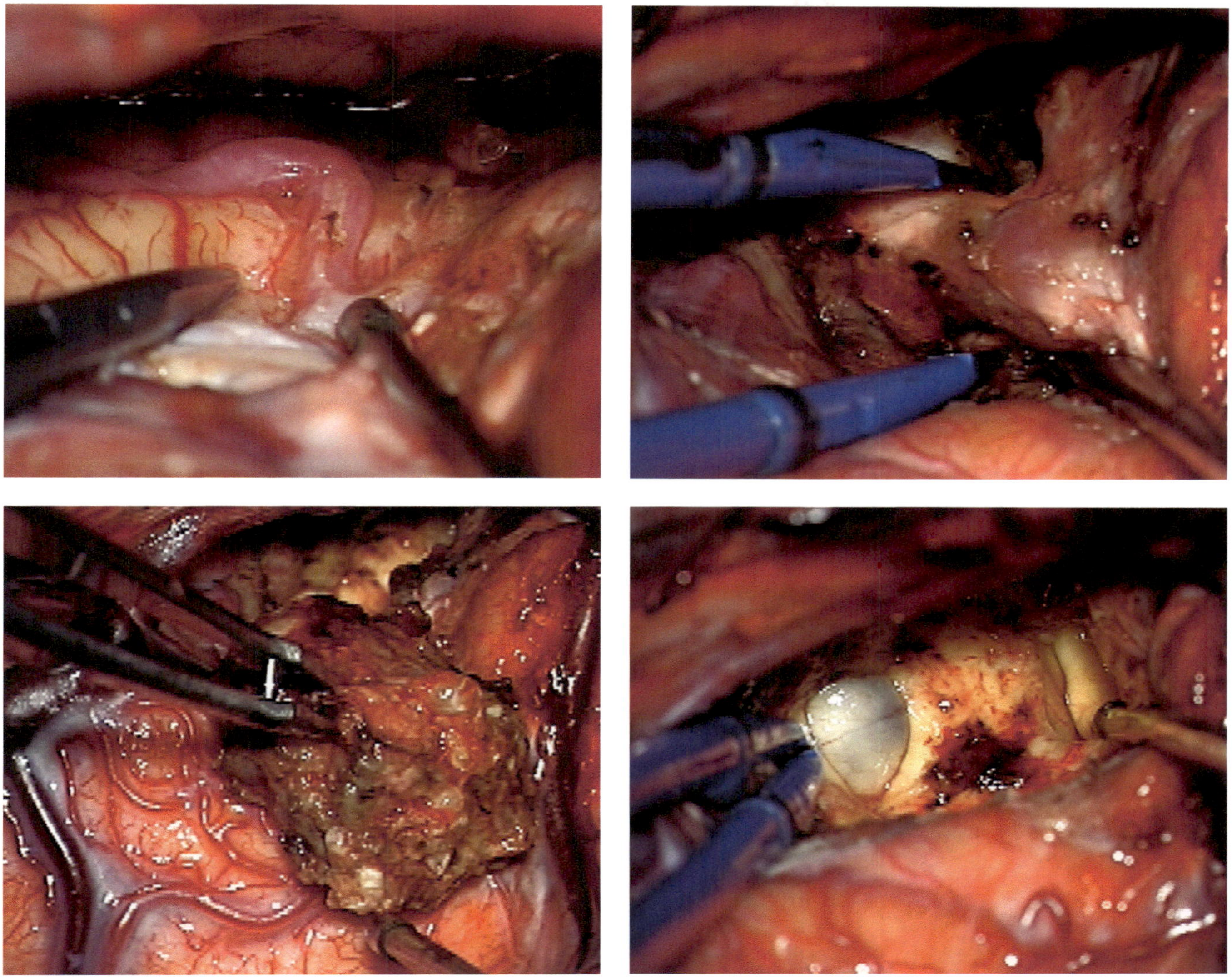

d e f g

Fig. 13.15 (*continued*) Feeding arteries adherent to the falx were (**d**) isolated anc (**e**) cauterized along the inferior margin of the AVM. (**f**) Gliotic planes and scarred nidus facilitated circumferential dissection and AVM removal, (**g**) which exposed a large radiation-induced cyst adjacent to the ventricle that was fenestrated and drained.

Paramedian Parieto-Occipital AVM Resection

The need to expose both the medial and lateral orthogonal surfaces prevents the use of gravity retraction with paramedian parieto-occipital AVMs. Instead of orienting the midline horizontally with the AVM down in the dependent position, the midline is oriented vertically for both interhemispheric dissection and lateral convexity dissection (**Fig. 13.16**). There are two different approaches to paramedian AVMs: parietal AVMs are approached "nose up," whereas occipital AVMs are approached "nose down." With parietal AVMs, the patient is positioned supine, the neck is flexed, and the head is rotated slightly away (20 degrees) from the AVM. With table rotation toward the AVM, the midline is vertical for interhemispheric access; and with table rotation away from the AVM, the midline is oriented at 45 degrees for lateral convexity access. Parietal AVMs are exposed with a biparietal or biparieto-occipital craniotomy eccentric to the side of the AVM.

With occipital AVMs, the patient is placed in the lateral position (or occasionally prone), and the head is rotated away from the AVM to bring the AVM up and the midline almost vertical. More table rotation aligns the midline vertically for interhemispheric access, and table rotation in the other direction aligns the midline at 45 degrees for lateral convexity access. Occipital AVMs are exposed with a torcular craniotomy that gets all the way around the paramedian occipital lobe, whereas parietal AVMs are exposed with a simpler biparietal or biparieto-occipital craniotomy (step 1). In both cases, crossing the SSS opens the interhemispheric fissure. Parietal AVMs are more common than occipital AVMs, and account for the 75% of paramedian AVMs.

Subarachnoid dissection includes both medial interhemispheric and lateral sulcal dissection (step 2). The absence of gravity retraction and the ability to maneuver freely around superficial convexity veins (PostCenV, ParV, and OccV) or medial draining veins (MedParV) makes them less obstructive than are medial AVMs (step 3). However, they are often

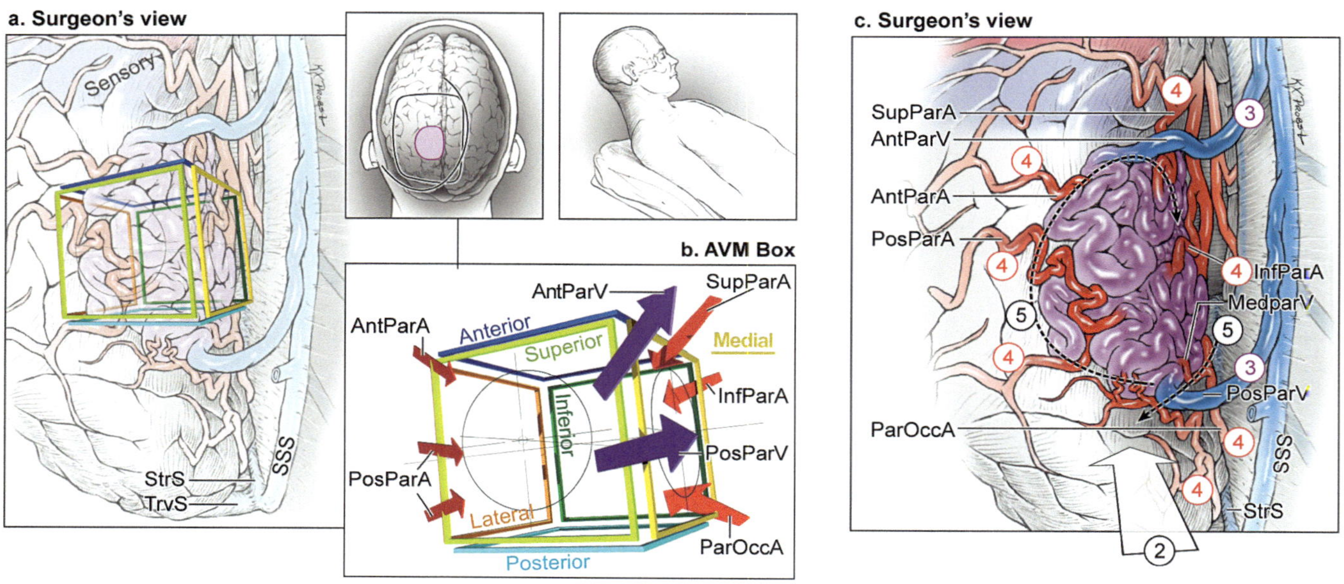

Fig. 13.16 Resection strategy for paramedian parieto-occipital AVMs. (**a**) Step 1, exposing the parietal AVM (surgeon's view) with a semicircular scalp incision (*left inset, dashed line*), bifrontal craniotomy (*left inset, solid line*), and posterior interhemispheric approach with the midline oriented vertically ("nose up," *right inset*). (**b**) AVM box showing arterial supply from the ACA, MCA, and PCA branches, and proximity to somatosensory cortex. (**c**) Step 2, dissecting AVM margins laterally in parietal sulci and opening the interhemispheric fissure; step 3, identifying draining veins laterally (AntParV and PosParV) and medially (MedParV); step 4, locating feeding arteries laterally (AntParA and PosParA), anteromedially (SupParA and InfParA), and inferomedially (ParOccA); and step 5, interrupting arterial fronts laterally along the SPL, anteriorly near cingulate gyrus, and inferiorly near the precuneus/cuneus (surgeon's view).

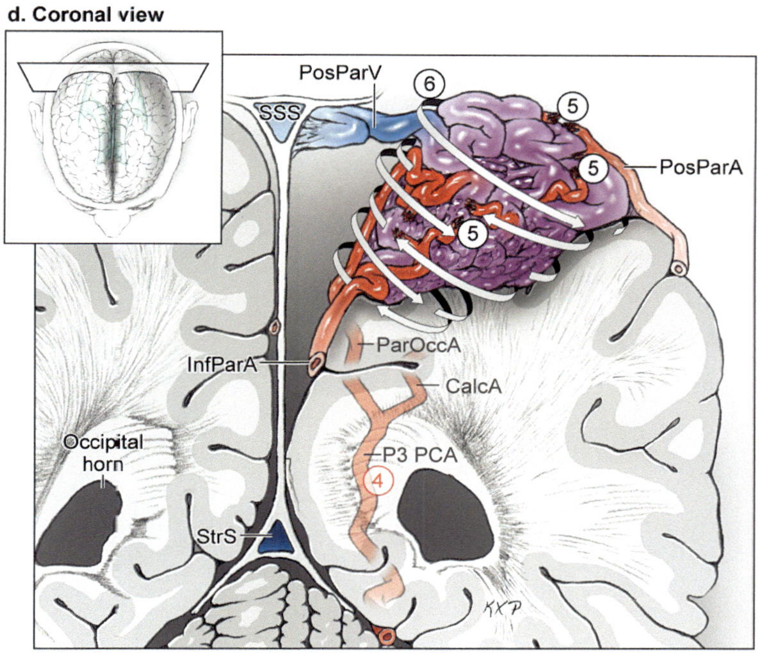

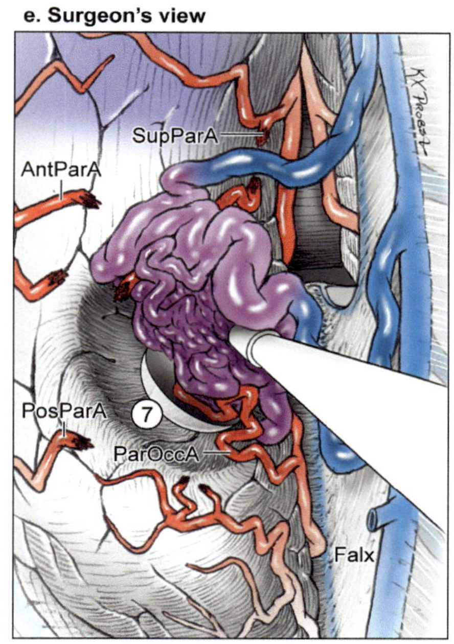

Fig. 13.16 (*continued*) (**d**) Step 6, circumdissecting into the parietal lobe (coronal cross-sectional view). (**e**) Step 7, mobilizing the AVM medially to dissect inferolaterally across the deep PCA, MCA, and ventricular feeding arteries (surgeon's view).

dilated and can be damaged with the dural opening or elevation of the dural flap. A sleeve of dura left on a draining vein with separate flaps on either side might improve medial access. If not, medial dissection may be deferred until the later stages of dissection. The watershed location of paramedian AVMs gives them a robust arterial supply from the MCA (AntParA and PosParA), ACA (SupParA and InfParA), and PCA (ParOccA and CalcA) (step 4), and creates fronts on the lateral (SPL and SOG), anterior (cingulate gyrus), and inferior (precuneus and cuneus) pial margins, respectively (step 5). The lateral, anterior, and inferior sides of the AVM receive major arterial inputs (step 6). Paramedian AVMs have parallel angles of attack when the operating table is aggressively rotated to bring the midline vertical or roll up the lateral convexity. The deep plane can reach the ventricle and receive deep inputs from MCA, PCA, and choroidal arteries, as well as outputs to deep atrial veins (step 7) (**Figs. 13.17** and **13.18**).

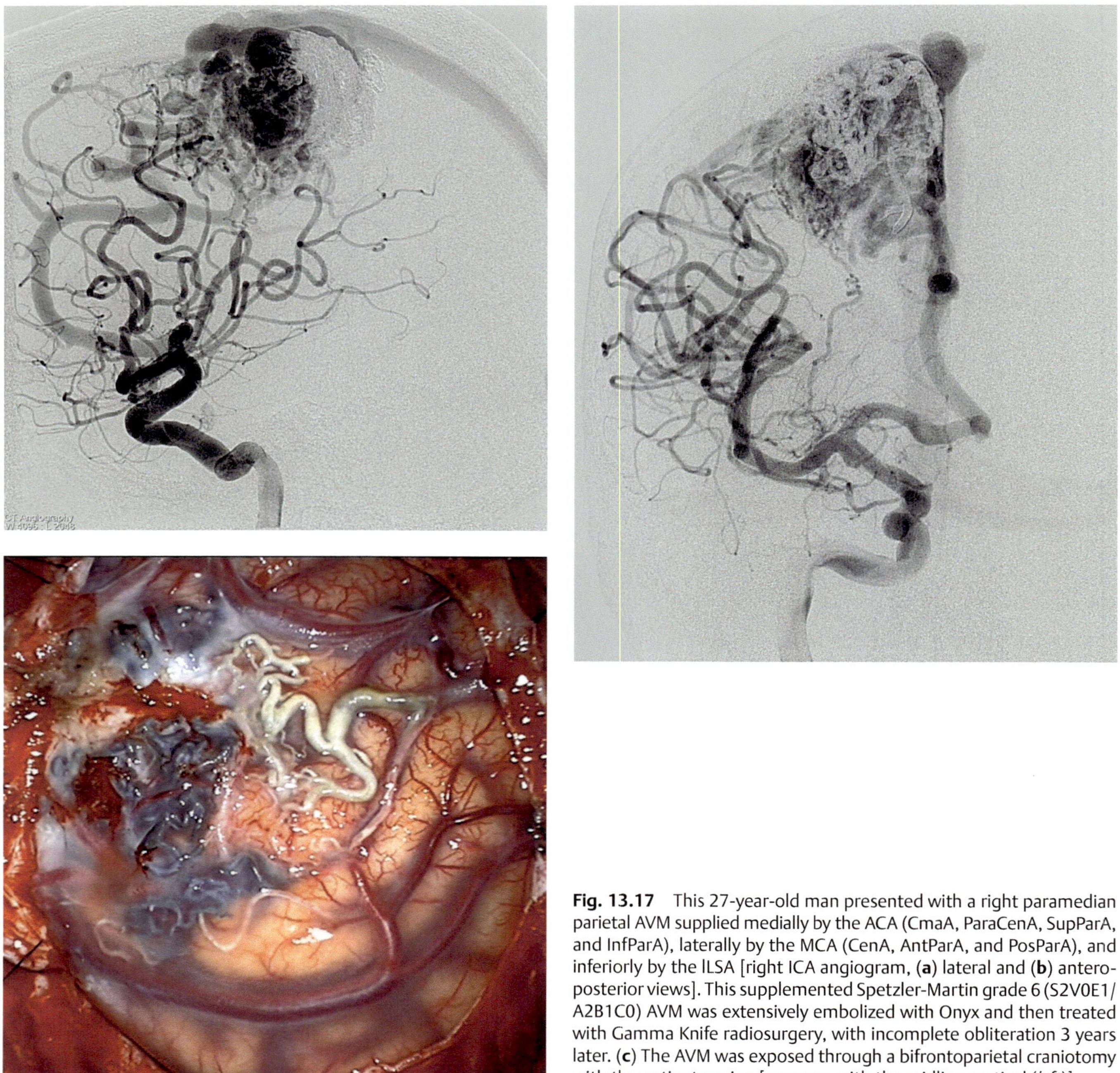

a b c

Fig. 13.17 This 27-year-old man presented with a right paramedian parietal AVM supplied medially by the ACA (CmaA, ParaCenA, SupParA, and InfParA), laterally by the MCA (CenA, AntParA, and PosParA), and inferiorly by the ILSA [right ICA angiogram, (**a**) lateral and (**b**) anteroposterior views]. This supplemented Spetzler-Martin grade 6 (S2V0E1/A2B1C0) AVM was extensively embolized with Onyx and then treated with Gamma Knife radiosurgery, with incomplete obliteration 3 years later. (**c**) The AVM was exposed through a bifrontoparietal craniotomy with the patient supine [nose up, with the midline vertical (*left*)].

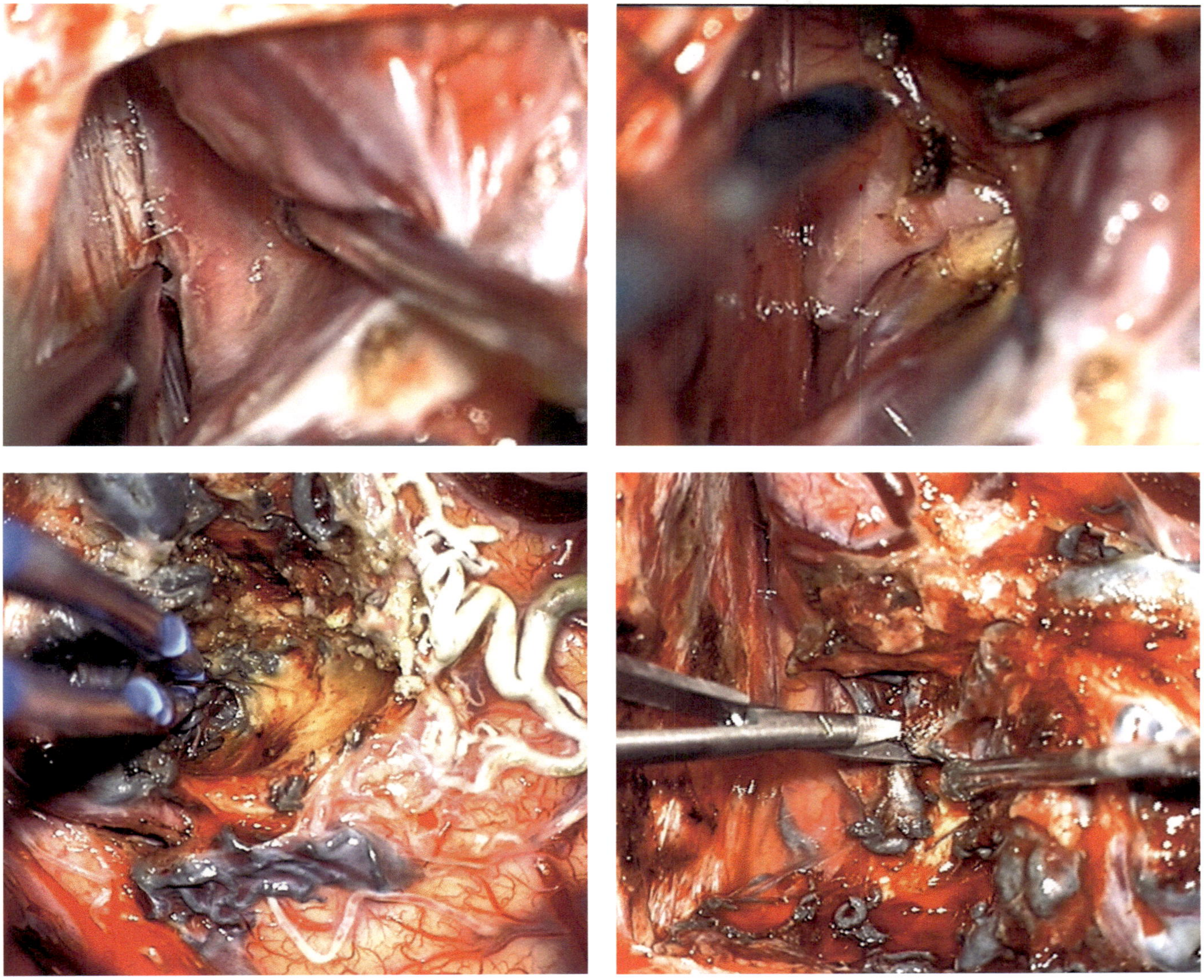

d e f g

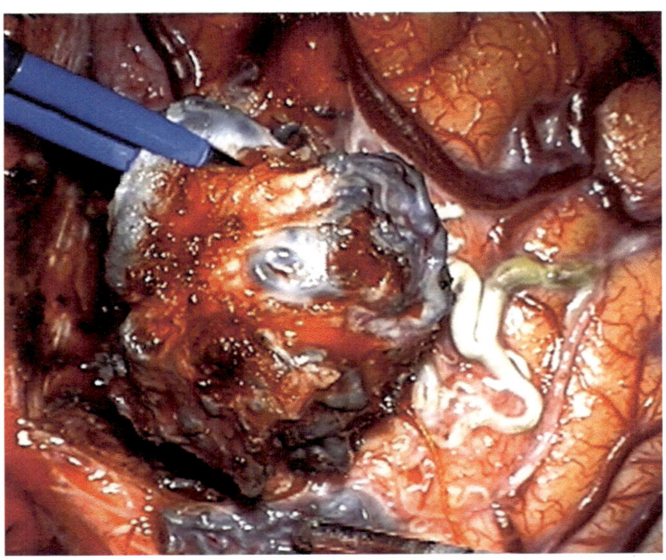

h

Fig. 13.17 (*continued*) (**d**) This exposure enabled access to the ACA feeders medially along the falx and (**e**) inferior to the nidus. (**f**) Lateral MCA feeders were also accessible, and radiosurgery created gliotic planes around the parenchymal sides. (**g**) The deep plane was dissected by mobilizing the AVM laterally away from the falx and dividing casted feeders inferiorly. (**h**) The AVM was resected and angiography showed no residual nidus.

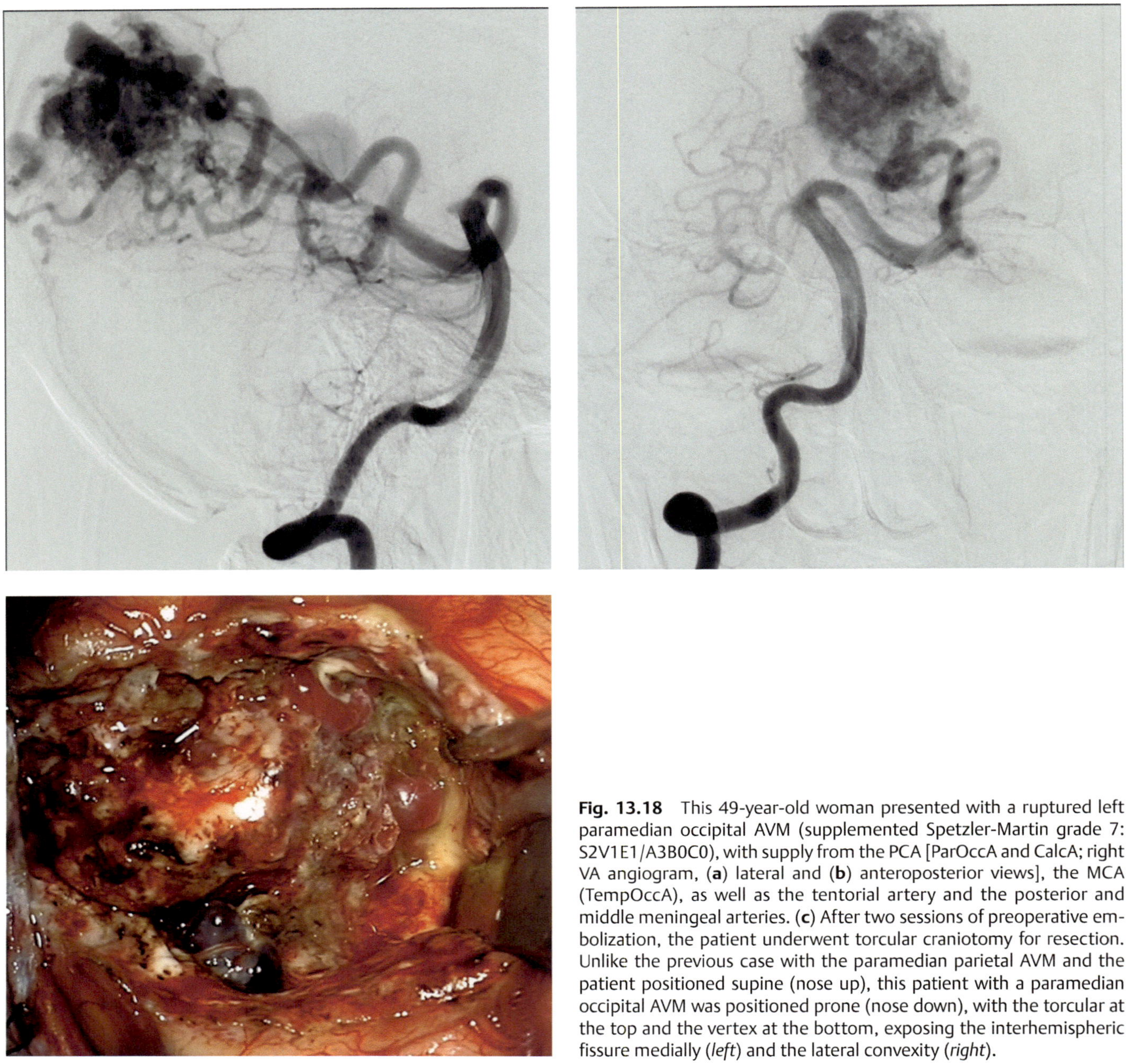

Fig. 13.18 This 49-year-old woman presented with a ruptured left paramedian occipital AVM (supplemented Spetzler-Martin grade 7: S2V1E1/A3B0C0), with supply from the PCA [ParOccA and CalcA; right VA angiogram, (**a**) lateral and (**b**) anteroposterior views], the MCA (TempOccA), as well as the tentorial artery and the posterior and middle meningeal arteries. (**c**) After two sessions of preoperative embolization, the patient underwent torcular craniotomy for resection. Unlike the previous case with the paramedian parietal AVM and the patient positioned supine (nose up), this patient with a paramedian occipital AVM was positioned prone (nose down), with the torcular at the top and the vertex at the bottom, exposing the interhemispheric fissure medially (*left*) and the lateral convexity (*right*).

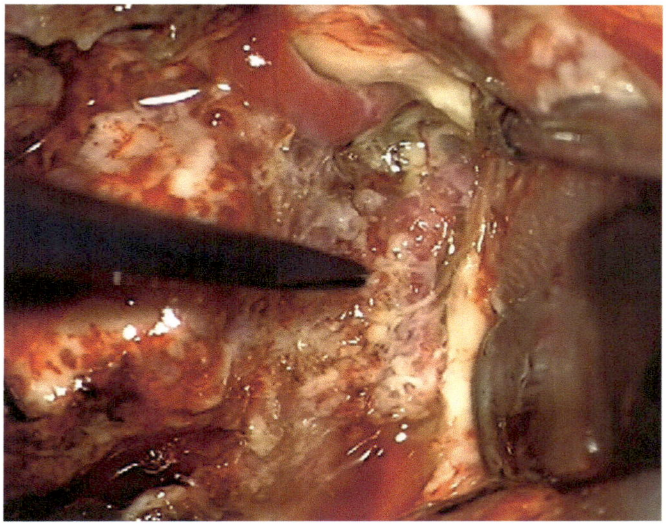

d

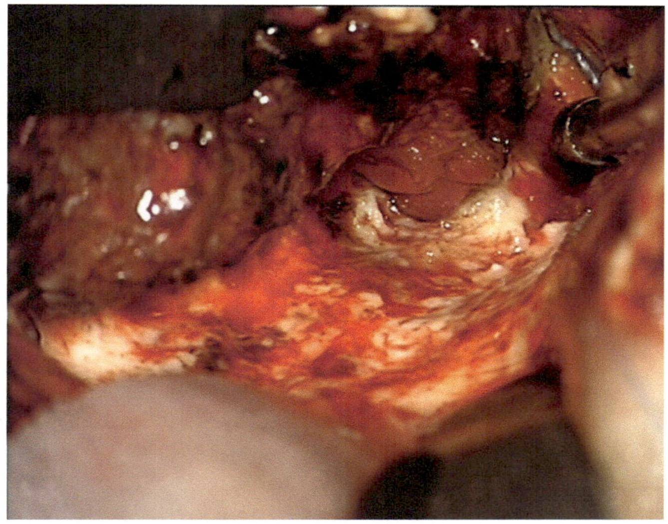

e

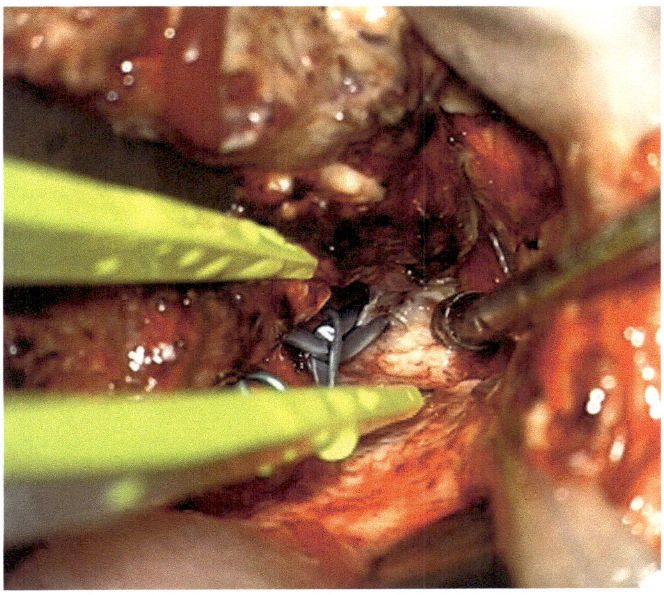

f

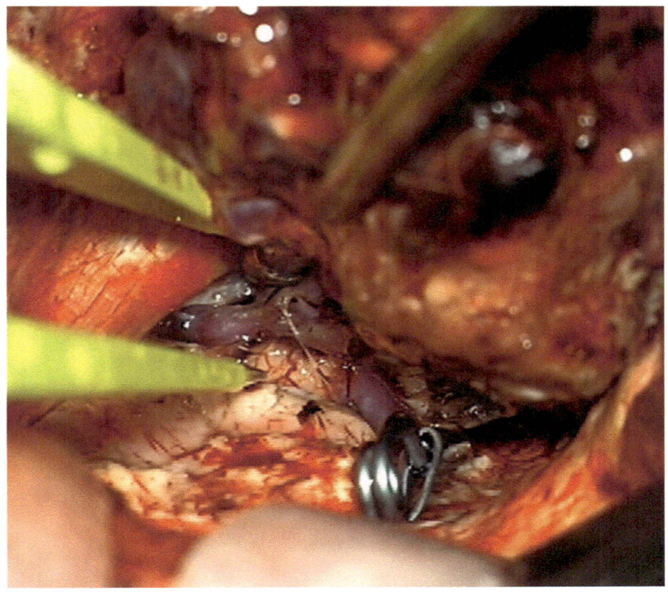

g

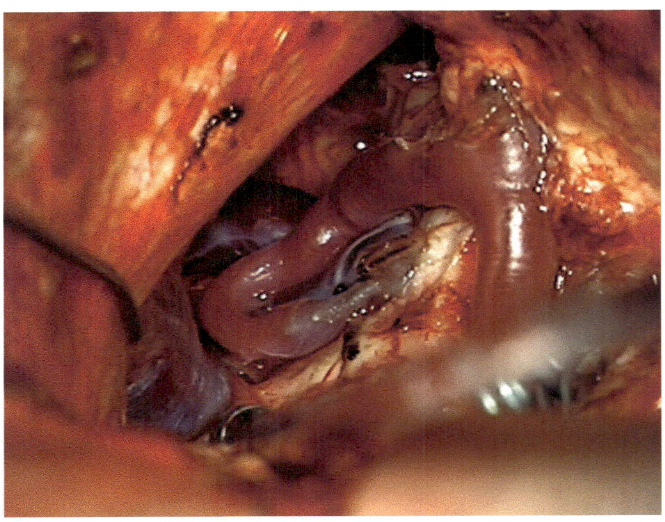

h

Fig. 13.18 (*continued*) (**d**) The PCA supply was identified at the inferolateral margin, (**e**) at the superolateral margin, and (**f**) clip occluded. (**g**) Additional supply was interrupted medially at the falcotentorial junction. (**h**) After resection, the stumps of medial PCA feeders were seen adjacent to the VoG (at the tip of the Rhoton No. 6 dissector).

Basal Occipital AVM Resection

Basal occipital AVMs are exposed with a craniotomy that crosses the TrvS to visualize the supratentorial-infraoccipital plane and undersurface of the occipital lobe (**Fig. 13.19,** step 1). Basal occipital AVMs that are medial in the lingula or OTG require a torcular craniotomy, whereas lateral AVMs in the lower part of the IOG require just an occipital-suboccipital craniotomy without torcular exposure. Patients are positioned laterally or prone with the "nose down," the AVM up, the midline vertical, and the head flexed to look down the axis of the tentorium, which rises as it deepens. By extending the craniotomy below transverse sinus and flapping the dura inferiorly, occipital retraction is minimized. Supratentorial-infraoccipital dissection leads to the AVM on the basal surface (step 2) or its draining vein, usually a posterior TempBasV or OccBasV (step 3). Dissection to the tentorial incisura allows CSF drainage from the quadrigeminal cistern and brain

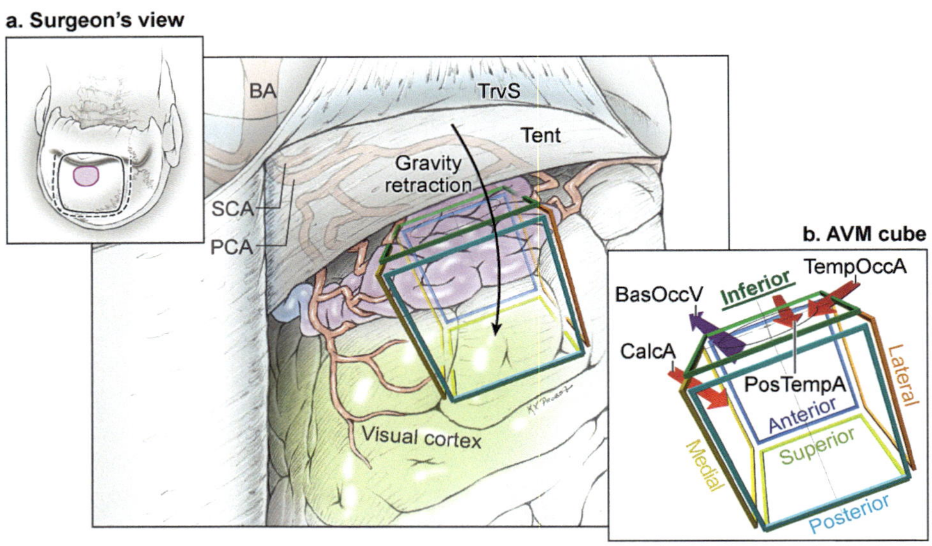

Fig. 13.19 Resection strategy for basal occipital AVMs. (**a**) Step 1, exposing the AVM with the patient positioned prone ("nose down"), a horseshoe scalp incision (*inset, dashed line*), torcular craniotomy eccentric to the AVM side (*inset, solid line*), and a supratentorial-infraoccipital approach (surgeon's view). A diagonal incision in the dura to the torcula creates two triangular dural flaps, one based on the SSS and the other based on the TrvS. (**b**) AVM box showing arterial supply from PosTempA with lesser contributions from CalcA and TempOccA, drainage to basal occipital veins, and proximity to visual cortex.

c. Surgeon's view

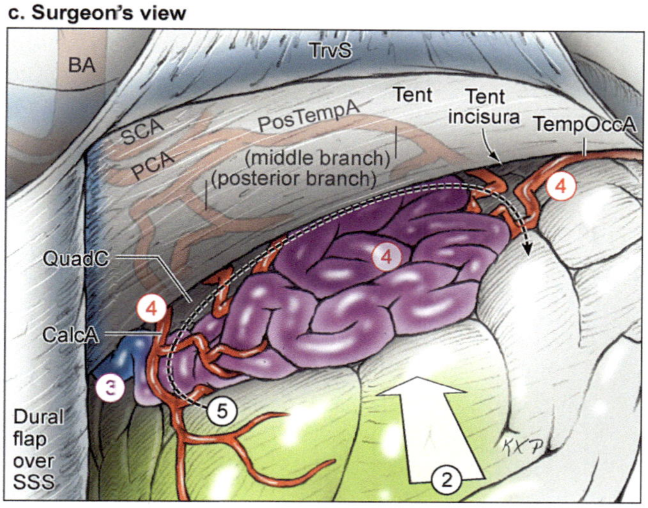

. Parasagittal view

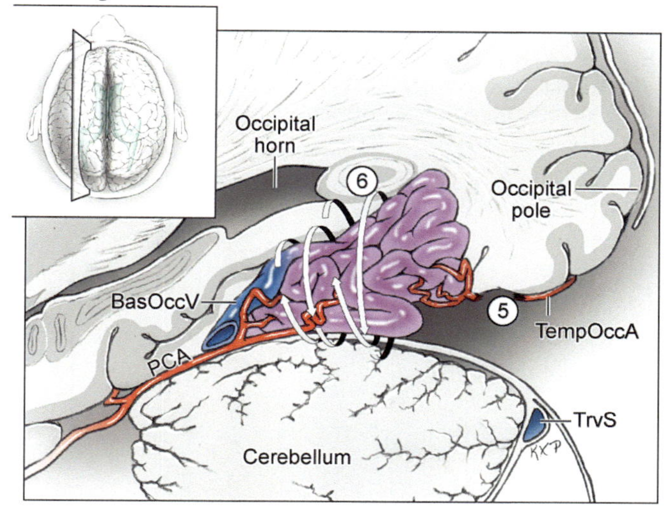

e. Surgeon's view

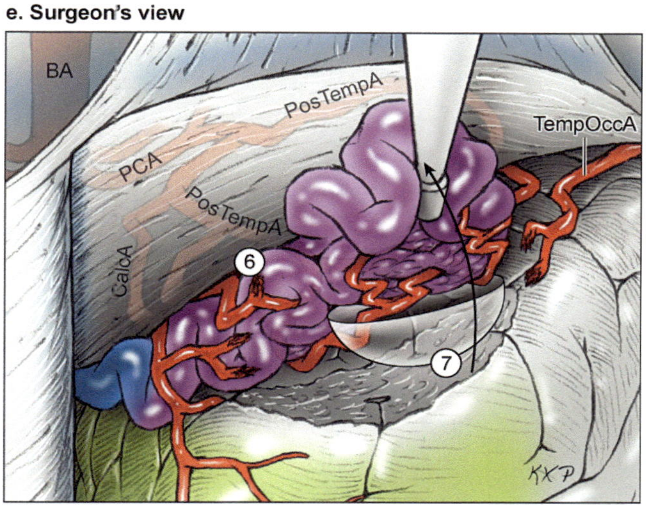

Fig. 13.19 (*continued*) (**c**) Step 2, opening the supratentorial-infra-occipital plane and releasing CSF from quadrigeminal cistern; step 3, identifying occipital basal veins; step 4, locating PCA feeding arteries (PosTempA); and step 5, interrupting the anterior front of arteries near fusiform gyrus and lingula (surgeon's view). (**d**) Step 6, circumdissecting superiorly into the occipital parenchyma (parasagittal cross-sectional view). (**e**) Step 7, mobilizing the AVM inferiorly to interrupt the PCA feeders supplying the superior side of the AVM (surgeon's view).

relaxation. PosTempA and CalcA supply these AVMs (step 4) at their anterior margin, and although they are deep to the nidus, they can be occluded in the pia early in their course along the tentorium at the OTG or lingula (step 5). Feeders that course in the sulci off the tentorium are occluded later, after circumdissecting the nidus and drawing it out of the occipital lobe, toward the tentorium and into the surgical corridor (step 6). Tight dissection planes spare the visual apparatus. Deep PCA feeders and deep veins (AntCalcV) are found during final ependymal dissection (step 7) (**Figs. 13.20** and **13.21**).

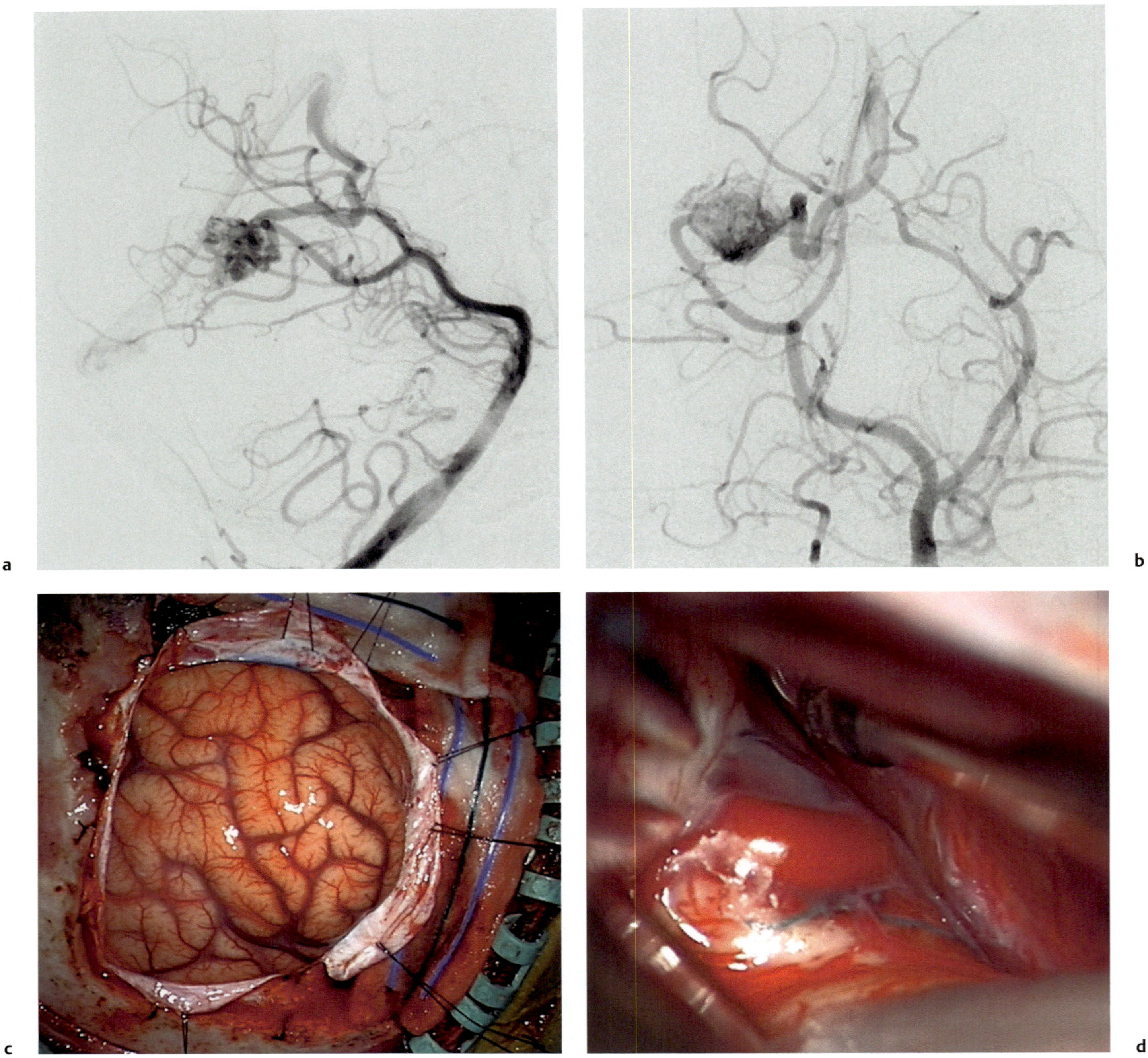

Fig. 13.20 This 15-year-old boy presented with a hemorrhage from a right basal occipital AVM (supplemented Spetzler-Martin grade 4: S1V1E1/A1B0C0), fed by a PCA branch (PosTempA) and draining to AntCalcV and VoG [right VA angiogram, (**a**) lateral and (**b**) anteroposterior views]. (**c**) The occipital lobe was exposed through a right torcular craniotomy with the patient in the lateral position, right side up, and the nose turned down (SSS vertical at right, and TrvS horizontal at top). (**d**) A supratentorial-infraoccipital approach arrived at the AVM's draining vein on the basal occipital surface, with some retraction on the occipital lobe (*bottom left*).

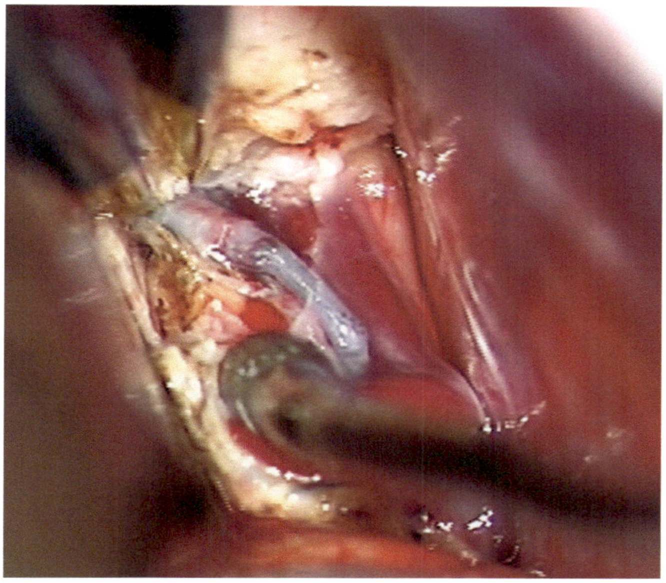

e

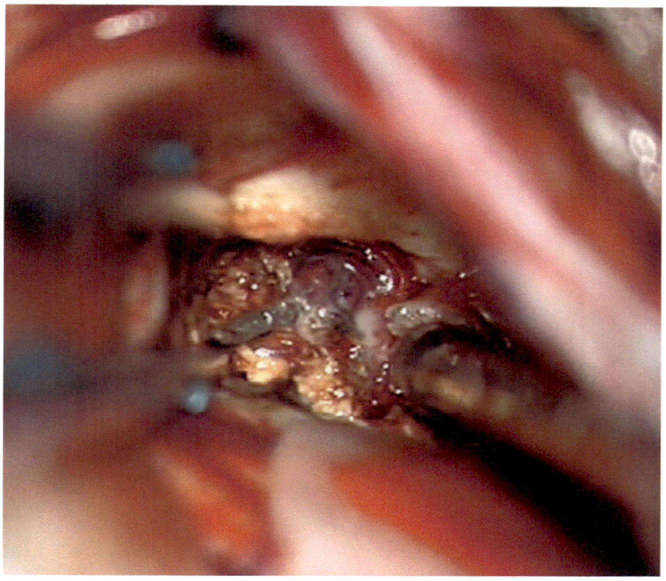

f

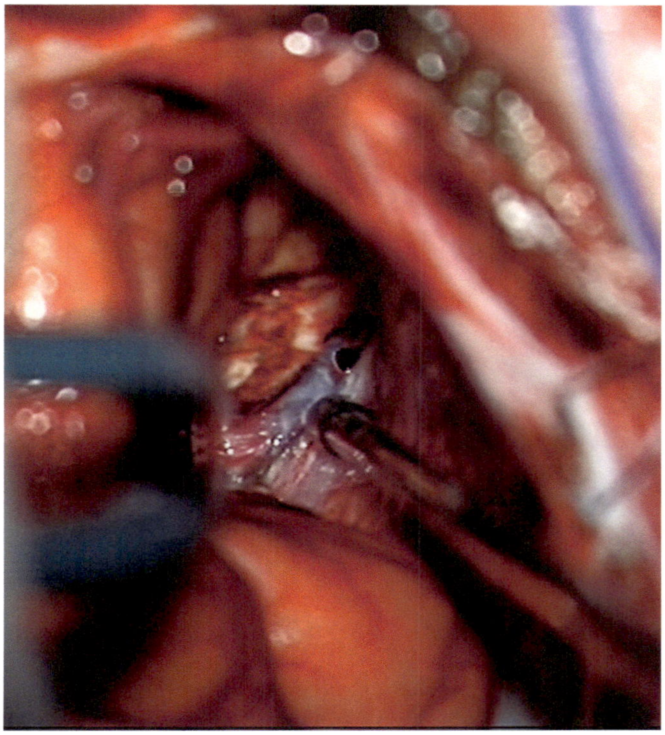

g

Fig. 13.20 (*continued*) (**e**) The PCA feeder was occluded and (**f**) the nidus was mobilized out of the occipital lobe toward the tentorium. The bipolars functioned as a dynamic retractor and allowed the fixed retractor to be removed. (**g**) This supratentorial-infraoccipital approach accessed the tentorial incisura (at the sucker tip) and the quadrigeminal cistern was drained for brain relaxation.

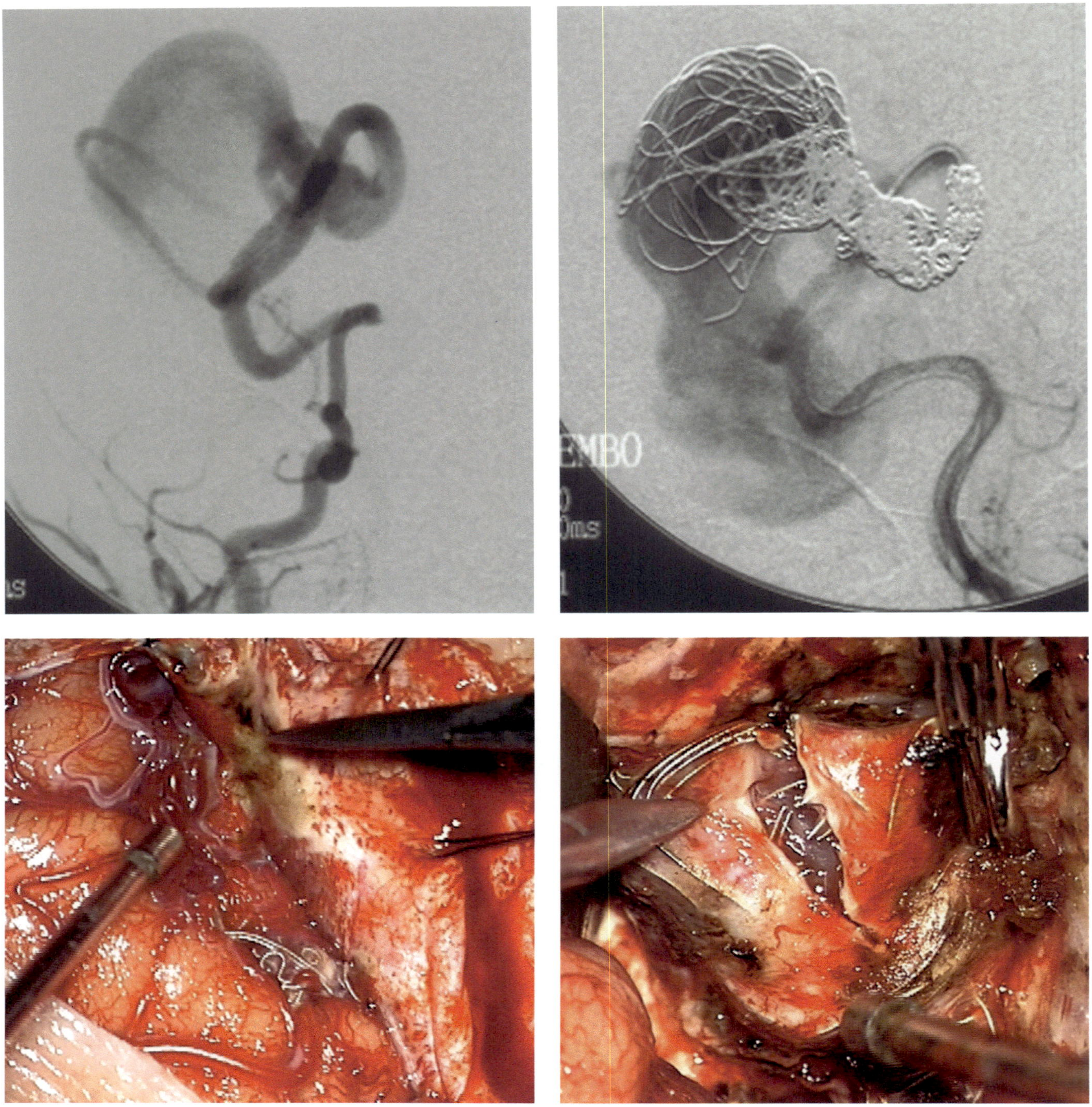

Fig. 13.21 This 3-year-old boy presented with this pial arteriovenous fistula located on the right basal occipital surface (supplemented Spetzler-Martin grade 2: S1V0E0/A1B0C0), supplied by two trunks of the PCA (PosTempA and CalcA) and drained by a giant varix [right VA angiogram, (**a**) anteroposterior view]. (**b**) The AVM was treated multiple times with coil embolization and incomplete obliteration (right VA angiogram, anteroposterior view). (**c**) The occipital lobe was exposed through a right torcular craniotomy with the patient in the lateral position, right side up, and the nose turned down, with the dural reflected along the lateral margin of an enlarged, triangular torcula (torcula at right, SSS vertical at right). A supratentorial-infraoccipital approach exposed the feeding arteries on the basal occipital surface, which were packed with coils (center). (**d**) After dividing these feeders, dissecting around the varix, and occluding its connection to the transverse sinus with clips, the varix was opened.

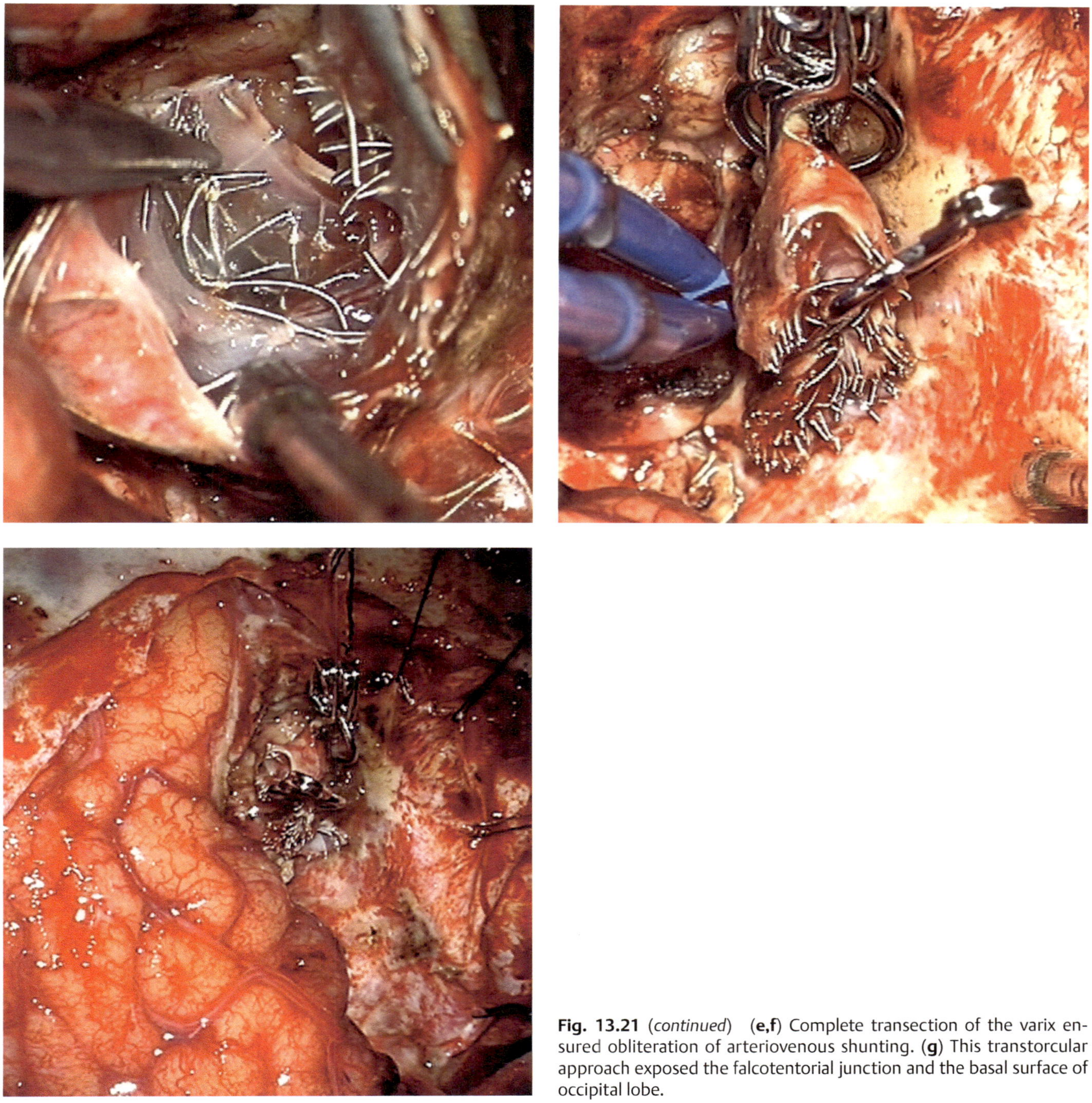

e f g

Fig. 13.21 (*continued*) (**e,f**) Complete transection of the varix ensured obliteration of arteriovenous shunting. (**g**) This transtorcular approach exposed the falcotentorial junction and the basal surface of occipital lobe.

Conclusion

Parieto-occipital AVMs differ from AVMs in the frontal and temporal lobes because of their more robust arterial supply from multiple territories and the difficulties in reaching the back of the head. Parieto-occipital AVMs require careful conceptualization of the craniotomy, exposure, and approach, in order to optimize patient position and gravity retraction. Convexity AVMs are common in the parieto-occipital lobe, as they are in the frontal and temporal lobes. As a whole, cerebral convexity AVMs account for nearly 30% of all AVMs, and when paramedian AVMs are included with lateral AVMs, this percentage rises to nearly 40%. This high frequency of convexity AVMs reflects the expanse of the cerebral hemispheres. Subsequent chapters delve into smaller, deeper regions beneath the hemisphere that account for fewer AVMs but require more complex exposures and techniques.

14 Ventricular and Periventricular Arteriovenous Malformations

Microsurgical Anatomy

Brain

The cerebrum separates neatly into frontal, temporal, and parieto-occipital lobes, and arteriovenous malformations (AVMs) located in the cerebral hemispheres are based on their cortical surfaces. The ventricles and deep structures of the central core lie at the center of the cerebrum and lack cortical surfaces, but have ependymal surfaces on which ventricular and periventricular AVMs are based. Although the central core is composed of neural structures (basal ganglia, thalamus, internal, external, and extreme capsules, to be covered in the following chapter), the ventricles are cavities whose contents are simply cerebrospinal fluid (CSF) and choroid plexus. Ventricular and periventricular AVMs reside in the choroid plexus and some of the structures that make up the ventricle's walls.

The lateral ventricle is composed of five parts: frontal horn, body, atrium, occipital horn, and temporal horn (**Fig. 14.1**). Choroid plexus is present only in the body, atrium, and temporal horn; its absence in the frontal and occipital horns accounts for the absence of AVMs there. Choroid plexus in the body of the lateral ventricle and the roof of the third ventricle are close and continuous, running through each foramen of Monro (FoM), turning around 180 degrees to hang as parallel strands into the third ventricle, and running to the suprapineal recess posteriorly.

The thalamus lies at the center of the cerebrum and the lateral ventricle wraps around it in a “C” shape. Three other C-shaped structures wrap around the thalamus superiorly, posteriorly, and inferiorly in the wall of the lateral ventricle: choroid plexus, fornix, and caudate nucleus. The fornix is composed of hippocampomammillary tract fibers that arise as fimbria on the ventricular surface of the hippocampal formation in temporal horn. They form the crus of the fornix, which courses posteriorly, wraps around the pulvinar of the thalamus, and joins the opposite crus in the body of the lat-

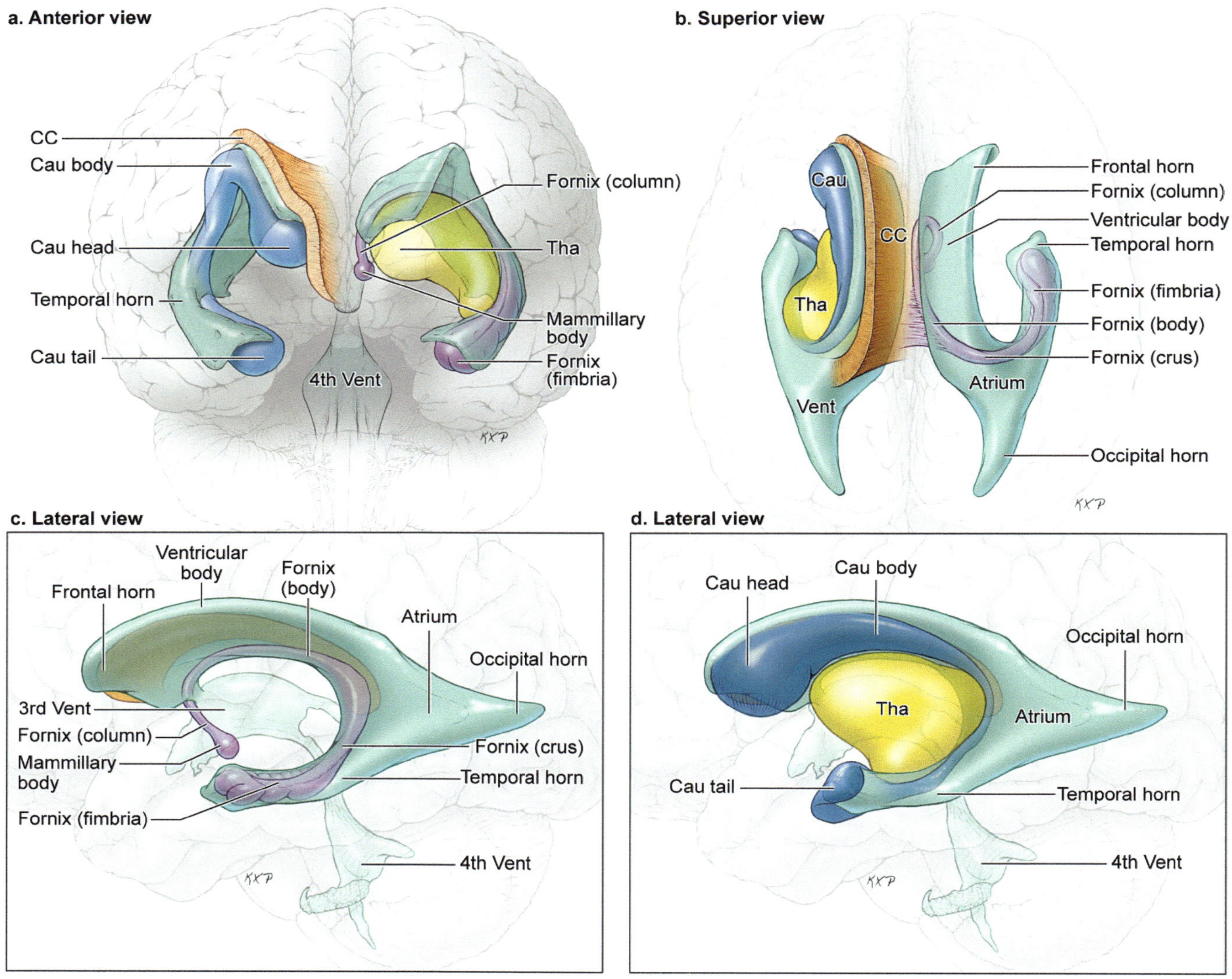

Fig. 14.1 Microsurgical anatomy of the ventricles and periventricular structures. Five parts of the lateral ventricle (frontal horn, ventricular body, atrium, temporal horn, and occipital horn) and five C-shaped structures wrapping around the thalamus (lateral ventricle, caudate nucleus, fornix, choroid plexus, and corpus callosum) are shown in (**a**) anterior, (**b**) superior, and (**c,d**) lateral views.

e. Coronal section

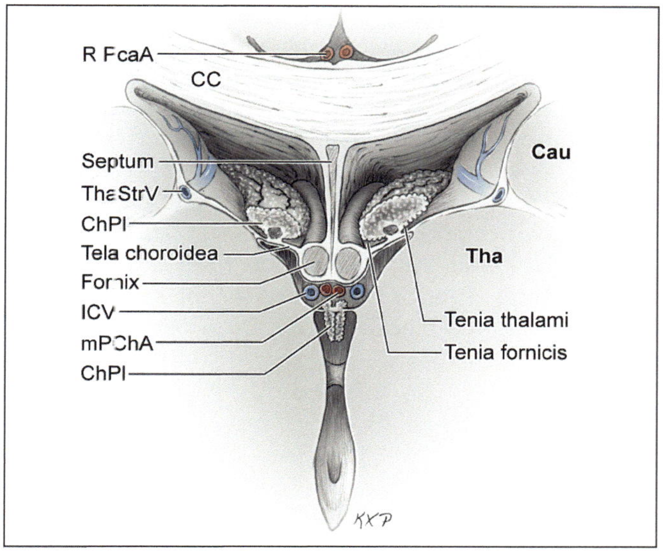

f. Axial section

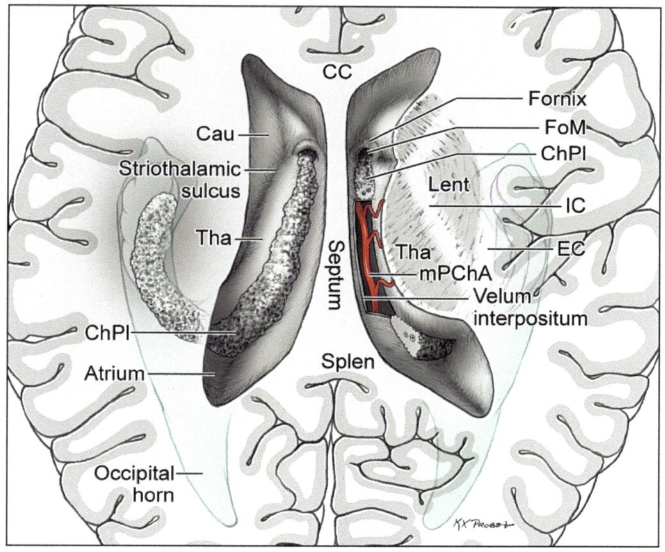

Fig. 14.1 (*continued*) Microsurgical anatomy of the ventricular body and choroidal fissure, (**e**) coronal and (**f**) axial cross-sectional views, with the tela choroidea cut and a portion of the choroid plexus removed from the right ventricular body to show the mPChA in the velum interpositum.

eral ventricle to become the body of fornix. The fornix continues forward along the superomedial thalami in the medial wall of the lateral ventricular body, splits anteriorly into two columns, and then dives into the anterior margin of the FoM to end in the mammillary bodies. The caudate nucleus forms the lateral wall of the lateral ventricle with its head bulging into the ventricle at the frontal horn and body, its body forming part of the lateral wall at the atrium, and its tail curving into the roof of the temporal horn.

The corpus callosum forms the largest part of the ventricular walls, and is made up of the rostrum and genu anteriorly, the body centrally, and the splenium posteriorly. The rostrum forms the floor of the frontal horn; the genu and body form the roof; and the splenium forms the medial wall of the atrium. The septum pellucidum separates the lateral ventricles in the midline. It is composed of two laminae that are normally fused (but may also be separated as a cavum septum pellucidum) and attach to the genu and rostrum in the frontal horn and to the body and fornix in the ventricular body.

The choroidal fissure is a narrow cleft between the fornix and thalamus where the choroid plexus attaches in the ventricular body, atrium, and temporal horn (**Fig. 14.1**). The choroidal fissure extends in a C-shaped arc from the FoM, around the thalamic surfaces, to the inferior choroidal point behind the head of hippocampus. The choroidal fissure is divided into the ventricular body and atrial and temporal parts. The tela choroidea is the clear membrane in which the choroid plexus arises, and the tela choroidea attaches to neural structures via small ridges called teniae: tenia thalami, tenia fornicis, and tenia fimbriae. The temporal part of the choroidal fissure is in the temporal horn between the fimbria of the fornix and thalamus. The body portion of the choroidal fissure opens into the velum interpositum and roof of third ventricle. The third ventricle is a narrow, funnel-shaped, midline cavity located below the body of the lateral ventricles between the two halves of thalamus and hypothalamus. Third ventricle communicates with each lateral ventricle through the FoM and with the fourth ventricle through the aqueduct of Sylvius. The roof of the third ventricle is composed of four layers: the fornix, two membranes of the tela choroidea, and a layer of blood vessels between the tela [the medial posterior choroidal artery (mPChA) and the internal cerebral vein (ICV)]. The velum interpositum is the space between the two layers of the tela in the roof of the third ventricle. Veins of the body and frontal horn converge on the ICV in the velum interpositum just behind the FoM. The confluence of arteries and veins traveling in the velum interpositum make this is an important region for ventricular AVMs.

Arteries

The ependyma and choroid plexus of the lateral and third ventricles are supplied by the anterior (AChA) and posterior choroidal arteries (mPChA and lateral posterior choroidal artery [lPChA]) (**Fig. 14.2**). The AChA arises from lateral supraclinoid internal carotid artery (ICA) as its last branch before its terminal bifurcation. Its initial "cisternal" segment has a characteristic posteromedial course, which on anteroposterior angiography is seen medial to the ICA. It passes below and medial to the optic tract to reach the lateral aspect of the cerebral peduncle and the crural cistern, where it runs between the cerebral peduncle and uncus. It climbs superiorly on the uncus to reach the choroidal fissure of the temporal lobe. This cisternal segment is bisected by the lateral geniculate body. The AChA's intraventricular "plexal" segment begins at the plexal point where it pierces the choroidal fissure, enters the temporal horn, and supplies the choroid plexus. It continues posteriorly along the medial border of the choroidal plexus in close relation to and anastomosing frequently with branches of the lPChA. Critical branches from the cisternal segment supply the optic tract, the middle third of the cerebral peduncle, the posterior limb of the internal capsule, the lateral geniculate body, the globus pallidus, and

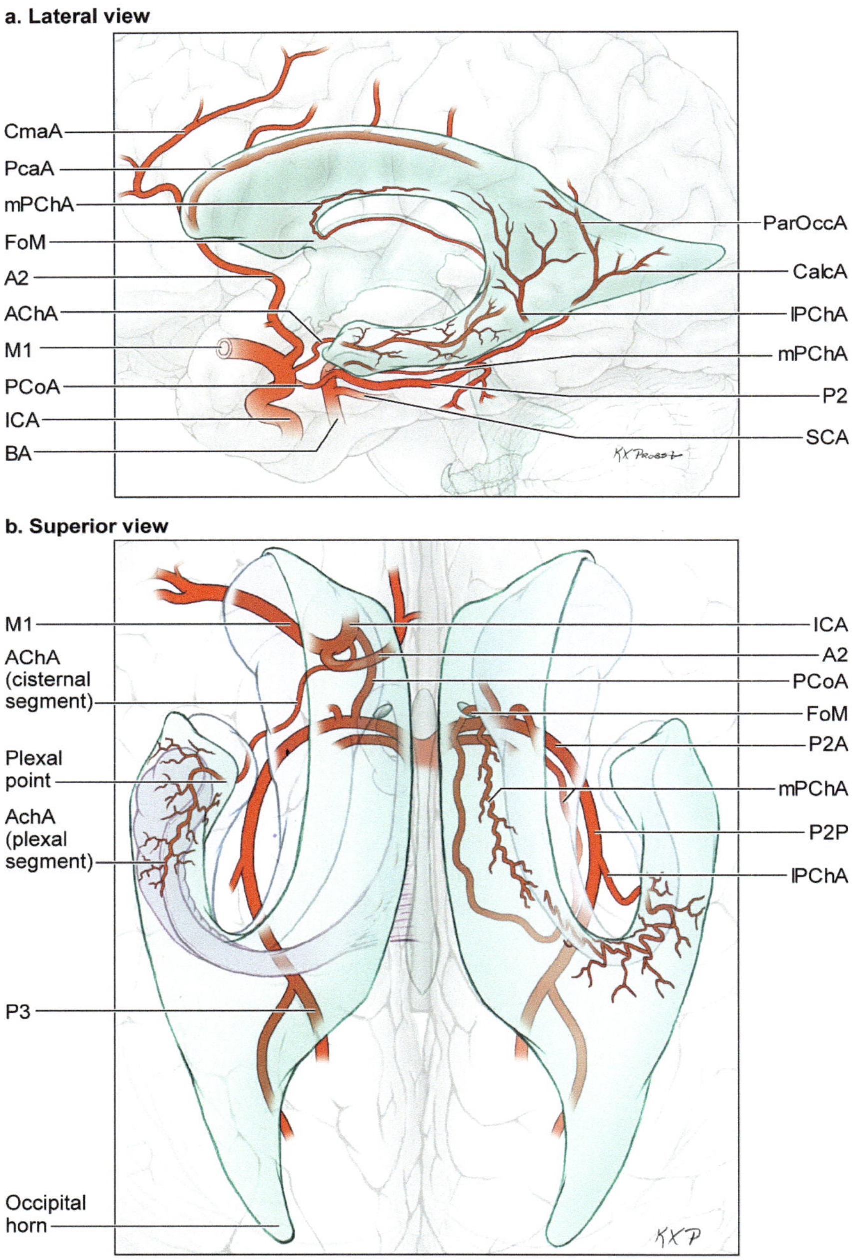

Fig. 14.2 Microsurgical anatomy of the ventricular arteries. The ependyma and choroid plexus of the lateral and third ventricles are supplied by choroidal arteries (AChA, mPChA, and lPChA), (**a**) lateral and (**b**) superior views. The AChA has cisternal and plexal segments divided by the plexal point, where it traverses the choroidal fissure of the temporal horn. The mPChA has a long course from the P2 PCA to the atrium, encircling the midbrain, coursing through the velum interpositum, and running along the lateral ventricular floor, with two complete reversals of direction along the way. The lPChA has a straight course from the distal P2 PCA to the atrium.

the origin of optic radiations, whereas branches from the plexal segment are usually non-eloquent.

The mPChA arises from the posterior cerebral artery (PCA) along its proximal P2 postcommunicating segment (crural segment, P2A) on its medial wall. It may also arise from the P3 quadrigeminal segment or from ParOccA or CalcA. The mPChA encircles the midbrain, paralleling the PCA trunk before curling forward at the superior colliculus and ascending next to the pineal gland to the roof of the third ventricle. There it enters the velum interpositum to course between the thalami to the FoM and the choroidal fissure. It makes a hairpin turn to enter the lateral ventricles and course posteriorly in the lateral ventricular floor. This course of the mPChA on angiography has been characterized as the "3 sign" from the curvature in the artery as it drapes over the superior colliculus and pineal gland. The course of the mPChA has two complete reversals of direction, one gradually around the pineal region posteriorly and the other sharply through the FoM anteriorly. The mPChA may be duplicated or rarely triplicated, and it sends branches along its course to the cerebral peduncle, tegmentum, geniculate bodies, colliculi, pulvinar, pineal gland, and medial thalamus.

The lPChA originates from the distal P2 segment (ambient segment, P2P), courses laterally through the ambient cistern, and enters the choroidal fissure of the lateral ventricle at the posterior part of the temporal horn and atrium. There are multiple lPChAs (four on average) that anastomose with the mPChA as its runs posteriorly toward the atrium and with the AChA as it runs posteriorly in the temporal horn. The lPChA sends branches to the cerebral peduncle, posterior commissure, fornix (crura and body), lateral geniculate body, pulvinar, dorsomedial thalamic nucleus, and body of caudate nucleus.

Corpus callosum is supplied by the anterior cerebral artery (ACA) and pericallosal artery (PcaA). Short callosal arteries from the PcaA penetrate the genu and body of the corpus callosum to supply these structures and the septum pellucidum, columns of fornix, and anterior commissure. Long callosal arteries run parallel to the PcaA and also supply the corpus callosum. Splenium is supplied by SplenA, which originates variously from ParOccA, CalcA, PosTempA, mPChA, or lPChA. SplenA anastomoses with the PcaA to complete the "limbic loop," a collateral circuit around the corpus callosum that connects the ACA and PCA circulations.

Veins

Ventricular veins on the lateral ventricular walls provide landmarks during intraventricular surgery that are often more orienting than the arteries, which are smaller, fewer in number, and buried below tufts of choroid plexus. Veins are easily visible in the ependyma (**Fig. 14.3**) and with AVMs, and are often dilated and tortuous. Anterior and posterior septal veins (SepV) drain the medial frontal horn and course to the FoM where they terminate in the ICV. Anterior and posterior caudate veins (CauV) drain the lateral frontal horn and terminate in the thalamostriate vein (ThaStrV) near the FoM. ThaStrV courses in the striothalamic sulcus between the caudate nucleus and thalamus. It makes a hairpin turn at the posterior margin of the FoM to enter the velum interpositum and join the ICV, a turn known angiographically as the "venous angle" on lateral views in the venous phase. The ICVs are paired, parallel veins running in the velum interpositum from the FoM to the vein of Galen (VoG). The two ICVs, two basal veins of Rosenthal (BVRs), and the precentral cerebellar vein converge on the VoG.

Medial atrial veins (AtrV) drain the medial wall of the atrium, passing through the fornix or choroidal fissure to the ICV in the velum interpositum. The lateral AtrV drains

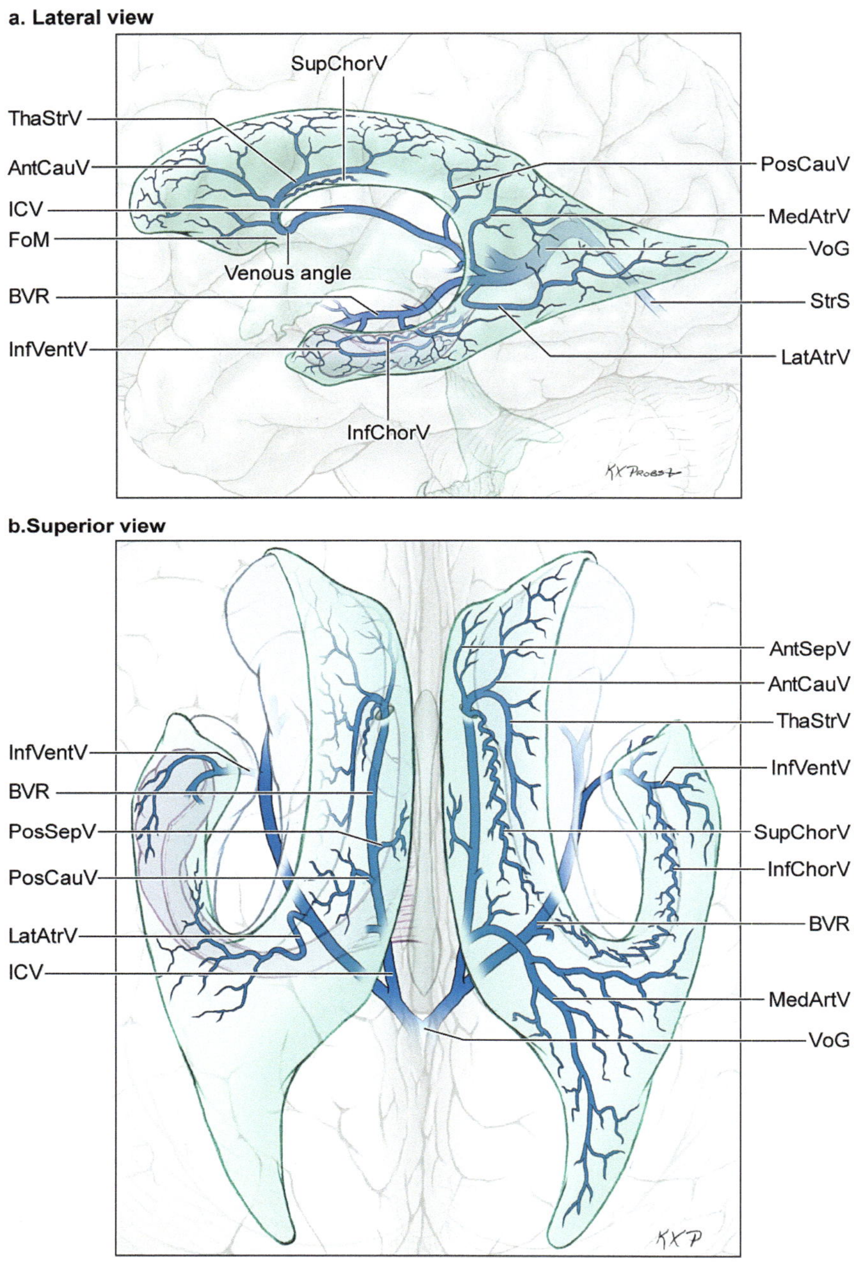

Fig. 14.3 Microsurgical anatomy of ventricular veins and deep venous system. (**a**) Veins of the lateral ventricle, lateral and (**b**) superior views.

the lateral wall of the atrium and passes through the choroidal fissure to reach the BVR in the ambient or quadrigeminal cisterns. The medial and lateral AtrV can join near the choroidal fissure to form a common trunk, the common atrial vein. The superior choroidal vein (ChorV), the largest of the choroidal veins, runs in the choroid plexus in the body of the lateral ventricle and terminates in ThaStrV in the FoM. The inferior ChorV runs in the temporal horn and terminates in the inferior ventricular vein or the amygdaloid vein, which then exits the choroidal fissure to join the BVR. The superior and inferior ChorVs anastomose in the glomus of the choroid plexus in the atrium.

Four Ventricular AVM Subtypes

Ventricular and periventricular AVM subtypes include callosal, ventricular body, atrial, and temporal horn AVMs.

The Callosal AVM

Callosal AVMs are located in the roof of the lateral ventricles (**Fig. 14.4**). This subtype was the most common, accounting for more than half of ventricular/periventricular AVMs. The classic AVM is entirely in the corpus callosum, but it can extend superiorly to involve some cingulate gyrus or inferiorly into the septum or lateral ventricle. Callosal AVM locations range from rostrum to splenium with important anatomic and surgical differences, but they are considered collectively because of their relative rarity (approximately 4% of all brain AVMs). They are supplied by the ACA and PcaA, which give rise bilaterally to short and long callosal arteries on their inferior and medial surfaces that descend into the corpus callosum and AVM. These feeding arteries are tiny in the absence of callosal AVMs but enlarge in their presence. Normal branches to the cingulate gyrus and medial frontal lobe can be differentiated from AVM feeders by their small size and their origin from PcaA's lateral surface. The PcaA is typically a transit artery that supplies the medial homunculus for the

Medial view

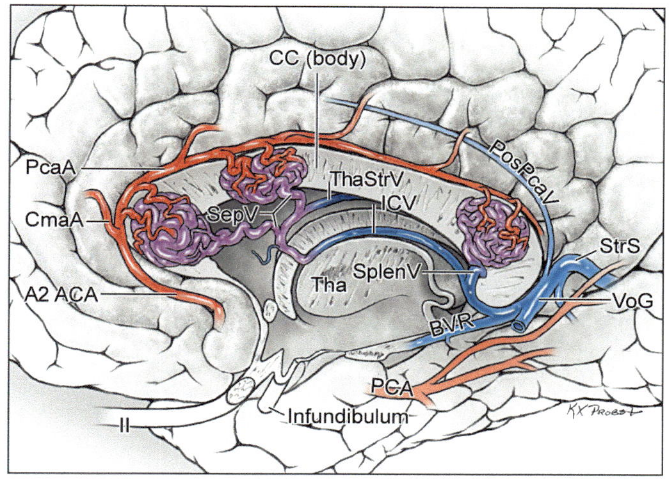

Fig. 14.4 The callosal AVM, medial view. Callosal AVMs are located in the corpus callosum and range from the rostrum to the splenium; three different callosal AVMs are shown in the genu, body, and splenium. They are supplied by long and short callosal arteries branching from the ACA and PcaA, and drain deeply to ventricular veins (SepV, CauV, and ThaStrV).

motor and sensory cortex distal to the AVM, and therefore must be preserved by skeletonization. Although anterior callosal AVMs in the genu and body are supplied by the PcaA, posterior callosal AVMs are also supplied by SplenA from the PCA. Callosal AVMs that extend laterally into the frontal white matter can get additional supply from the medial lenticulostriate artery (mLSA) or lateral lenticulostriate artery (lLSA). Although they are included with ventricular AVMs, callosal AVMs do not involve the choroid plexus and are not supplied by the choroidal arteries. Callosal AVMs drain deep into ventricular veins (SepV, CauV, ThaStrV, and ICV). Splenial AVMs also drain deep to the VoG, either via SplenV that remains extraventricular or through MedAtrV that descends to the ICV distal to the FoM. Callosal AVMs are not strictly eloquent, but the splenium has been implicated in calculation and visuospatial processing.

The Ventricular Body AVM

The ventricular body AVM is a midline AVM located in the center of the lateral ventricular system at the complex intersection of the thalamus, caudate nucleus, fornix, septum, velum interpositum, choroid plexus, and choroidal fissure (**Fig. 14.5**). Ventricular body AVMs include those in the septum, body of fornix, velum interpositum, and choroid plexus of the ventricular body or third ventricle. Ventricular body AVMs do not include those in the lateral wall, lateral floor, or roof of the ventricular body. The caudate nucleus forms the lateral wall, and AVMs here are included in the basal ganglial subtype of deep AVMs; the thalamus forms the lateral floor, and AVMs here are included in the thalamic subtype of deep AVMs; and the corpus callosum forms the roof of the ventricular body and AVMs here are included in the callosal subtype. Ventricular body AVMs are uncommon, accounting for only 12% of ventricular/periventricular AVMs. They are challenging because they are deeper than callosal AVMs and accessible only through a small opening in the corpus callosum and choroidal fissure. The mPChA runs through the center of the region and is the major feeder to these AVMs. The lPChA supply is usually minimal. The PcaA contributes to AVMs in the septum. The mLSA and anterior communicating artery (ACoA) perforators can supply septal AVMs anterior to the FoM. The ICV also runs through the center of the region and drains these AVMs. The fornix is intimately related to these AVMs, forming the medial border of the choroidal fissure and also descending in the anterior aspect of the FoM. Even though the ventricular body AVM is surrounded by CSF rather than parenchyma, forniceal manipulation can cause debilitating memory and cognitive impairment, making it an eloquent AVM that requires careful handling.

Medial view

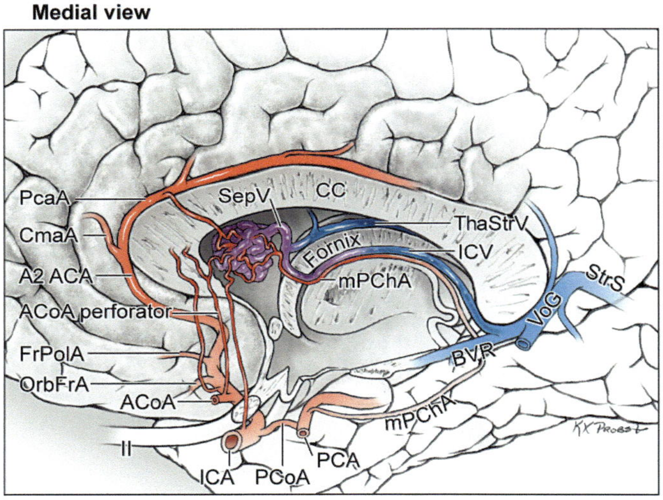

Fig. 14.5 The ventricular body AVM, medial view. Ventricular body AVMs include those in the septum, body of fornix, velum interpositum, and choroid plexus of the ventricular body and the roof of third ventricle. The mPChA is a consistent supplier to these AVMs, with additional supply from the PcaA, ACoA perforators, mLSA, and lPChA, depending on location. Venous drainage collects in the internal cerebral vein.

The Ventricular Atrium AVM

The atrial AVM resides in the atrium, posterior and lateral to the ventricular body (**Fig. 14.6**). Callosal and ventricular body AVMs are midline, whereas atrial and temporal horn AVMs have laterality. The C-shaped structures that wrap around the thalamus (i.e., caudate nucleus, crus of fornix, and choroid plexus) deviate laterally as they course around its posterior surface toward the temporal horn, and atrial

Axial section

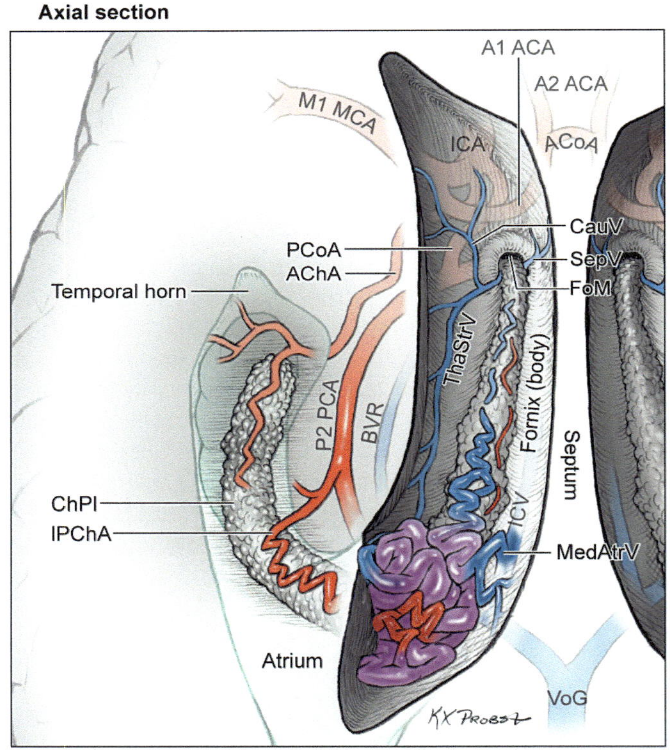

Fig. 14.6 The ventricular atrium AVM, axial cross-sectional view. This AVM is located in the atrium of the lateral ventricle, supplied by the lPChA, and drained by atrial veins (medial to the ICV and lateral to the BVR).

AVMs are in the middle zone between the ventricular body and temporal horn. They were the second most common ventricular/periventricular subtype and accounted for around 20%. Atrial AVMs are supplied by the lPChA, which enters the ventricle at the atrial portion of the choroidal fissure. Collateral connections within the choroid plexus enable the AChA to supply these AVMs from below via the temporal horn's plexus, and the mPChA to supply them from anteriorly via the ventricular body's plexus. Atrial AVMs drain through the medial and lateral AtrVs that course through the choroidal fissure of the atrium and connect to the ICV and BVR, respectively. Atrial AVMs sit on the pulvinar surface, which has no eloquence, but the crus of the fornix lies medial to the choroid plexus. Atrial AVMs differ from thalamic AVMs that may protrude into the atrium, but are deeply embedded in the thalamus, extend close to the posterior limb of the internal capsule, are supplied by thalamoperforators rather than choroidal arteries, and are exquisitely eloquent.

The Temporal Horn AVM

The temporal horn AVM is based on the choroid plexus in the temporal horn (**Fig. 14.7**). This AVM differs from the medial temporal AVM that lies medial to the temporal horn in the uncus, hippocampus, and parahippocampus. Temporal horn AVMs are surrounded almost entirely by ependyma. When they present with hemorrhage, the bleeding is intraventricular rather than intraparenchymal. Their primary supply is the plexal segment of the AChA, which is enlarged. The lPChA can also contribute to these AVMs through the choroidal fissure and collateral connections from the atrium. The choroidal fissure of the medial temporal lobe forms a stalk of arterial supply to the nidus medially. Venous drainage is via the inferior ChorV, which exits the choroidal fissure via the inferior ventricular vein and joins the BVR in the ambient cistern. Temporal horn AVMs typically respect ependymal boundaries and spare eloquent hippocampal structures.

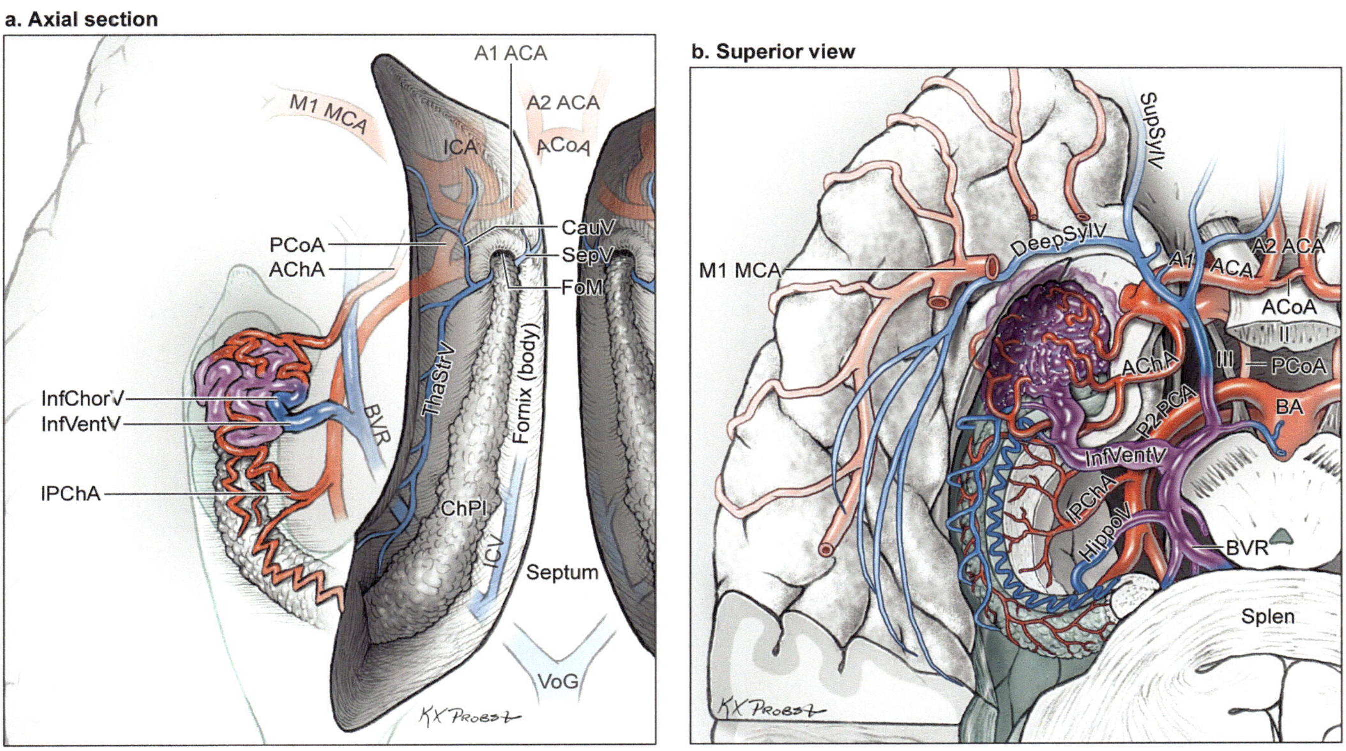

Fig. 14.7 The temporal horn AVM: (**a**) axial cross-sectional and (**b**) superior views, with the temporal horn unroofed. This AVM is located in the choroid plexus and choroidal fissure of the temporal horn, supplied by the AChA and to a lesser degree the lPChA, and drained by the inferior choroidal and inferior ventricular veins.

Ventricular/Periventricular AVM Resection Strategies

Callosal AVM Resection

The callosal AVM is exposed with a bifrontal craniotomy and gravity retraction to open the anterior interhemispheric fissure (**Fig. 14.8,** step 1). The AVM's midline location allows for a right-sided approach down the interhemispheric fissure that avoids a craniotomy over and the bridging veins on the dominant hemisphere. The patient is positioned supine with the left shoulder bolstered, the head turned 90 degrees to the right, the midline aligned horizontally, and the neck flexed laterally to bring the vertex up 45 degrees. A C-shaped scalp incision begins at the widow's peak, courses posteriorly slightly to the left of midline, and then arcs laterally and anteriorly. The craniotomy is positioned two thirds anterior and one third posterior to coronal suture, crossing the superior sagittal sinus (SSS) to remove any bone that might overhang the interhemispheric fissure. The SSS is crossed carefully with the craniotome, establishing its epidural location visually by aiming light into the cut of bone and irrigating to see intact dura before crossing the sinus. If a dural tear is detected, the flap is taken in two pieces. The craniotomy flap can be raised as one flap in younger patients with nonadherent dura and in many women with a shallow bony sulcus around the SSS. However, this flap is raised in two pieces in elderly patients or those with adherent dura. The first piece is a unilateral frontal flap taken up to, but not across, the SSS. After removing this bone flap, dura-containing SSS is dissected from the inner table of the skull under direct visualization and the second portion of the craniotomy safely crosses the SSS twice with the dura retracted. The dura is opened with a semicircular flap based on the SSS anterior to the bridging frontal veins. A vein that fuses with the dura before reaching the SSS can be saved by dividing the dural flap on both sides of the vein and elevating two flaps, fashioning a sleeve of dura over the vein.

After releasing arachnoid adhesions and granulations adjacent to the SSS, gravity pulls the hemisphere away from the falx and opens the interhemispheric fissure without a retractor (step 2). Dissection along the falx continues to its free edge. The corpus callosum cistern is opened and dissection along an ascending branch from the callosomarginal artery (CmaA) identifies the subarachnoid plane that separates the medial frontal lobes. Dissection deepens the PcaA and widens anteriorly and posteriorly along the PcaA to get around the AVM. The callosal AVMs drain inferiorly into the ventricular veins (SepV, CauV, ThaStrV, and ICV) that are not visualized until after dissecting through the corpus callosum into the ventricle (step 3). Similarly, posterior drainage to SplenV may not be seen until after dissecting the back end of the nidus. Bilateral PcaAs course on top of the nidus and supply the AVM's superior margin (step 4), giving an overview of feeding callosal arteries that facilitates skeletonization. Distal-to-proximal (posterior-to-anterior) skeletonization helps preserve the distal PcaA trunk that nourishes the downstream sensorimotor cortex. Short callosal feeding arteries are coagulated along a superior front as they originate from the PcaA's inferior surface, and long callosal feeding arteries are coagulated along an anterior front as they travel to the nidus (step 5). Parenchymal dissection proceeds transcallosally with planes developed laterally on both sides of the corpus callosum and posteriorly (step 6). Transcallosal dissection has a parallel angle of attack, but transcingulate dissection outside the interhemispheric fissure for larger callosal AVMs that extend laterally might require mobiliza-

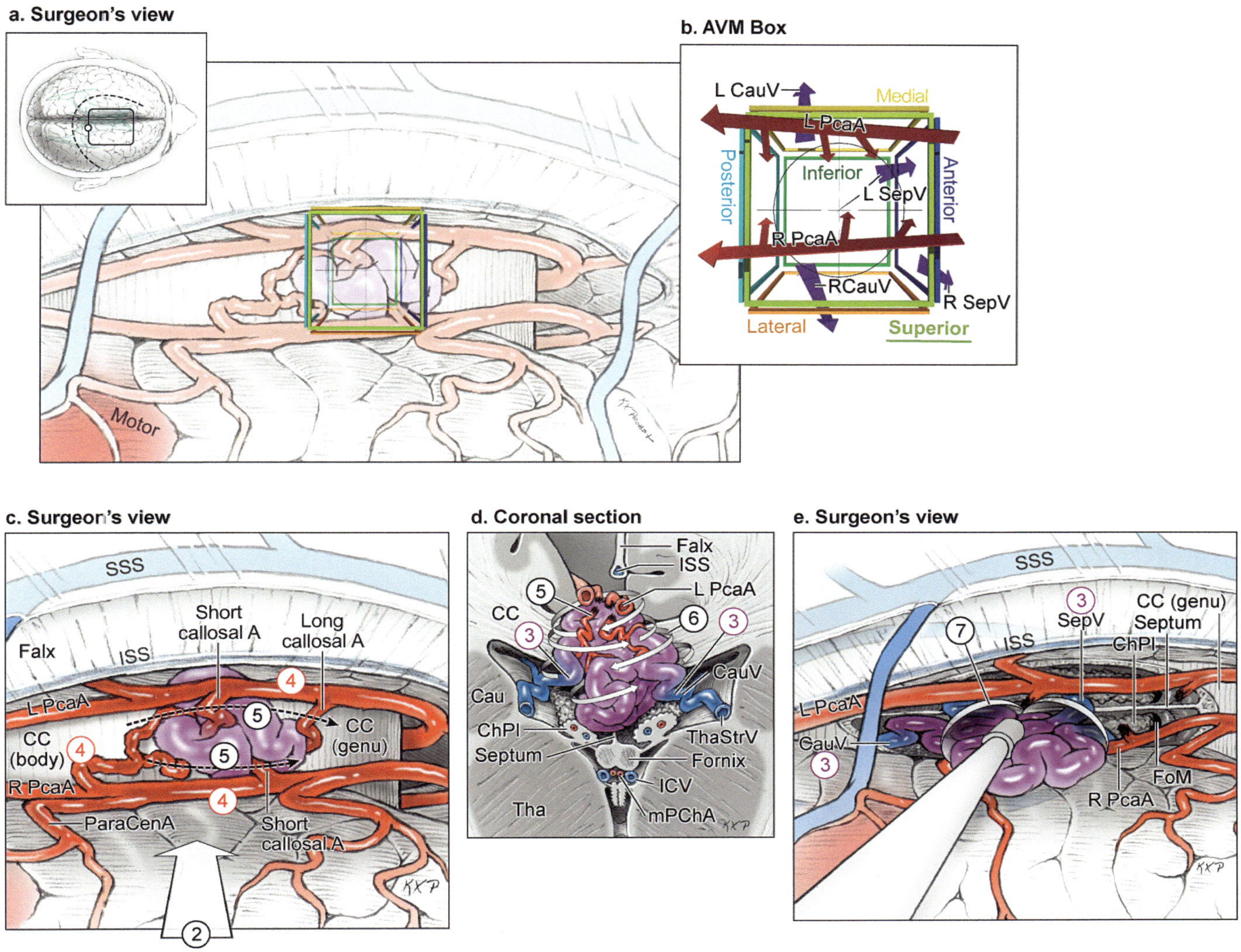

Fig. 14.8 Resection strategy for callosal AVMs. (**a**) Step 1, exposing the AVM with a semicircular scalp incision (*inset, dashed line*), bifrontal craniotomy (*inset, solid line*), and anterior interhemispheric approach with the midline oriented horizontally for gravity retraction of the right hemisphere (surgeon's view). (**b**) AVM box showing arterial supply from short and long callosal branches from the pericallosal arteries, descending drainage to the ventricular veins (SepV and CauV), and proximity to the motor cortex (red). Note that the AVM's superficial surface is depicted with a circle on its base side and that side's label is underlined. The AVM's axis is depicted with a line through the box. Arterial and venous anatomy are superimposed on the box with red inflow arrows and blue outflow arrows, respectively. (**c**) Step 2, widely opening the interhemispheric fissure down to the corpus callosum (broad white arrow, surgeon's view). Although the dura has been resected in this illustration to view venous connections to the SSS, it is elevated medially as a flap that requires release of arachnoidal adhesions and preservation of the bridging veins. Step 3, draining veins are not visualized until after dividing the corpus callosum; step 4, identifying the feeding callosal arteries originating from the PcaA bilaterally; and step 5, interrupting the anterior front of long callosal arteries and skeletonizing the superior front of short callosal arteries in a distal-to-proximal direction (*dashed black lines*). (**d**) Step 6, dissecting transcallosally into the lateral ventricles (*encircling arrows,* coronal cross-sectional view). (**e**) Step 7, identifying draining veins and dissecting ependymal planes in ventricles and across septum (spherical scoops, surgeon's view).

tion of the nidus toward the midline. Ependymal dissection of callosal AVMs is the easiest of all AVMs because the deep side is surrounded by CSF and one needs only to enter the ventricle (step 7). This side connects with septal arteries and ventricular veins that are not visualized until the ventricle is opened, and they are both carefully divided because of the danger of interventricular bleeding. Before closing, an intraventricular clot that might obstruct the FoM is evacuated. Most callosal AVMs are in the body of the corpus callosum (**Figs. 14.9** and **14.10**), but those in the rostrum, genu, and

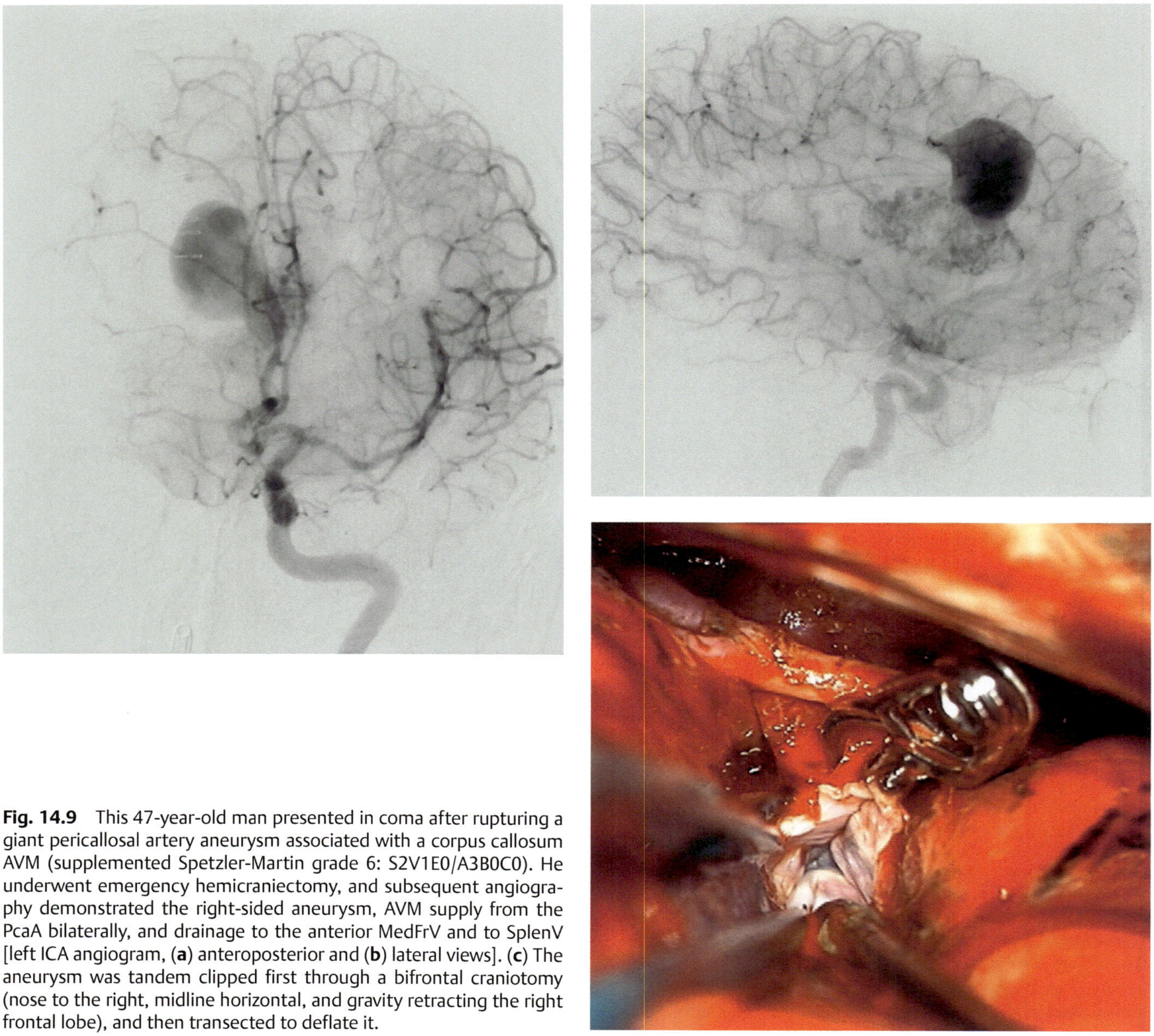

a b c

Fig. 14.9 This 47-year-old man presented in coma after rupturing a giant pericallosal artery aneurysm associated with a corpus callosum AVM (supplemented Spetzler-Martin grade 6: S2V1E0/A3B0C0). He underwent emergency hemicraniectomy, and subsequent angiography demonstrated the right-sided aneurysm, AVM supply from the PcaA bilaterally, and drainage to the anterior MedFrV and to SplenV [left ICA angiogram, (**a**) anteroposterior and (**b**) lateral views]. (**c**) The aneurysm was tandem clipped first through a bifrontal craniotomy (nose to the right, midline horizontal, and gravity retracting the right frontal lobe), and then transected to deflate it.

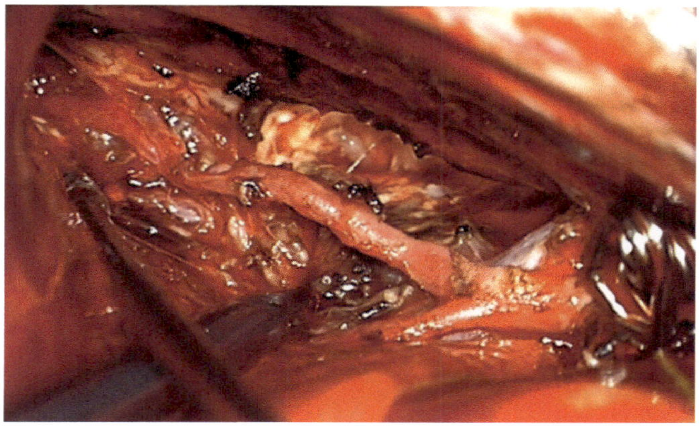
d

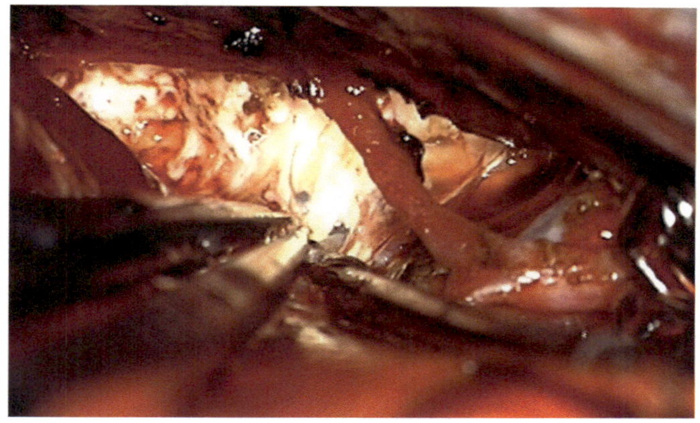
e

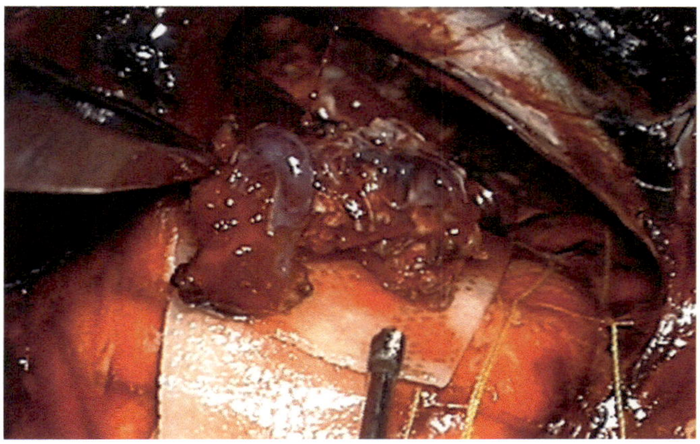
f

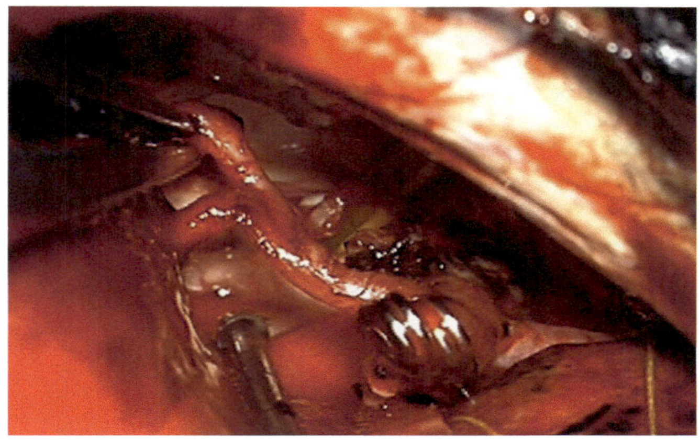
g

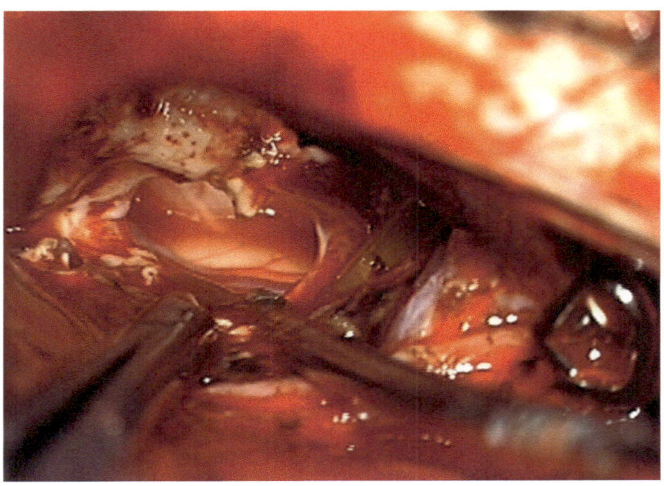
h

Fig. 14.9 (*continued*) (**d**) The efferent artery from the aneurysm (R PcaA) coursed on top of the AVM and was skeletonized to detach it from the AVM. (**e**) The left lateral margin of the AVM was dissected through corpus callosum and into lateral ventricle. (**f**) The AVM was removed, (**g**) with preservation of the distal PcaA. (**h**) Entry into the ventricle was necessary to interrupt all callosal feeders. Note the tip of the ventriculostomy catheter to the right of the sucker.

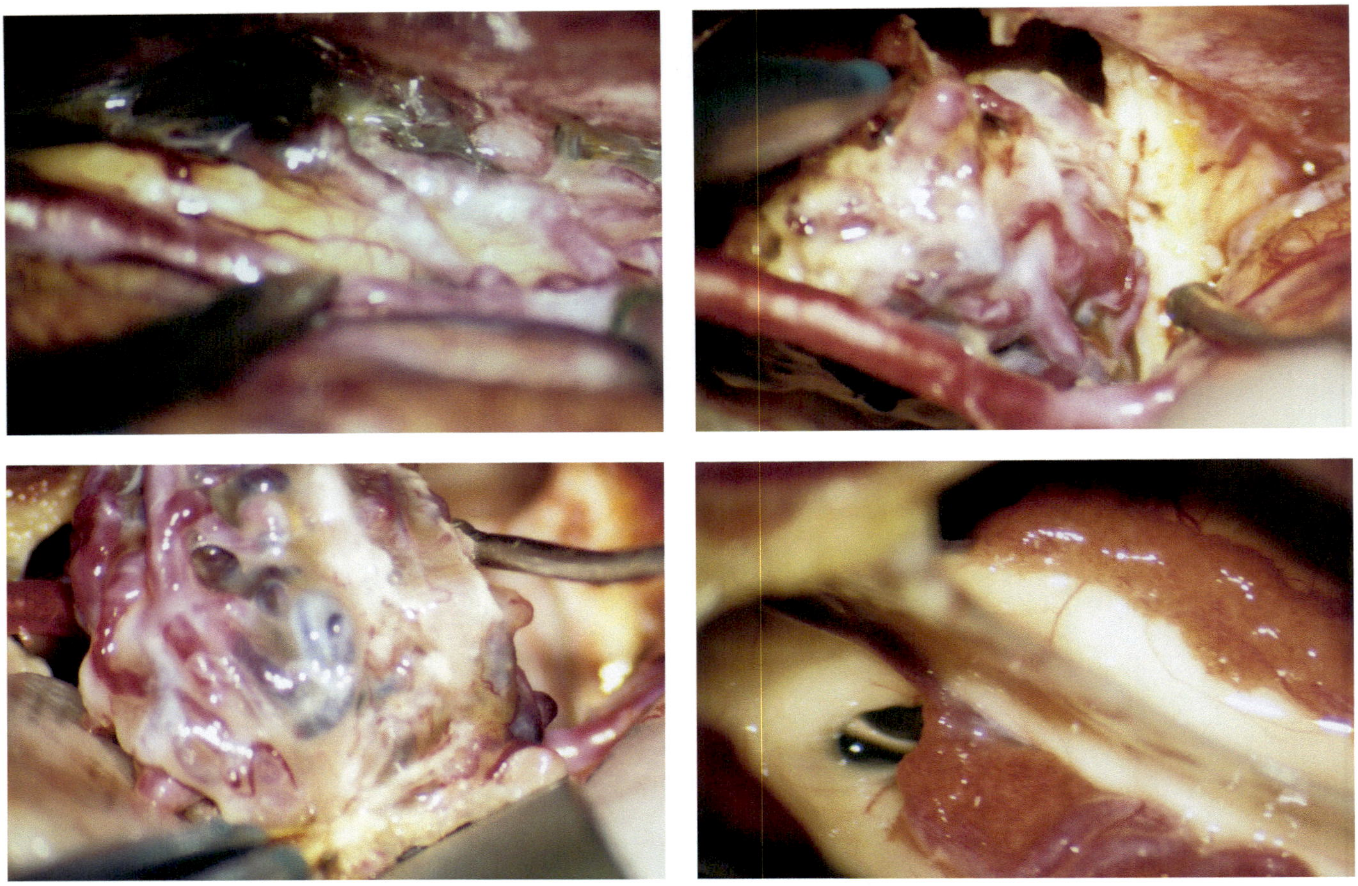

Fig. 14.10 This 58-year-old man presented with a corpus callosum AVM (supplemented Spetzler-Martin grade 6: S1V1E0/A3B1C0) fed by the left PcaA. (**a**) A bifrontal craniotomy eccentric to the left exposed the interhemispheric fissure (nose to the left, midline horizontal, gravity retracting the left frontal lobe). (**b**) The left PcaA running on top of the AVM was skeletonized and the AVM was circumferentially dissected through the corpus callosum. (**c**) The AVM was removed, (**d**) unroofing the lateral ventricles to reveal the choroid plexus, mPChA, foramen of Monro, and septum.

splenium are approached the same way, except that the trajectory to rostrum and genu AVMs is more anterior and to the splenium is more posterior. Splenial AVMs fed by SplenA with minimal ACA input are better approached through a torcular craniotomy and posterior interhemispheric approach that also uses gravity retraction (**Figs. 14.11** and **14.12)**

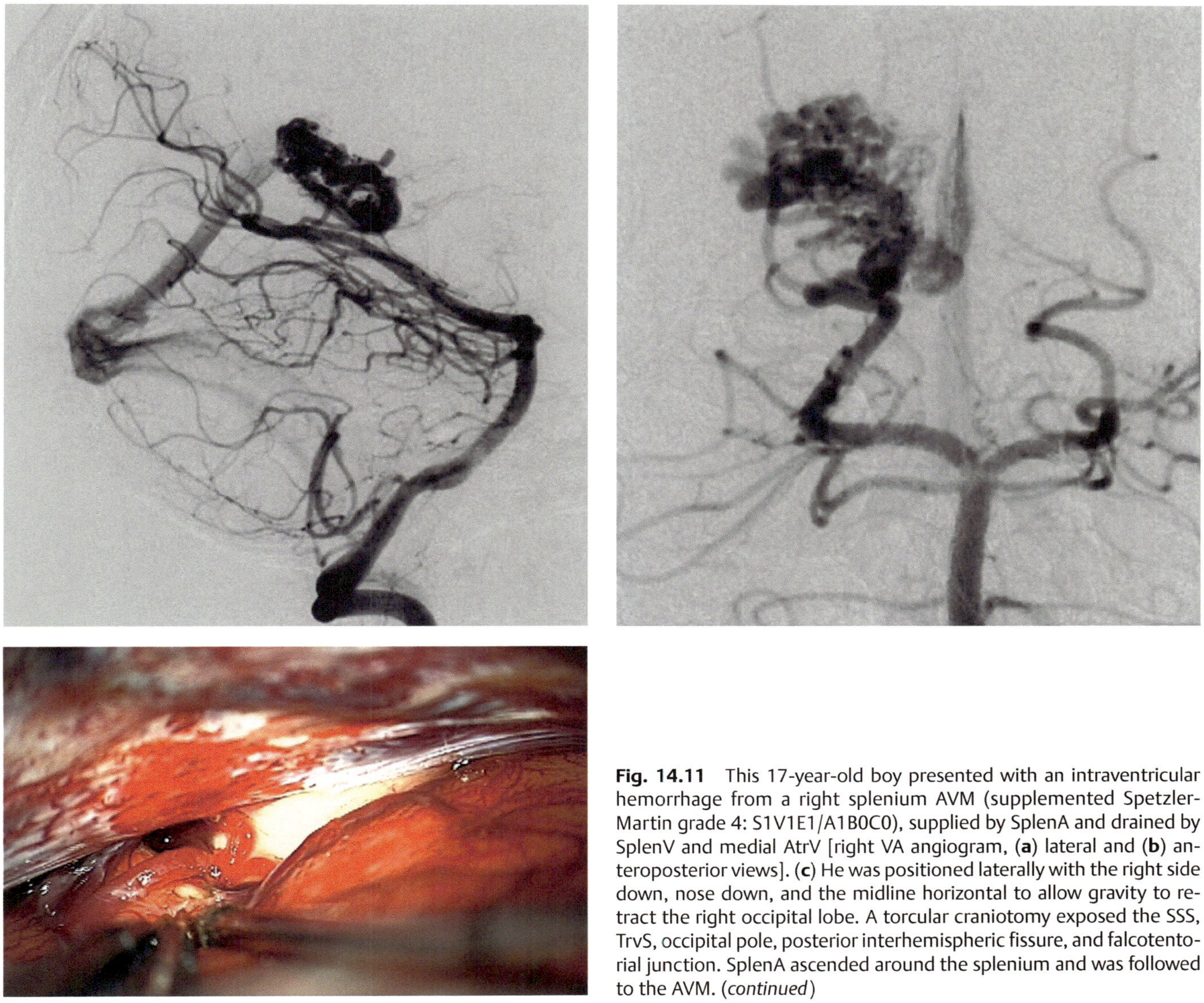

a b c

Fig. 14.11 This 17-year-old boy presented with an intraventricular hemorrhage from a right splenium AVM (supplemented Spetzler-Martin grade 4: S1V1E1/A1B0C0), supplied by SplenA and drained by SplenV and medial AtrV [right VA angiogram, (**a**) lateral and (**b**) anteroposterior views]. (**c**) He was positioned laterally with the right side down, nose down, and the midline horizontal to allow gravity to retract the right occipital lobe. A torcular craniotomy exposed the SSS, TrvS, occipital pole, posterior interhemispheric fissure, and falcotentorial junction. SplenA ascended around the splenium and was followed to the AVM. (*continued*)

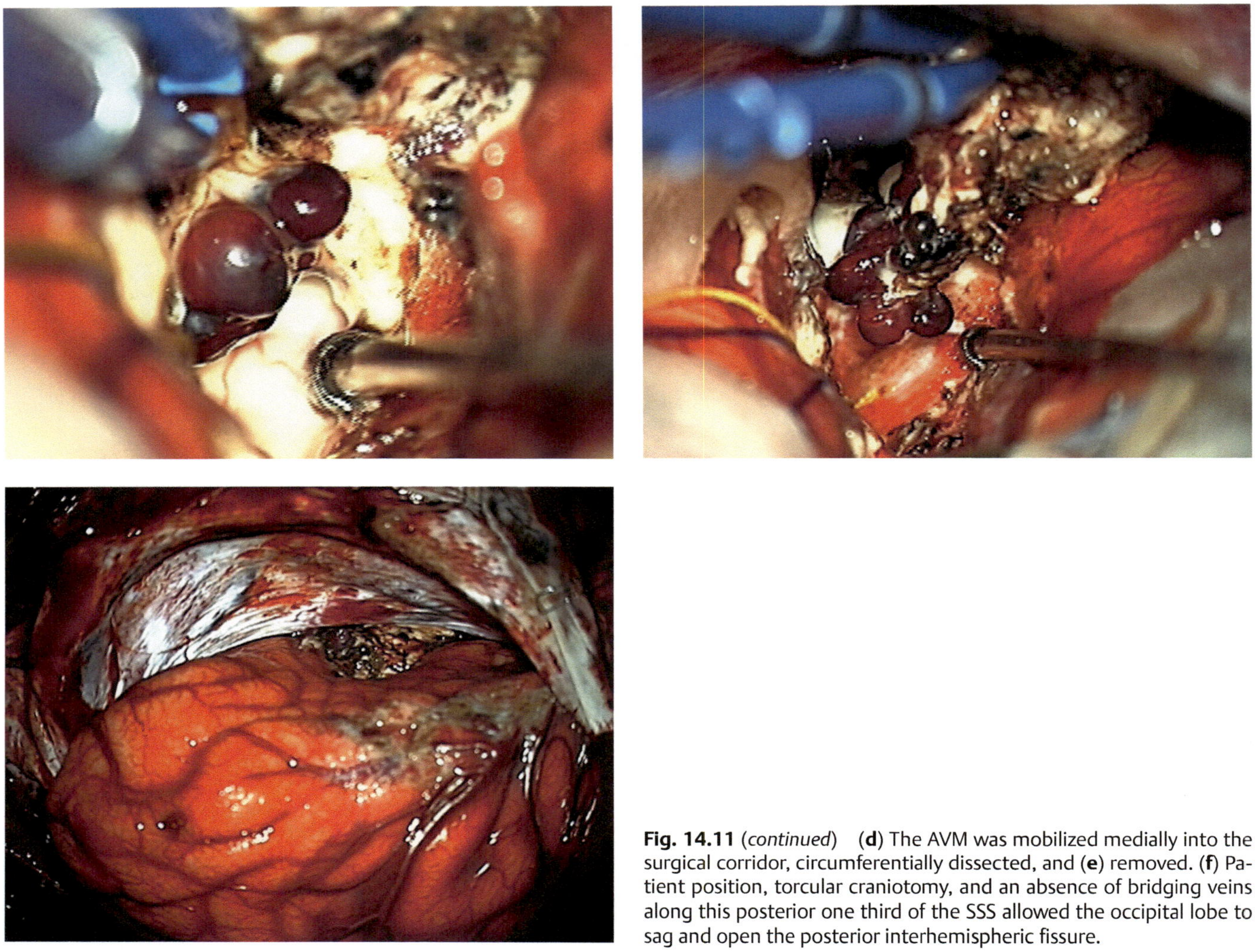

d e f

Fig. 14.11 (*continued*) (**d**) The AVM was mobilized medially into the surgical corridor, circumferentially dissected, and (**e**) removed. (**f**) Patient position, torcular craniotomy, and an absence of bridging veins along this posterior one third of the SSS allowed the occipital lobe to sag and open the posterior interhemispheric fissure.

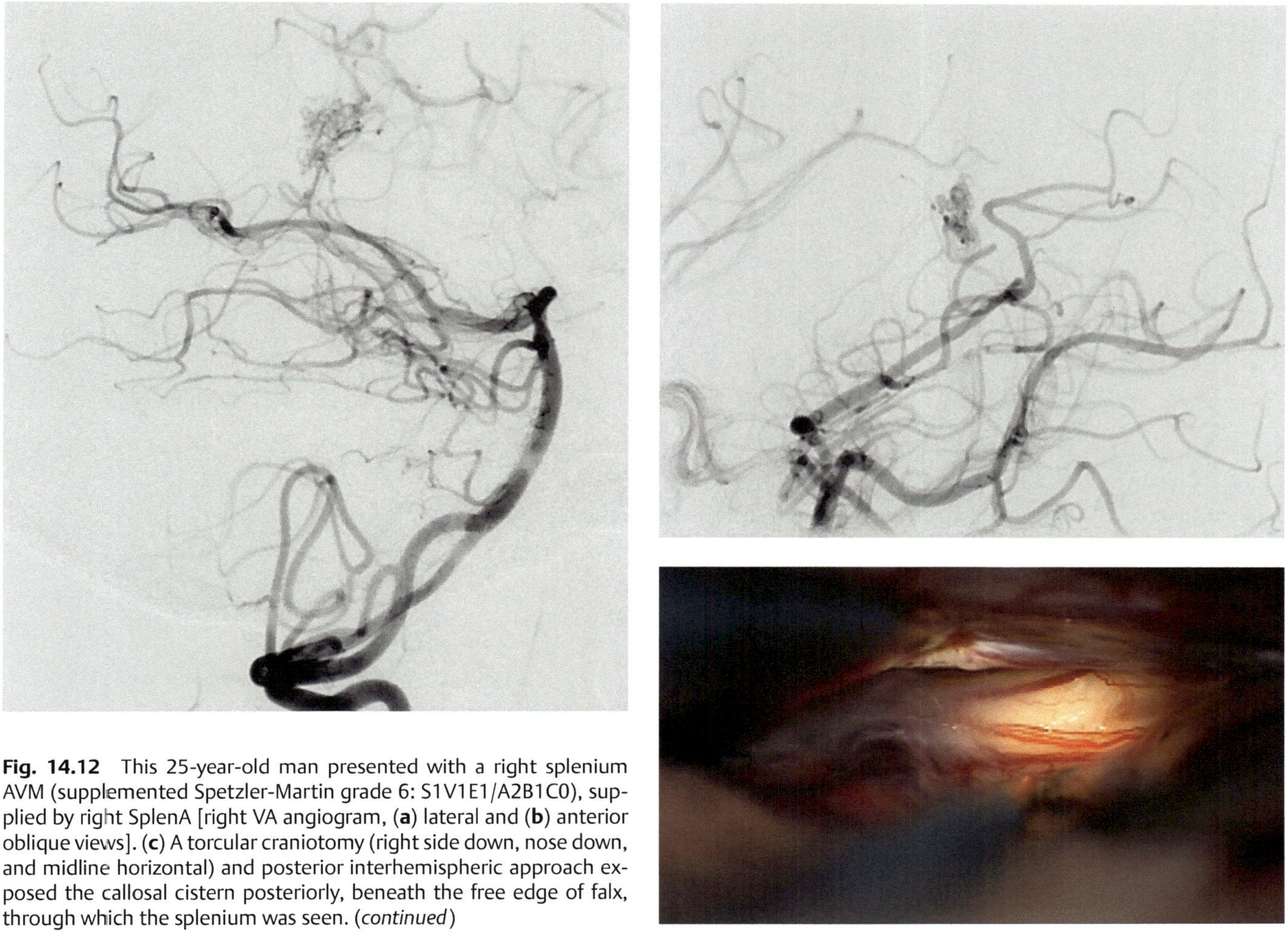

a b c

Fig. 14.12 This 25-year-old man presented with a right splenium AVM (supplemented Spetzler-Martin grade 6: S1V1E1/A2B1C0), supplied by right SplenA [right VA angiogram, (**a**) lateral and (**b**) anterior oblique views]. (**c**) A torcular craniotomy (right side down, nose down, and midline horizontal) and posterior interhemispheric approach exposed the callosal cistern posteriorly, beneath the free edge of falx, through which the splenium was seen. (*continued*)

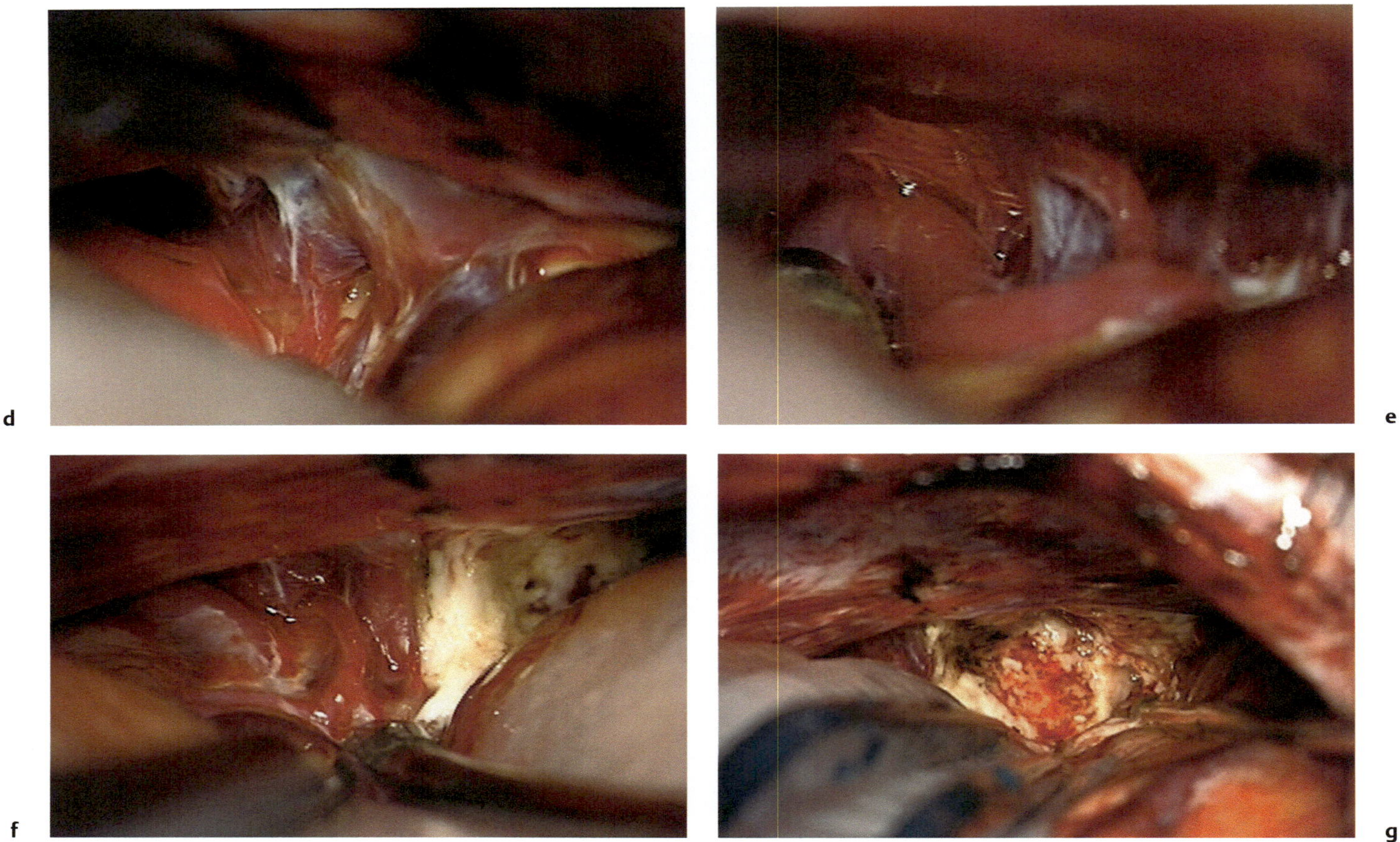

Fig. 14.12 (*continued*) (**d**) The VoG was seen after entering the cistern, (**e**) as was the SplenA. (**f**) The AVM sat in the splenium and extended to the roof of the ventricle, and (**g**) was removed completely.

Ventricular Body AVM Resection

Ventricular body AVMs are exposed with a bifrontal craniotomy (**Fig. 14.13,** step 1) and anterior interhemispheric-transcallosal approach (step 2), exactly like that used for callosal AVMs. The approach is to the right side of the falx to protect the veins in the dominant hemisphere, even when the AVM is in the left ventricle (contralateral transcallosal approach). The subarachnoid dissection steps are the same, but the AVM is not visualized until after dividing the corpus callosum and entering the lateral ventricle. Ventricular body AVMs drain to the ICV (step 3), which is exposed through choroidal fissure by enlarging the FoM posteriorly and opening into the velum interpositum. This exposure also accesses the mPChA, which is a major supplier to these AVMs (step 4). Transchoroidal fissure dissection sweeps the ventricular body's choroid plexus laterally, incises the tela choroidea between the choroid plexus laterally and fornix medially (tenia fornicis), and traces ThaStrV through the FoM into its convergence with the ICV. The anteromedial aspect of the ThaStrV-ICV junction is followed and may require interruption of the anterior SepV or CauV. Sacrifice of these small tributaries is tolerable when ThaStrV and ICV are preserved. Posterior dissection between the paired ICVs extends the opening into the roof of the third ventricle as far back as the posterior commissure, where the crus of the fornix crosses on its lateralizing course around the thalamus. Arterial input from the mPChA is interrupted proximally in the velum interpositum at the AVM's posteroinferior margin (step 5). A second front of arterial input can be found anteri-

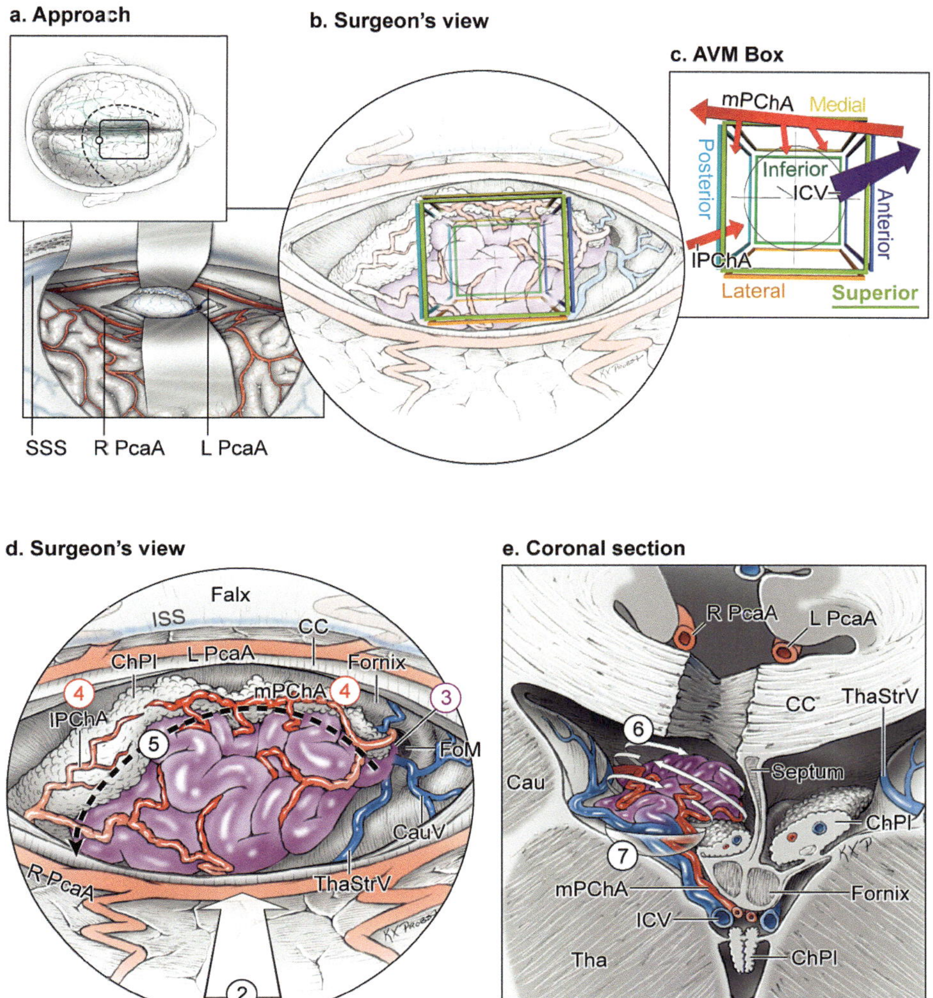

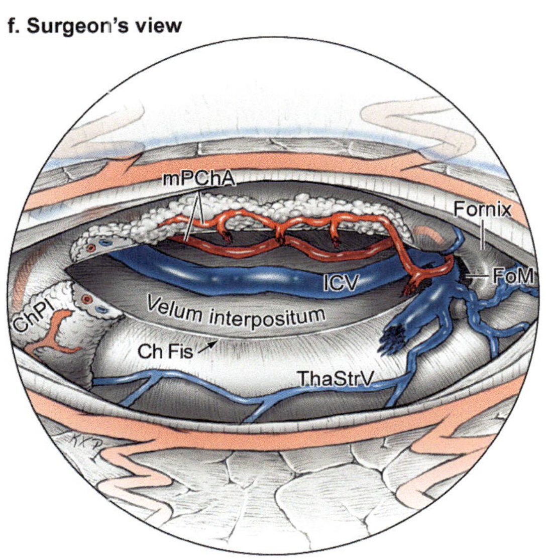

Fig. 14.13 Resection strategy for ventricular body AVMs. (**a**) Step 1, exposing the AVM with a semicircular scalp incision (*inset, dashed line*), bifrontal craniotomy (*inset, solid line*), and transcallosal approach with the midline oriented horizontally for gravity retraction of the right hemisphere (surgeon's view). (**b**) Division of corpus callosum accesses the ventricular body and exposes the AVM on the ventricular floor. (**c**) AVM box showing arterial supply from the mPChA and to a lesser degree the lPChA, and venous drainage to the internal cerebral vein. (**d**) Step 2, approaching the AVM with an interhemispheric-transcallosal dissection into the ventricle; step 3, identifying drainage to the ICV at the foramen of Monro; step 4, identifying supply from the mPChA and lPChA; and step 5, interrupting the anterior and posterior fronts of the choroidal arteries. (**e**) Step 6, an intraventricular location minimizes circumdissection, but the fornix is carefully protected; and step 7, mobilizing the AVM out of the choroidal fissure to interrupt the deep supply from the mPChA in the velum interpositum and from the ACoA plus the mLSA perforators anterior to the FoM. (**f**) Dissection through choroidal fissure opens the velum interpositum to access the deep feeders from the mPChA and additional connections to the draining vein (ICV).

orly in the septum between the columns of the fornix and the rostrum from the mLSA (A1 ACA), ACoA, and A2 ACA. Parenchymal dissection is limited to the nidus located in the septum, preserving the columns of the fornix as they descend through the FoM (step 6). Access is parallel but exposure is limited by the long surgical corridor, the tight confines of the choroidal fissure, and the fornix. The deep plane receives ascending supply from the ACoA perforators and mLSA, and also transmits the ICV posteriorly out of view (step 7). In addition, the thalamus lies inferolateral to the velum interpositum and may transmit some thalamoperforator supply (**Figs. 14.14** and **14.15**).

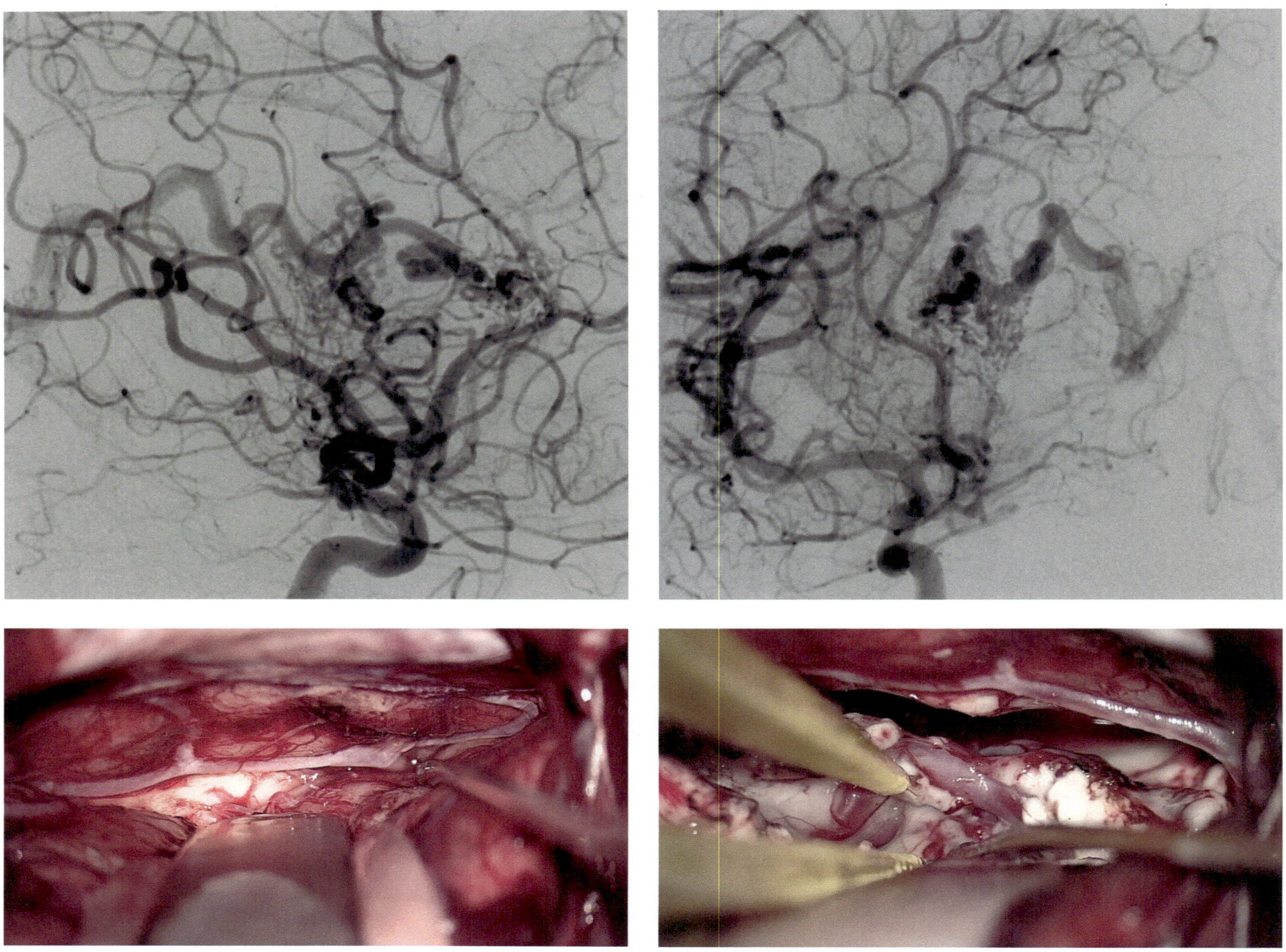

a b c d

Fig. 14.14 This 23-year-old woman presented with an intraventricular hemorrhage from a ventricular body (septal) AVM, with supplemented Spetzler-Martin grade 5: S2V1E0/A2B0C0. She underwent Gamma Knife radiosurgery and it hemorrhaged again 4 years later. The AVM was supplied by the ACA/PcaA branches, ACoA perforators, and mPChA [right ICA angiogram, (**a**) lateral and (**b**) anterior oblique views]. (**c**) The interhemispheric fissure was opened through a bifrontal craniotomy (nose to the right, midline horizontal, with gravity retracting the right hemisphere), exposing the corpus callosum, CmaA, and PcaA. (**d**) A 2.5-cm section of corpus callosum was resected to expose the AVM in the septum, and the left ACA was skeletonized.

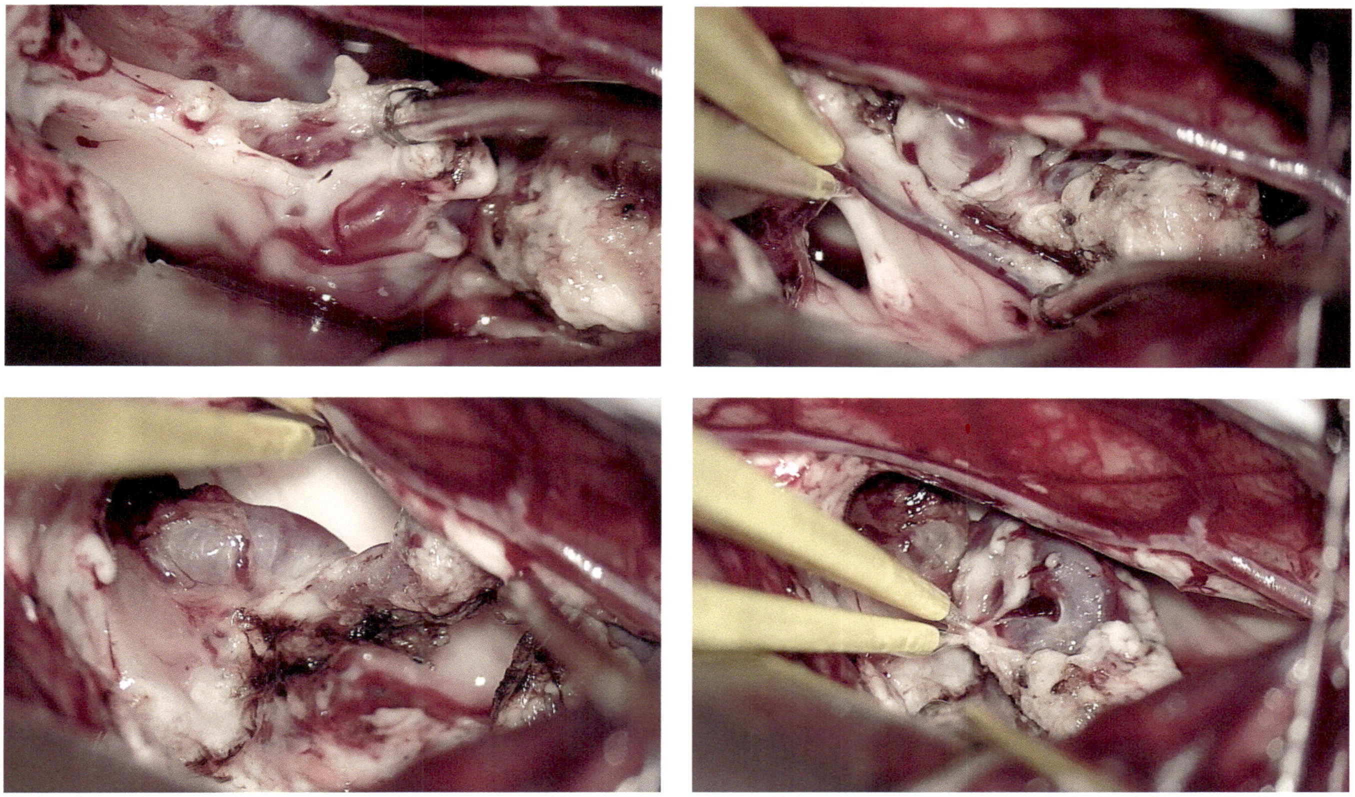

e f g h

Fig. 14.14 (*continued*) (**e**) The posterior margin of the AVM was mobilized anteriorly away from the fornix. (**f**) The foramen of Monro, fornix, and right SepV were preserved at the base of the septum. (**g**) The draining vein darkened and (**h**) was coagulated as it joined ICV. The AVM was resected completely.

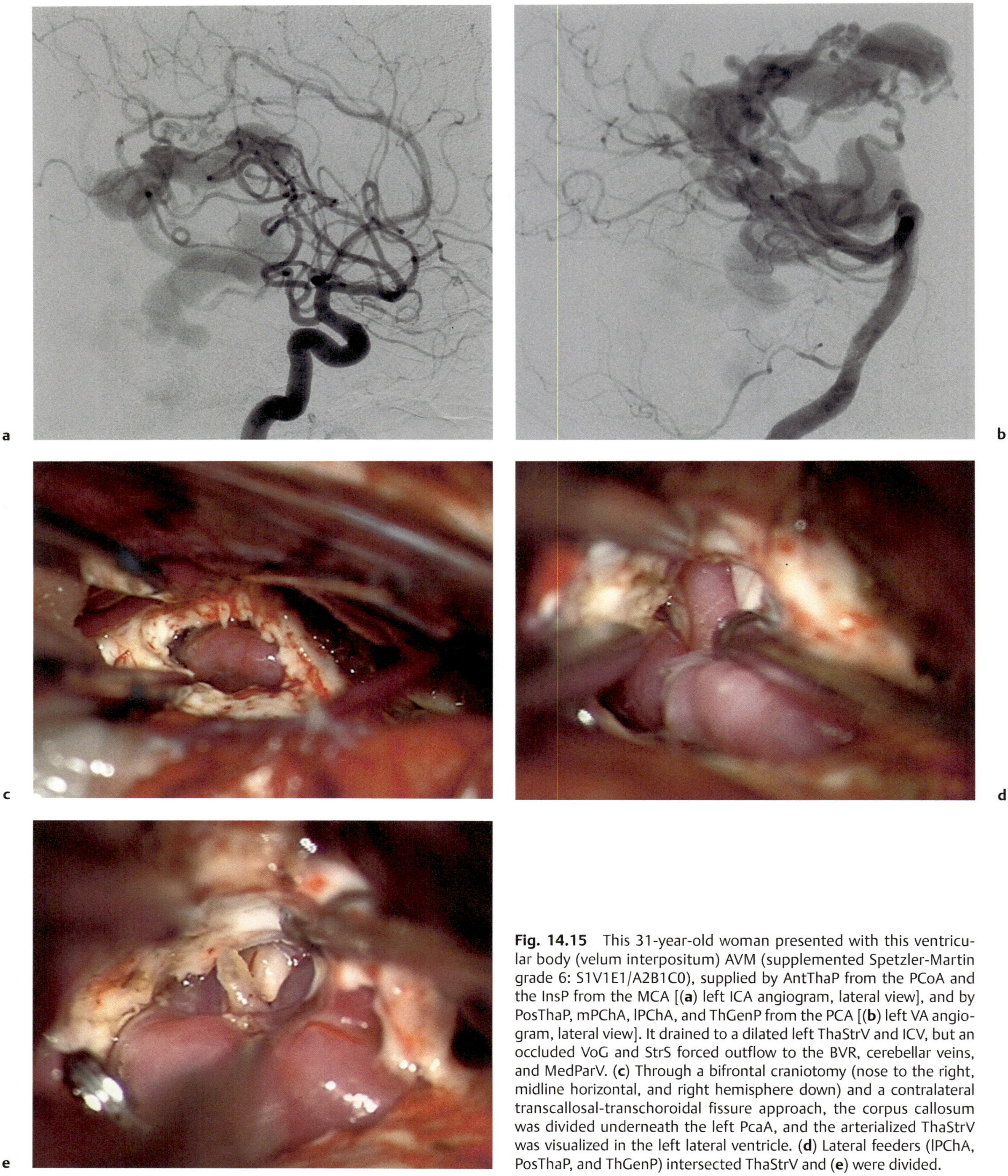

Fig. 14.15 This 31-year-old woman presented with this ventricular body (velum interpositum) AVM (supplemented Spetzler-Martin grade 6: S1V1E1/A2B1C0), supplied by AntThaP from the PCoA and the InsP from the MCA [(**a**) left ICA angiogram, lateral view], and by PosThaP, mPChA, lPChA, and ThGenP from the PCA [(**b**) left VA angiogram, lateral view]. It drained to a dilated left ThaStrV and ICV, but an occluded VoG and StrS forced outflow to the BVR, cerebellar veins, and MedParV. (**c**) Through a bifrontal craniotomy (nose to the right, midline horizontal, and right hemisphere down) and a contralateral transcallosal-transchoroidal fissure approach, the corpus callosum was divided underneath the left PcaA, and the arterialized ThaStrV was visualized in the left lateral ventricle. (**d**) Lateral feeders (lPChA, PosThaP, and ThGenP) intersected ThaStrV and (**e**) were divided.

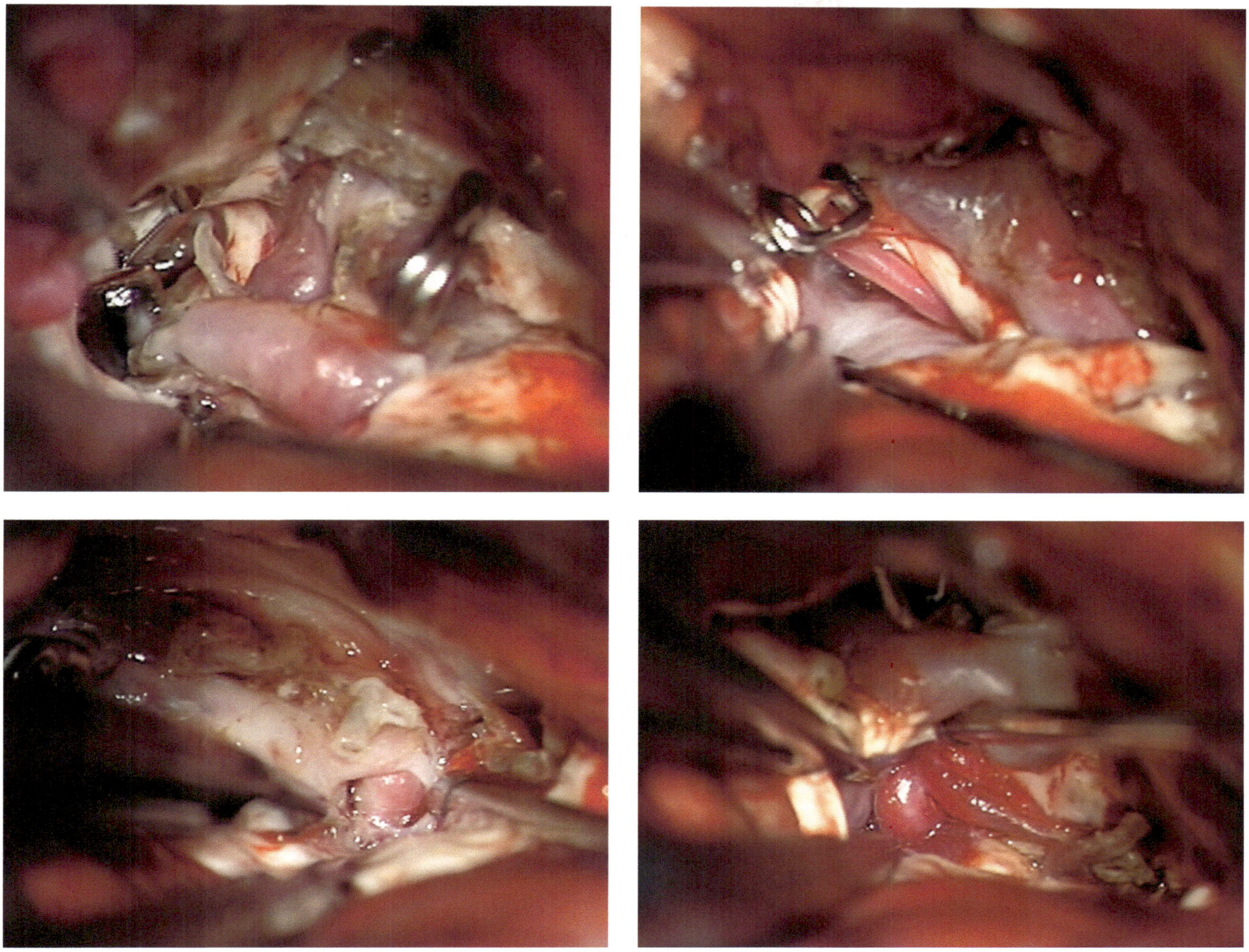

f g h i

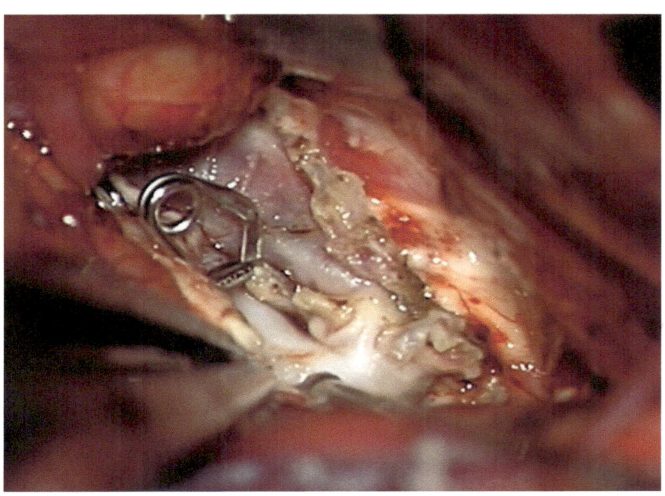

j

Fig. 14.15 (*continued*) (**f**) After skeletonizing ThaStrV, (**g**) the choroidal fissure was opened and ICV was followed into velum interpositum where mPChA feeders were exposed posteriorly. (**h**) Anterior feeders (AntThaP and InsP) were exposed in the venous angle and (**i**) under ICV. (**j**) The draining venous complex darkened after all arterial feeders were occluded.

Ventricular Atrium AVM Resection

Atrial AVMs are resected through a parietal craniotomy and superior parietal lobule approach (**Fig. 14.16**). The patient is positioned laterally with the head turned toward the floor to bring the parietal convexity uppermost in the field. A trajectory through the superior parietal lobule (SPL) to the atrium is selected using frameless stereotactic navigation. Alternatively, an entry point is selected that is between 6 and 9 cm above the inion and between 3 and 5 cm lateral to the midline. A C-shaped scalp incision is centered over this entry point, and a parietal craniotomy flap is elevated (step 1). A transcortical corridor is opened through the SPL to the atrium (step 2). The atrial portion of the choroidal fissure lies between the crus of the fornix posteriorly and the pulvinar and caudate body anteriorly. Draining veins include AtrV (medial and lateral), ChorV (superior and inferior), and posterior CauV, which all converge on the choroidal fissure and collect in the ICV and BVR en route to the VoG (step 3). This venous anatomy as well as arterial supply from the lPChA (step 4) is accessed by opening the choroidal fissure. Like the transchoroidal fissure dissection into velum inter-

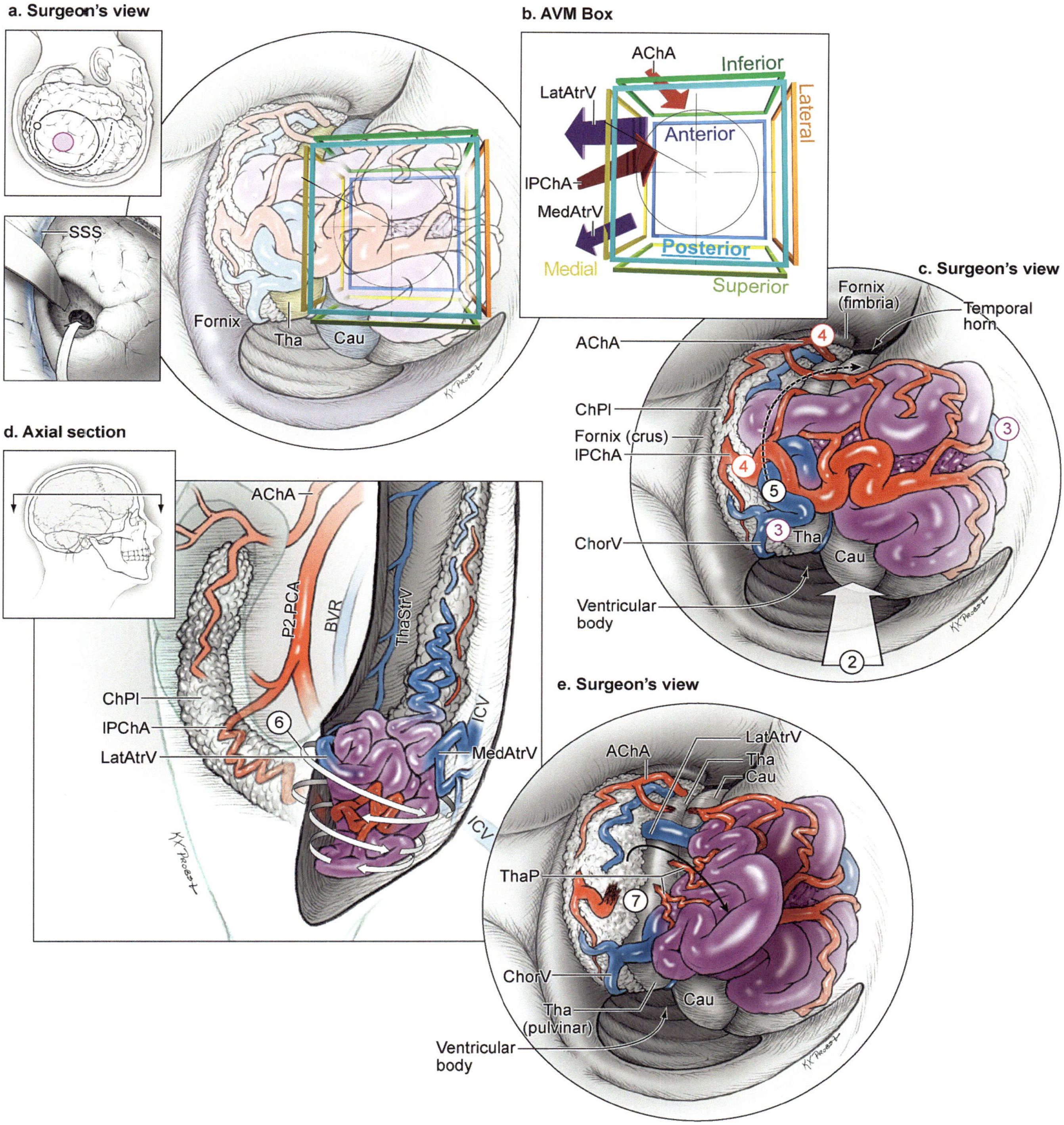

Fig. 14.16 Resection strategy for ventricular atrium AVMs. (**a**) Step 1, exposing the AVM with a semicircular scalp incision (*top inset, dashed line*), parietal craniotomy (*top inset, solid line*), and a superior parietal lobule approach (*bottom inset*) that traverses parietal cortex to enter the atrium (surgeon's view). (**b**) AVM box showing supply from the lateral posterior choroidal artery, drainage to the medial and lateral atrial veins, and proximity to the thalamus, caudate nucleus, and fornix. (**c**) Step 2, entering the atrium with a transcortical approach through the SPL; step 3, identifying draining veins as they converge on the choroidal fissure; step 4, identifying arterial supply from the lPChA and AChA; and step 5, interrupting the inferior front along the choroidal fissure (surgeon's view). (**d**) Step 6, circumdissection is intraventricular without parenchymal planes (axial cross-sectional view). (**e**) Step 7, mobilizing the AVM laterally to divide deep supply from thalamoperforators on the pulvinar surface and lenticulostriates on the caudate surface, and also visualize atrial veins as they exit the choroidal fissure (spherical scoop, surgeon's view).

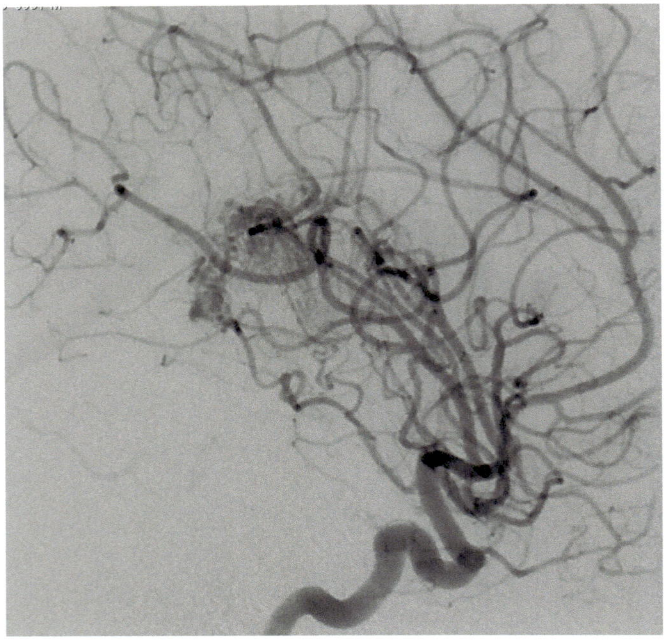

a

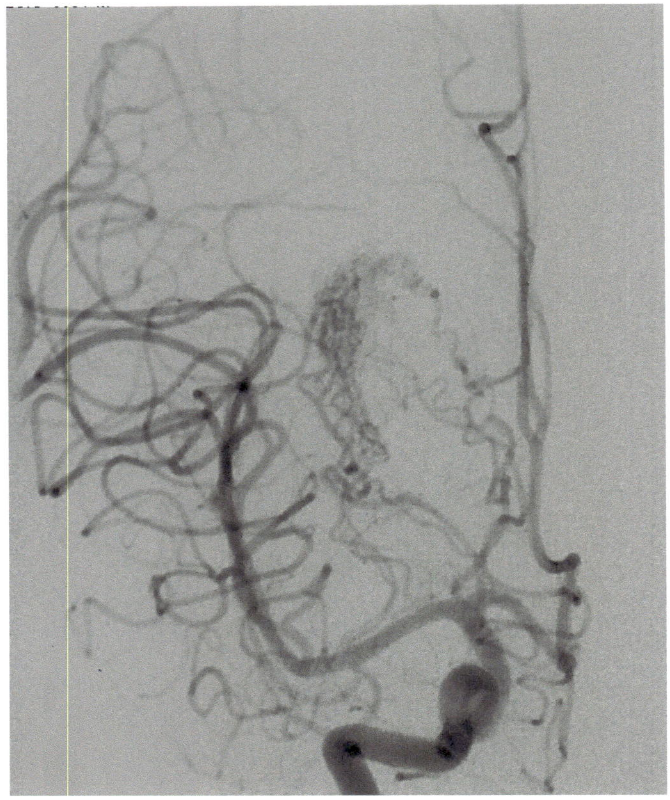

b

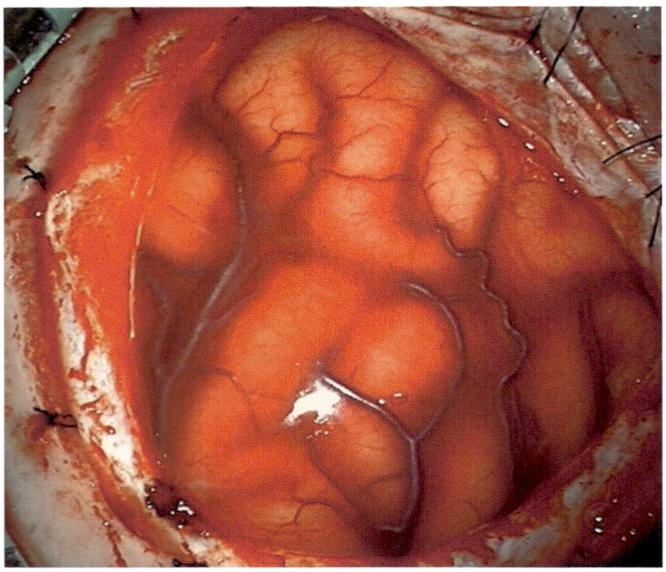

c

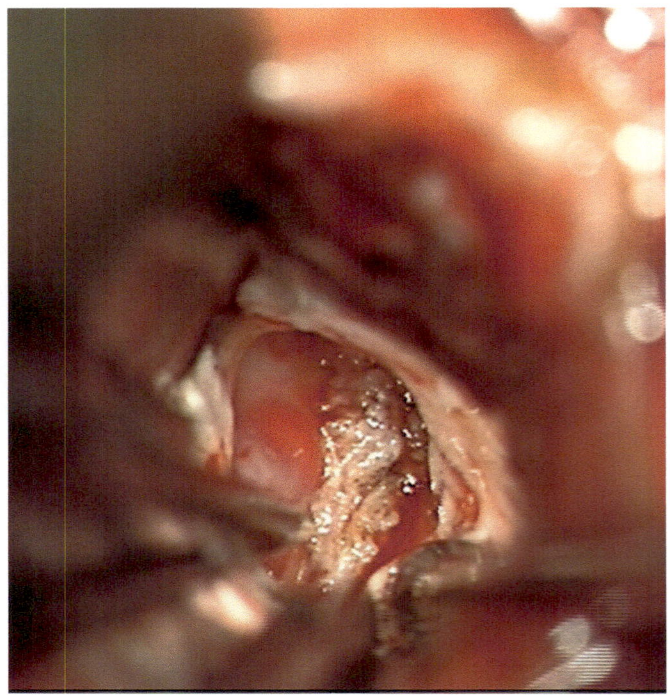

d

Fig. 14.17 This 3-year-old boy presented with intraventricular hemorrhage from a right atrial AVM (supplemented Spetzler-Martin grade 5: S2V1E0/A1B0C1), supplied by the AChA and lLSA and drained by MedAtrV and ICV [right ICA angiogram, (**a**) lateral and (**b**) anteroposterior views]. (**c**) A right parietal craniotomy exposed the superior parietal lobule (lateral position, midline horizontal, nose to the left). (**d**) A transcortical approach through the SPL accessed the atrium of the lateral ventricle, where the choroid plexus was cauterized adjacent to an enlarged AChA.

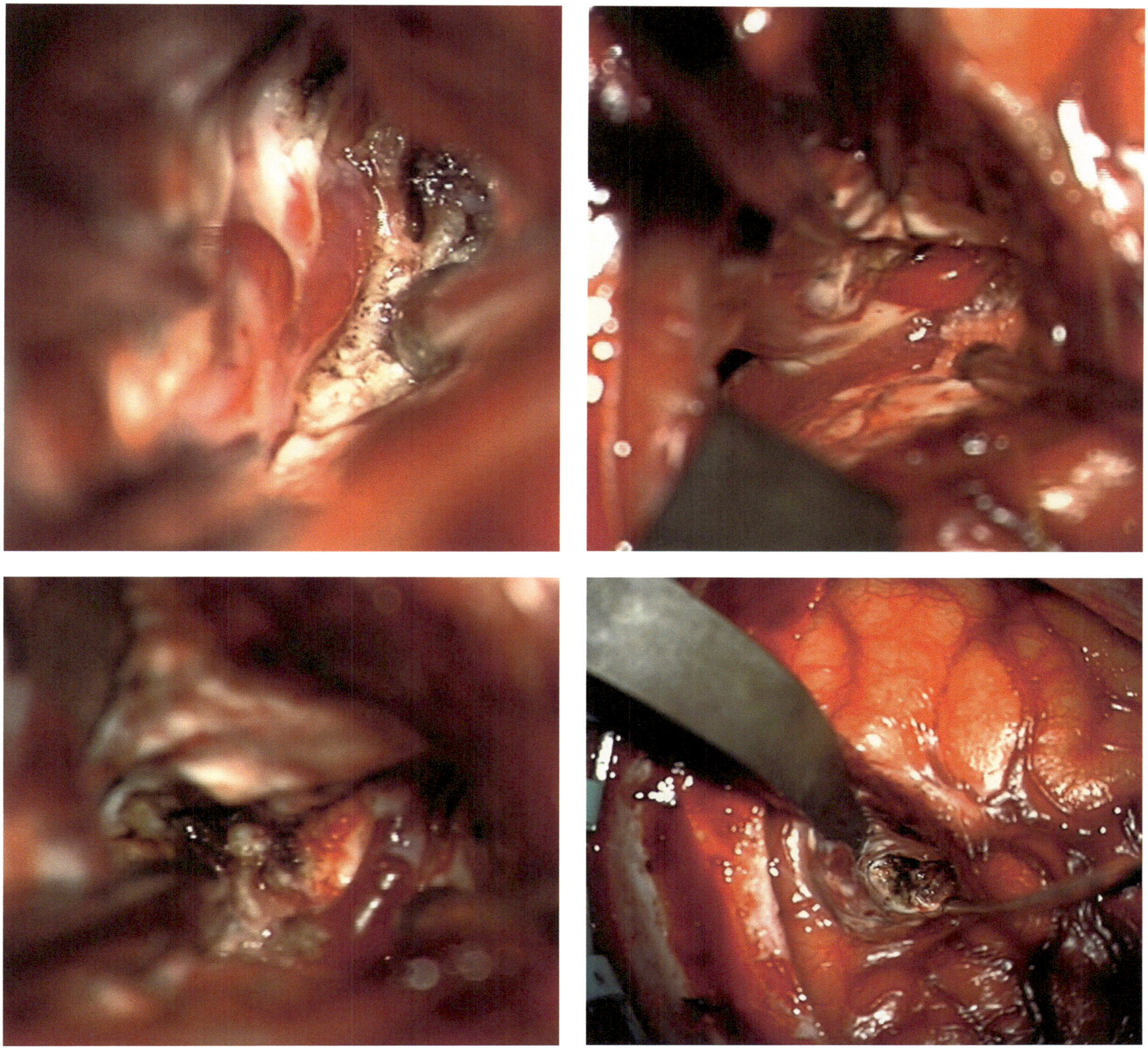

e f g h

Fig. 14.17 (*continued*) (**e**) The AChA was followed from the temporal horn to the undersurface of the thalamus to the AVM, where it was interrupted. (**f**) The draining vein was visualized on the posterior thalamus in the superior atrium. (**g**) After cauterizing small transthalamic feeding arteries on the thalamic surface, the draining vein darkened and the AVM was removed. (**h**) This transcortical corridor was long and narrow, but well tolerated clinically.

positum, the tela choroidea is opened on the fornix side of the choroid plexus (tenia fornicis) to avoid the thalamus. The arterialized vein is identified as it exits the choroidal fissure, and lPChA feeders are coagulated at the AVM's inferior margin (step 5). Circumdissection has no parenchymal planes and is parallel, albeit deep (step 6). Widening the choroidal fissure expands the view of the draining atrial veins, the AChA input from the temporal horn, and the normal PCA along its ambient segment. There may be some thalamoperforator supply on the pulvinar surface or lLSA on the caudate body that is interrupted at the ependyma (step 7). Although not strictly eloquent, atrial AVMs are adjacent to the posterior thalamus, caudate body, and crus of fornix (**Fig. 14.17**).

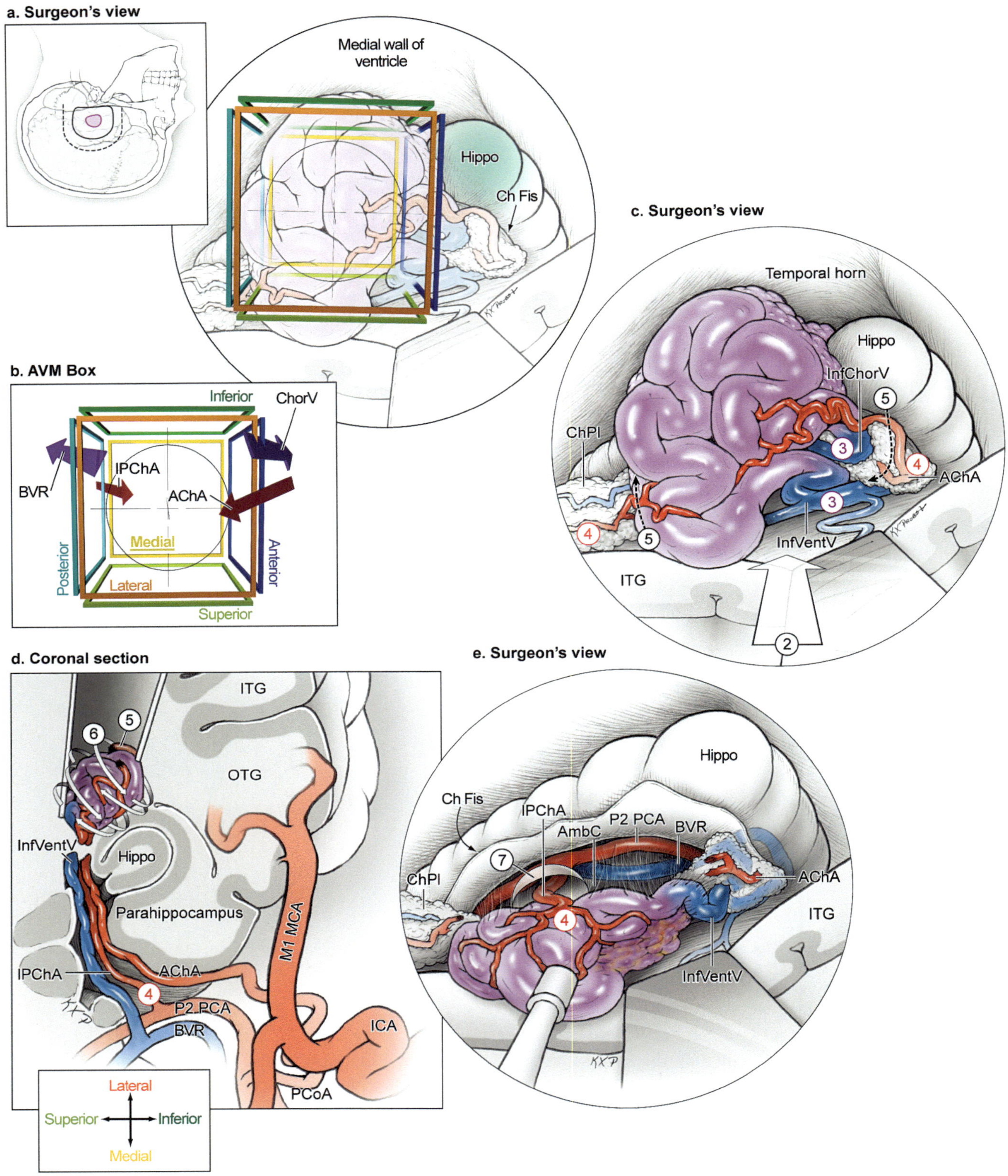
a. Surgeon's view
Medial wall of ventricle
Hippo
Ch Fis
b. AVM Box
Inferior
ChorV
BVR
IPChA
AChA
Medial
Posterior
Anterior
Lateral
Superior
c. Surgeon's view
Temporal horn
Hippo
InfChorV
ChPl
AChA
InfVentV
ITG
d. Coronal section
ITG
OTG
InfVentV
Hippo
Parahippocampus
M1 MCA
IPChA
AChA
P2 PCA
BVR
ICA
PCoA
Lateral
Superior
Inferior
Medial
e. Surgeon's view
Hippo
Ch Fis
IPChA
AmbC
P2 PCA
BVR
ChPl
AChA
ITG
InfVentV

Fig. 14.18 (*opposite*) Resection strategy for temporal horn AVMs. (**a**) Step 1, exposing the AVM with a horseshoe scalp incision (*inset, dashed line*), temporal craniotomy (*inset, solid line*), and transcortical approach through the inferior temporal gyrus. (**b**) AVM box showing arterial supply from the AChA and lPChA, venous drainage medially to the BVR, and proximity to the dominant hemisphere's hippocampus. (**c**) Step 2, entering the temporal horn with a transcortical approach through the ITG; step 3, identifying draining choroidal and ventricular veins (the BVR is not visible until later); step 4, identifying the AChA in the choroidal fissure anteriorly; and step 5, interrupting the anteromedial front in the proximal choroidal fissure. (**d**) Step 6, dissecting along the choroidal fissure from proximal to distal (coronal cross-sectional view). (**e**) Step 7, mobilizing the AVM out of the choroidal fissure to divide the lPChA supply and identify the BVR in ambient cistern.

Temporal Horn AVM Resection

Temporal horn AVMs are resected like basal temporal AVMs through a temporal craniotomy (**Fig. 14.18,** step 1) and transcortical approach through the inferior temporal gyrus (ITG). The patient is positioned supine, head turned 90 degrees laterally, and the vertex lowered to gain an upward angle toward the temporal horn. A horseshoe incision and the temporal craniotomy are based over the ear. The approach enters low in the ITG and angles up to the ventricle, staying beneath the optic radiations in Meyer's loop that passes over the temporal horn (step 2). Navigation helps aim this transcortical route. Once entered, the horn is opened longitudinally along its axis for a full view of the AVM. The inferior ChorV and BVR (step 3) are not visible until the end of the dissection. The AChA is identified proximally in the choroidal fissure at the plexal point anteriorly, and the lPChA supply is identified distally in the choroidal fissure past the nidus (step 4). The AChA inputs are interrupted initially (step 5), but additional choroidal supply persists on the medial margin. Dissection down the choroidal fissure from proximal to distal interrupts these choroidal feeders, requiring an anterior attack and some AVM mobilization laterally (step 6). The choroidal fissure is preferentially opened inferiorly, through the tela choroidea between the choroid plexus and the fimbria of the fornix (tenia fimbriae), avoiding the tail of the caudate and the inferior thalamus on the superior side. The final stages of dissection reach the venous connections to the BVR and remaining inputs from the lPChA (step 7). Although not strictly eloquent, but like other ventricular AVMs, temporal horn AVMs are adjacent to the thalamus, caudate nucleus (tail), fornix (fimbria), and hippocampus (**Fig. 14.19**).

a 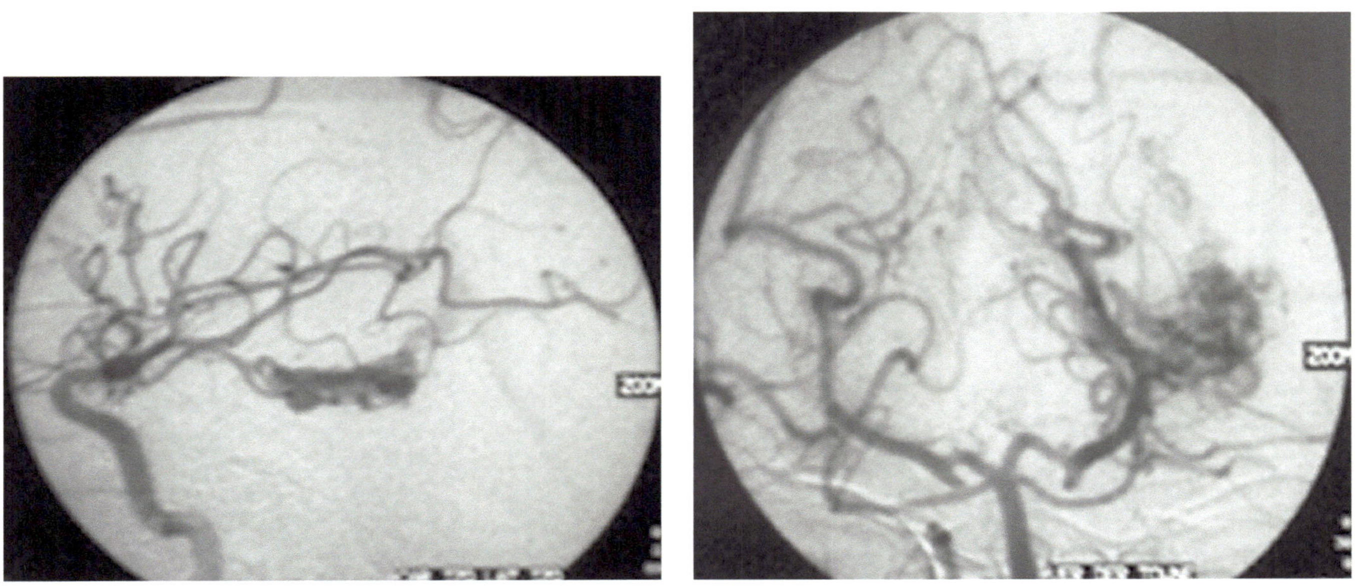 b

Fig. 14.19 This 19-year-old man presented in a coma with an intraventricular hemorrhage from a left temporal horn AVM (supplemented Spetzler-Martin grade 4: S1V1E1/A1B0C0), supplied by the AChA [(**a**) left ICA angiogram, lateral view] and lPChA [(**b**) left VA angiogram, anteroposterior view]. The AVM was incompletely resected, and the patient was referred 3 months later for complete resection. (*continued on next page*)

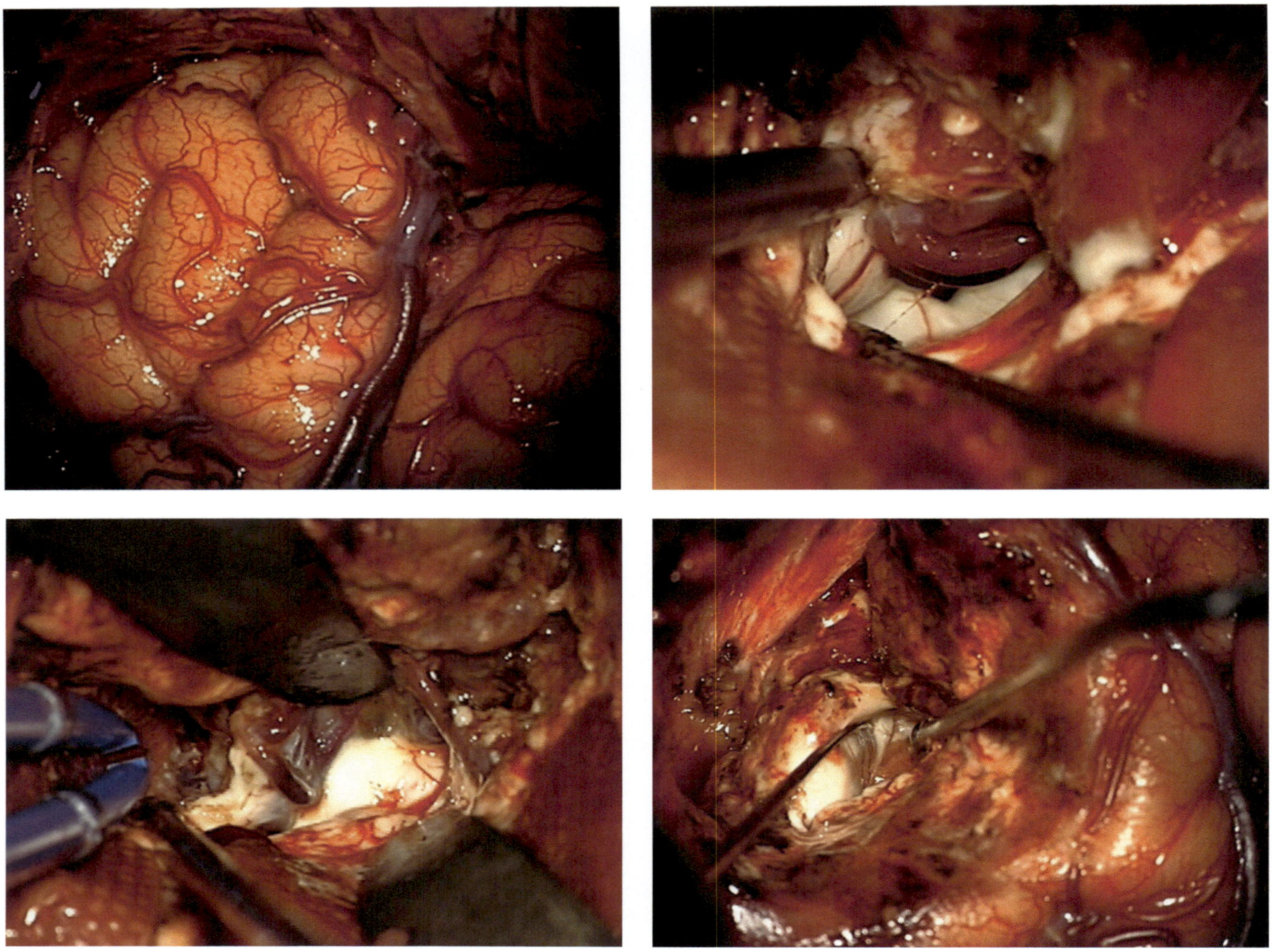

c d e f

Fig. 14.19 (*continued*) (**c**) The left pterional craniotomy was reopened to expose the anterior temporal lobe, and (**d**) the prior transcortical approach through the inferior temporal gyrus was followed to the temporal horn. (**e**) The AChA entered the horn through the choroidal fissure to supply the AVM anteriorly and the lPChA supplied the AVM posteriorly. (**f**) Transcortical exposure through the ITG enabled complete AVM resection with good exposure of temporal horn.

■ Conclusion

Ventricular and periventricular AVMs are special. They reside in ventricular chambers "floating" in CSF and are easier than all other AVMs to circumdissect. These features make them completely different from parenchymal AVMs and from deep AVMs in the adjacent central core (to be covered in the next chapter). At the same time, the deep location of ventricular/periventricular AVMs raises their Spetzler-Martin grades while lengthening and limiting their surgical corridors. They are generally favorable for surgery and associated with excellent results, provided that the fornix and thalamus are handled gently and with respect. Unfortunately, these are uncommon AVMs, second in rarity to brainstem AVMs (7% of this experience overall).

15 Deep Arteriovenous Malformations

■ Microsurgical Anatomy

Brain

Deep arteriovenous malformations (AVMs) are situated in the insula and central core of the hemisphere. Although these areas lie beneath portions of frontal, temporal, and parieto-occipital lobes, they are discussed separately in this book from lobar AVMs because their depth and anatomy make them completely different surgically. Deep AVMs are discussed separately from ventricular AVMs because they are based in brain parenchyma rather than in ventricles.

The insula is a triangular-shaped structure covering the lateral surface of the central core, with the triangle's base under the frontal operculum and its apex directed anteriorly and inferiorly toward the limen insulae (**Fig. 15.1a**). The insula is divided into anterior and posterior parts by the central sulcus of the insula, which runs parallel and deep to the central sulcus of the convexity. The anterior insula is composed of three to five short gyri, and the posterior insula is composed of two long gyri. These gyri course radially from the limen insulae in a posterosuperior direction. The limen insulae, a slightly raised area overlying the uncinate fasciculus and the lateral border of the anterior perforated substance, marks the junction of the sphenoidal and insular compartments of the sylvian fissure, and the division between the M1 and M2 segments of the middle cerebral artery (MCA), where the artery turns upward. The insula is separated from the sylvian surfaces of the frontal, parietal, and temporal lobes by the limiting sulcus (circular sulcus).

a.

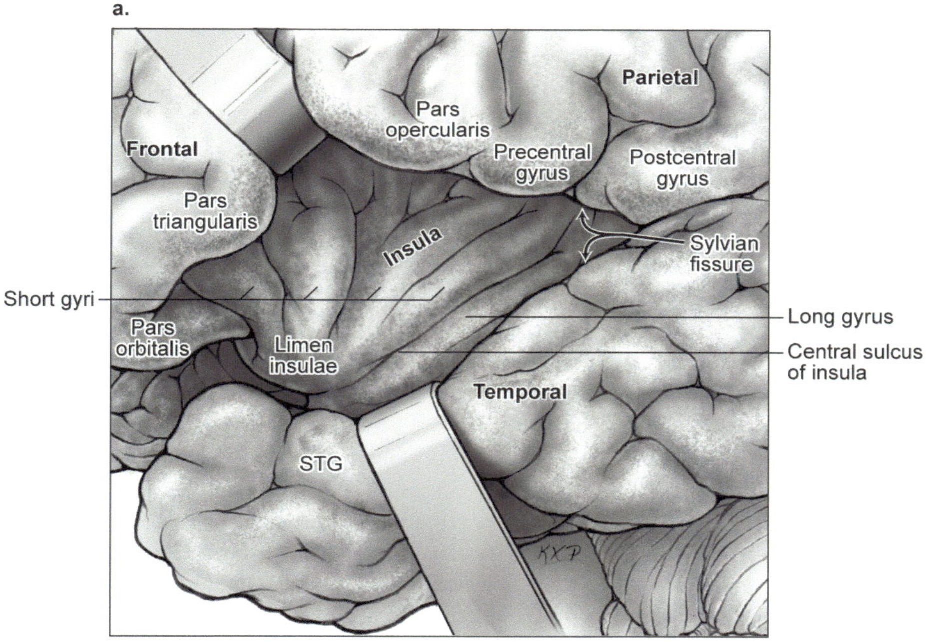

Fig. 15.1 (**a**) Microsurgical anatomy of the insula, as seen laterally through the left operculum. (*continued on next page*)

b.

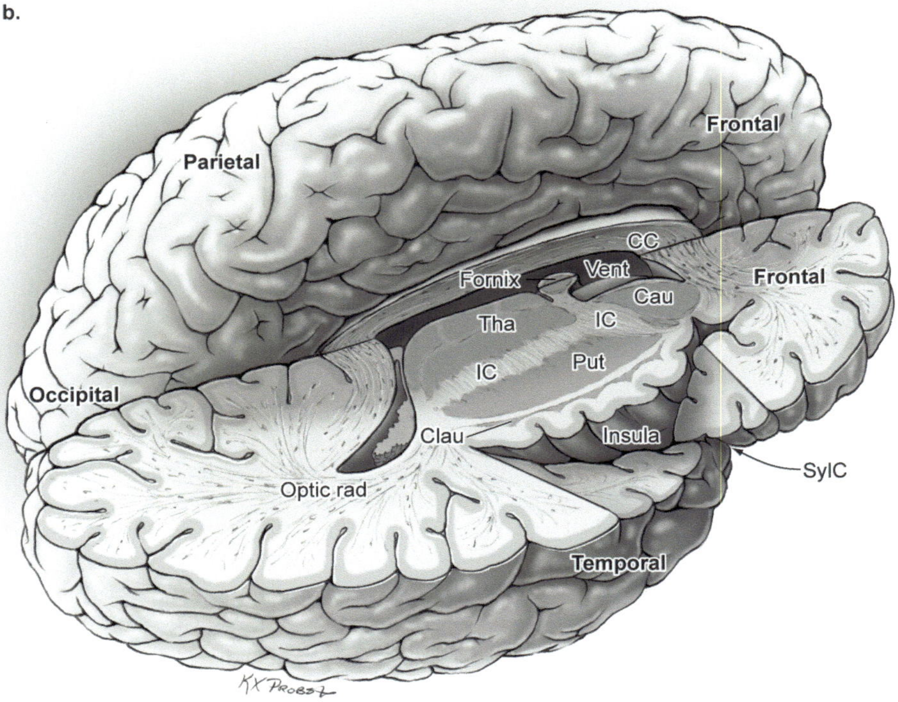

Fig. 15.1 *(continued)* (**b**) Cross-sectional anatomy of the central core (horizontal section through the right hemisphere).

The central core is situated between the insula and the midline, and is composed of the basal ganglia (putamen, globus pallidus, and caudate nucleus); thalamus; fornix; internal, external, and extreme capsules; and claustrum (**Fig. 15.1b**). The central core is attached to the rest of the hemisphere by an anterior and posterior isthmus. All information passing between the cortex and the brainstem and spinal cord is relayed in or carried by fibers passing through the central core.

Arteries

The central core and insula are supplied by perforating arteries: small end-arteries that terminate in critical deep structures (**Fig. 15.2**). Although enlarged cortical feeders to AVMs appear most threatening, they are superficial and often easy to identify, cauterize, and control. In contrast, small perforators that are often overlooked angiographically are deep and difficult to cauterize; they traverse vital white matter tracts, persistently supply the nidus long after the cortical feeders are interrupted, and are accessible only after arriving at the last margin of the AVM. Therefore, they warrant special respect.

The lateral lenticulostriate arteries (lLSA) are the MCA's perforators. On average, 10 perforators originate from the M1 segment along its superior-posterior surface proximal to its bifurcation, although an early bifurcation results in their postbifurcation origin. The lLSA penetrates the brain at the anterior perforated substance, passes through the putamen, and supplies the upper part of the internal capsule, globus pallidus, and caudate nucleus (head and body).

The medial lenticulostriate arteries (mLSA) are the anterior cerebral artery's (ACA) perforators. On average, eight perforators arise from the A1 segment, concentrated more proximally (laterally) than distally (medially). The mLSA enters the anterior perforated substance to supply the suprachiasmatic part of the hypothalamus and third ventricle, as well as the dorsal surfaces of the optic chiasm, nerve, and tract. The recurrent artery of Heubner (RAH) is the most medial mLSA, originating from the A1-A2 ACA junction directly lateral to the anterior communicating artery (ACoA) and slightly on the A2 side. It doubles back on itself, parallel-

Fig. 15.2 *(opposite)* (**a**) Insular arteries from MCA trunks are unnamed stem arteries (M2 segments) that acquire names when they reach the cortical surface (M4 segment). (**b**) The central core is supplied by perforating arteries, including lenticulostriate arteries (lLSA, mLSA, and RAH), insular perforators (InsP), thalamoperforators (AntThaP and PosThaP), thalamogeniculate arteries (ThGenP), peduncular perforators (PedP), and circumflex perforators (CirP) (lateral view). (**c**) Perforating arteries from the anterior circulation and (**d**) the posterior circulation (coronal cross-sectional views through the basal ganglia and thalamus, respectively).

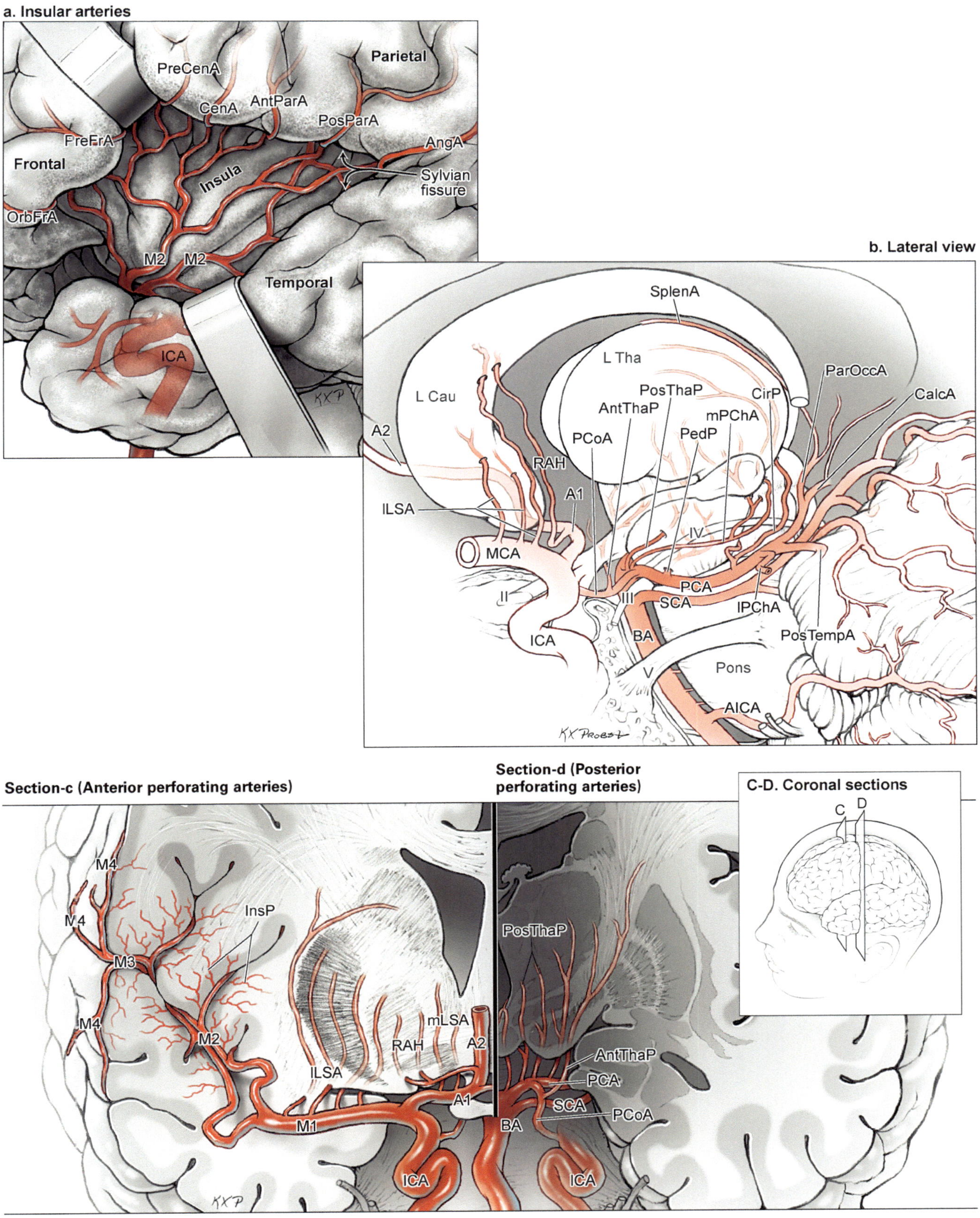
a. Insular arteries
PreCenA
Parietal
CenA
AntParA
PosParA
PreFrA
AngA
Frontal
Insula
Sylvian fissure
OrbFrA
M2
M2
Temporal
ICA
b. Lateral view
SplenA
L Tha
ParOccA
L Cau
PosThaP
CirP
CalcA
AntThaP
mPChA
A2
PCoA
PedP
RAH
A1
ILSA
IV
MCA
PCA
II
III
SCA
IPChA
ICA
BA
PosTempA
Pons
V
AICA
Section-c (Anterior perforating arteries)
Section-d (Posterior perforating arteries)
C-D. Coronal sections
C
D
M4
InsP
M4
PosThaP
M3
M4
mLSA
M2
RAH
A2
AntThaP
ILSA
PCA
A1
SCA
M1
PCoA
BA
ICA
ICA

ing the A1 segment and coursing above the internal carotid artery (ICA) terminus and M1 MCA to the proximal sylvian fissure. It enters the anterior perforated substance with other lLSAs to supply the head of caudate nucleus and adjacent internal capsule, and may also supply the anterior putamen and globus pallidus.

Insular perforators (InsPs) are poorly described in normal anatomic specimens. As is often the case, arteries that are insignificant in the absence of arteriovenous pathology become significant in the presence of such pathology. The InsP supplies AVMs in the sylvian fissure, insula, and lateral basal ganglia. It arises from the M2 segment distal to the limen insulae, which differentiates it from the lLSA arising from the M1 segment. The InsP ascends with M2 stem arteries before penetrating the insular cortex and central core laterally, whereas the lLSA penetrates the central core inferiorly.

Anterior thalamoperforators (AntThaPs) originate from the posterior communicating artery (PCoA) along its superior and lateral surfaces. There are, on average, eight anterior thalamoperforators, the largest of which is the premammillary artery, which penetrate the third ventricle in front of or beside the mammillary bodies. AntThaP supplies the posterior hypothalamus, ventral thalamus, optic tract (anterior third), posterior limb of internal capsule, posterior perforated substance, and subthalamic nucleus.

Posterior thalamoperforators (PosThaPs) originate from the P1 segment of the posterior cerebral artery (PCA), typically from its middle third along the superior and posterior surfaces. The number of thalamoperforators varies from one (artery of Percheron) to 12, with an average of four. PosThaP ascends to the posterior perforated substance and the upper part of the interpeduncular fossa, and supplies the thalamus, posterior hypothalamus, subthalamus, and the medial part of midbrain.

Peduncular perforators (PedPs) arise from the P2 segment and pass directly into the cerebral peduncle, supplying corticospinal and corticobulbar tracts, substantia nigra, red nucleus, and tegmentum. Circumflex perforators (CirPs) encircle the brainstem variable distances (short and long) before penetrating the brain. They arise from the P1 and P2 PCA segments and course around the midbrain medial to the parent PCA. The short CirP penetrates at or before the geniculate bodies, and the long CirP travels back to the quadrigeminal cistern to supply the collicular plate, superior colliculi primarily. The anterior peduncle is typically supplied by the PedP whereas the lateral peduncle is supplied by the CirP.

Thalamogeniculate arteries (ThGenPs) originate from the P2 PCA beneath the lateral thalamus and ascend to the geniculate bodies in the roof of the ambient cistern (AmbC). On average, two or three ThGenPs arise at the P2A-P2P junction to supply the posterior half of the lateral thalamus, posterior limb of internal capsule, and optic tract.

Veins

The deep venous system collects from veins in the basal cisterns and ventricles, which were discussed in Chapter 14. Important veins include the lateral ones draining the ventricular surface of the central core (**Fig. 15.3**): the anterior and posterior caudate vein (CauV) draining the caudate nucleus and terminating in ThaStrV; ThaStrV coursing in the striothalamic sulcus between the caudate nucleus and thalamus; the internal cerebral vein (ICV), a paired vein running in the velum interpositum from the foramen of Monro (FoM) to the vein of Galen (VoG); the VoG, which collects from the two ICVs, two basal veins of Rosenthal (BVRs), and the precentral cerebellar vein; and lateral atrial vein (AtrV), which drains the lateral wall of the atrium, posterior thalamus, and caudate body, and then passes through the choroidal fissure to reach the BVR in the ambient or quadrigeminal cisterns. The insula is drained by insular veins, which collect in DeepSylV and the BVR.

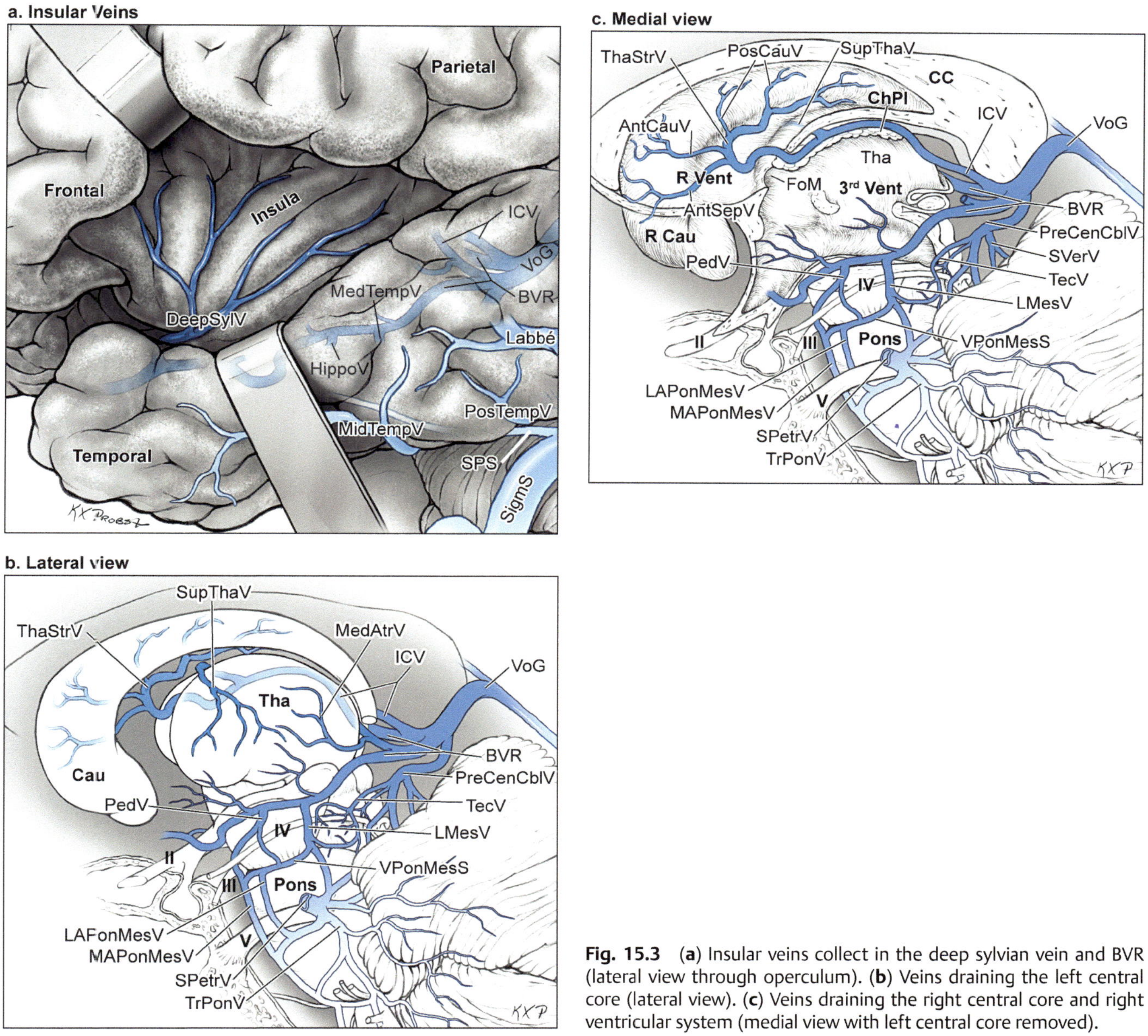

Fig. 15.3 (**a**) Insular veins collect in the deep sylvian vein and BVR (lateral view through operculum). (**b**) Veins draining the left central core (lateral view). (**c**) Veins draining the right central core and right ventricular system (medial view with left central core removed).

Four Deep AVM Subtypes

The Pure Sylvian AVM

Deep AVM subtypes include the pure sylvian, insular, basal ganglial, and thalamic AVMs (**Fig. 15.4**). The pure sylvian AVM, as introduced by Sugita in his classification of AVMs in the sylvian fissure, is located in the fissure without a parenchymal base on the frontal, temporal, or insular cortex (**Fig. 15.5**). Unlike most other AVMs that are based in brain tissue, pure sylvian AVMs are entirely in the subarachnoid space. The AVM splays the fissure, displacing the superior temporal gyrus down on the temporal side and the precentral gyrus, pars opercularis, and pars triangularis up on the frontal side. There are few other such AVMs whose parenchymal planes are replaced by arachnoidal planes: VoG AVMs, pial brainstem AVMs, and some ventricular AVMs. Pure sylvian AVMs are particularly clean because the dissection is subarachnoid without pial or parenchymal transgression. Furthermore, the location is superficial with excellent exposure. Pure sylvian AVMs are supplied by MCA stem arteries arising from both superior and inferior trunks along their M2 and M3 segments. The nidus resides laterally in the operculum, which situates feeding MCA branches deep to the nidus. Feeders are typically large terminal arteries with high-flow intranidal shunts, which frequently enlarge draining veins into varices. SupSylV and DeepSylV provide drainage, with superficial veins more dominant than deep veins. The sylvian AVMs that do not respect the opercular surfaces of the frontal lobe, temporal lobe, or insula are categorized as sylvian frontal, sylvian temporal, or insular AVMs, respectively. Pure sylvian AVMs were the least common of the deep AVMs (14%), which attests more to their rarity than their operability.

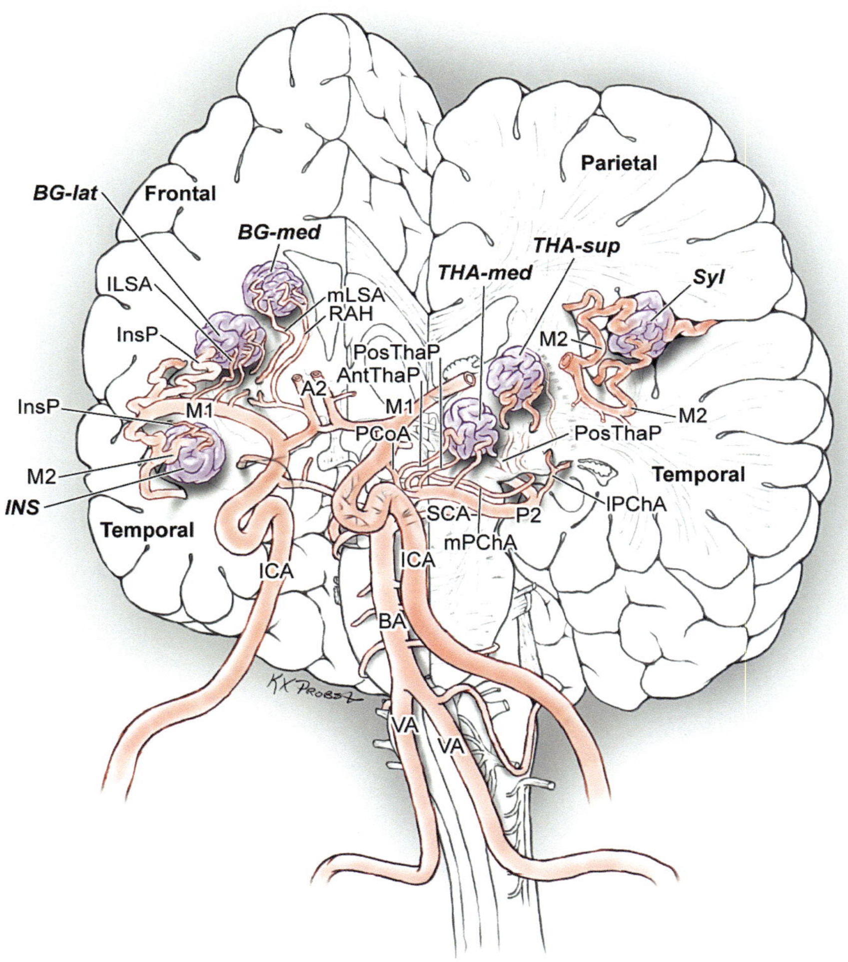

Fig. 15.4 Overview of deep AVM subtypes, which include pure sylvian (SYL), insular (INS), basal ganglial [lateral (BG-lat), and medial (BG-med)], and thalamic [superior (THA-sup) and medial (THA-med)], as seen in an anterior oblique, coronal cross-sectional view.

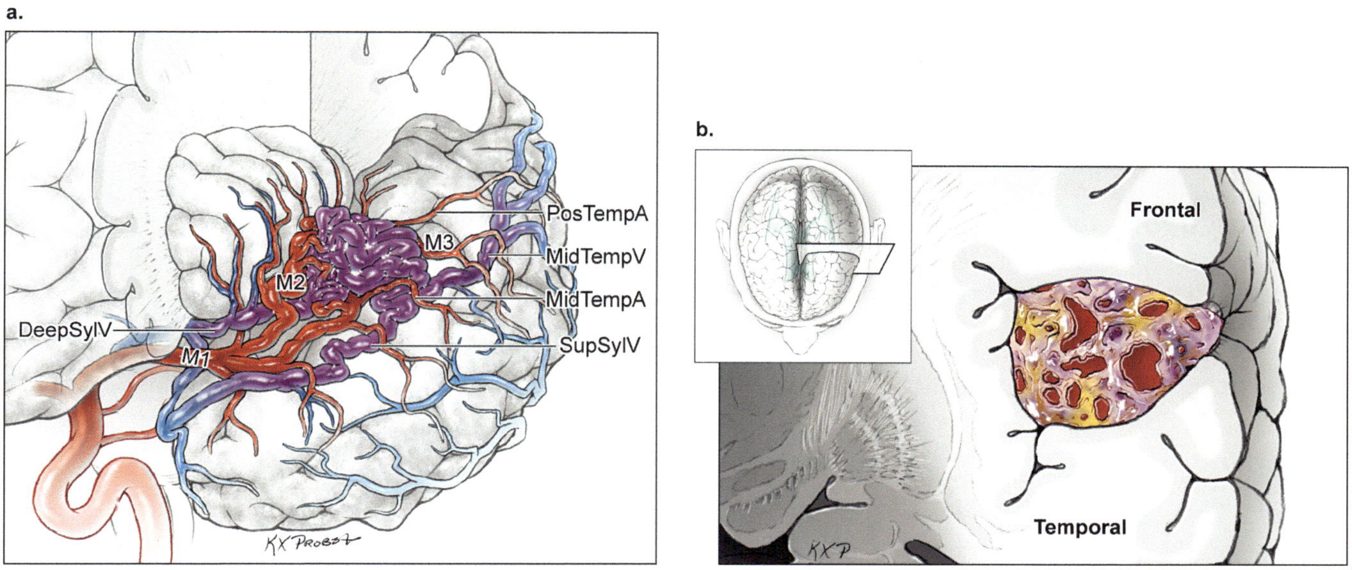

Fig. 15.5 The pure sylvian AVM subtype, viewed anteriorly (**a**) with the frontal and parietal lobes removed partially, and (**b**) in coronal cross section. This AVM is located in the subarachnoid spaces of the sylvian cistern without a parenchymal base in the frontal, temporal, or insular cortex. It is supplied by MCA stem arteries (M2 and M3 segments) and drained by sylvian veins (SupSylV and DeepSylV).

The Insular AVM

Insular AVMs sit in the limen insulae, short gyri, and long gyri on the insular surface, but lateral to the basal ganglial structures and respectful of the claustrum (**Fig. 15.6**). Insular AVMs were included in Sugita's classification of sylvian fissure AVMs and described as deep sylvian AVMs. Insular AVMs were the most common of the deep AVM in my practice, accounting for nearly half (45%) of those treated surgically. The M2 segments supply insular AVMs and course above or lateral to the nidus, requiring the resection to proceed between these arteries. Feeders are large stem arteries and the InsP. Sylvian veins drain these AVMs, with DeepSylV more dominant than SupSylV. Although the role of the insular cortex in speech processing and in conduction between Wernicke's and Broca's areas is unclear, it is consid-

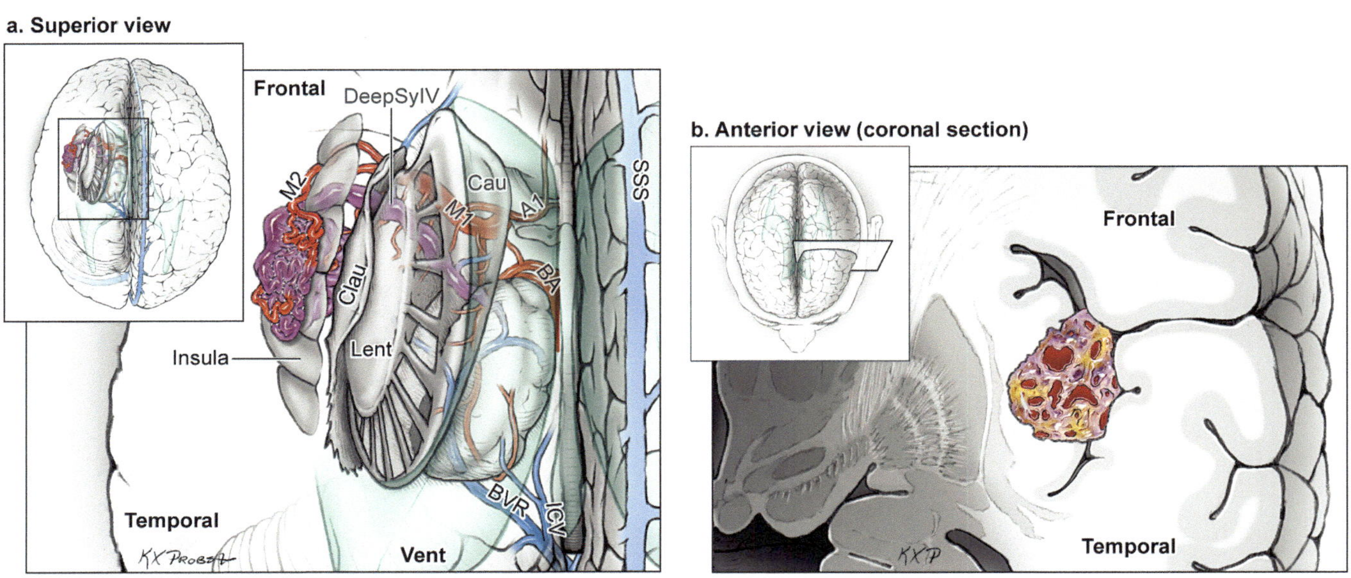

Fig. 15.6 The insular AVM subtype: (**a**) superior and (**b**) coronal cross-sectional views. This AVM is located in insular cortex, supplied by MCA stem arteries (M2 segment) and insular perforators (InsP), and drained by DeepSylV.

ered non-eloquent. However, insular AVM exposure in the dominant hemisphere requires dissection adjacent and deep to speech areas in both the frontal and temporal lobes.

The Basal Ganglial AVM

The basal ganglia AVM is deep to the insular cortex in the putamen (**Fig. 15.7**), globus pallidus, anterior limb of the internal capsule, or caudate nucleus (**Fig. 15.8**). It sits lateral to the posterior limb of the internal capsule, whereas the thalamic AVM sits medial to the posterior limb. Basal ganglial AVMs have no cortical representation whatsoever and can be reached only laterally through a nonanatomic, transcortical route created either surgically or by hemorrhage. Consequently, basal ganglial AVMs located laterally in the putamen are the most favorable for resection (lateral variant). Some located in the caudate head can be reached medially through a transependymal route through the lateral ventricle (medial variant). The AVMs in other basal ganglial locations are less favorable for surgery. Lateral basal ganglial AVMs are deeper than insular AVMs and are fed by the InsP and lLSA rather than MCA stem arteries. Medial basal ganglial AVMs receive inputs from the mLSA and RAH. Drainage collects in the deep system via DeepSlyV (lateral variant) or CauV and ThaStrV (medial variant). Basal ganglial circuits are eloquent, and proximity to the internal capsule makes these AVMs dangerous.

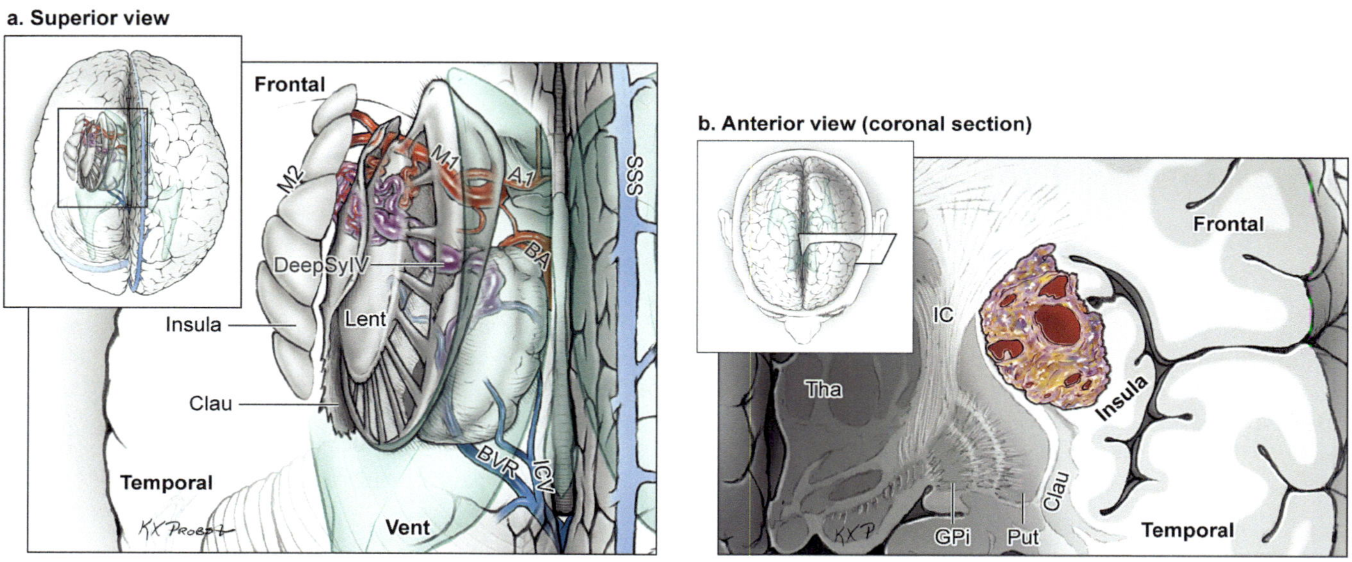

Fig. 15.7 The basal ganglial AVM subtype in the putamen: (**a**) superior and (**b**) coronal cross-sectional views. This lateral variant is located beneath the insular cortex in the putamen or globus pallidus, supplied by lLSA and InsP, and drained by DeepSylV.

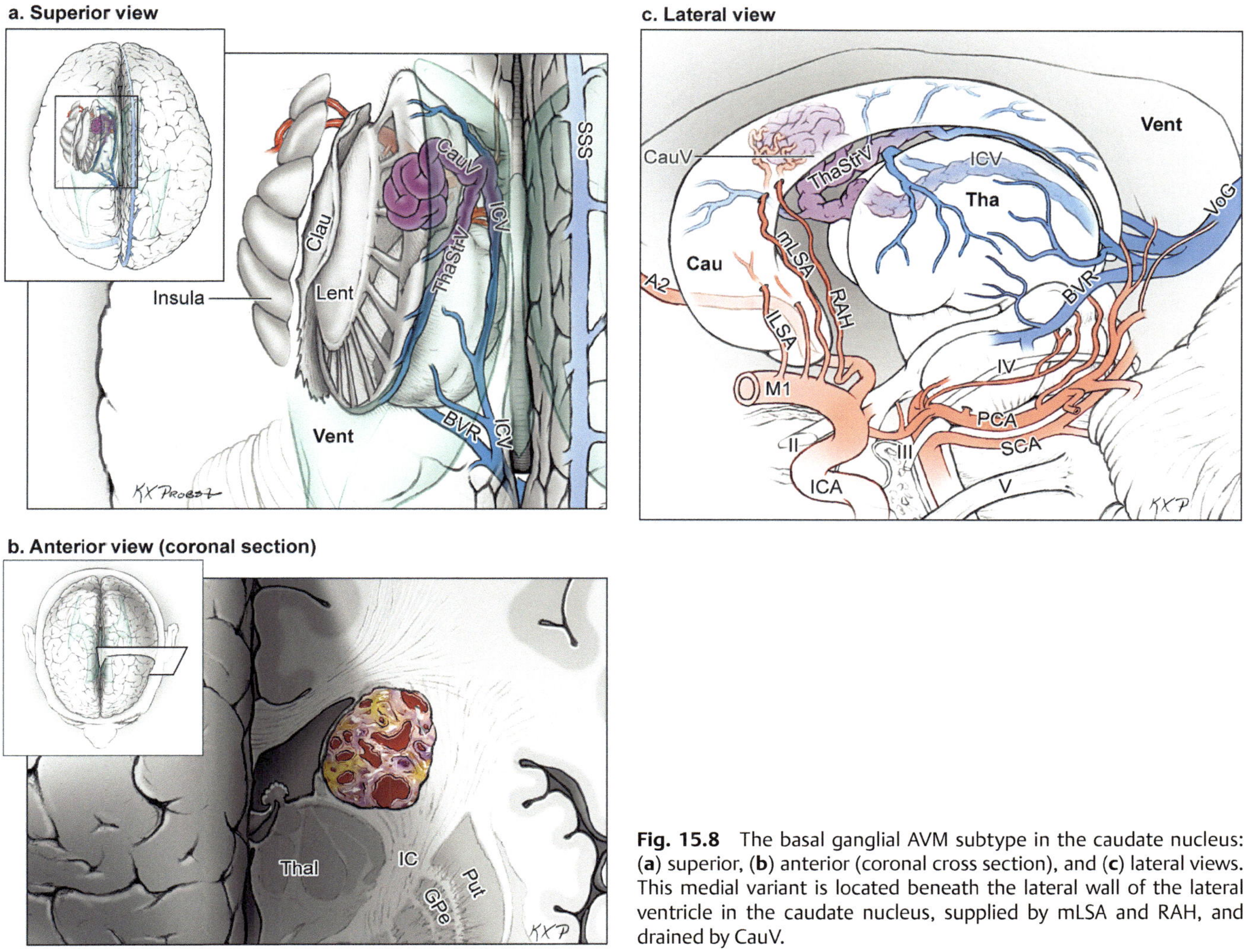

Fig. 15.8 The basal ganglial AVM subtype in the caudate nucleus: (**a**) superior, (**b**) anterior (coronal cross section), and (**c**) lateral views. This medial variant is located beneath the lateral wall of the lateral ventricle in the caudate nucleus, supplied by mLSA and RAH, and drained by CauV.

The Thalamic AVM

Together with the hypothalamus and brainstem, the thalamus is one of the inviolable brain structures that inspires caution. Compelling indications are needed to operate on a thalamic AVM: hemorrhage, significant preexisting deficits, failure of stereotactic radiosurgery, and young age. Thalamus does not tolerate much transgression, and operable AVMs must be small and superficially located on surgically accessible surfaces. Two such surfaces are (1) the superior thalamic surface that forms the floor of the ventricular body, behind the FoM, between the body of the fornix and the body of the caudate nucleus, and deep to the choroid plexus (superior variant, **Fig. 15.9**); and (2) the medial thalamic surface that forms the lateral wall of the third ventricle deep to the FoM (medial variant, **Fig. 15.10**). These surfaces are accessible through transcallosal and transcallosal-transchoroidal fissure approaches, respectively. Importantly, AVMs in these entry zones avoid the medial knee of internal capsule. Thalamic AVMs are supplied from below by AntThaP (from PCoA) and PosThaP (from P1 PCA), and from above by lPChA and mPChA. Thalamic AVMs on the superior wall drain ventricularly to the ICV, whereas medial wall drain cisternally to the BVR.

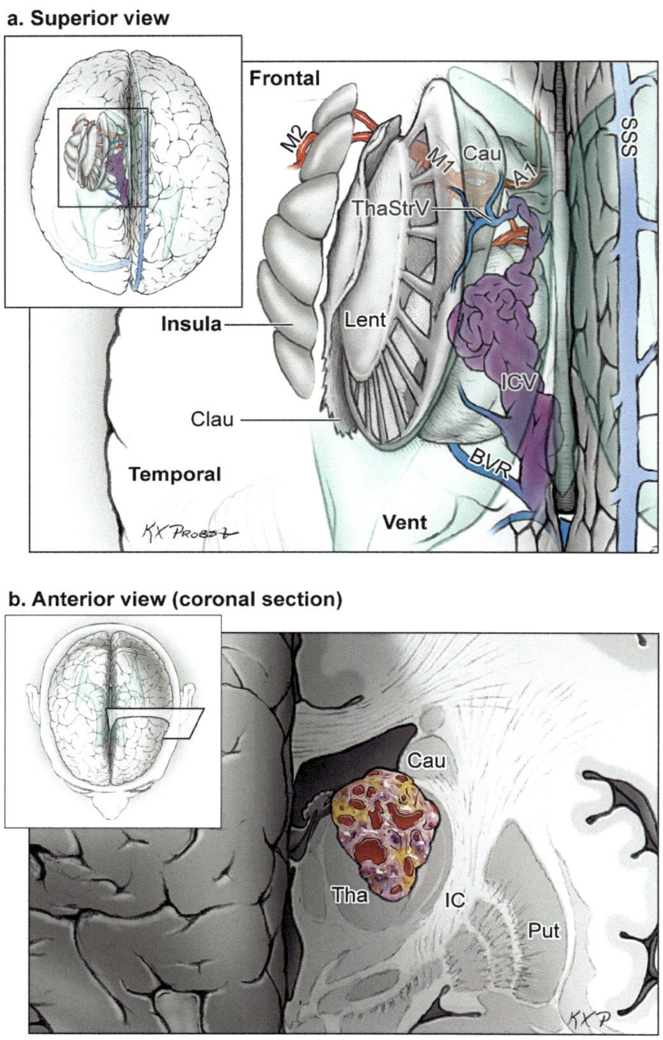

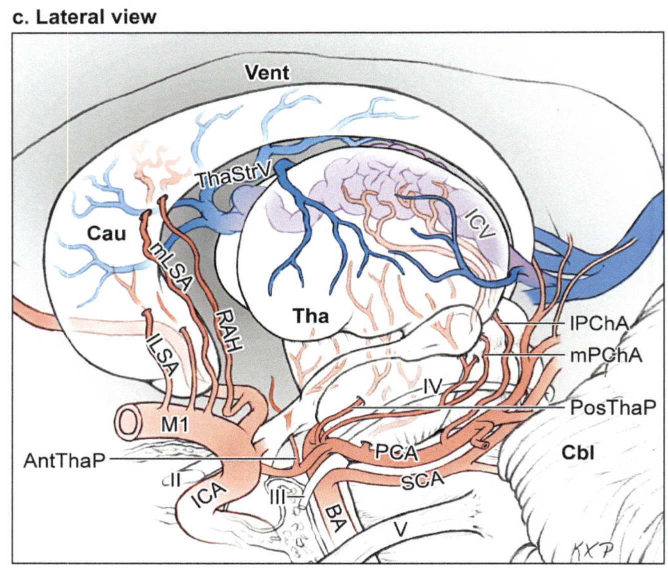

Fig. 15.9 The superior thalamic AVM subtype, viewed (**a**) superiorly, (**b**) anteriorly (coronal cross section), and (**c**) laterally. This superior variant is located on the superior thalamic surface, supplied by PosThaP and the posterior choroidal arteries (mPChA and lPChA), and drained by the ICV.

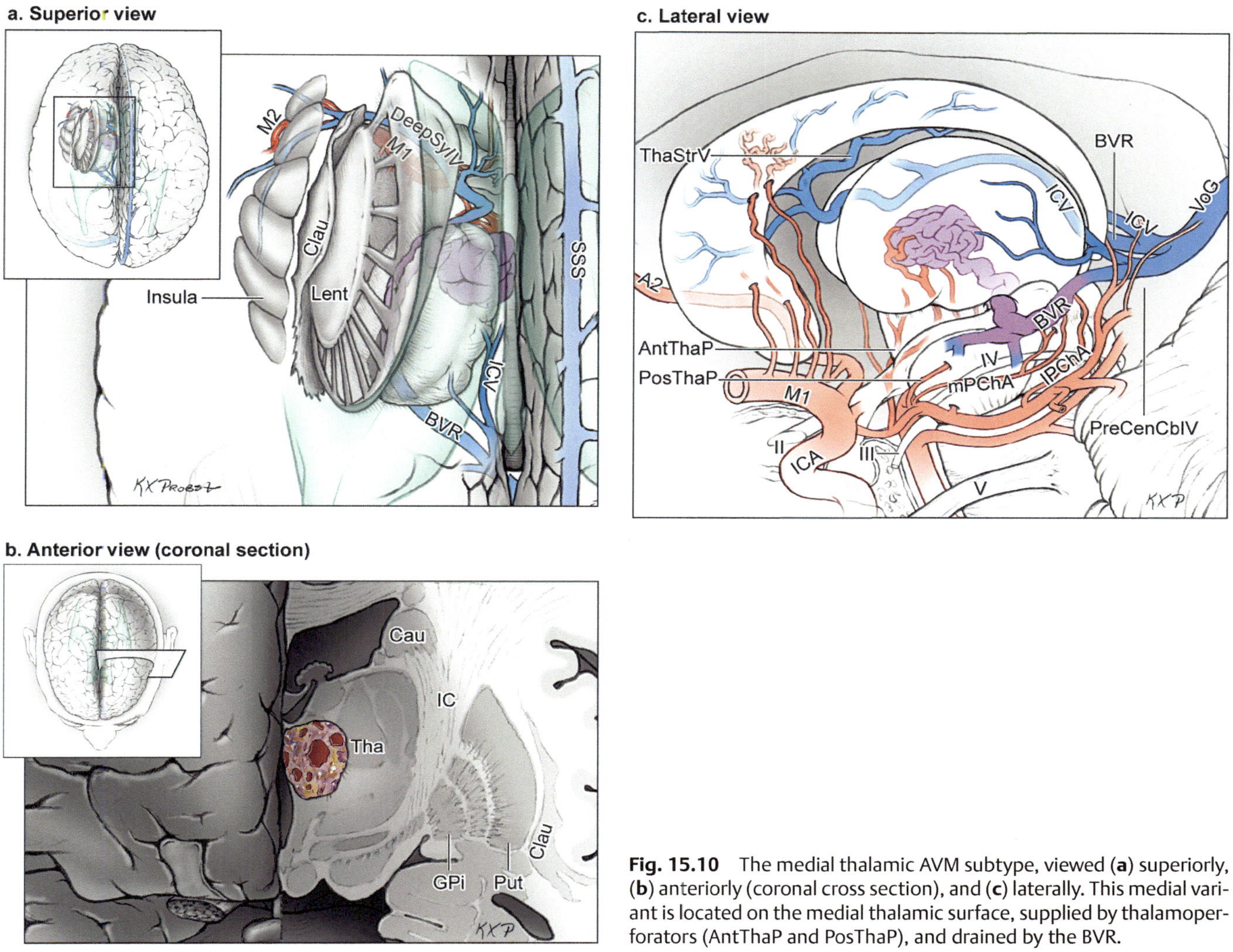

Fig. 15.10 The medial thalamic AVM subtype, viewed (**a**) superiorly, (**b**) anteriorly (coronal cross section), and (**c**) laterally. This medial variant is located on the medial thalamic surface, supplied by thalamoperforators (AntThaP and PosThaP), and drained by the BVR.

Resection Strategies for Deep AVMs

Pure Sylvian AVM Resection

Pure sylvian AVMs are exposed with a pterional craniotomy and transsylvian approach (**Fig. 15.11**). The patient is positioned supine with the head turned 20 to 30 degrees away from the AVM and extended 20 degrees, as for an MCA aneurysm, allowing the frontal and temporal lobes to fall naturally to either side of the fissure like pages in a book resting on its binding. The scalp incision and craniotomy extend around the posterior AVM margin, which might require a hairline incision and standard pterional craniotomy for anterior AVMs and a question mark incision and additional parietal/posterior temporal expansion for posterior AVMs (step 1). Pure sylvian AVMs are exposed and circumdissected

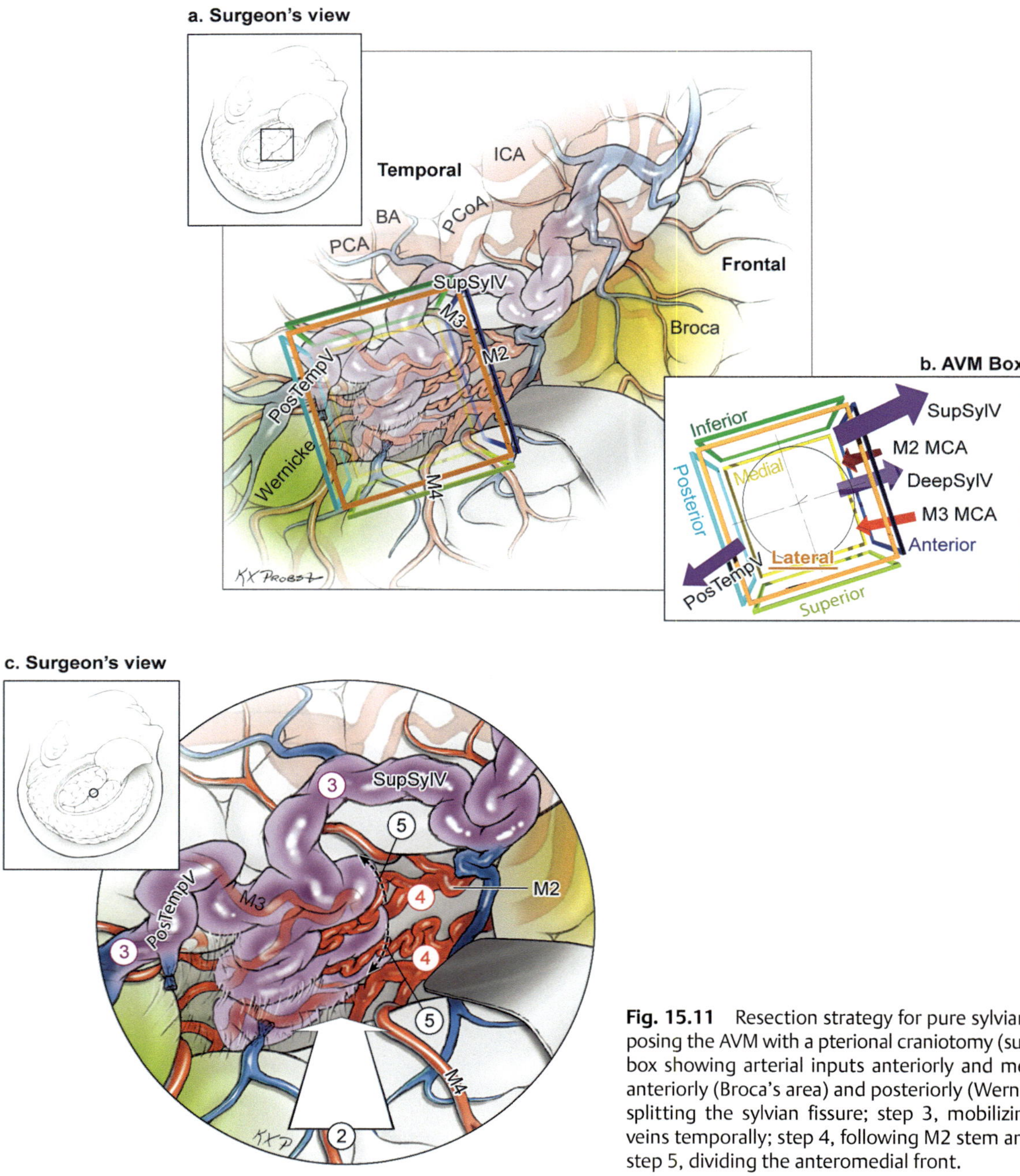

Fig. 15.11 Resection strategy for pure sylvian AVMs. (**a**) Step 1, exposing the AVM with a pterional craniotomy (surgeon's view). (**b**) AVM box showing arterial inputs anteriorly and medially, and eloquence anteriorly (Broca's area) and posteriorly (Wernicke's area). (**c**) Step 2, splitting the sylvian fissure; step 3, mobilizing superficial draining veins temporally; step 4, following M2 stem arteries to the AVM; and step 5, dividing the anteromedial front.

d. Coronal view

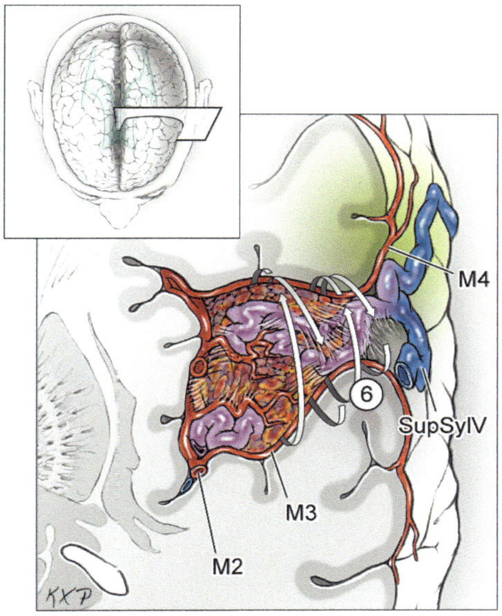

Fig. 15.11 (*continued*) (**d**) Step 6, circumdissecting within the subarachnoid spaces of the sylvian fissure (coronal cross-sectional view). (**e**) Step 7, dividing terminal M2/M3 feeding arteries, skeletonizing stem arteries en passage (distal to proximal), mobilizing the AVM out of the sylvian fissure (surgeon's view), and (**f**) accessing deep feeding arteries along insular cortex (coronal cross-sectional view).

e. Surgeon's view

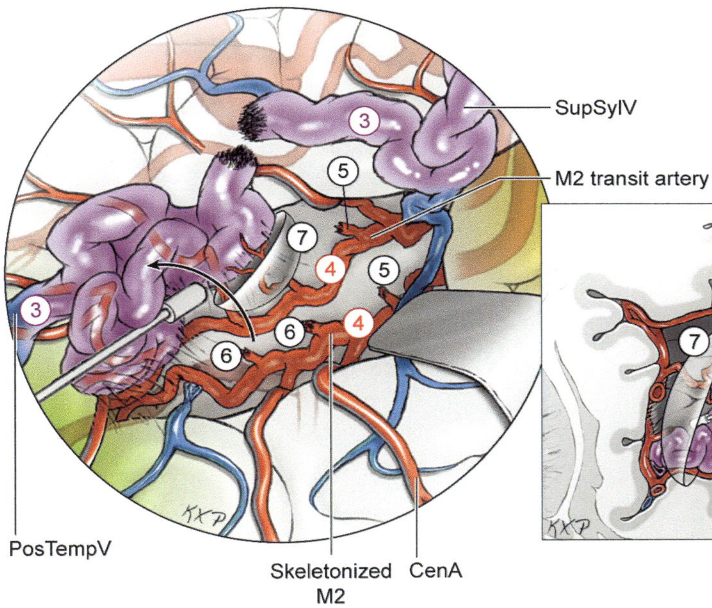

f. Coronal view

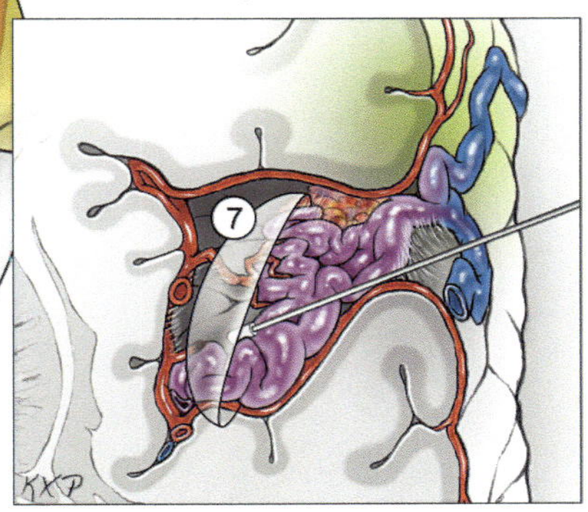

in the subarachnoid phase of dissection without pial, parenchymal, or ependymal dissection. Sylvian fissure arachnoid is incised below the pars triangularis where the distal fissure is widest, SupSylV is mobilized to the temporal side of the fissure, and the fissure is split from distal to proximal (step 2). Drainage through an enlarged or variceal SupSylV remains centered over the nidus throughout the dissection (step 3). Supply originates from the insular M2 and opercular M3 segments of MCA stem arteries and from both superior and inferior trunks (step 4). These feeding arteries are situated underneath the nidus on both the frontal and temporal sides, forming an anteromedial front (step 5). Sylvian arteries are a mixture of terminal feeding arteries, transit arteries, and bystander arteries. High-flow terminal feeders are identified in the proximal fissure on the inferomedial AVM margin as large pipes that frequently require occlusion with aneurysm clips rather than cautery. Transit arteries require skeletonization in a distal-to-proximal direction to interrupt their smaller nidal inputs and also preserve cortical arteries that continue en passage. Uninvolved bystander arteries are separated from the nidus and mobilized temporally or frontally. Meticulous arachnoidal dissection in the sylvian cistern maintains pial integrity and no parenchymal transgression is needed for circumdissection (step 6). Deep dissection exposes the full course of the M2 and M3 stem arteries, DeepSylV drainage, and insula cortex (step 7). Pure sylvian AVMs are extraparenchymal and therefore non-eloquent, but are adjacent to speech areas in the dominant frontal and temporal lobes (**Figs. 15.12** and **15.13**).

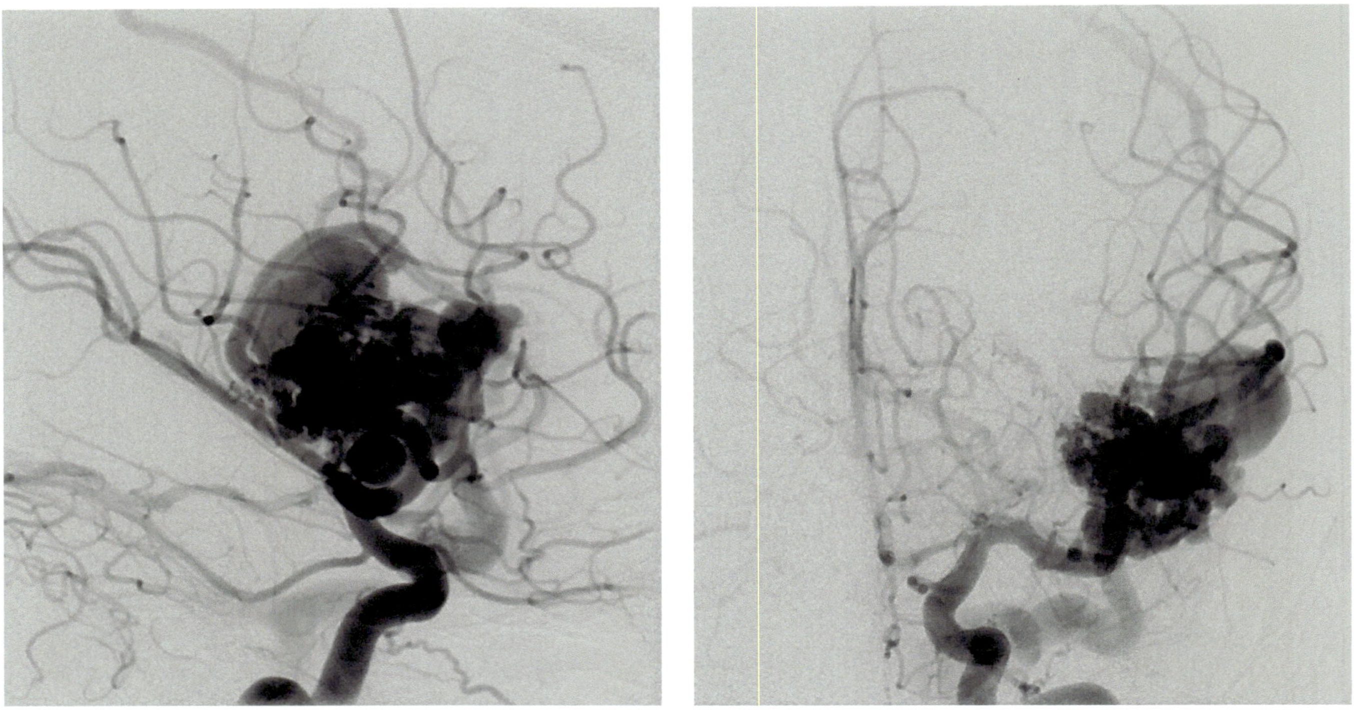

a

b

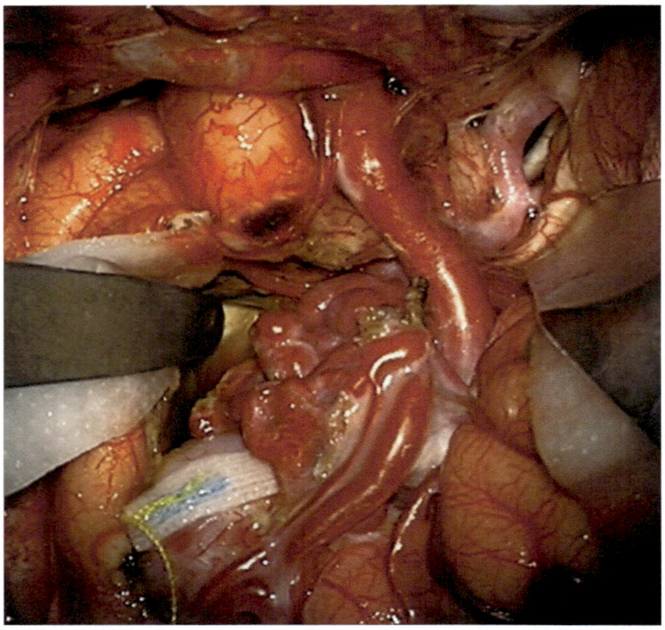

c

Fig. 15.12 This 20-year-old woman presented with a remote hemorrhage and seizures from a left pure sylvian AVM (supplemented Spetzler-Martin grade 4: S1V1E1/A1B0C0), supplied by M2 MCA trunks and drained by DeepSylV and SupSylV [left ICA angiogram, (**a**) lateral and (**b**) anteroposterior views]. (**c**) The AVM was exposed through a pterional craniotomy and resided entirely in the sylvian fissure.

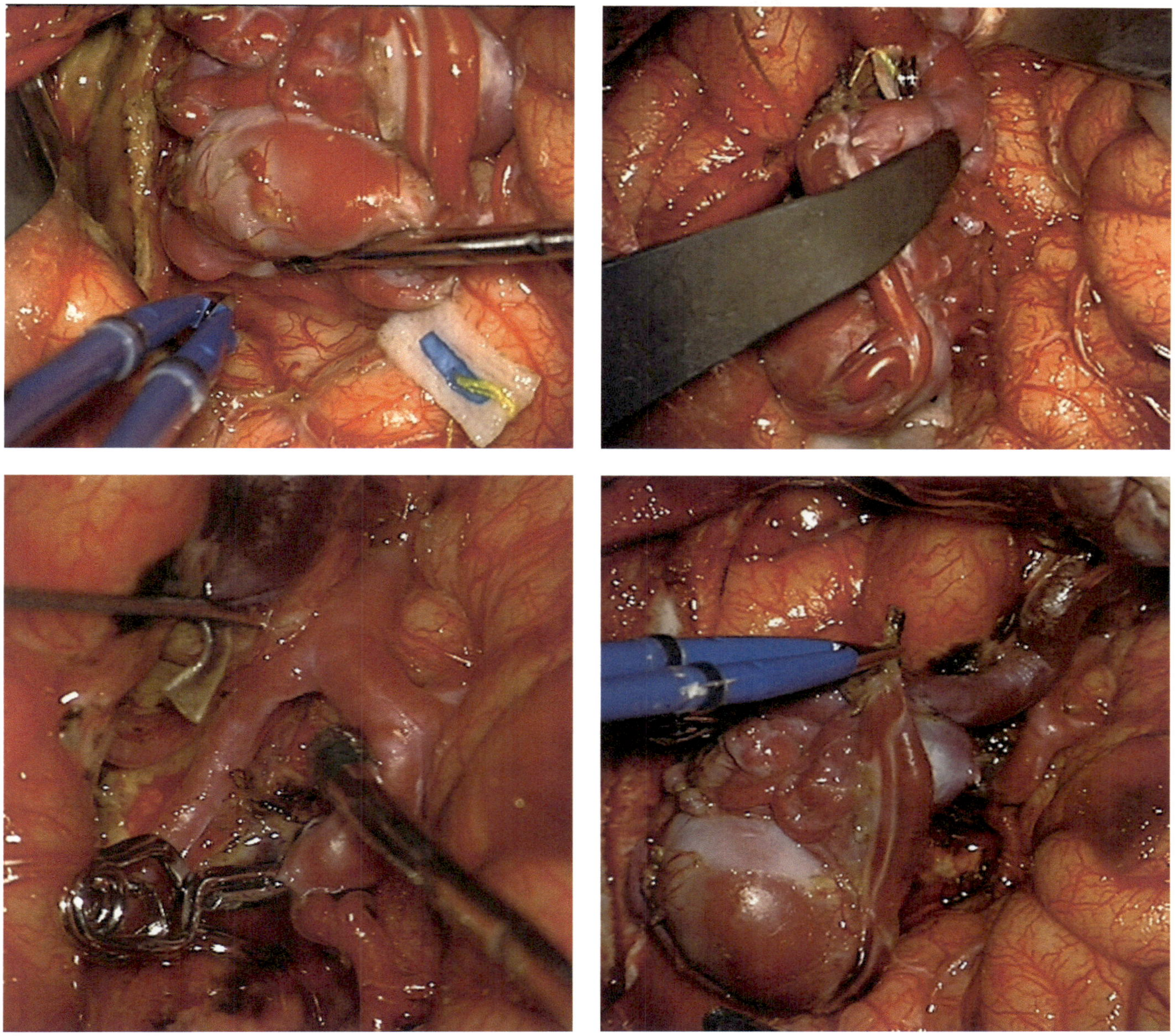

d e f g

Fig. 15.12 (*continued*) Arachnoidal planes were dissected inferiorly, (**d**) posteriorly, and (**e**) superiorly, with intact pia on the temporal and frontal opercula and angular gyrus. (**f**) A large feeding artery from the frontal trunk was clip occluded, (**g**) after which the AVM darkened and was resected.

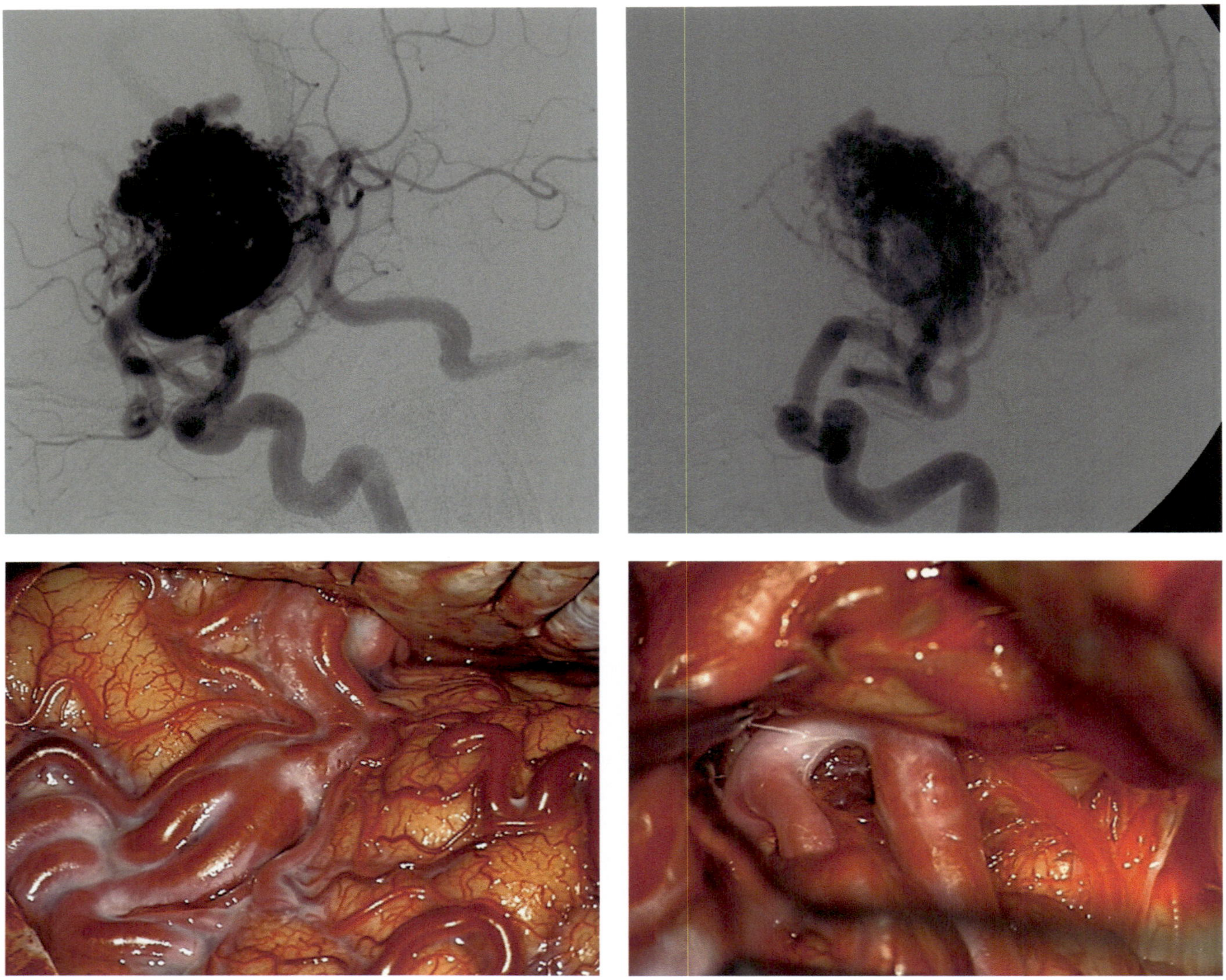

a b c d

Fig. 15.13 This 53-year-old man presented with a left pure sylvian AVM (supplemented Spetzler-Martin grade 8: S2V1E1/A3B1C0), supplied by M2 MCA branches [left ICA angiogram, (**a**) lateral and (**b**) anteroposterior views]. Despite its high grade, he insisted on having it removed. (**c**) The sylvian fissure was covered by a complex of arterialized SupSylVs, and (**d**) proximal sylvian fissure dissection exposed the feeding arteries.

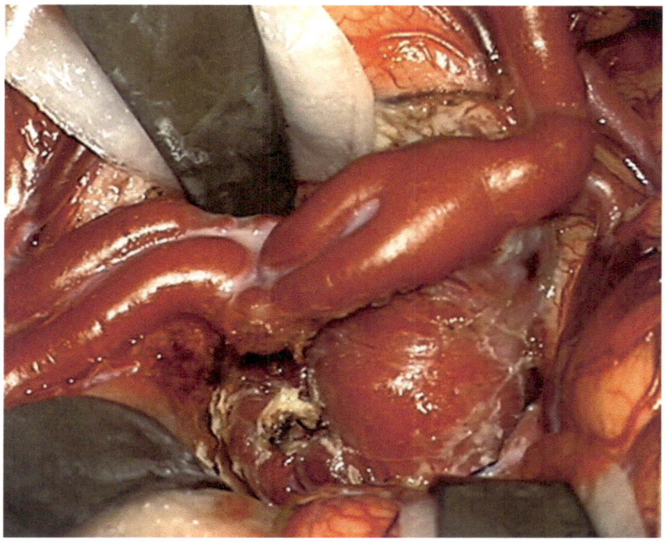

e

Fig. 15.13 (*continued*) (**e**) The AVM coalesced on a large varix in the sylvian cistern, (**f**) which darkened with distal-to-proximal skeletonization of the M3 and M2 MCA segments. (**g**) The AVM was rolled out of the sylvian fissure after separating the MCA stem arteries from the nidus.

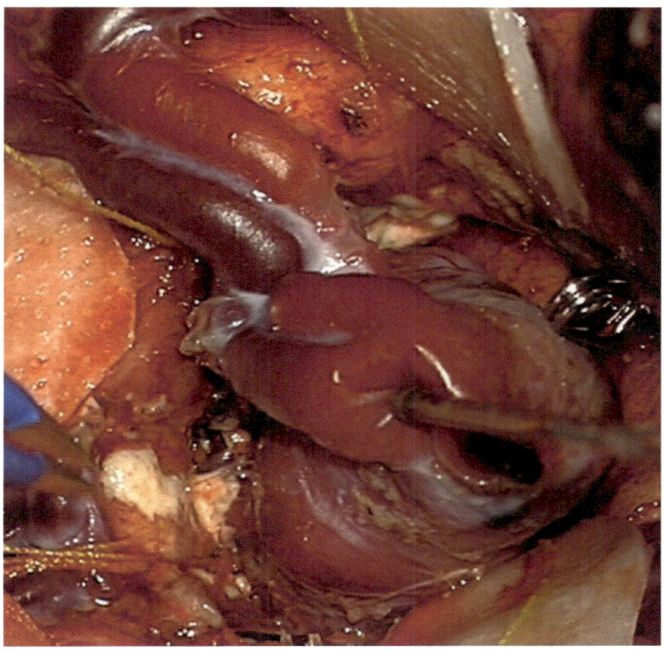

f

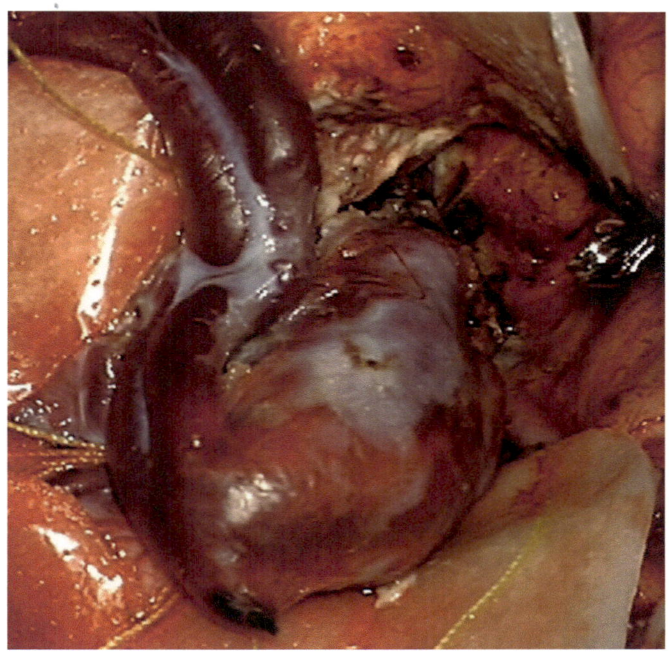

g

Insular AVM Resection

Insular AVMs are also resected through a pterional craniotomy and transsylvian approach (**Fig. 15.14**), with patient position, scalp incision, and craniotomy, as with pure sylvian AVMs (step 1). Insular AVMs require a more extensive sylvian split and deeper dissection to visualize the nidus (step 2). After opening the cortical arachnoid and mobilizing SupSylV temporally, a cortical artery is followed into the operculum to develop the separation plane between the frontal and temporal lobes. Opercular arteries are followed down to the insular arteries and the MCA trunks at the bi- or trifurcation. Spreading dissection from inside-out separates the frontal and temporal lobes, and smaller arterial branches are mobilized frontally or temporally. The limen insulae and short gyri are then exposed through the M2 segments. A posterior transsylvian-transinsular approach is needed for AVMs in the long gyri. With this posterior approach, dissection typically begins at the same place as with the anterior approach, but proceeds in the opposite direction. Cortical

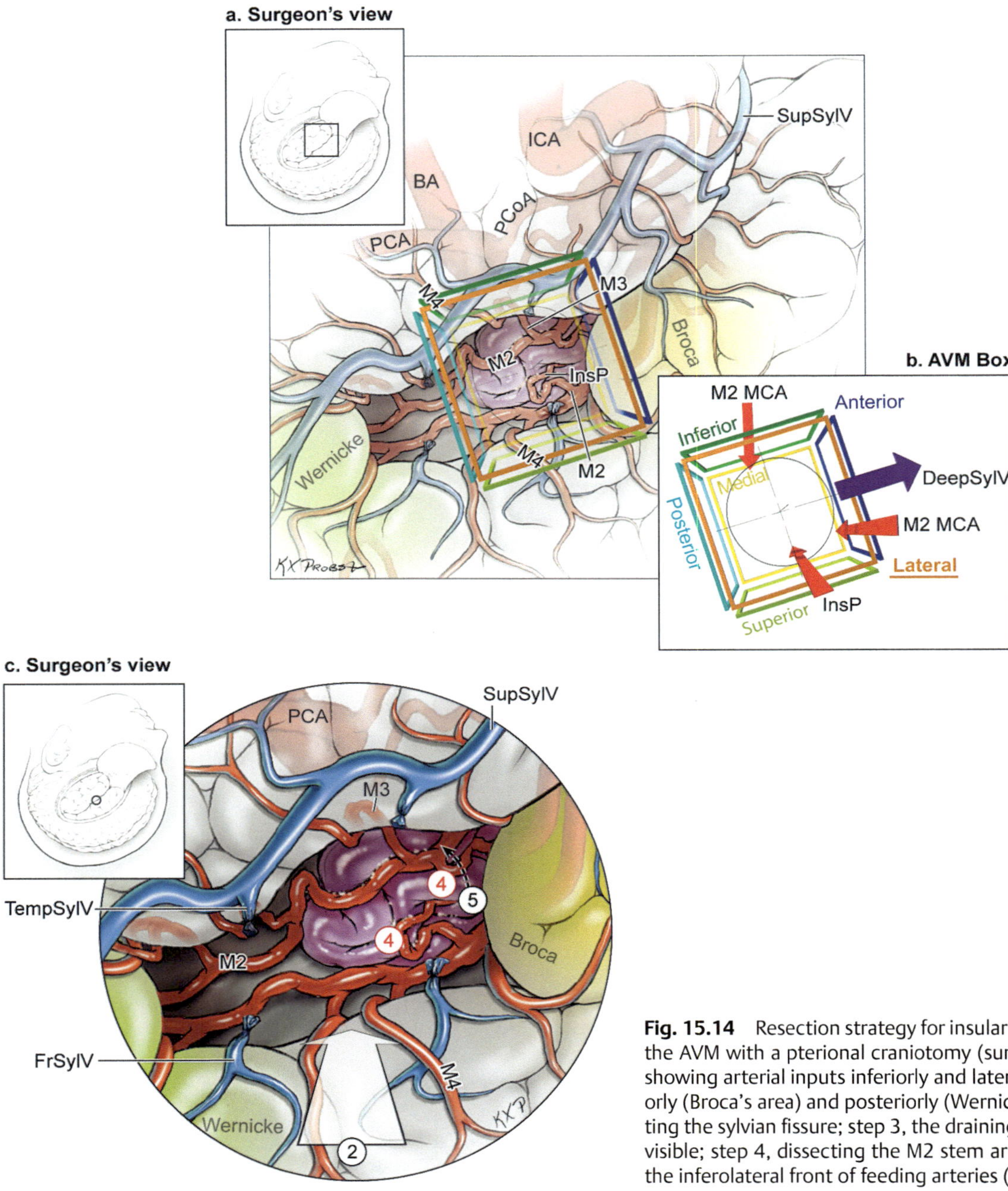

Fig. 15.14 Resection strategy for insular AVMs. (**a**) Step 1, exposing the AVM with a pterional craniotomy (surgeon's view). (**b**) AVM box showing arterial inputs inferiorly and laterally, and eloquence anteriorly (Broca's area) and posteriorly (Wernicke's area). (**c**) Step 2, splitting the sylvian fissure; step 3, the draining vein (DeepSylV) is not yet visible; step 4, dissecting the M2 stem arteries; and step 5, dividing the inferolateral front of feeding arteries (M2 and InsP).

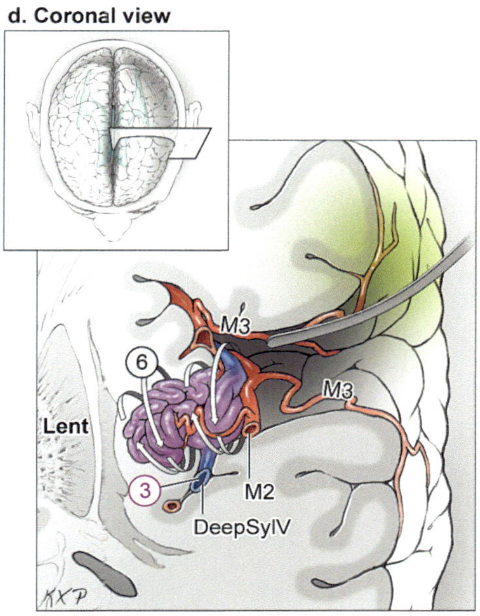

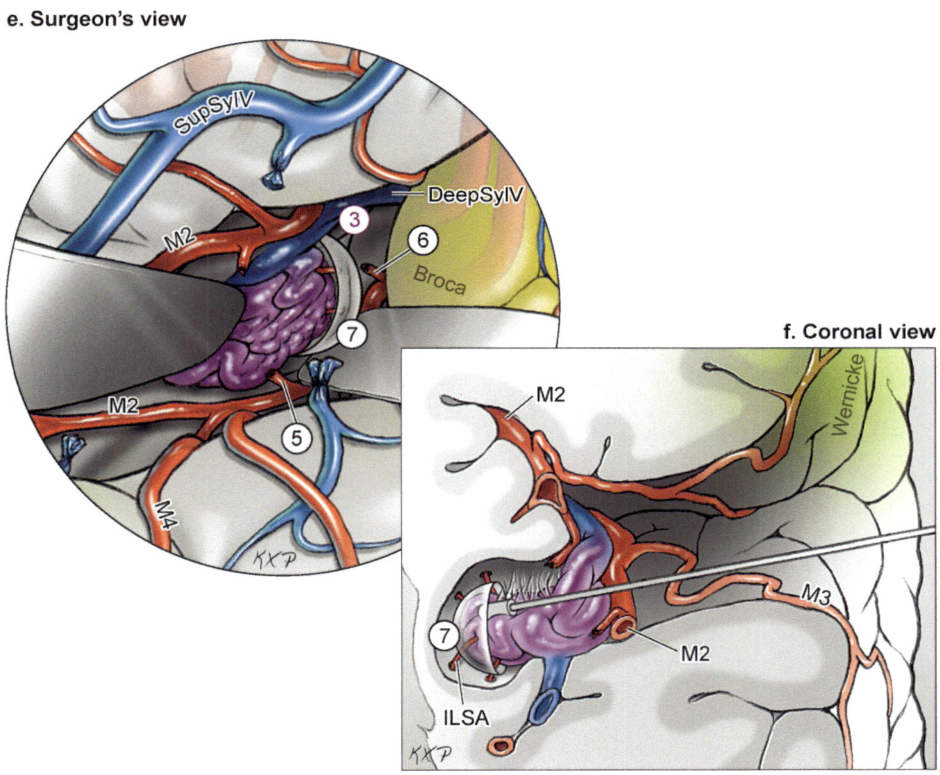

Fig. 15.14 (*continued*) (**d**) Step 6, circumdissecting between and deep to the M2 arteries and identifying the draining vein (coronal cross-sectional view). (**e**) Step 7, skeletonizing the M2 transit arteries, mobilizing the AVM into the sylvian fissure (surgeon's view), and (**f**) interrupting the deep supply from the ILSA (coronal cross-sectional view).

arachnoid is incised posteriorly, following the fissure below the pars triangularis, pars opercularis, precentral gyrus, and the gyral bridge between the lower ends of pre- and postcentral gyri. Dissection proceeds from proximal to distal, mobilizing veins and following cortical arteries down into the fissure. Separation of frontal and temporal lobes is more difficult distally than proximally because the sylvian cistern ends and opercular surfaces are adherent. The opening may be facilitated by splitting the proximal fissure first and extending posteriorly into the distal fissure, but overlying veins often prevent continuous dissection without venous sacrifice. Opercular arteries are followed down to the depths of the opercular cleft to reach the long gyri. The distal sylvian fissure is narrow and constrained, and unlike with the proximal sylvian fissure, often requires a retractor.

Insular AVMs drain through insular veins and DeepSylV (step 3), and arterialization offers a landmark to those AVMs beneath the insular cortex. Stem arteries and the InsP supplying AVM overlie the nidus (step 4). Feeders intersect the AVM inferolaterally and are occluded with a pial incision along this margin of superficial insular AVMs (step 5). Deeper AVMs require a transinsular incision, resecting overlying cortex, and following the arterialized vein into insula. Circumdissection proceeds perpendicularly between superficial M2 segments and closes arterial inputs on the lateral and inferior sides (step 6). The AVM is drawn into the surgical corridor to visualize the superior and medial sides. The medial margin adjacent to basal ganglia (caudate head and putamen) may have some lLSA supply and a deep vein (CauV) that courses through the basal ganglia to the lateral ventricle (step 7). Transinsular dissection is deep to eloquent speech areas in the dominant frontal and temporal lobes, but requires careful splitting of the sylvian fissure and gentle retraction if fixed retractors are used (**Figs. 15.15** and **15.16**).

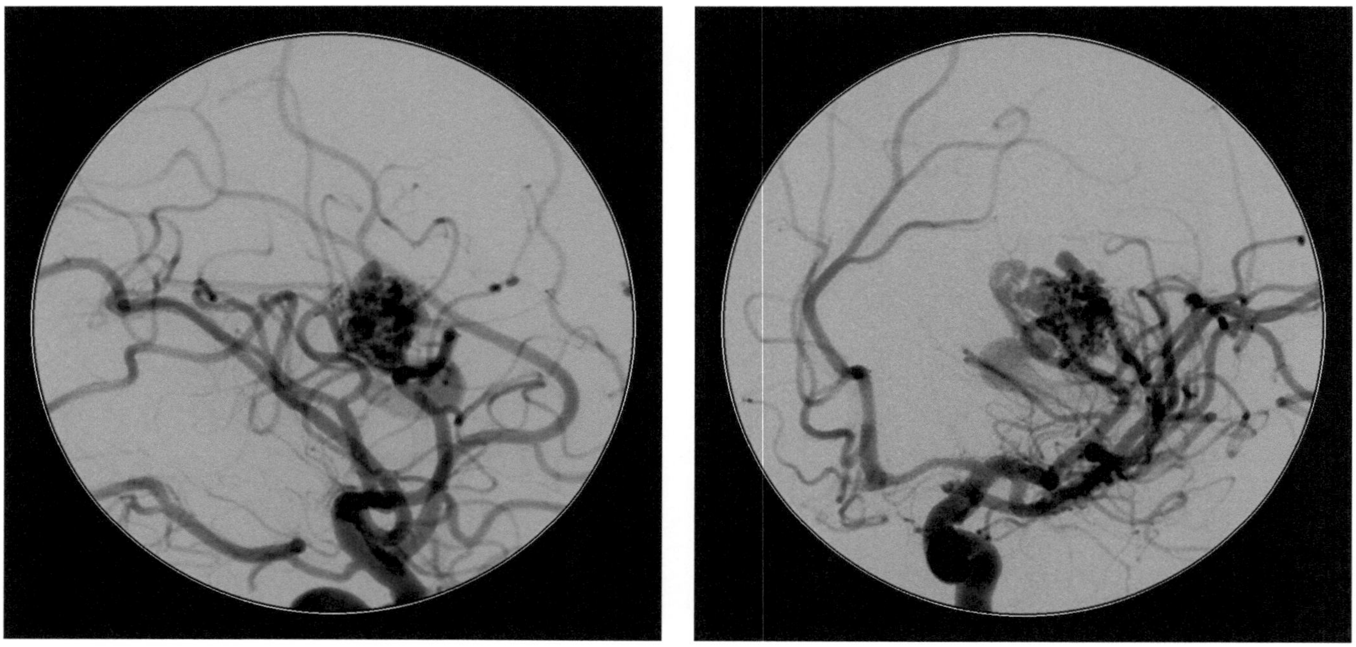

a b

Fig. 15.15 This 40-year-old man presented with this left insular AVM (supplemented Spetzler-Martin grade 5: S1V0E1/A2B1C0), supplied by two M2 stem arteries originating from the superior trunk and draining to DeepSylV [left ICA angiogram, (**a**) lateral and (**b**) anteroposterior views].

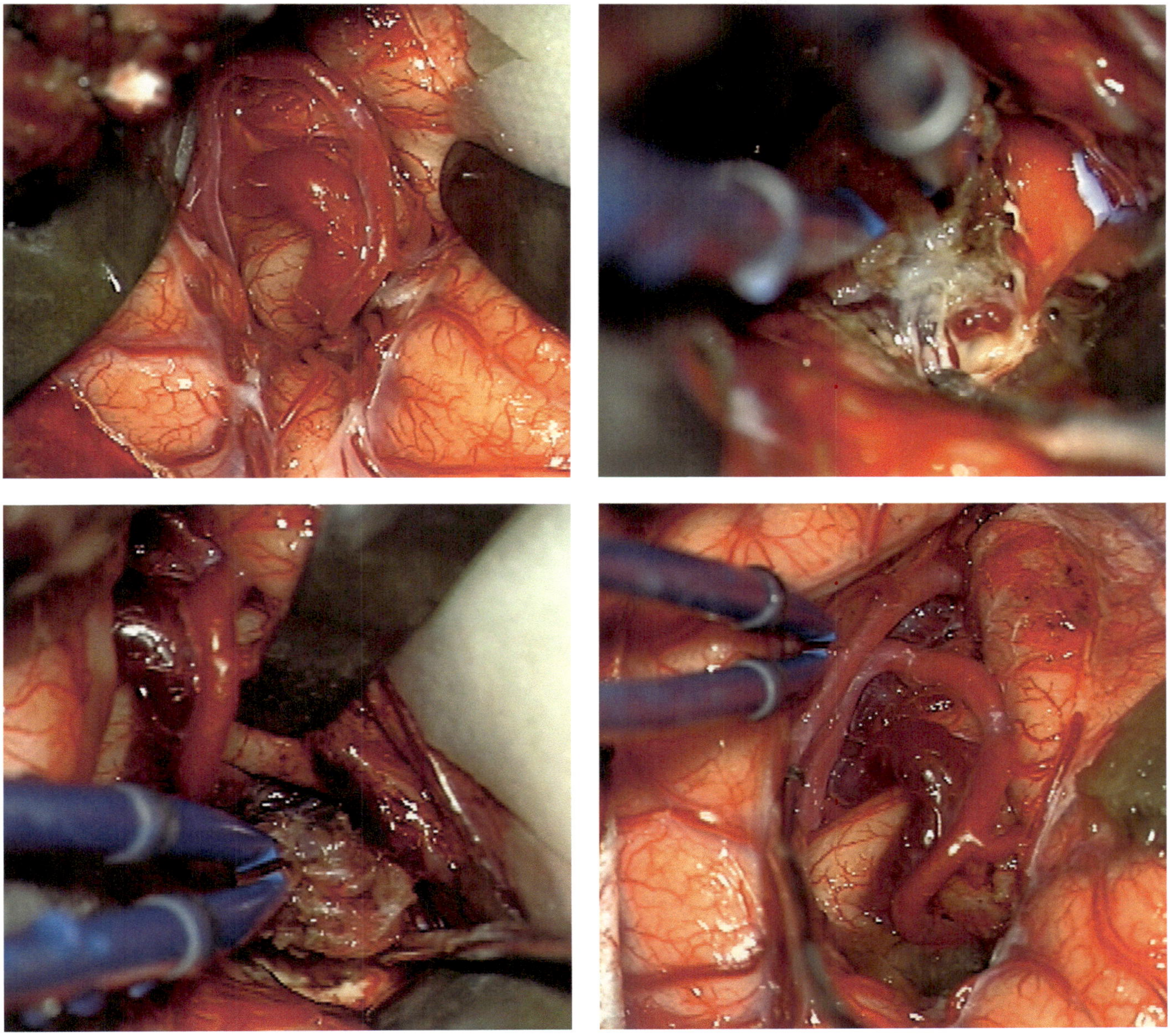

Fig. 15.15 *(continued)* (**c**) The short gyri of the insula were exposed with a wide sylvian fissure split and the arterialized draining vein was visualized [pterional craniotomy with retractors on the temporal (left) and frontal (right) opercula]. The draining vein and the adjacent M2 stem artery led to the AVM, (**d**) which was mobilized down into the sylvian cistern. (**e**) The AVM was removed, (**f**) preserving normal branches of the MCA and the darkened DeepSylV.

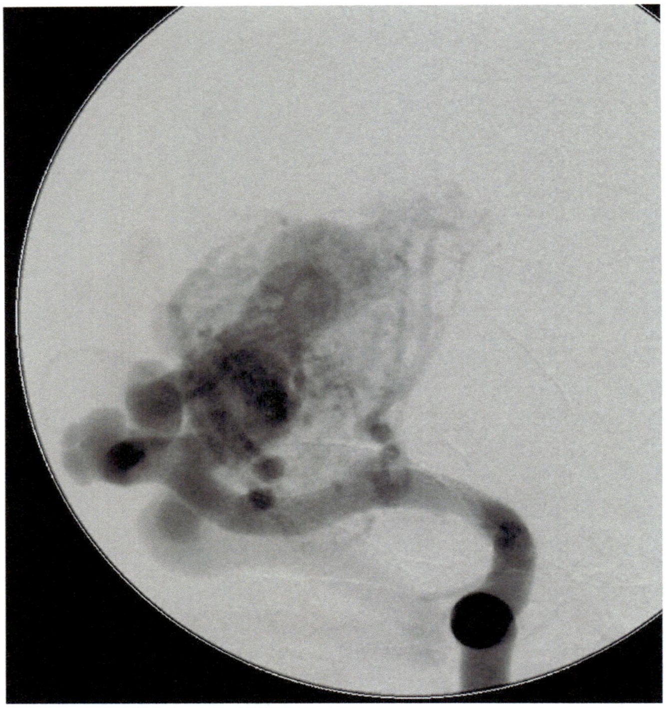

a

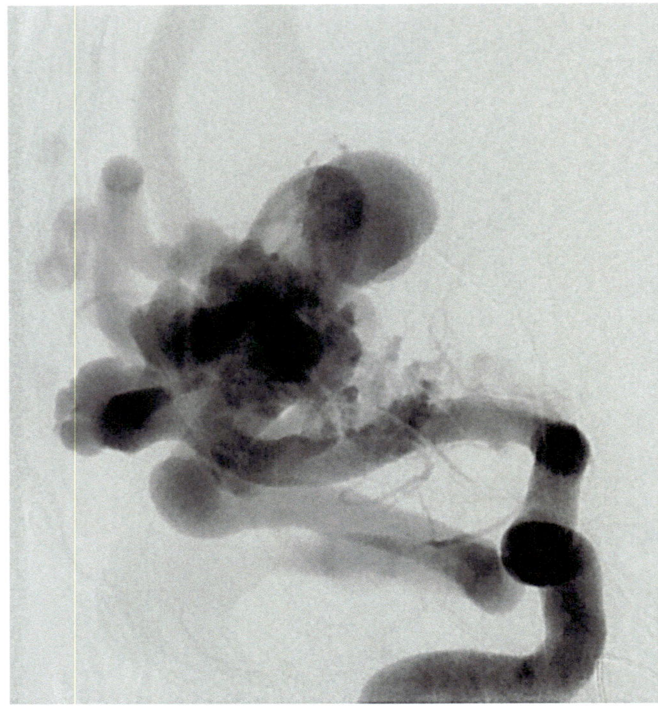

b

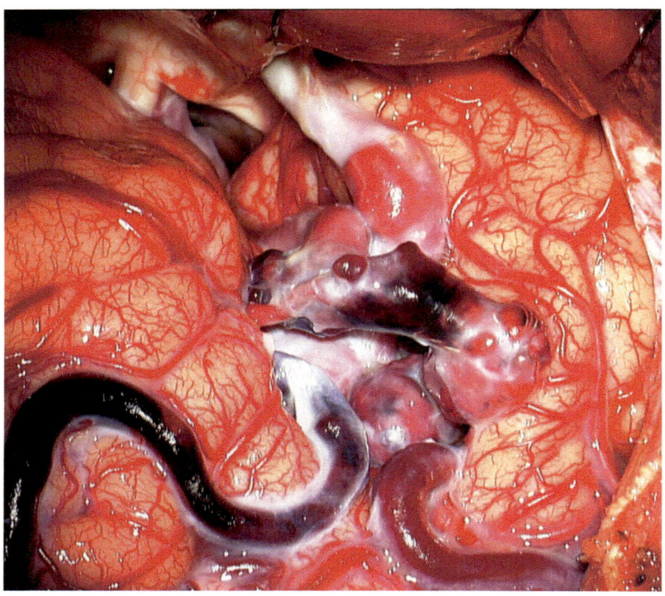

c

Fig. 15.16 This 15-year-old boy presented with a complex AVM that had a sylvian arteriovenous (AV) fistula and a right insular AVM (supplemented Spetzler-Martin grade 6: S2V1E1/A1B1C0), supplied by the InsP and lLSA [(**a**) right ICA angiogram, anteroposterior view]. Treatment with Gamma Knife radiosurgery reduced the insular AVM volume [(**b**) right ICA angiogram, anteroposterior view], but the fistula persisted. The AV fistula was coiled with incomplete occlusion of the shunt, and (**c**) then exposed in the sylvian fissure through a pterional craniotomy.

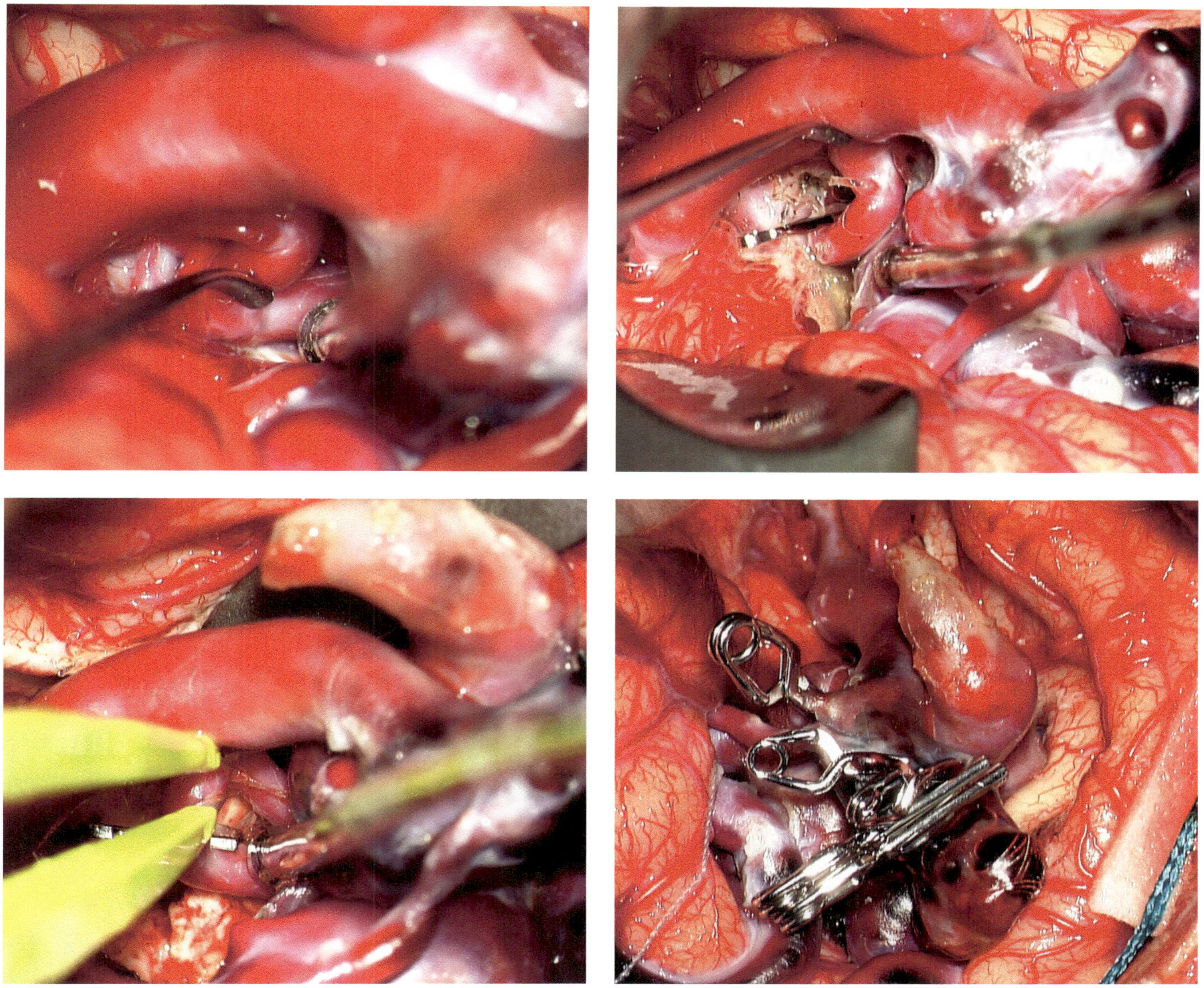

d e f g

Fig. 15.16 (*continued*) (**d**) The InsPs from the proximal M2 segments feeding the AVM (**e,f**) were skeletonized. (**g**) The fistula was occluded with stacked clips proximal to the coils and distal to a normal frontal branch, and an associated aneurysm was also clipped.

Basal Ganglial AVM Resection

The AVMs in the basal ganglia that are favorable for surgery are either lateral in the putamen or medial in the caudate nucleus. Lateral basal ganglial AVM resection is an extension of insular AVM resection, and medial basal ganglial AVM resection is an extension of ventricular body AVM resection. The lateral basal ganglial AVM is resected through a pterional craniotomy and a transsylvian-transinsular approach (**Fig. 15.17,** step 1). Sylvian fissure dissection might require an anterior split, a posterior split, or both, depending on the AVM's size and its anteroposterior location in the putamen (step 2). Drainage to the lateral ventricular veins (CauV and ThaStrV) or the BVR is not visualized until the end of the dissection (step 3). These AVMs are supplied by perforators (InsP and ILSA; step 4). The InsP is identified on M2 stem arteries and occluded on the way through the insula (lateral front, step 5). The insula overlying the AVM is resected to reach the nidus or an associated hematoma is traversed. With no veins and few anatomic landmarks to guide the transinsular approach,

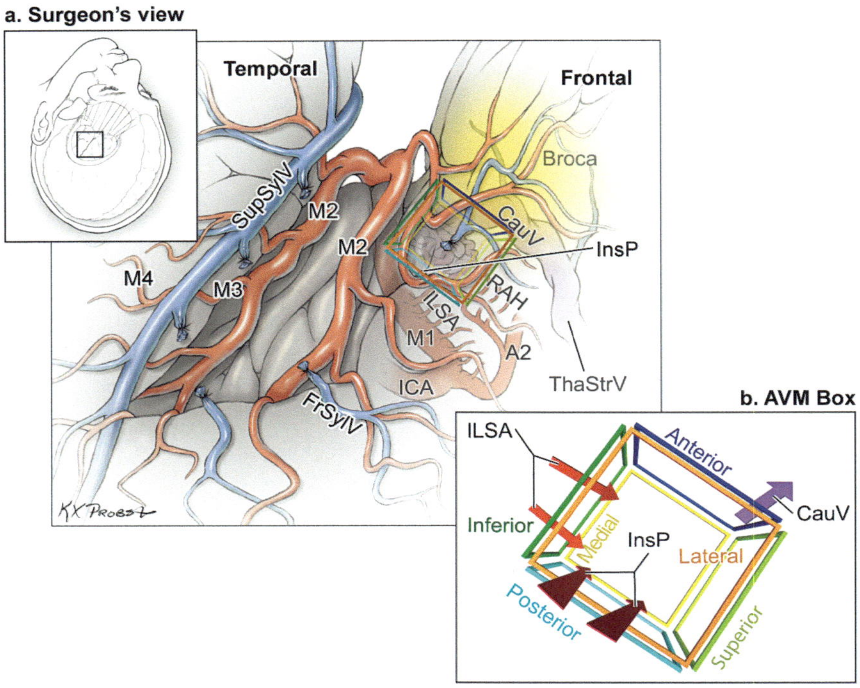

Fig. 15.17 Resection strategy for lateral basal ganglial AVMs. (**a**) Step 1, exposing the AVM with a pterional craniotomy (surgeon's view). (**b**) AVM box showing InsP input on the lateral side and ILSA input on the inferior side, and eloquence anterolaterally (Broca's area, yellow).

c. Surgeon's view

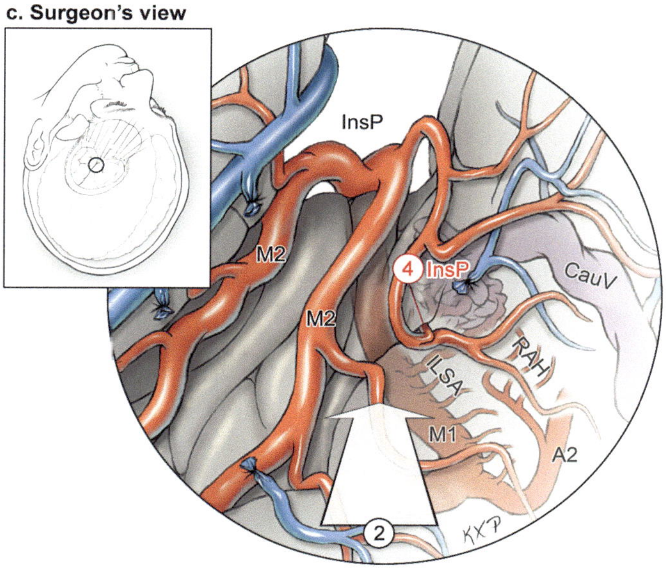

Fig. 15.17 *(continued)* (**c**) Step 2, splitting the sylvian fissure; step 3, the draining vein is not yet visible (CauV); and step 4, identifying feeders from M2 stem arteries (InsP). (**d**) Step 5, dividing the lateral front of the InsP deep to the M2 arteries; and step 6, dissecting transcortically through the insula to access and circumdissect the AVM (coronal cross-sectional view). (**e**) Step 7, mobilizing the AVM laterally, interrupting deep lenticulostriate arteries (lLSA and mLSA), and exposing the ventricular vein (CauV).

d. Coronal view

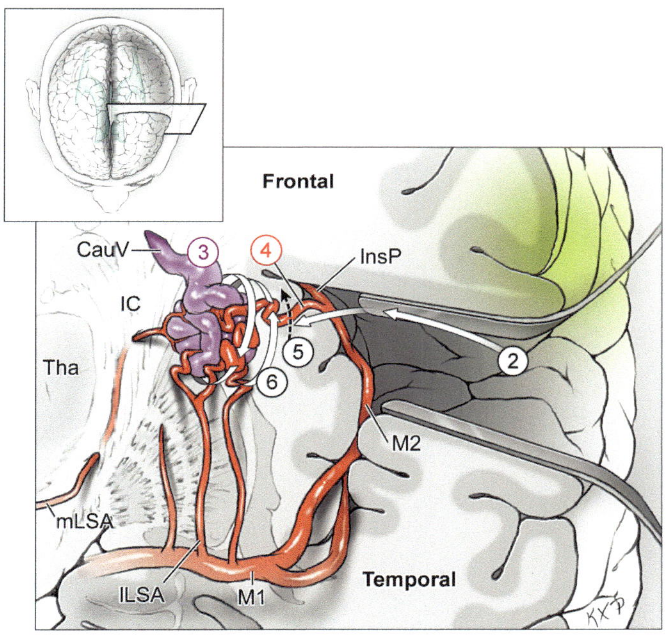

e. Surgeon's view

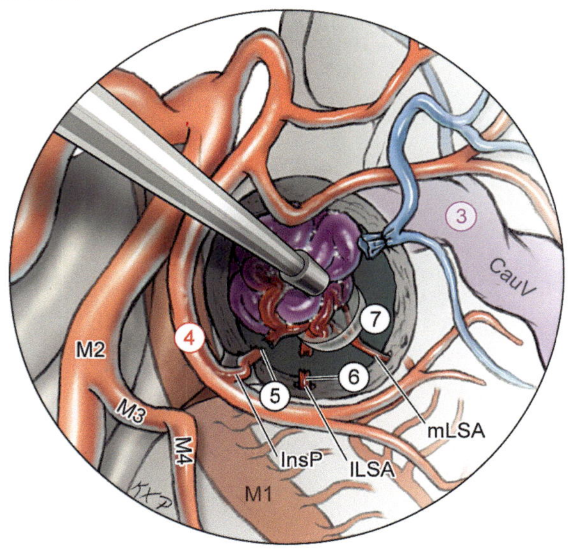

navigation and a hemosiderin stain are helpful. Parenchymal dissection is deep, perpendicular, and confined, which makes the presence of a hematoma or encephalomalacia advantageous. The inferior side receives arterial input from the lLSA and the lateral side receives input from the InsP (step 6). The deep medial side is next to the internal capsule, and perforator supply is meticulously controlled with microclips and cautery to avoid bleeding that might need to be chased into white matter (step 7). The draining vein is identified to confirm the absence of arterialization (**Figs. 15.18, 15.19, 15.20**).

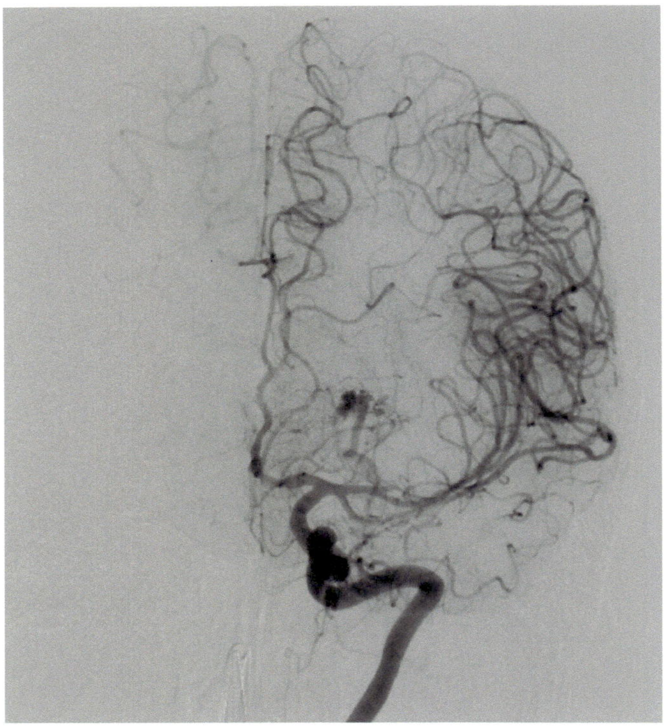

a

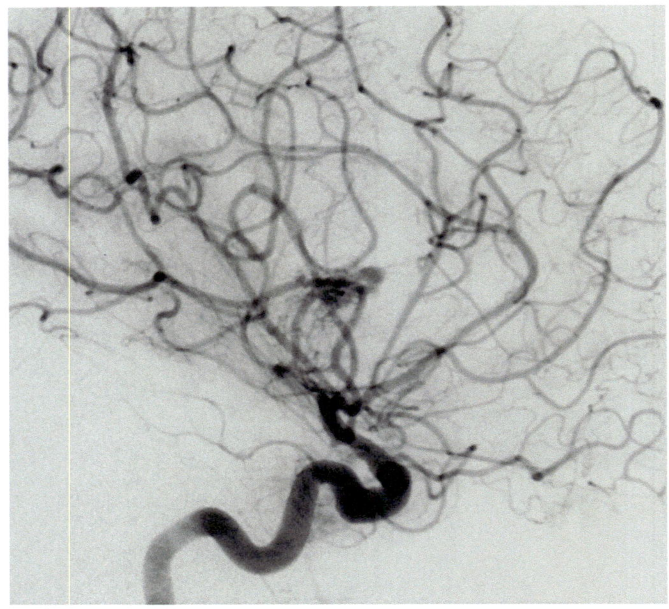

b

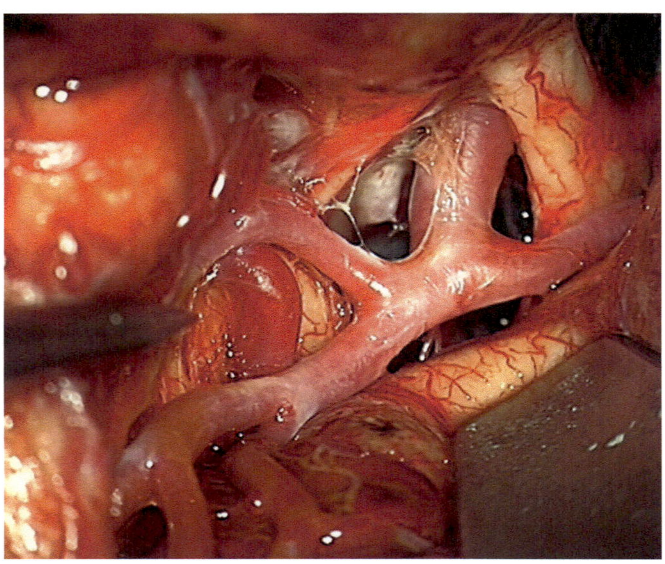

c

Fig. 15.18 This 68-year-old woman presented with a left basal ganglial AVM and an associated hematoma (supplemented Spetzler-Martin grade 5: S1V0E1/A3B0C0), supplied by lLSA [left ICA angiogram, (**a**) anteroposterior and (**b**) lateral views]. (**c**) Transsylvian exposure laid out the MCA branches and the draining DeepSylV below the M1 segment.

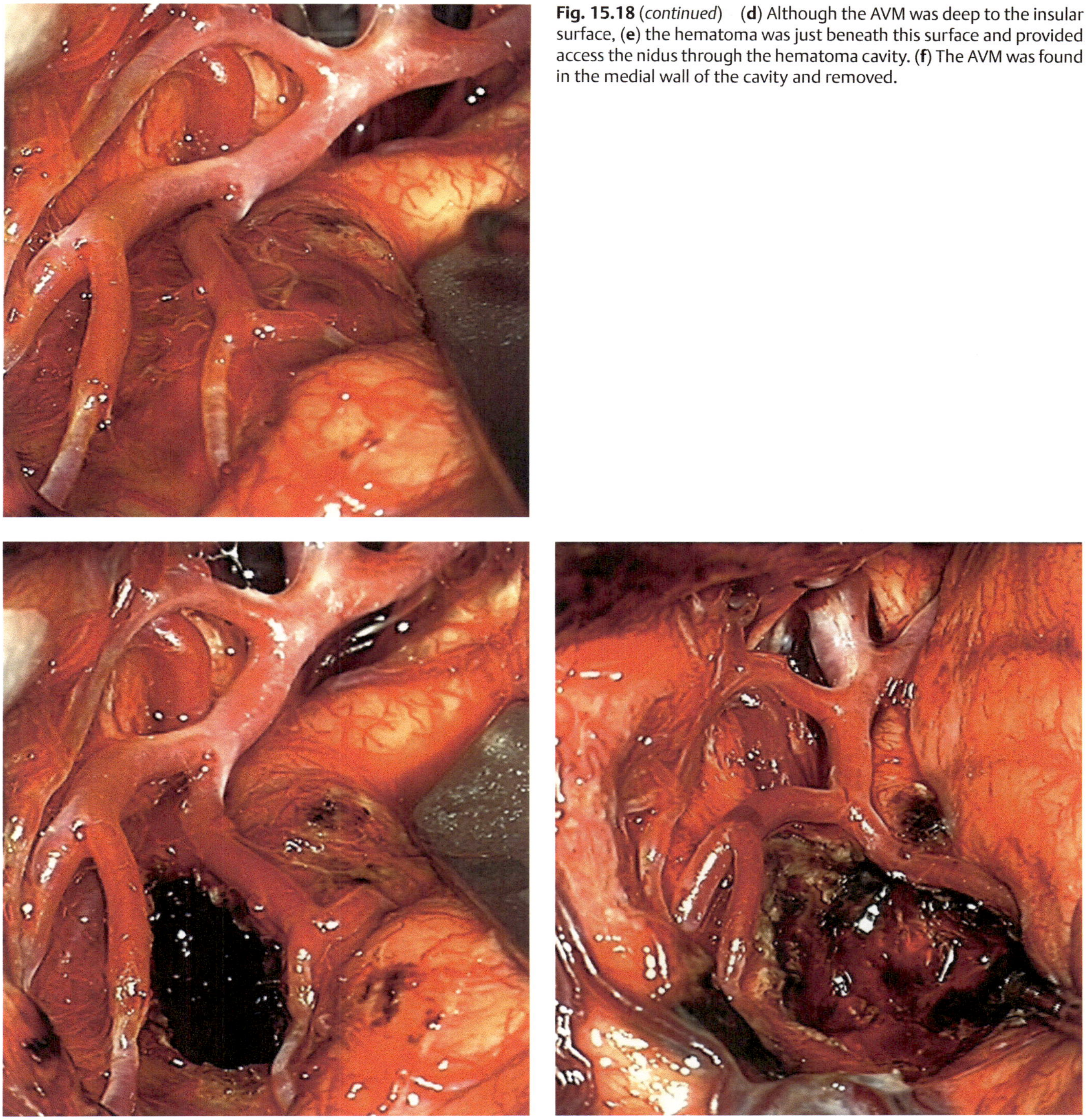

d e f

Fig. 15.18 (*continued*) (**d**) Although the AVM was deep to the insular surface, (**e**) the hematoma was just beneath this surface and provided access the nidus through the hematoma cavity. (**f**) The AVM was found in the medial wall of the cavity and removed.

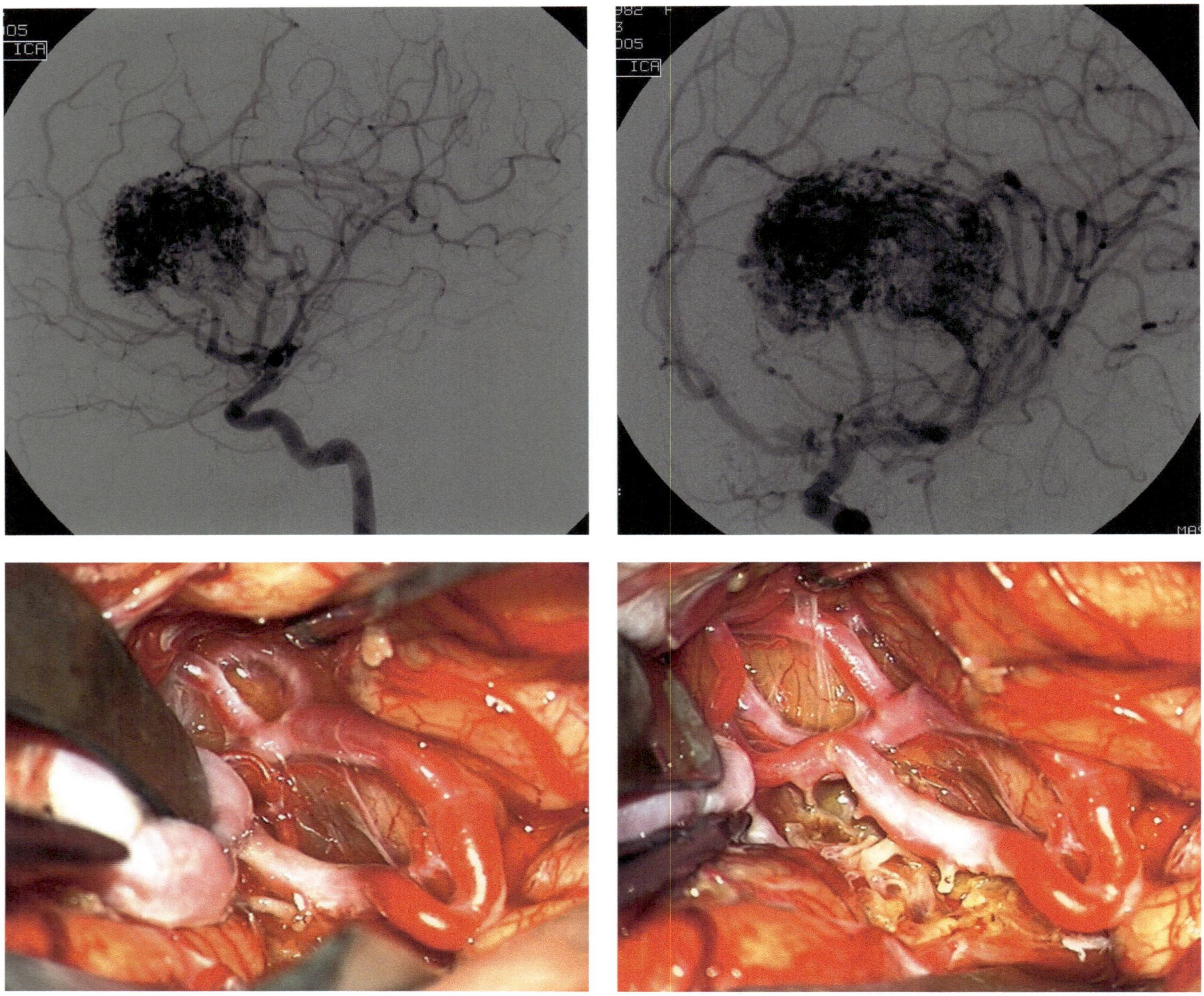

a b c d

Fig. 15.19 This 22-year-old woman presented in a coma from a ruptured left basal ganglial (caudate head) AVM (supplemented Spetzler-Martin grade 5: S2V0E1/A2B0C0), supplied by M2 MCA stem arteries, ILSA, and InsP [left ICA angiogram, (**a**) lateral and (**b**) anterior oblique views]. She was treated with hemicraniectomy and later with Gamma Knife radiosurgery, with reduction in AVM volume. (**c**) An anterior transsylvian approach exposed the MCA bifurcation and feeding arteries originating from the superior trunk, (**d**) which was skeletonized. There were no feeding arteries from the inferior trunk.

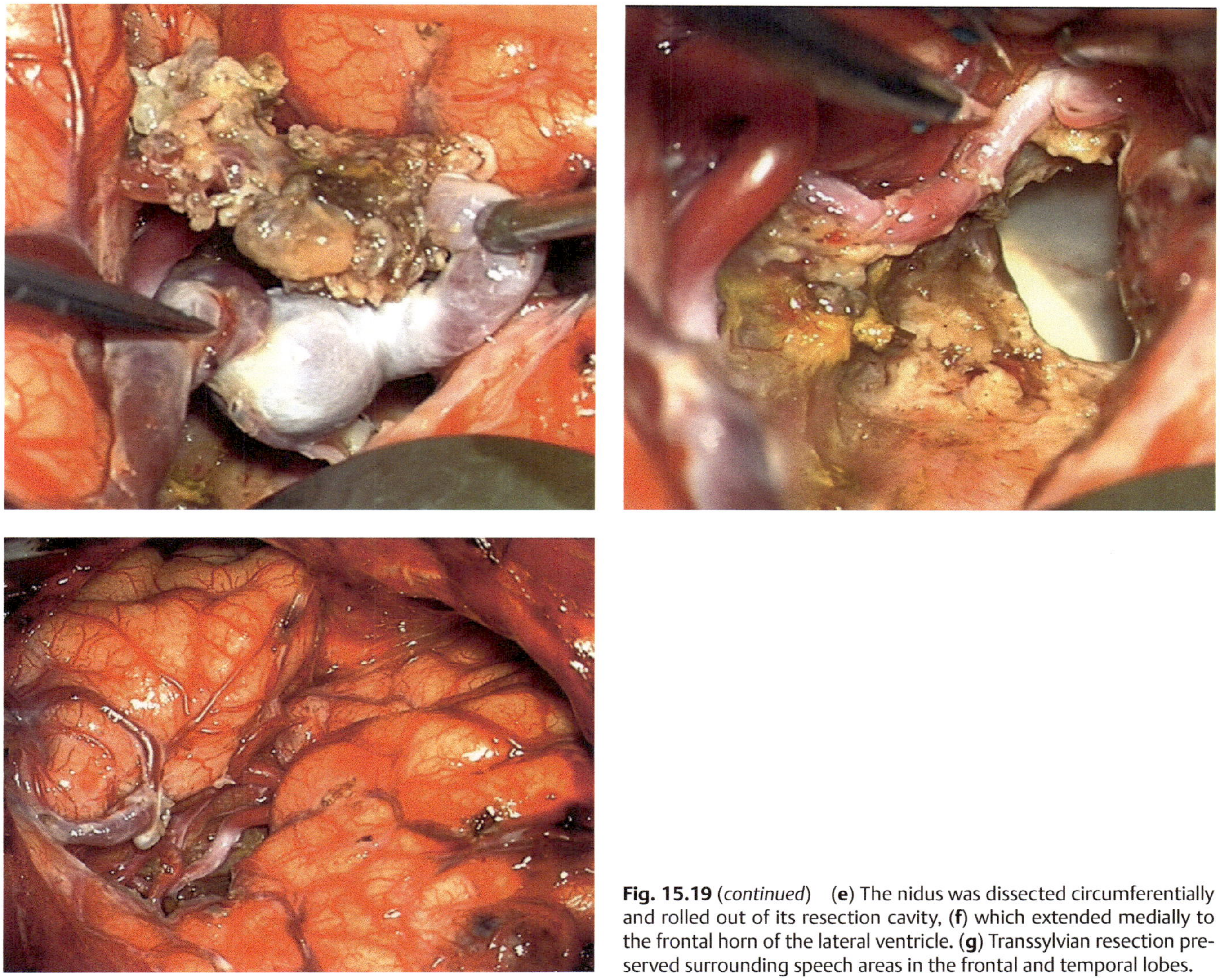

e f g

Fig. 15.19 (*continued*) (**e**) The nidus was dissected circumferentially and rolled out of its resection cavity, (**f**) which extended medially to the frontal horn of the lateral ventricle. (**g**) Transsylvian resection preserved surrounding speech areas in the frontal and temporal lobes.

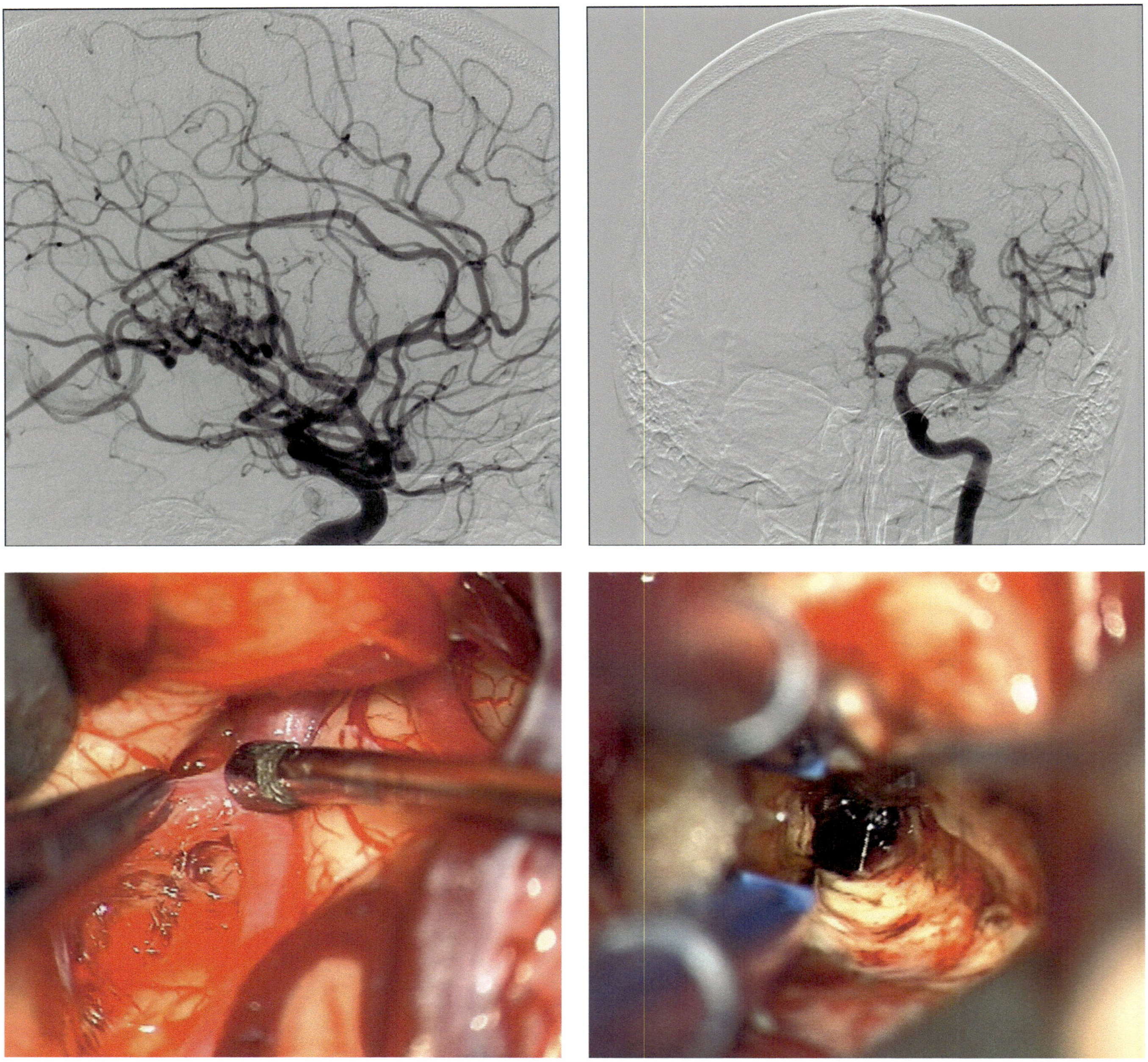

a b c d

Fig. 15.20 This 26-year-old man presented with a left putamenal hemorrhage from this basal ganglial AVM (supplemented Spetzler-Martin grade 5: S1V1E1/A2B0C0), supplied by lLSA and InsP and drained by ThaStrV [left ICA angiogram, (**a**) lateral and (**b**) anteroposterior views]. (**c**) A posterior transsylvian approach exposed the long gyri of the insula and the distal M2 segments. (**d**) Using intraoperative navigation to localize the hematoma, a transinsular corridor was opened to access the hematoma cavity.

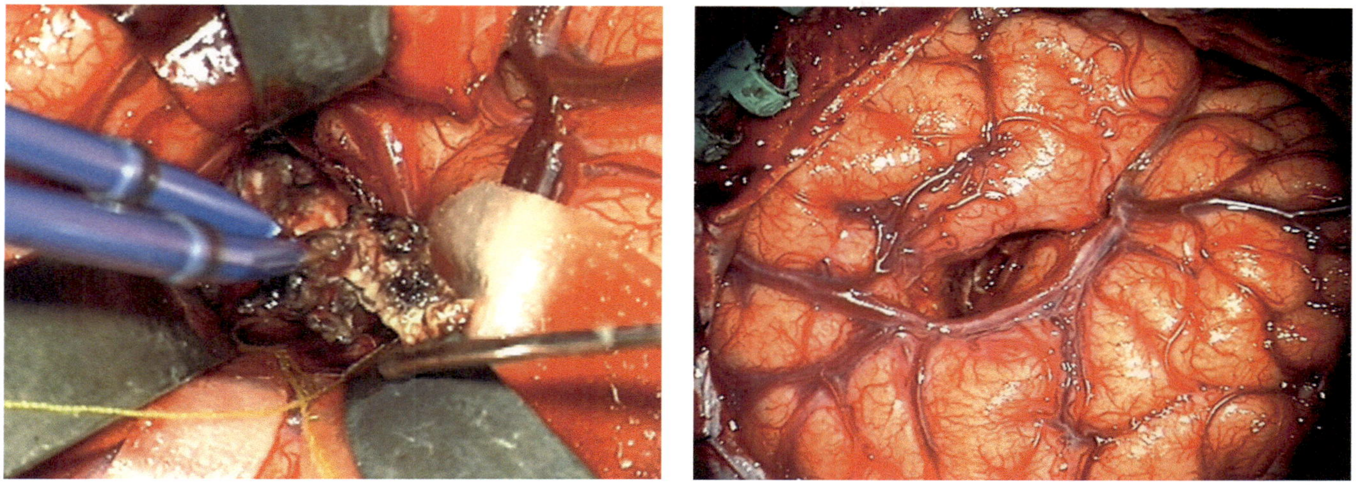

e f

Fig. 15.20 (*continued*) (**e**) This small AVM was circumdissected and removed. (**f**) Language areas adjacent to the distal sylvian fissure were preserved, and the patient had no speech deficits.

The medial basal ganglial AVM is resected through a bifrontal craniotomy (**Fig. 15.21**, step 1) and contralateral transcallosal approach with gravity retraction. With the contralateral approach, the head is positioned with the midline oriented horizontally and the AVM on the upside, allowing gravity to retract the opposite hemisphere. The trajectory begins in the interhemispheric fissure contralateral to the AVM but ends in the ventricle ipsilateral to the AVM. This crossing trajectory maximizes lateral exposure in the ventricle to access the caudate nucleus. Therefore, the "subarachnoid" route includes an interhemispheric fissure split, division of the corpus callosum under the ipsilateral pericallosal artery (PcaA) to enter the ipsilateral ventricle, and transventricular dissection to arrive at the caudate nucleus (step 2). Like lateral basal ganglia AVMs, medial basal ganglial AVMs drain to the CauV and ThaStrV, but unlike with lateral AVMs, these veins are superficial in the surgical field and identified early (step 3). Arterial feeders consist of the mLSA and RAH (step 4). Ependymal dissection circumscribes the AVM on the lateral ventricular wall and accesses the inferomedial front of perforators (step 5). The nidus is mobilized down into the ventricle with circumdissection, and arterial supply on the inferior side is interrupted (step 6). Upward retraction on the falx and corpus callosum helps visualize the deep lateral plane that receives the remaining mLSA feeders (step 7). Anterior limb and genu of internal capsule adjacent to caudate head are protected during the resection.

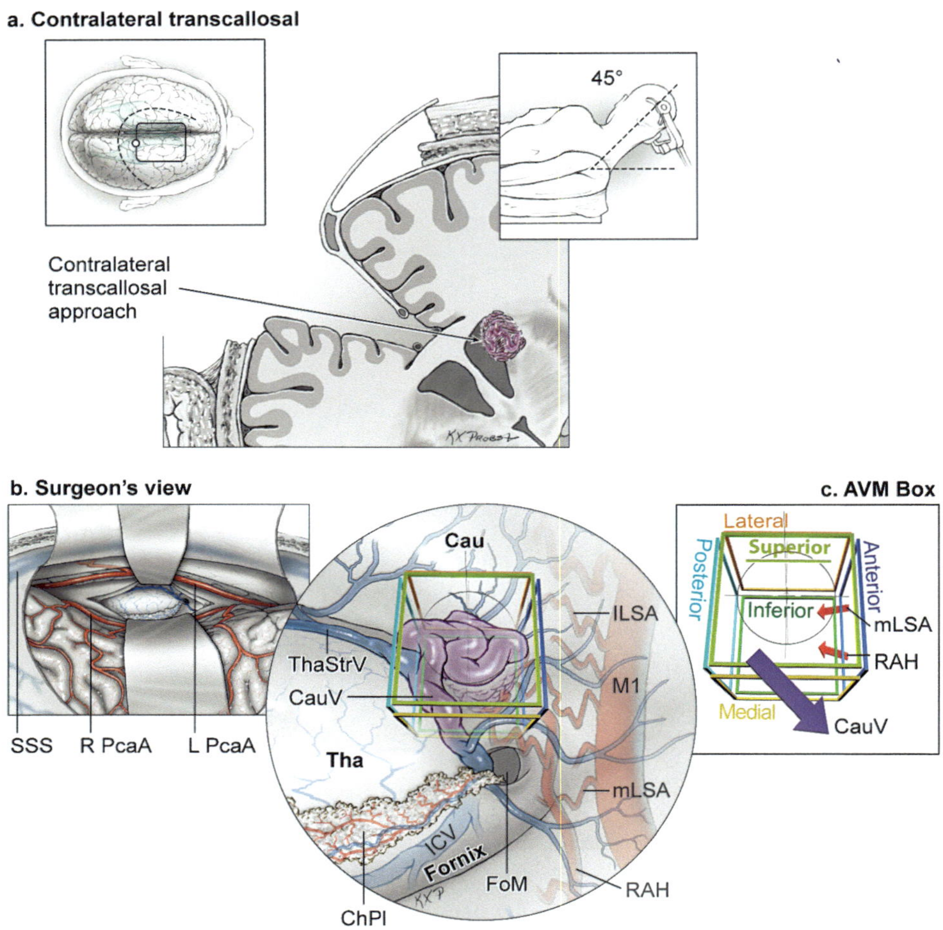

Fig. 15.21 Resection strategy for medial basal ganglial AVMs. (**a**) Step 1, exposing the AVM with a semicircular scalp incision (*dashed line*), bifrontal craniotomy eccentric to the right (*solid line*), and contralateral transcallosal approach with the left AVM on the upside, gravity retracting the right frontal lobe (midline horizontal and head angled upward 45 degrees), and the trajectory crossing the interhemispheric fissure to the left ventricle. (**b**) The dural flap elevates the SSS and a callosal incision under the left PcaA enters the left ventricle. These AVMs sit in the caudate nucleus lateral to the foramen of Monro and ThaStrV. (**c**) AVM box showing inferior supply from lenticulostriate arteries (mLSA and RAH) and medial drainage to the CauV.

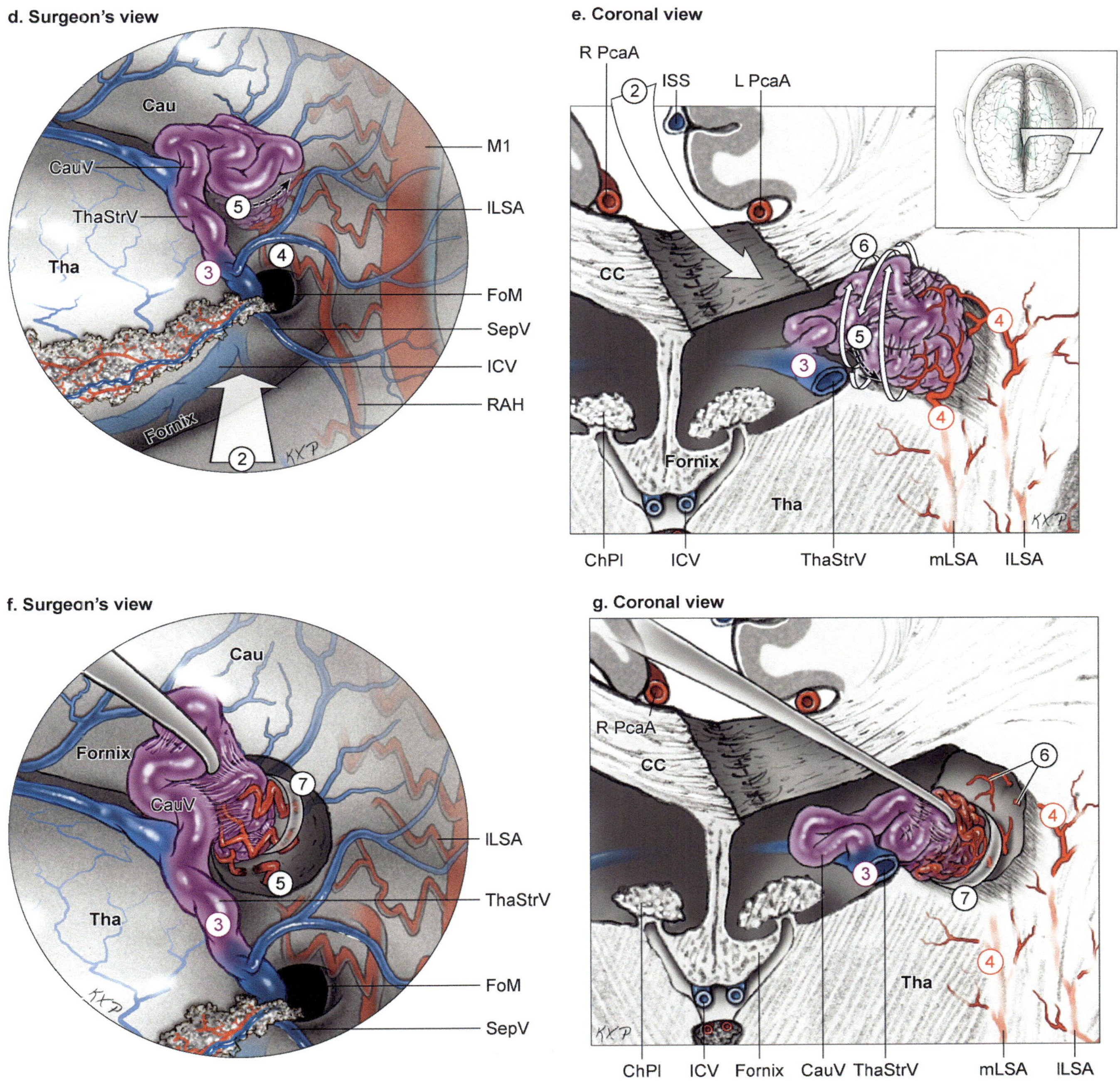

Fig. 15.21 (*continued*) (**d**) Step 2, exposing lateral ventricular wall; step 3, identifying venous drainage at the venous angle; and step 4, identifying arterial supply in the ependyma (surgeon's view). (**e**) Step 5, dividing the inferior front of lenticulostriates medially under the caudate head; and step 6, circumdissecting into the caudate nucleus (coronal cross-sectional view). (**f**) Step 7, mobilizing AVM into the ventricle and interrupting inferolateral feeding arteries (lLSA) [surgeon's and (**g**) coronal cross-sectional views].

Thalamic AVM Resection

The thalamus is encircled by the lateral ventricles, and its two halves are separated by the third ventricle. Therefore, the ventricular system is used to access most thalamic AVMs. There are seven surgical routes to thalamic AVMs (**Fig. 15.22**): transcallosally, with either an anterior-ipsilateral approach (1) or anterior-contralateral approach (2) for AVMs in the superior thalamus; a posterior-ipsilateral approach (3) for AVMs in the posterior thalamus; or transcallosal-transchoroidal approach (4) for AVMs in the medial thalamus; and transcortically, either transfrontal (5), transtemporal (6), or transparietal (7) approaches. The anterior transcallosal approaches (ipsi- and contralateral) offer a direct view of the floor of the lateral ventricle and superior thalamus. The contralateral transcallosal approach's steeper viewing angle across to the lateral wall of the ventricle is not necessary for thalamic AVMs, but this approach avoids the dominant hemi-

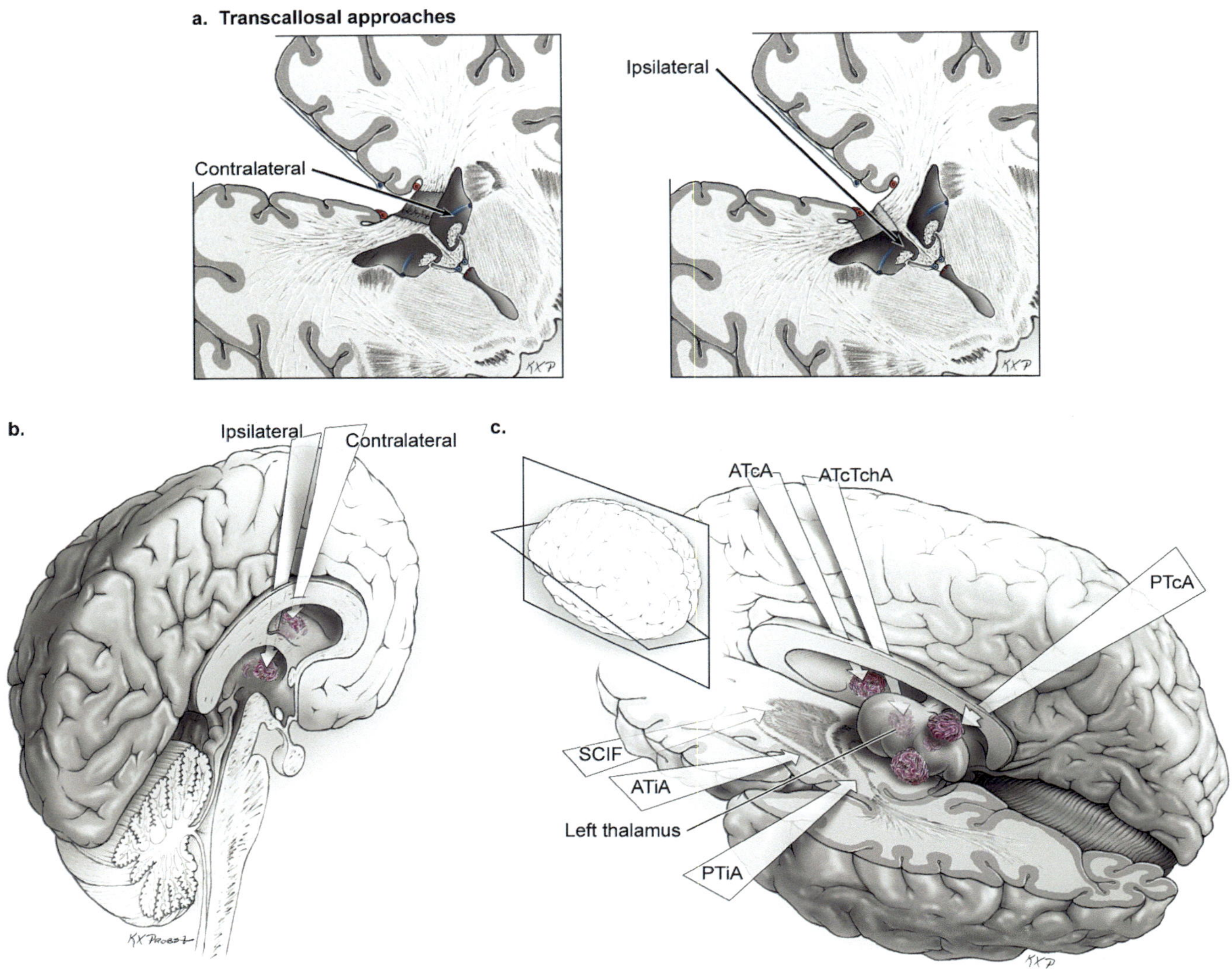

Fig. 15.22 Surgical approaches to deep AVMs. (**a**) Anterior transcallosal approaches (ATcA) are contralateral (craniotomy and AVM on opposite sides) for medial basal ganglial AVMs and ipsilateral (craniotomy and AVM on the same side) for superior thalamic AVMs (coronal cross-sectional views). (**b**) The crossing trajectory of the contralateral approach visualizes the lateral wall of the lateral ventricle (posterior oblique view of medial left hemisphere). (**c**) The anterior transcallosal approach extends into the third ventricle by opening the choroidal fissure and velum interpositum for medial thalamic AVMs (ATcTchA, anterior transcallosal-transchoroidal approach). The posterior transcallosal approach (PTcA) uses a torcular craniotomy and posterior interhemispheric dissection for posterior thalamic AVMs. Transsylvian approaches (TSyl) include the anterior transinsular approach (ATiA), posterior transinsular approach (PTiA), and supracarotid-infrafrontal approach (SCIF). Transsylvian approaches are used for pure sylvian, insular, and lateral basal ganglial AVMs, whereas the supracarotid-infrafrontal approach is used for inferior basal ganglial AVMs.

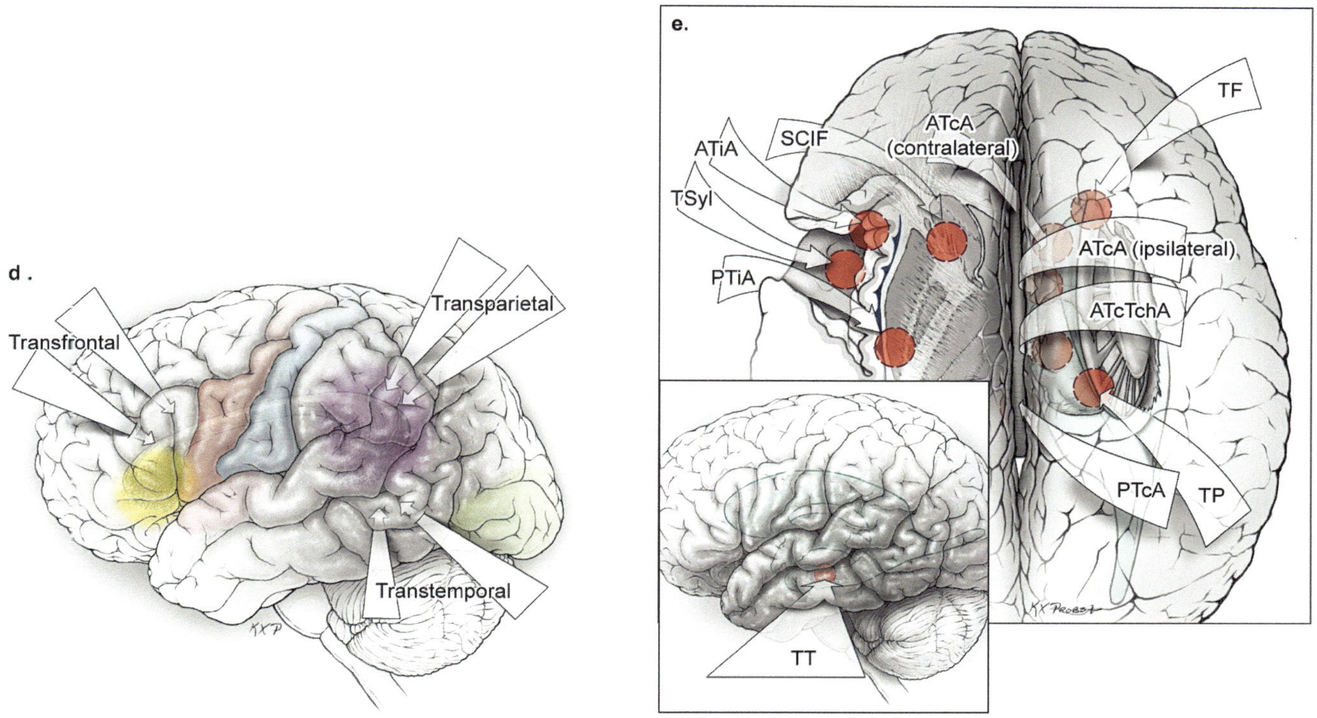

Fig. 15.22 (*continued*) (**d**) Transcortical approaches are used instead of subarachnoid and transventricular routes when hematomas or encephalomalacia create direct, nonanatomic corridors to deep AVMs. These transfrontal (TF), transparietal (TP), and transtemporal (TT) approaches are either transcortical or transsulcal. (**e**) Summary of approaches to deep AVMs, as viewed superiorly and laterally (*inset*).

sphere with left-sided AVMs. The transcallosal-transchoroidal approach deepens the exposure by opening the tela choroidea of the choroid plexus, following ThaStrV and ICV into velum interpositum, unroofing the third ventricle, and widening the FoM to enter the third ventricle (as described for ventricular body AVMs). This approach accesses medial thalamic AVMs. The posterior transcallosal approach transgresses the splenium for a more posterior view of the superior thalamus, as well as posterior feeding arteries and draining veins. All of the transcallosal variations require a craniotomy that crosses the midline to expose the superior sagittal sinus (SSS), with the anterior approaches using a bifrontal craniotomy and the posterior approach using a torcular craniotomy. All of the transcallosal variations use gravity retraction to drop the dependent hemisphere and open the interhemispheric fissure. The anterior approaches use a supine position with the head turned to align the midline horizontally, and the posterior approach uses a lateral position also with the head turned to align the midline horizontally.

Transcortical approaches are used when hematoma or encaphalomalacia from prior hemorrhage creates an extra-anatomical corridor to the AVM that would otherwise not exist. These cavities reach thalamic AVMs with minimal additional transgression through the cortex. Transcortical routes can also be used in the absence of hematoma or encephalomalacia, but can produce new neurologic deficits for which the neurosurgeon is responsible. The SPL approach is one such approach (described for atrial AVMs), entering the atrium of the lateral ventricle and exposing the posterior thalamus. These corridors are long, confining, and without anatomic landmarks, necessitating neuronavigation and brain retraction. In summary, the neurosurgeon should exploit direct, nonanatomic corridors to thalamic AVMs when they already exist and otherwise select anatomic corridors through

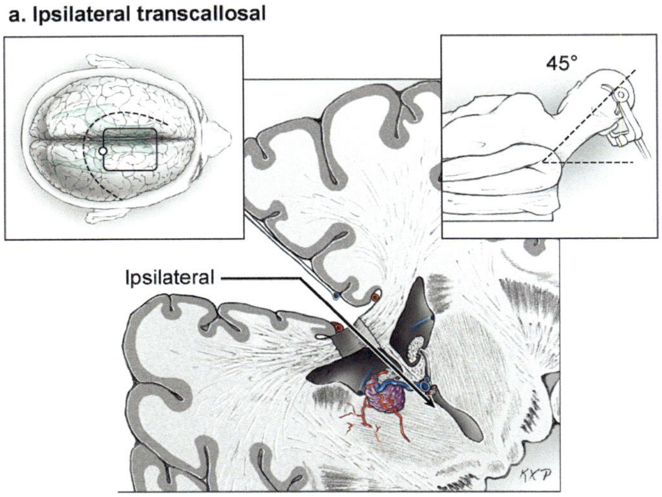

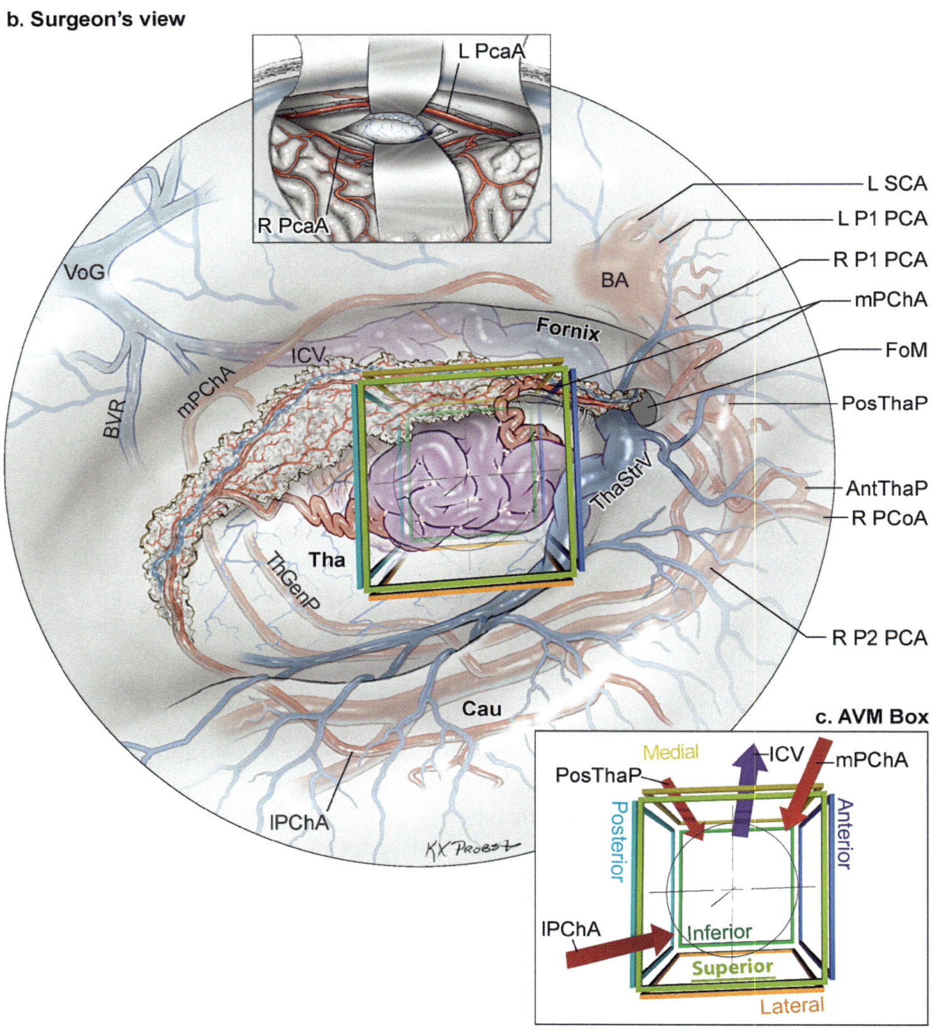

Fig. 15.23 Resection strategy for superior thalamic AVMs. (**a**) Step 1, exposing the AVM with a semicircular scalp incision (*dashed line*), bifrontal craniotomy eccentric to the right (*solid line*), and ipsilateral transcallosal approach with the right AVM on the downside, gravity retracting the right frontal lobe (midline horizontal and head angled upwards 45 degrees), and the trajectory entering the right ventricle. (**b**) The dural flap elevates the SSS and a callosal incision under the right PcaA enters the right ventricle (*inset*). These AVMs sit on the superior thalamic surface behind the foramen of Monro and ThaStrV. (**c**) AVM box shows supply superiorly from the choroidal arteries (mPChA and lPChA) and inferiorly from the thalamoperforators (PosThaP).

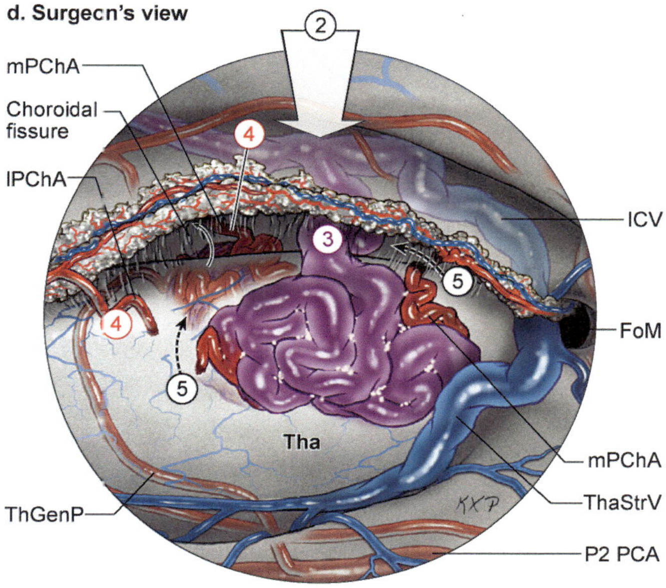

Fig. 15.23 (*continued*) (**d**) Step 2, exposing the AVM in the ventricular body; step 3, locating the vein medially in the choroidal fissure draining to the ICV; step 4, identifying choroidal feeders (mPChA and lPChA); and step 5, interrupting the superomedial arterial front along the choroidal fissure (surgeon's view). (**e**) Step 6, circumdissecting into the thalamus (coronal cross-sectional view). (**f**) Step 7, mobilizing the AVM upward out of the thalamus and into the lateral ventricle, and dividing the inferior feeding arteries (PosThaP and ThGenP, surgeon's view).

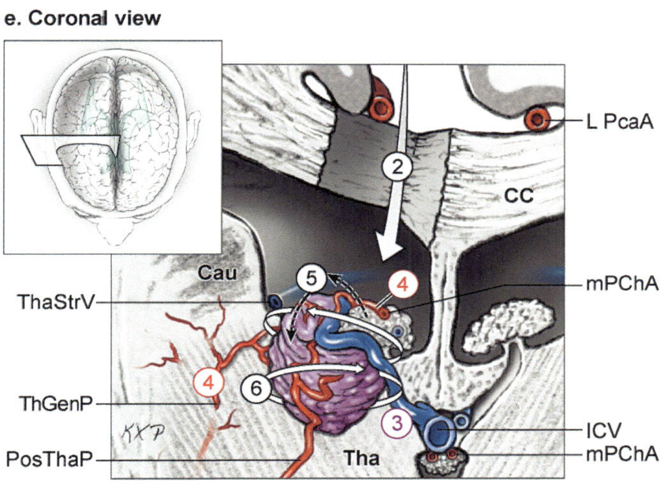

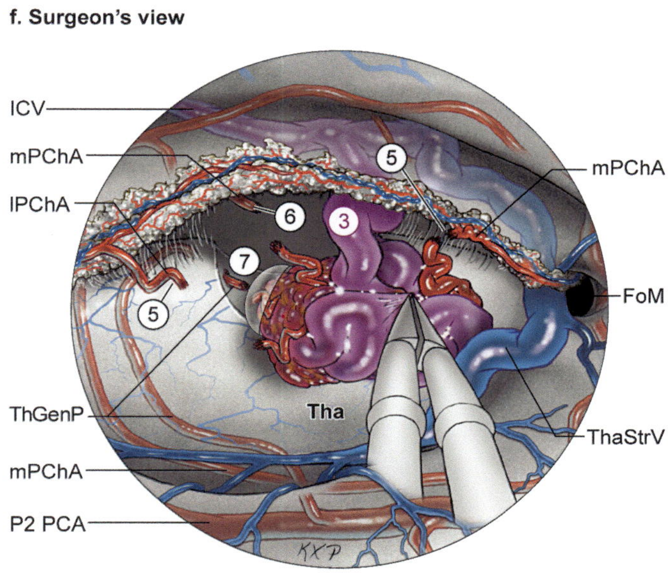

subarachnoid and ventricular spaces that minimize brain transgression.

The most common approaches to thalamic AVMs were the anterior transcallosal and transcallosal-transchoroidal approaches for superior thalamic and medial thalamic AVMs, respectively. A bifrontal craniotomy (**Fig. 15.23**, step 1) and an interhemispheric-transcallosal dissection (step 2) enter the lateral ventricle and expose the superior thalamic surface. Drainage into ThaStrV is seen on the floor of the ventricular body, whereas direct drainage into the ICV is seen after opening the choroidal fissure and following ThaStrV around its arc into the ICV (step 3). Superior thalamic AVMs are supplied by posterior choroidal arteries (mPChA and lPChA) and thalamoperforators (PosThaP), whereas medial thalamic AVMs are supplied only by thalamoperforators (AntThaP and PosThaP) (step 4). The mPChA and lPChA are occluded on the superomedial margin of the superior thalamic AVM, and PosThaPs are occluded on the superolateral margin (step 5). Additional perforating artery supply is occluded on anterior, lateral, and posterior sides as the nidus is drawn toward the midline and into the lateral ventricle (step 6). The last of the perforator supply is found on the inferior margin, as are any drainage connections to the BVR (step 7) (**Figs. 15.24, 15.25, 15.26**).

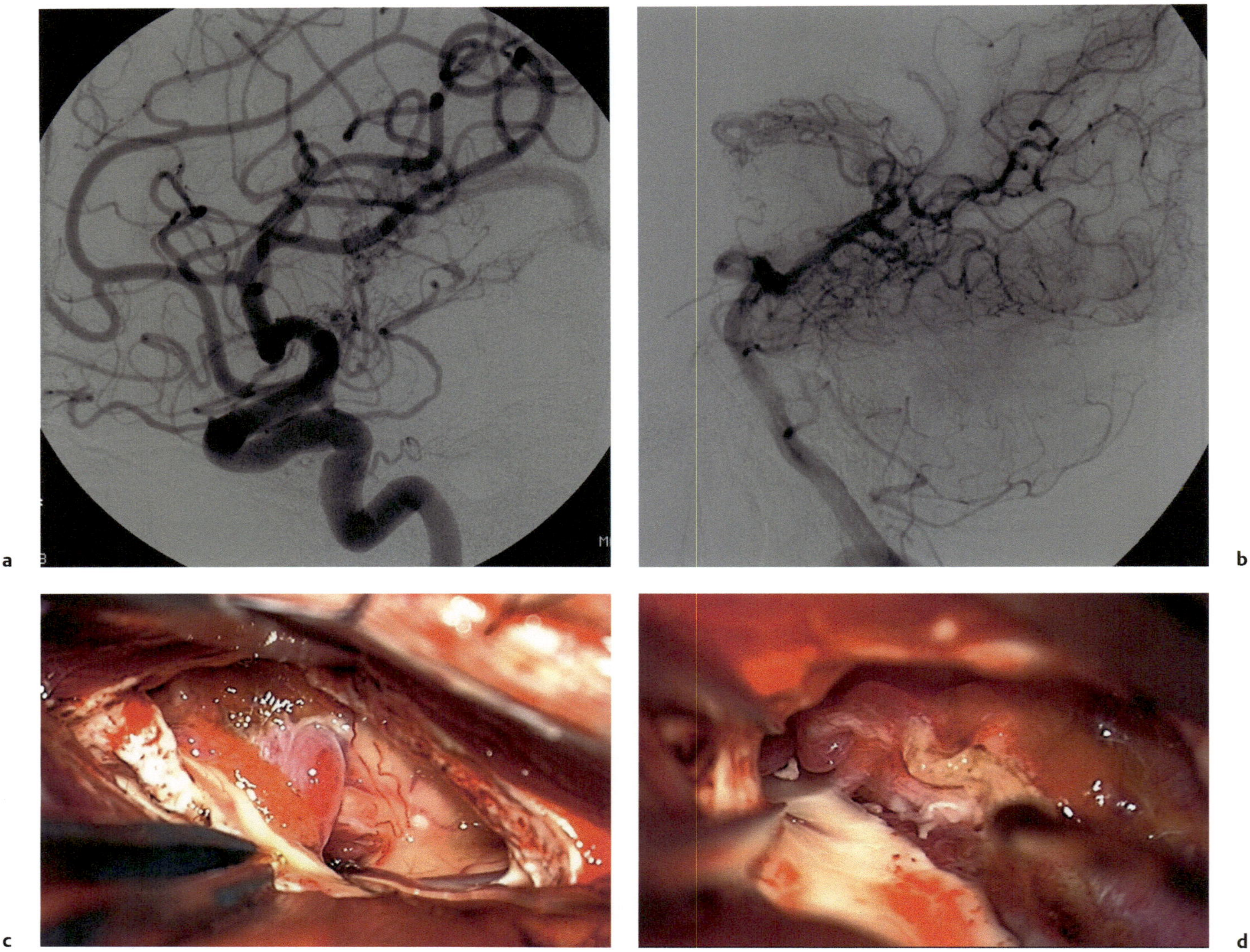

Fig. 15.24 This 51-year-old man presented with a thalamic and intraventricular hemorrhage from this left superior thalamic AVM (supplemented Spetzler-Martin grade 6: S1V1E1/A3B0C0), supplied by AntThaP [(**a**) left ICA angiogram, lateral view], PosThaP, and mPChA [(**b**) left VA angiogram, lateral view], and drained by ThaStrV and ICV. (**c**) The left ventricle was entered using a bifrontal craniotomy (nose to the right, midline horizontal, and right hemisphere down) and a contralateral transcallosal-transchoroidal fissure approach. The contralateral approach eliminated risk to the bridging veins in the dominant hemisphere. The septum mobilized inferiorly (at tip of bipolar forceps) and the foramen of Monro was visualized (at tip of sucker) with the dilated, arterialized ThaStrV coursing into the venous angle. (**d**) The choroidal fissure was opened into the velum interpositum by mobilizing the choroid plexus laterally and incising the taenia fornicis along the lateral edge of fornix.

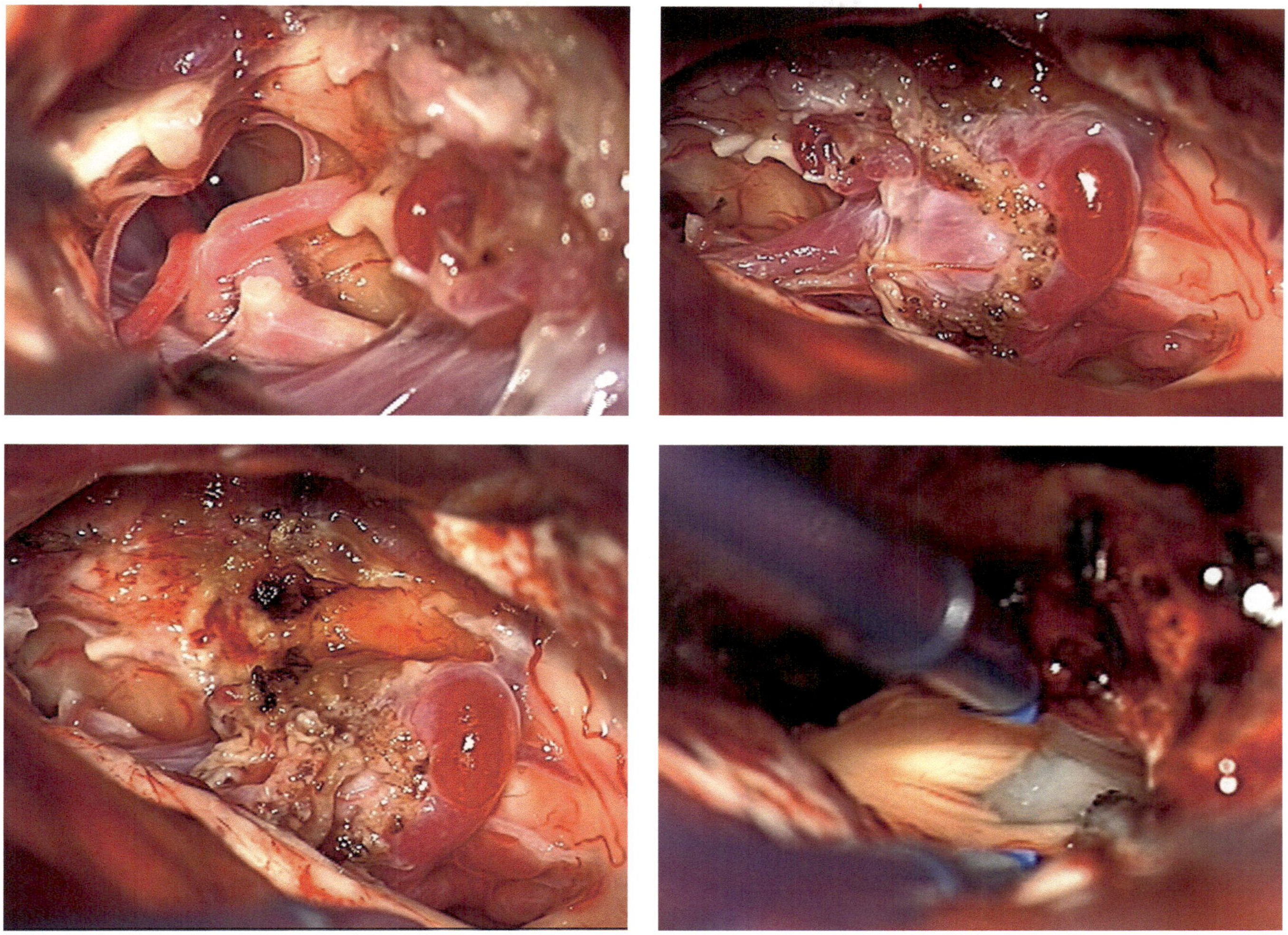

e f g h

Fig. 15.24 *(continued)* (**e**) The mPChA feeders were identified posteriorly in the velum interpositum lateral to the ICV. (**f**) Extensive opening of the choroidal fissure along the medial border of the ICV exposed the AVM's base on the superomedial surface of the thalamus. Note the course of the coagulated ChPl across the AVM, ThaStrV, and ICV. (**g**) Interruption of AntThaP and PosThaP on the AVM's lateral margin darkened the vein and separated it from the thalamus. (**h**) After removing the AVM, the mammillary bodies, floor of the third ventricle, and medial thalamus were seen from above.

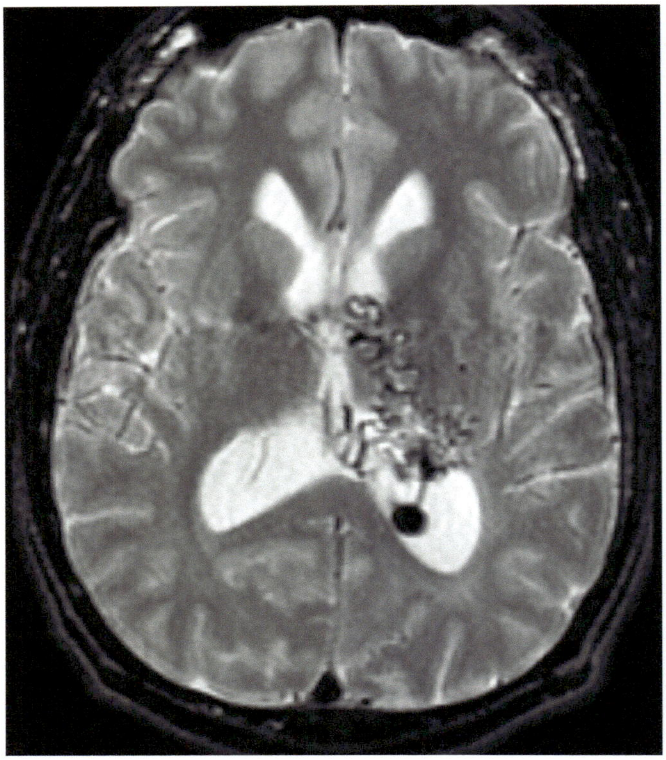

a

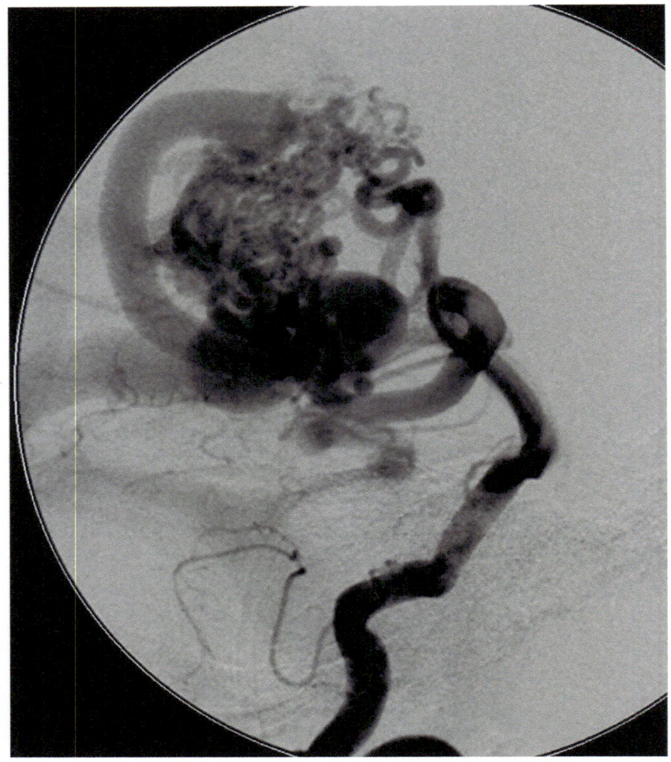

b

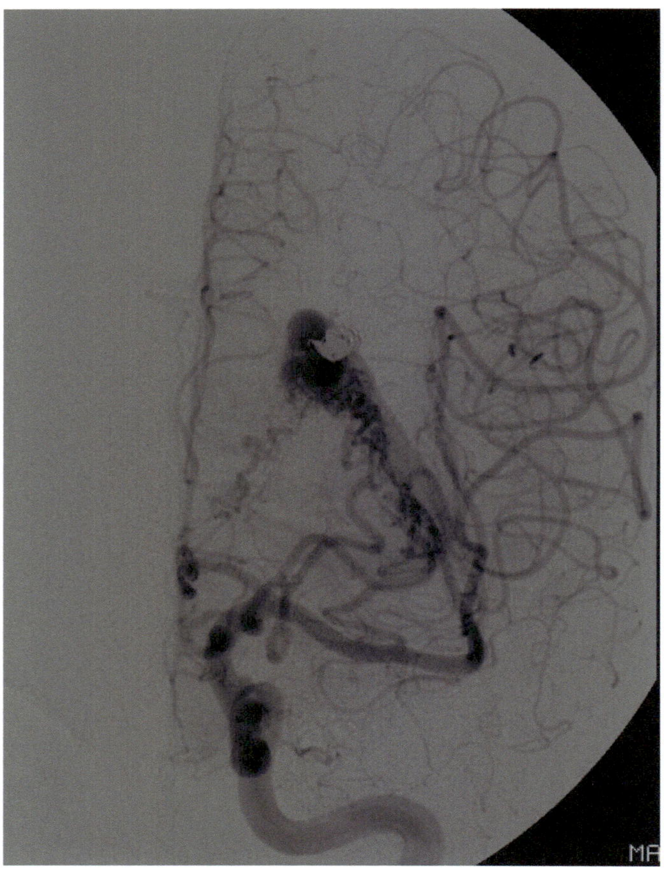

c

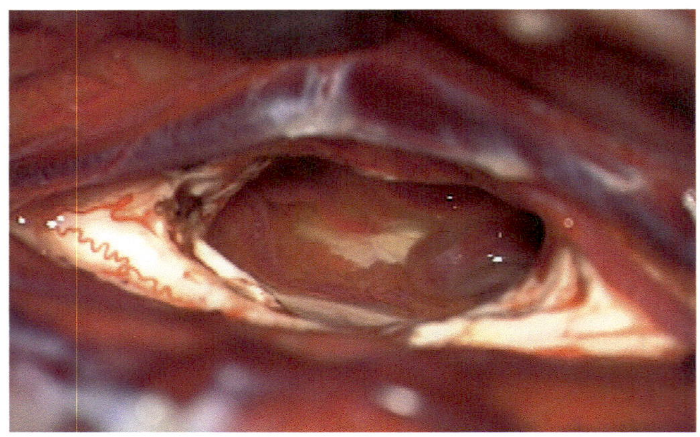

d

Fig. 15.25 This 30-year-old man presented with a minor intraventricular hemorrhage from a left superior thalamic AVM (supplemented Spetzler-Martin grade 6: S2V1E1/A2B0C1), situated in the posterosuperior thalamus with transthalamic supply [(**a**) axial T2-weighted MRI]. (**b**) The AVM was supplied by PosThaP, mPChA, and lPChA and drained to MedAtrV and ICV, as well as to LatAtrV and a cerebellar vein (left VA angiogram, lateral view). He was treated with Gamma Knife radiosurgery in two stages with reduction in AVM volume, as seen on a postembolization angiogram that demonstrated its supply from AntThaP, AChA, and lLSA [(**c**) left ICA angiogram, anteroposterior view]. (**d**) The AVM was approached through a bifrontal craniotomy (nose to the right, midline horizontal, and right hemisphere down) and a contralateral transcallosal approach, using the crossing trajectory to view into the atrium. The only retractor was on the falx to elevate the ISS, with gravity opening the interhemispheric fissure.

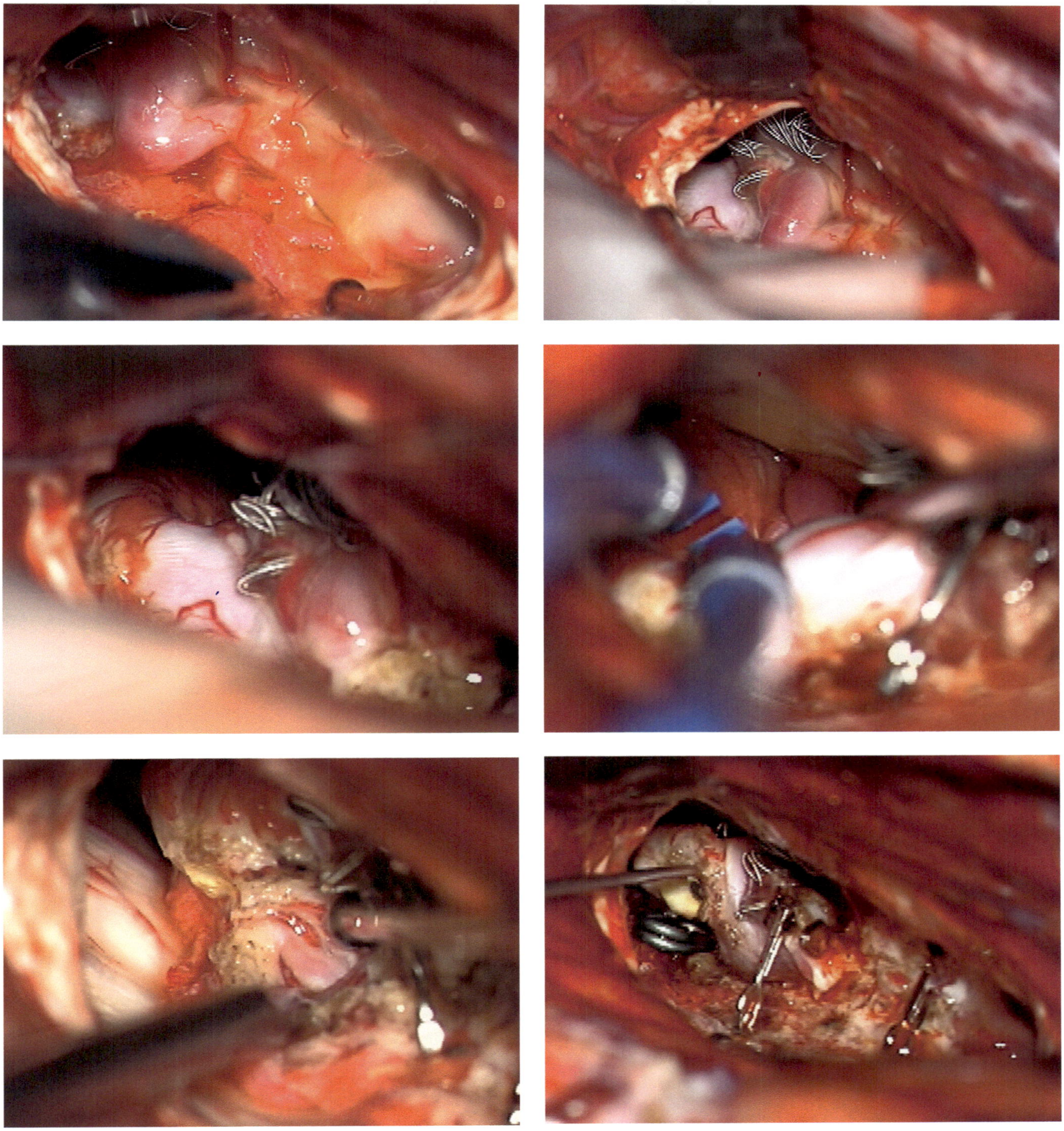

Fig. 15.25 (*continued*) (**e**) Dilated feeders on the superior surface of thalamus were followed posteriorly (**f**) to coils that were embolized through the lPChA. (**g**) LatAtrV arced around the posterior aspect of thalamus toward the temporal horn, (**h**) where the AChA supply ascended to the nidus. (**i**) Additional supply from the mPChA was found medial to LatAtrV in the atrium. (**j**) The choroidal supply to the AVM was interrupted completely, but deep plane of dissection across the thalamus was not clean enough to interrupt thalamoperforator supply and allow safe resection. The nidus was left in situ and a faint shunt from thalamoperforator supply was treated radiosurgically.

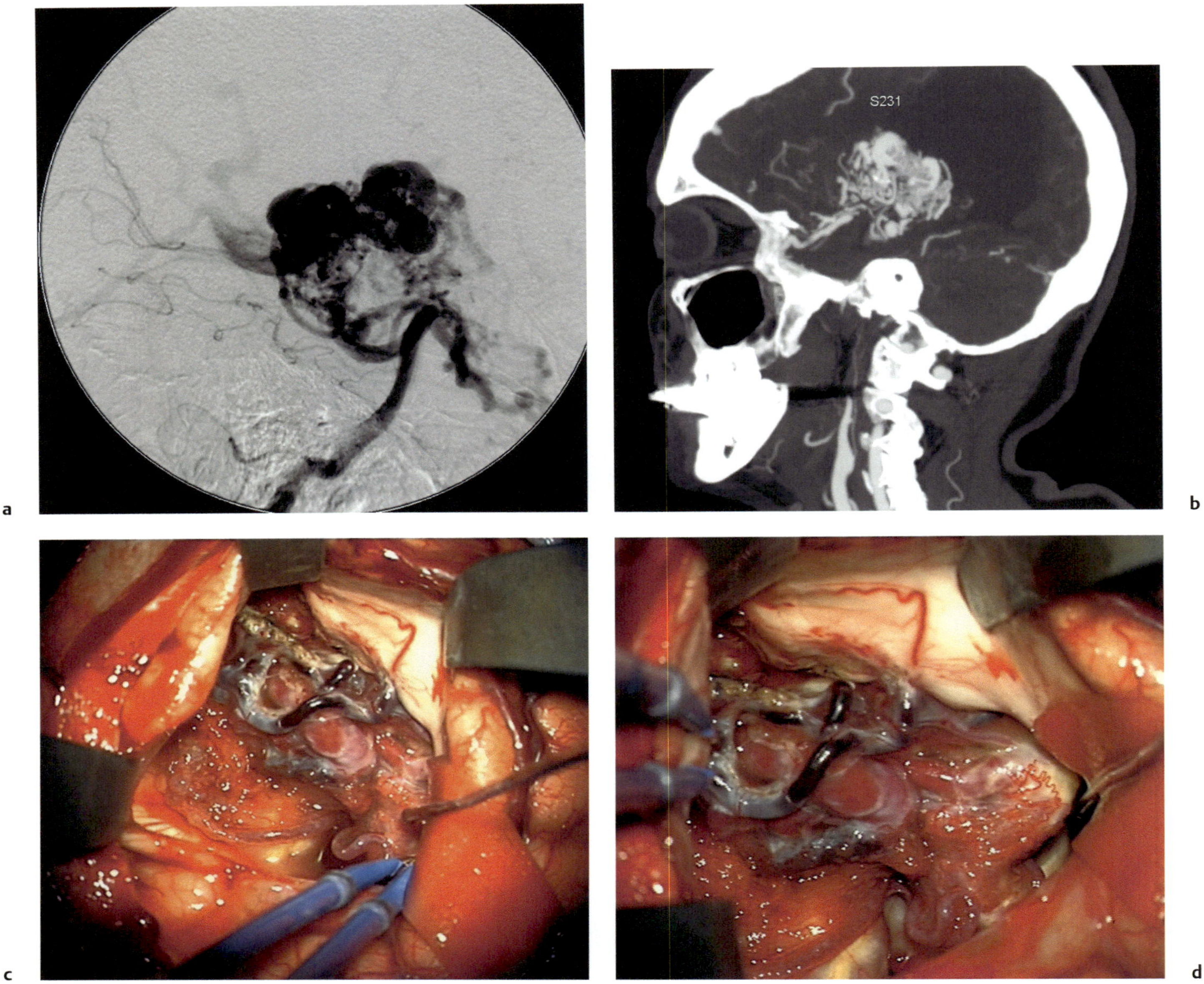

Fig. 15.26 This 60-year-old woman presented with an intraventricular hemorrhage from a left thalamic AVM that had been followed conservatively for years (supplemented Spetzler-Martin grade 7: S2V1E1/A3B0C0). (**a**) Like the previous case, it was supplied by PosThaP, mPChA, and lPChA (left VA angiogram, lateral view) as well as AntThaP, AChA, and lLSA (not shown). (**b**) A prior stroke from a left ICA occlusion resulted in a large encephalomalacia cavity (computed tomography angiogram, sagittal view), (**c**) which was used to access the atrium transcortically (lateral position, left side up, nose to the right, and midline horizontal). (**d**) The AVM was widely exposed on the posterior thalamus.

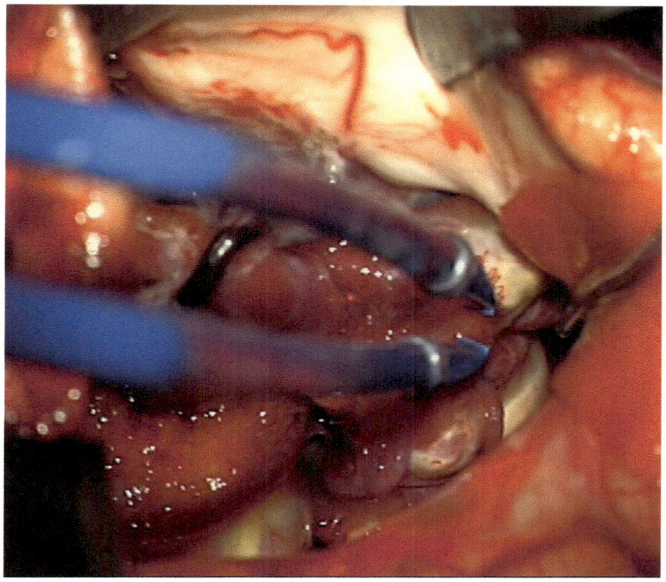

e

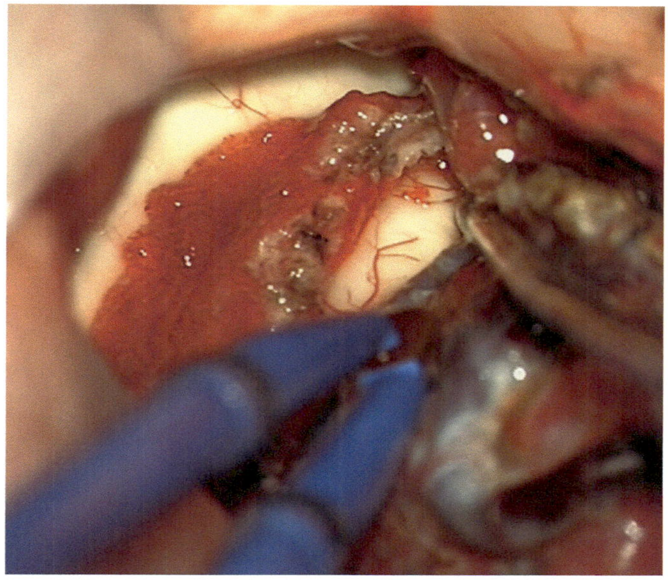

f

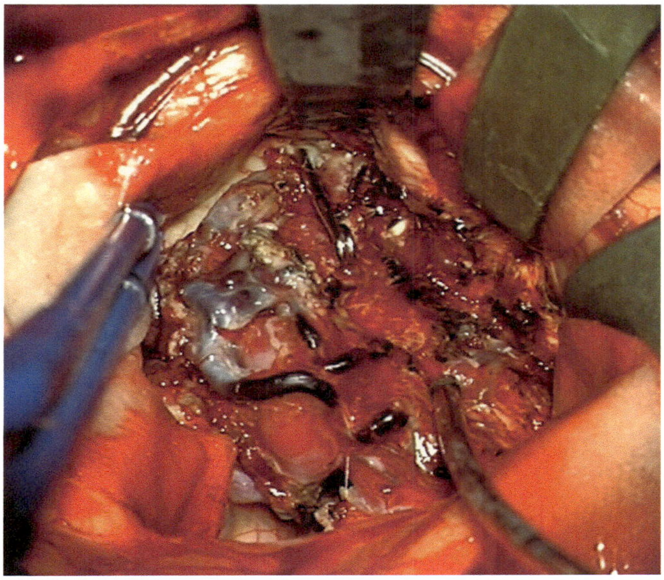

g

Fig. 15.26 (*continued*) (**e**) Supply from the mPChA was interrupted anteriorly and (**f**) supply from the AChA in the temporal horn (at sucker tip) was interrupted inferiorly. (**g**) Thalamoperforator supply could not be interrupted safely, and the de-arterialized nidus was left in situ for treatment subsequently with radiosurgery.

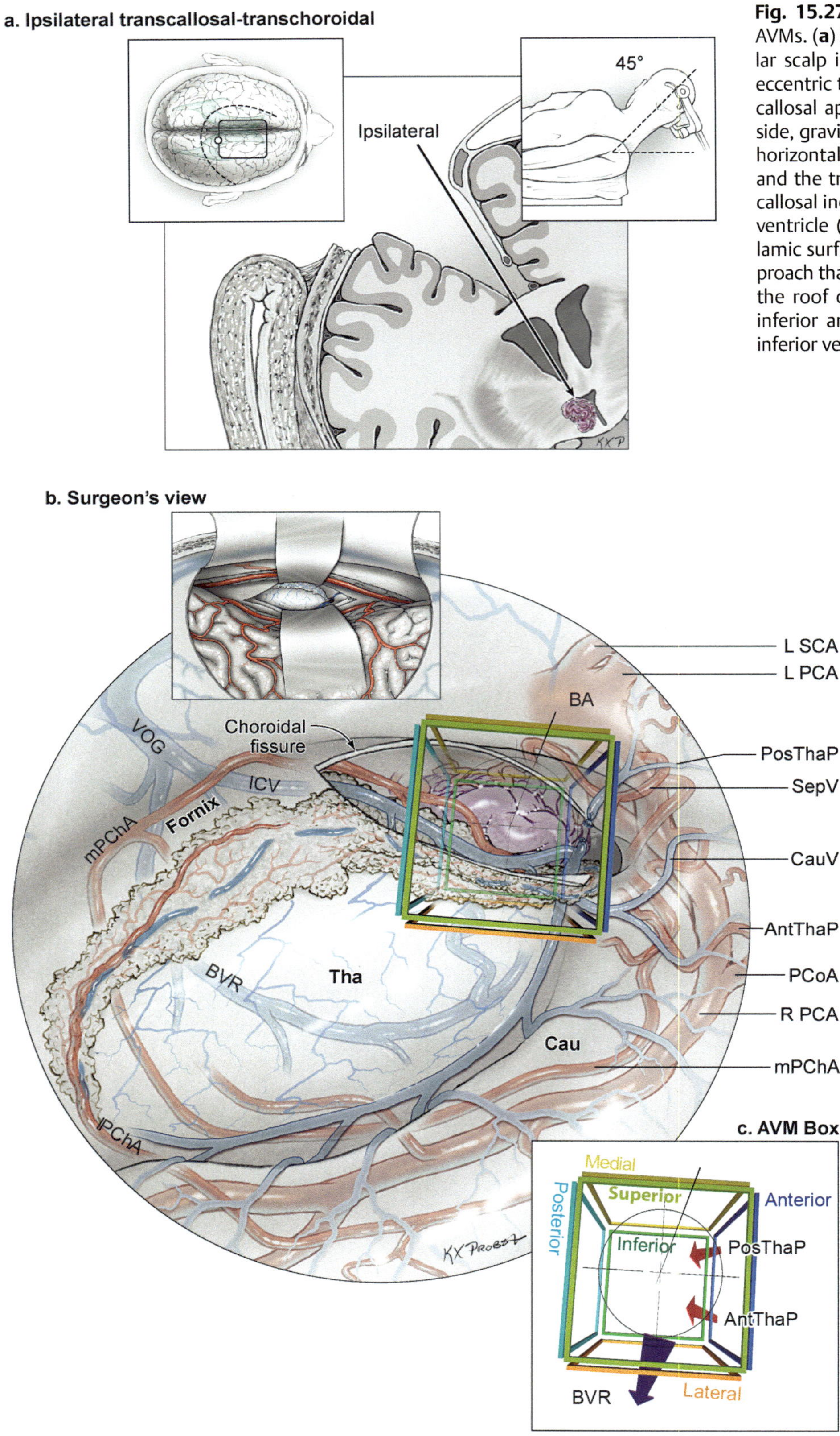

Fig. 15.27 Resection strategy for medial thalamic AVMs. (**a**) Step 1, exposing the AVM with a semicircular scalp incision (*dashed line*), bifrontal craniotomy eccentric to the right (*solid line*), and ipsilateral transcallosal approach with the right AVM on the downside, gravity retracting the right frontal lobe (midline horizontal and head angled upwards 45 degrees), and the trajectory entering the right ventricle. (**b**) A callosal incision under the right PcaA enters the right ventricle (*inset*). These AVMs sit on the medial thalamic surface and require a transchoroidal fissure approach that enlarges the foramen of Monro and opens the roof of the third ventricle. (**c**) AVM box shows inferior arterial supply (AntThaP and PosThaP) and inferior venous drainage (BVR).

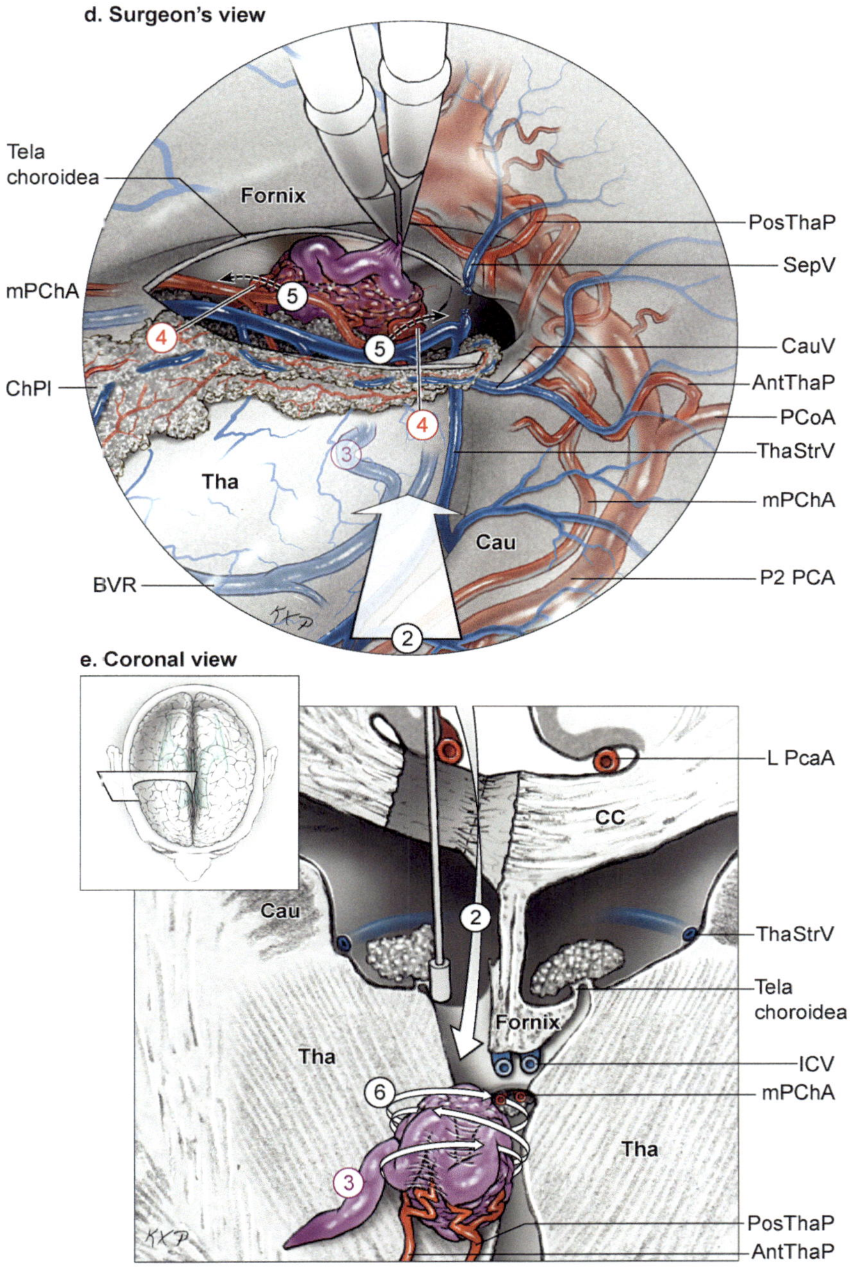

Fig. 15.27 (*continued*) (**d**) Step 2, opening the choroidal fissure by dividing the SepV, sweeping the choroid plexus laterally, incising the tela choroidea along fornix, following ThaStrV as it turns into the ICV, entering the velum interpositum, and dividing the tela choroidea in the third ventricular roof. Step 3, drainage to the BVR is deep and not visible; step 4, identifying thalamoperforator inputs; and step 5, interrupting thalamoperforator feeders along the superior margin (surgeon's view). (**e**) Step 6, circumdissecting into the thalamus (coronal cross-sectional view). (*continued on next page*)

f. Coronal view

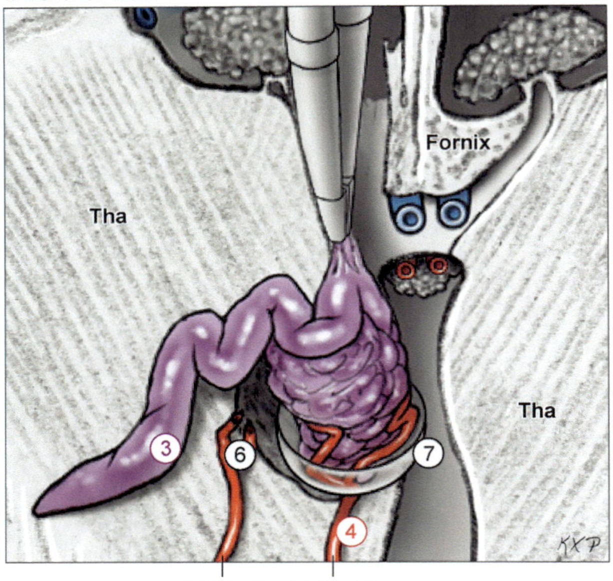

Fig. 15.27 (*continued*) (**f**) Step 7, mobilizing the AVM out of thalamus and into third ventricle, interrupting the inferior thalamoperforator supply, and dividing the draining vein (coronal cross-sectional view).

The medial thalamic AVM has similar dissection steps (**Fig. 15.27**), but access is limited through the FoM and the posterior opening into the velum interpositum. The dissection is even more perpendicular, requiring the nidus to be mobilized medially from the thalamus and into the third ventricle (step 6). Medial thalamic AVMs are supplied inferiorly, and this supply is not disrupted until the end of the dissection (step 7). Similarly, descending drainage to the BVR is not seen until the end. Working in and through the FoM is done gently because the genu of the internal capsule nears the thalamic surface just lateral to the foramen, and the columns of fornix descend anteromedially in the foramen. Thalamoperforator supply is meticulously controlled with cautery and microclips to avoid bleeding that might escape into the thalamus (**Fig. 15.28**).

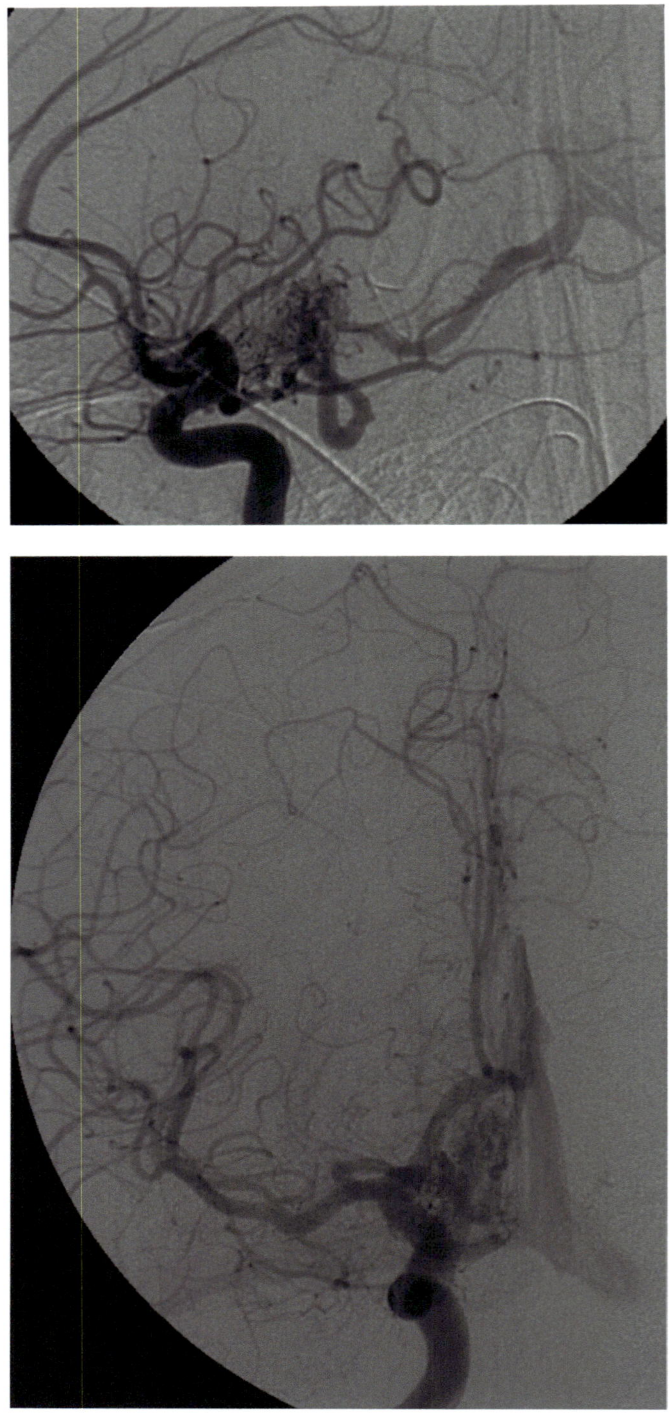

a

b

Fig. 15.28 This 54-year-old woman presented with intraventricular hemorrhage from a right medial thalamic AVM (supplemented Spetzler-Martin grade 6: S1V1E1/A3B0C0), supplied by AntThaP and drained by BVR [right ICA angiogram, (**a**) lateral and (**b**) anteroposterior views].

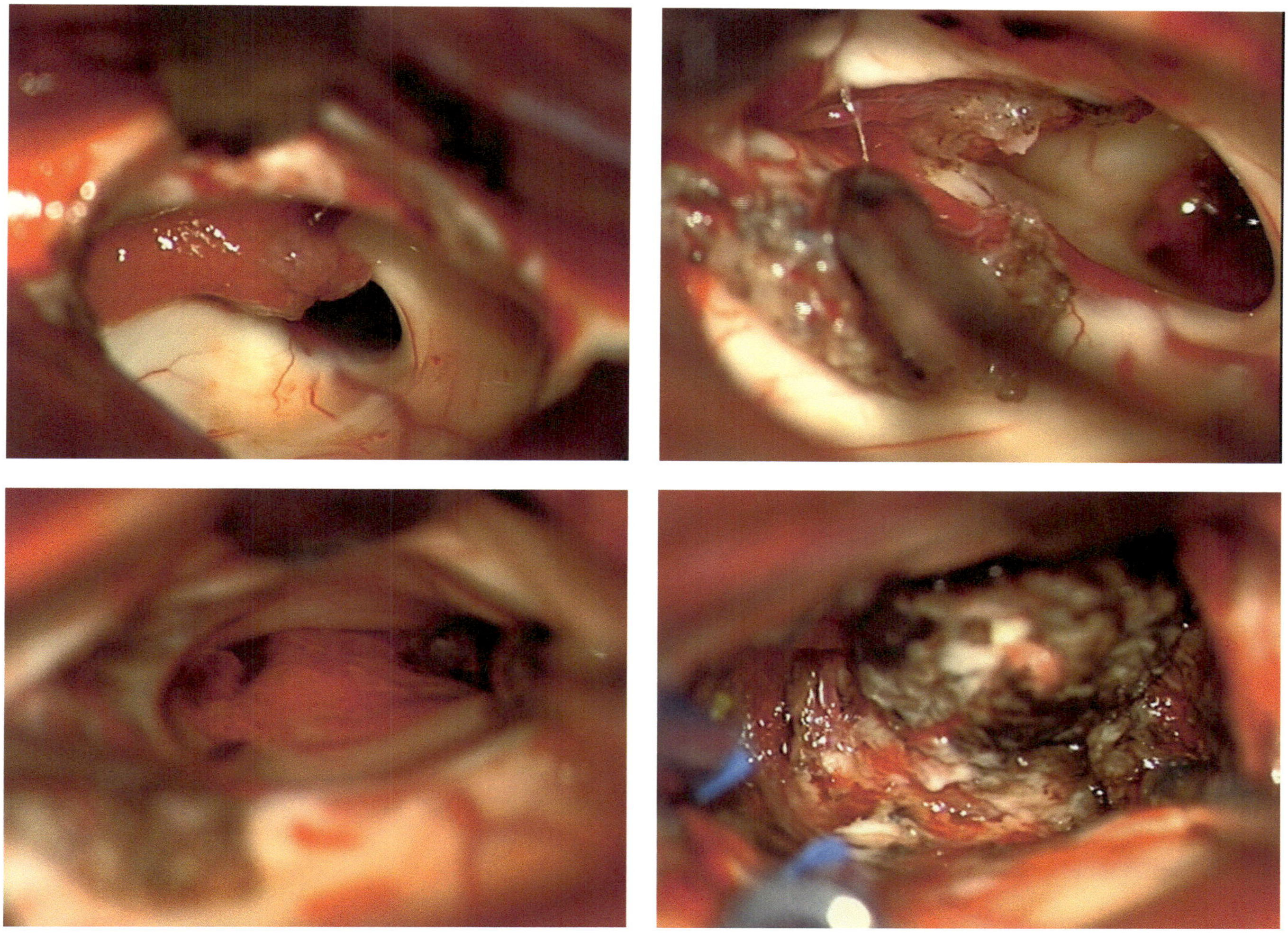

c d e f

Fig. 15.28 (*continued*) (**c**) The right ventricle was entered through a bifrontal craniotomy (nose to the right, midline horizontal, and right hemisphere down) and an ipsilateral transcallosal-transchoroidal fissure approach. There was no ThaStrV at the foramen of Monro, and only SepV and a small CauV. (**d**) Choroid plexus was coagulated and mobilized laterally to expose tenia fornicis, which was incised posteriorly along the lateral edge of the fornix to enlarge the FoM and enter the velum interpositum. Note the mPChA in the velum interpositum and hematoma in the third ventricle. (**e**) The AVM was visible in the medial wall of thalamus where it bled into third ventricle. (**f**) The nidus was circumferentially dissected, mobilizing it medially into the ventricle. (*continued on next page*)

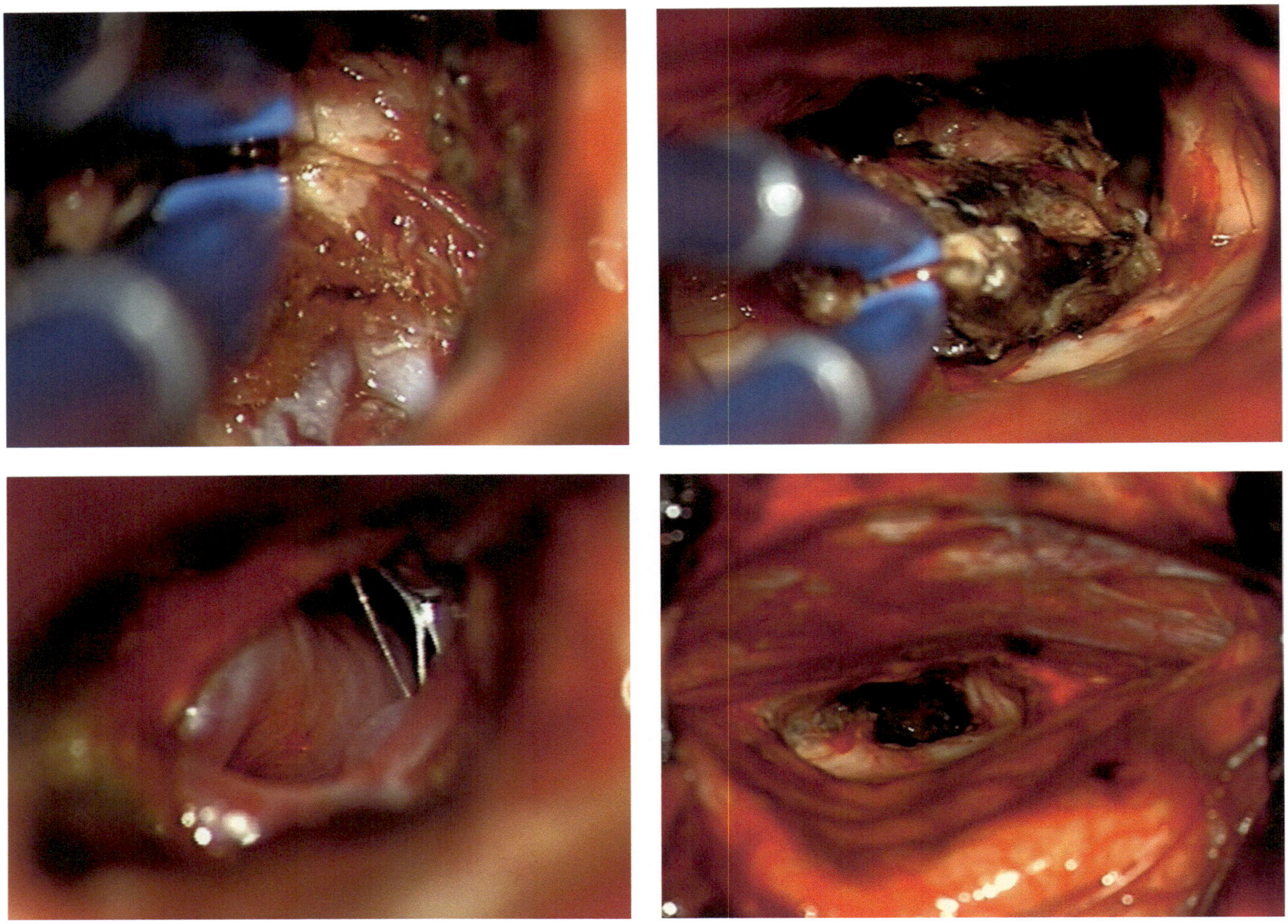

g h i j

Fig. 15.28 (*continued*) (**g**) The draining vein was encountered along the deep side as it exited through the floor of third ventricle. (**h**) After removing the AVM, (**i**) the basilar artery was visualized down its trunk through the opening in the ventricular floor. (**j**) This remarkable exposure capitalized on anatomic planes through the interhemispheric fissure and ventricular system, which were opened widely with subarachnoid dissection, gravity retraction, brain relaxation, and CSF release.

Conclusion

Deep AVMs are intimidating, prompting many neurosurgeons to treat them radiosurgically or not at all. Anatomic complexity and elegant surgical approaches make resection tempting, but the selection threshold must be high. Small AVMs with hemorrhagic presentation, secondary neurologic deficits, hematoma/encephalomalacia cavities, or incomplete radiosurgical obliteration should not be considered inoperable, and favorable results can be expected with surgery.

16 Brainstem Arteriovenous Malformations

■ Microsurgical Anatomy

Brain

Structures in the posterior fossa occur in "3's." The brainstem is composed of midbrain, pons, and medulla; superior, middle, and inferior cerebellar peduncles connect the brainstem and cerebellum; brainstem and cerebellum are divided by cerebellomesencephalic, cerebellopontine, and cerebellomedullary fissures; the cerebellum has tentorial, petrosal, and suboccipital surfaces; and brainstem and cerebellum are supplied by the superior cerebellar artery, anterior inferior cerebellar artery, and posterior inferior cerebellar artery. Three neurovascular complexes are defined with one of the three brainstem parts, one of the three cerebellar surfaces, one of the three peduncles, one of the three major fissures, and one of the three cerebellar arteries (**Fig. 16.1**). In addition, each neurovascular complex contains a group of cranial nerves: the upper complex contains the oculomotor, trochlear, and trigeminal nerves; the middle complex contains the abducens, facial, and vestibulocochlear nerves; and the lower complex contains the glossopharyngeal, vagus, accessory, and hypoglossal nerves.

In summary, the upper complex includes the superior cerebellar artery (SCA), midbrain, cerebellomesencephalic fissure, superior cerebellar peduncle, tentorial cerebellar surface,

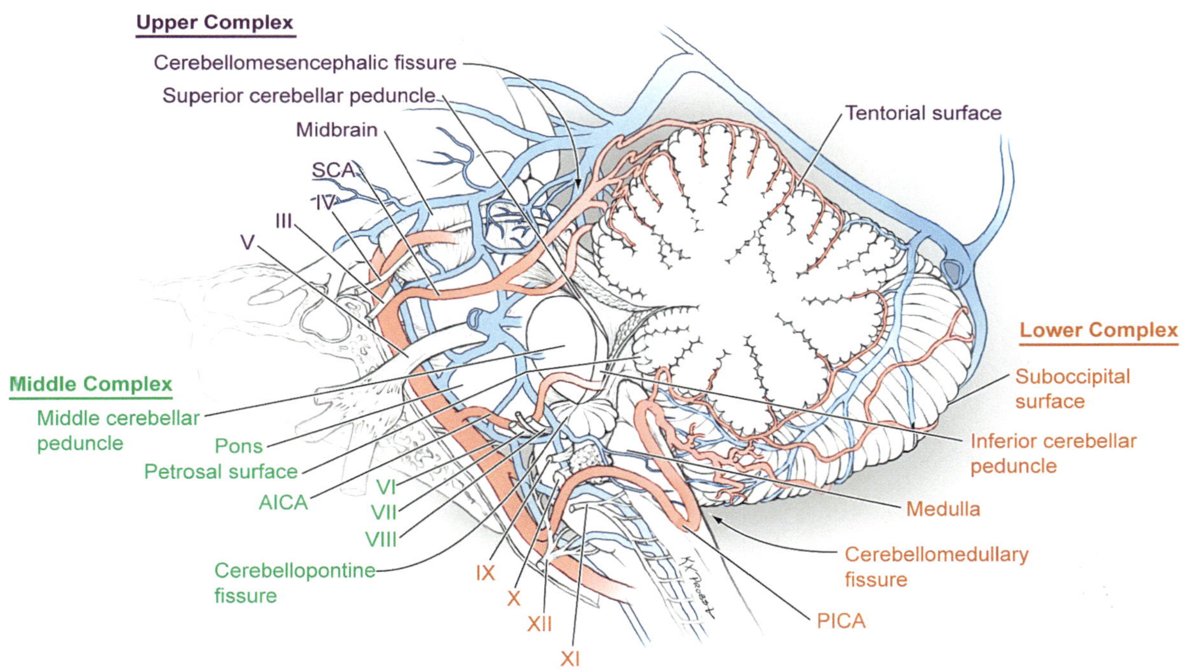

Fig. 16.1 Microsurgical anatomy of the three neurovascular complexes of the posterior fossa [upper (purple), middle (green), and lower (orange) complexes], each defined by a brainstem part, cerebellar surface, cerebellar peduncle, major fissure, cerebellar artery, and cranial nerve bundle (lateral view with sagittal cross section through the vermis).

and cranial nerves (CN) 3/4/5. The SCA arises in front of the midbrain and passes below CN3 and CN4 and above CN5 to reach the cerebellomesencephalic fissure, where it runs on the superior cerebellar peduncle and terminates by supplying the tentorial surface. The middle complex includes the anterior inferior cerebellar artery (AICA), pons, middle cerebellar peduncle, cerebellopontine fissure, petrosal surface, and CN6/7/8. The AICA arises at the pontine level, courses under CN6 and along CN7/8 to reach the surface of the middle cerebellar peduncle, where it courses along the cerebellopontine fissure and terminates by supplying the petrosal surface. The lower complex includes the posterior inferior cerebellar artery (PICA), medulla, inferior cerebellar peduncle, cerebellomedullary fissure, suboccipital surface, and CN9/10/11/12. The PICA arises at the medullary level, encircles the medulla, passing in relationship to lower CNs to reach the surface of the inferior cerebellar peduncle, where it dips into the cerebellomedullary fissure and terminates by supplying the suboccipital surface.

Surface anatomy provides landmarks for brainstem arteriovenous malformations (AVMs) (**Fig. 16.2**). Midbrain landmarks include the cerebral peduncles, CN3, interpeduncular fossa, posterior perforated substance, and pontomesencephalic fissure on the anterior surface; the cerebral peduncle, lateral geniculate body (LGB), lemniscal trigone, and CN4 on the lateral surface; and the pineal gland, tectum (superior and inferior colliculi), and CN4 on the posterior surface. Pontine landmarks include the basilar sulcus, pontomedullary sulcus, and CN6 on the anterior surface; the middle cerebellar peduncle, CN5 (sensory and motor roots), CN7/8 on the lateral surface; and the upper half of the fourth ventricular floor (above stria medullaris) on the posterior surface. Medullary landmarks include the pyramids, anteromedian sulcus between the pyramids, anterolateral sulcus, and CN12 rootlets arising from the anterolateral sulcus on the anterior surface; the olive, anterolateral (preolivary) sulcus, posterolateral (postolivary) sulcus, and CN9/10/11 rootlets arising from posterolateral sulcus on the lateral surface; and the pos-

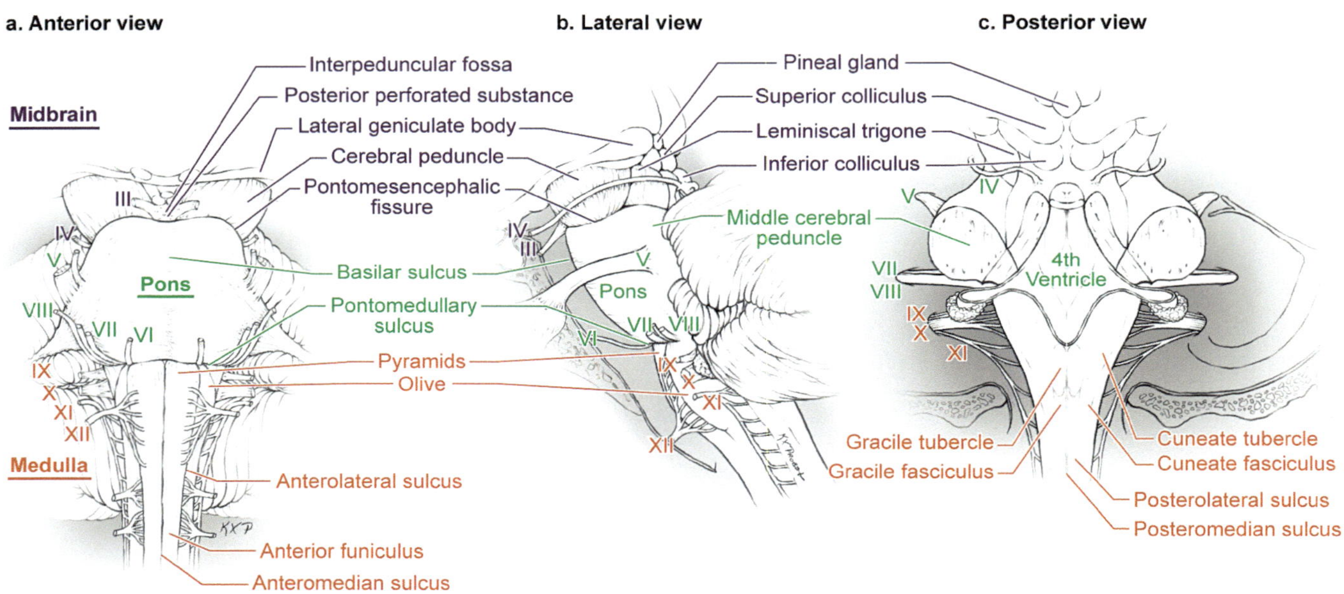

Fig. 16.2 Surface anatomy of the midbrain (purple), pons (green), and medulla (orange), seen in (**a**) anterior, (**b**) lateral, and (**c**) posterior views.

teromedian sulcus, gracile fasciculus and tubercle medially, cuneate fasciculus and tubercle laterally, posterior intermediate sulcus between them, inferior cerebellar peduncles, and the lower half of the fourth ventricular floor (below stria medullaris) on the posterior surface.

The fourth ventricular floor (a.k.a., rhomboid fossa) has three parts (**Fig. 16.3**): a pontine part extending from the cerebral aqueduct triangularly down to an imaginary line connecting the lower margin of the cerebellar peduncles; a junctional part forming a strip between the lateral recesses; and a medullary part extending triangularly down to the obex. Surface landmarks in the fourth ventricular floor include the median sulcus, facial colliculus, superior fovea, locus ceruleus, stria medullaris, inferior fovea, hypoglossal triangle, vagal triangle, and area postrema. The median sulcus divides the floor longitudinally in the midline, and the median eminence is a raised strip that parallels the median sulcus. The median eminence contains the facial colliculus rostrally and three triangular areas caudally—the hypoglossal triangle, vagal triangle, and area postrema—collectively forming the calamus scriptorius, named for its resemblance to a feather or pen nib. The sulcus limitans is another longitudinal sulcus on the lateral border of the median eminence. The locus ceruleus is a bluish gray area at the rostral end of the sulcus limitans in the lateral margin of the floor, and the superior and inferior foveae are dimples in the sulcus limitans, the superior one just lateral to the facial colliculus in the pons and the inferior one just lateral to the hypoglossal trigone in the medulla. The facial colliculus overlies the abducens nucleus and the ascending root of CN7. The hypoglossal trigone overlies the hypoglossal nucleus, and just below it, the vagal trigone overlies the dorsal nucleus of the vagus nerve. The area postrema is at the lower limit of the median eminence immediately rostral to the obex. The striae medullaris, which are white strands traversing the junctional part of the floor from the lateral recess to the sulcus limitans, overlie the vestibular area and the underlying vestibular nuclei.

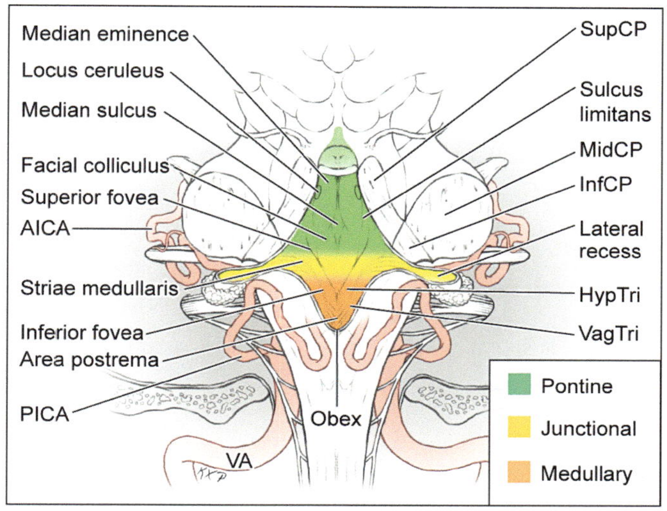

Fig. 16.3 Surface anatomy of the fourth ventricular floor, which forms the posterior surface of the pons and half of the medulla.

Liliequist's membrane separates the chiasmatic and interpeduncular cisterns and demarcates the boundary between the supra- and infratentorial cisterns (**Fig. 16.4**). The midbrain is surrounded by the interpeduncular, ambient, and quadrigeminal cisterns. The pons is surrounded by the prepontine and cerebellopontine cisterns. The medulla is surrounded by the premedullary and cerebellomedullary cisterns, and the cisterna magna. Midline cisterns are unpaired (IpC, PonC, MedC, QuadC, and MagnC), whereas lateral cisterns are paired (AmbC, CbPonC, and CbMedC). Anterior and posterior spinal cisterns surround the cord below the foramen magnum.

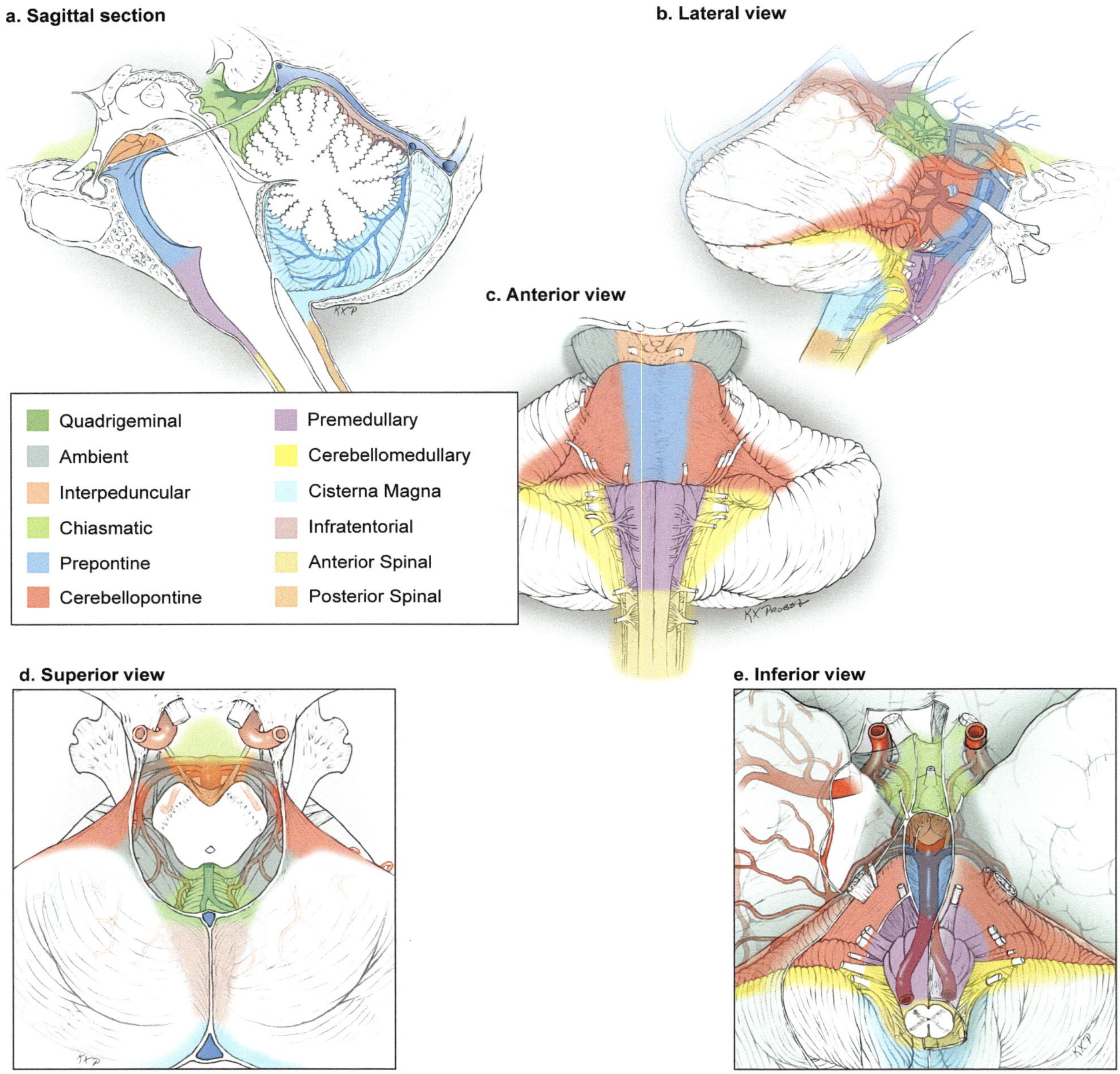

Fig. 16.4 Microsurgical anatomy of the posterior fossa cisterns: (**a**) sagittal cross-sectional, (**b**) lateral, (**c**) anterior, (**d**) superior, and (**e**) inferior views. The midbrain is surrounded by the interpeduncular, ambient, and quadrigeminal cisterns. The pons is surrounded by the prepontine and cerebellopontine cisterns. The medulla is surrounded by the premedullary and cerebellomedullary cisterns, and the cisterna magna.

Arteries

The SCA is divided into four segments (**Fig. 16.5**): anterior pontomesencephalic, lateral pontomesencephalic, cerebellomesencephalic, and cortical segments. The anterior pontomesencephalic segment (s1) begins at the SCA origin, courses underneath CN3, and ends at the anterolateral brainstem, medial to the tentorial edge. The lateral pontomesencephalic segment (s2) begins at the anterolateral brainstem, dips caudally to the trigeminal root, and terminates at the entrance to the cerebellomesencephalic fissure. The cerebellomesencephalic segment (s3) courses posteriorly within this fissure, following CN4 and the superior cerebellar peduncle. A series of hairpin curves leads deep into the fissure and then upward to reach the anterior edge of the tentorium. The cortical segment (s4) begins as distal branches exit the cerebellomesencephalic fissure and supply the cerebellum's tentorial surface.

The AICA is divided into four segments (**Fig. 16.5**): anterior pontine, lateral pontine, flocculopeduncular, and cortical segments. The anterior pontine segment (a1) begins at the AICA's origin from the basilar trunk and ends at the level of a line drawn through the long axis of the inferior olive extended upward on the pons. This segment courses below CN6 as it ascends to Dorello's canal. The lateral pontine segment (a2) begins at the anterolateral margin of the pons and passes through the cerebellopontine angle alongside CN7/8, the internal auditory meatus, lateral recess, and choroid plexus protruding from the foramen of Luschka. The labyrinthine artery, recurrent perforating arteries, and subarcuate artery arise from this segment. The flocculopeduncular segment (a3) begins as the artery passes the flocculus and middle cerebellar peduncle, and ends as it reaches the cerebellopontine fissure. It commonly bifurcates near CN7/8 into rostral and caudal trunks. The cortical segment (a4) supplies the petrosal surface distal to the cerebellopontine fissure.

The PICA has five segments (**Fig. 16.5**): anterior medullary, lateral medullary, tonsillomedullary, telovelotonsillar, and cortical segments. The anterior medullary segment (p1) begins at the PICA's origin, lies anterior to the medulla, and extends past the hypoglossal rootlets at the medial edge of the inferior olive. The lateral medullary segment (p2) extends from the most prominent point of the inferior olive to the rootlets of CN9/10/11 at the lateral edge of the olive. The tonsillomedullary segment (p3) begins where the PICA passes under or between the rootlets of CN9/10/11, descends to the inferior pole of the cerebellar tonsil, reverses course in the caudal or infratonsillar loop, and ascends along the medial tonsil to its midpoint. The telovelotonsillar segment (p4) begins at the midpoint of the PICA's ascent, continues toward the roof of the fourth ventricle, turns around again to form a cranial or supratonsillar loop, and courses downward and posteriorly to the tonsillobiventral fissure. This segment de-

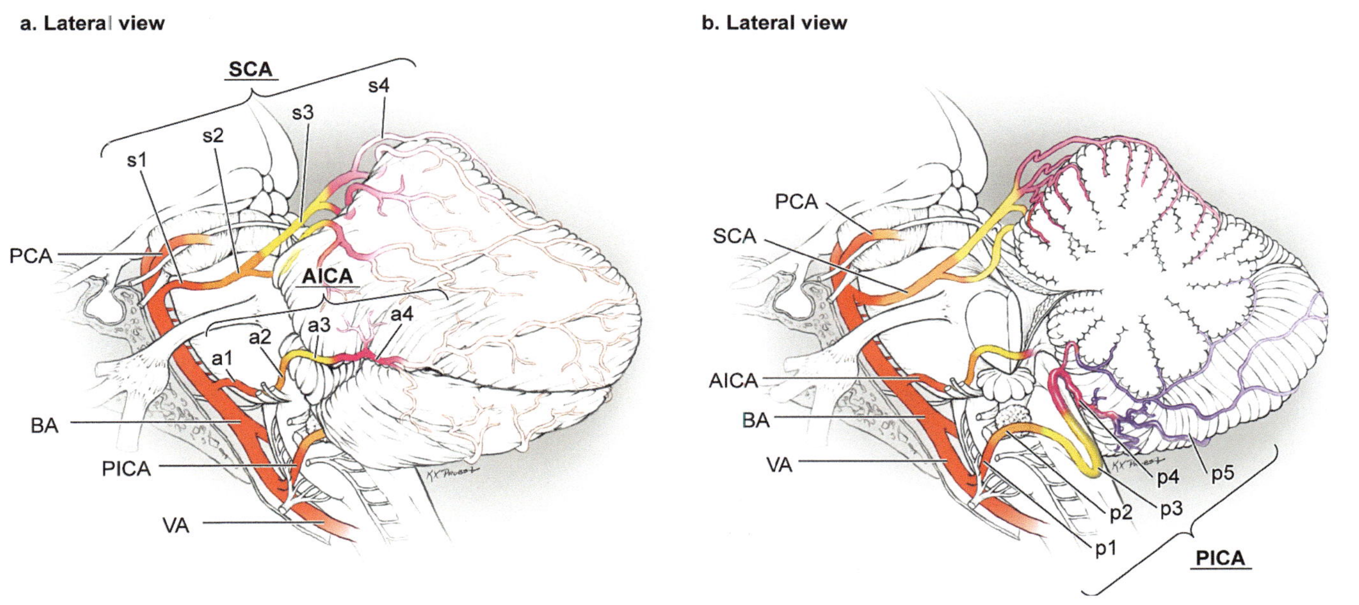

Fig. 16.5 Microsurgical anatomy of the brainstem and cerebellar arteries. Brainstem surfaces are supplied by the first three segments of the cerebellar arteries, with the anterior surfaces supplied by the first segments (s1 anterior pontomesencephalic, a1 anterior pontine, and p1 anterior medullary segments), the lateral surfaces supplied by the second segments (s2 lateral pontomesencephalic, a2 lateral pontine, and p2 lateral medullary segments), and the posterior surfaces supplied by the third segments (s3 cerebellomesencephalic, a3 flocculopeduncular, and p3 tonsillomedullary segments), shown in lateral views (**a**) with and (**b**) without the left cerebellum (sagittal section through the vermis).

rives its name from its branches to the choroid plexus of the fourth ventricle (tela choroidea) and its association with the roof of the fourth ventricle (inferior medullary velum). Cortical segment (p5) begins as the PICA emerges from the tonsillobiventral fissure where the tonsil, vermis, and biventral lobule meet. This segment has a medial trunk supplying the vermian surface and a lateral trunk supplying the tonsillar and hemispheric surfaces.

Veins

Brainstem veins are named according to the division of the brainstem, the surface, and their course longitudinally or transversely (**Fig. 16.6**). Longitudinal veins include the median anterior pontomesencephalic vein (MAPonMesV), median anterior medullary vein (MAMedV), lateral anterior pontomesencephalic vein (LAPonMesV), lateral anterior medullary vein (LAMedV), lateral mesencephalic vein (LMesV), lateral medullary vein (LMedV), and retro-olivary veins (ReOlvV). Transverse veins are the vein of the pontomesencephalic sulcus (VPonMesS), vein of the pontomedullary sulcus (VPonMedS), transverse pontine vein, transverse medullary vein, peduncular vein, and posterior communicating vein (PComV). Veins draining the brainstem bridge across the subarachnoid spaces to reach the dural sinuses. The peduncular, PComV, and tectal vein (TecV), as well as the longitudinal veins, ascend to the basal vein of Rosenthal (BVR) en route to the vein of Galen (VoG). Anterior brainstem veins course laterally to the superior petrosal (SPetrV, or Dandy's vein) and inferior petrosal veins (IPetrV) that drain to the petrosal sinuses (SPS and IPS, respectively).

Six Brainstem AVM Subtypes

The brainstem is one of the inviolable areas packed densely with cranial nerve nuclei and tracts. All brainstem AVMs are eloquent and drain deeply, raising their Spetzler-Martin grades to at least grade III. Fortunately, brainstem AVMs are rare (4% of AVMs in my surgical experience [25 patients] and 2% to 6% in published series) and many sit on the brainstem surface rather than in the parenchyma (70% in my surgical experience). This pial or "epipial" location makes them different from cerebral and cerebellar AVMs. The categorization of brainstem AVMs is based on the brainstem level and surface, as with other AVMs. Half were located in pons, one fourth in the midbrain, and one fourth in the medulla.

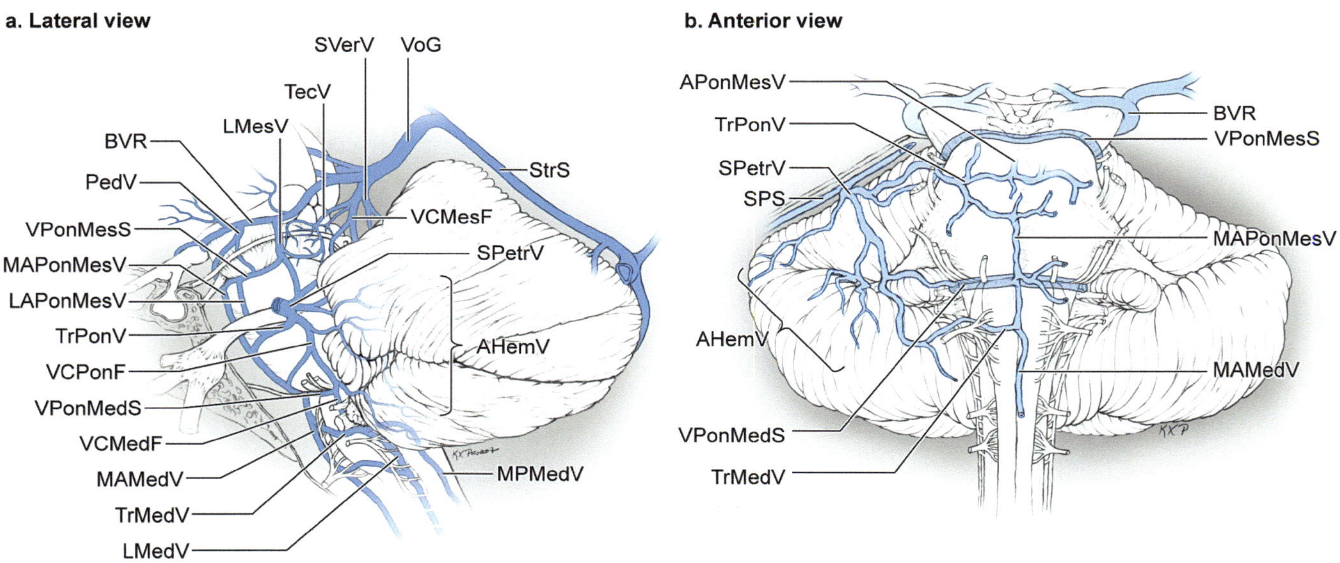

Fig. 16.6 Microsurgical anatomy of the brainstem veins. (**a**) Veins of the lateral brainstem (lateral view). (**b**) Veins of the anterior brainstem and cerebellum (anterior view). Brainstem veins are named according to the division of the brainstem (mesencephalon, pons, or medulla), the surface (anterior, lateral, or posterior), and their course (longitudinal or transverse).

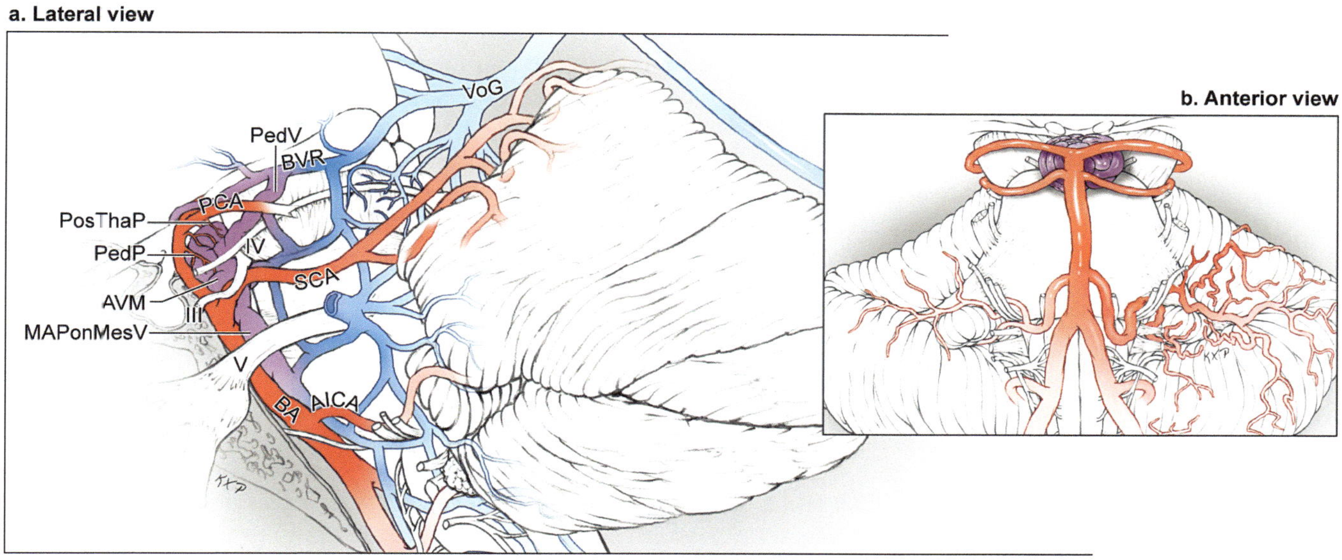

Fig. 16.7 The anterior midbrain AVM: (**a**) lateral and (**b**) anterior views. This AVM is located on the anterior midbrain surface on, in, or between the cerebral peduncles, is supplied by P1 PCA branches (PosThaP and PedP), and is drained by anterior veins (MAPonMesV, PedV, and PComV).

The Anterior Midbrain AVM

The anterior midbrain AVM is located on the anterior midbrain surface on, in, or between the cerebral peduncles (**Fig. 16.7**). This subtype is associated with CN3 and lies behind the P1 posterior cerebral artery (PCA) and PosThaP in the interpeduncular fossa. Portions of the AVM sit in the interpeduncular cistern. Perforating arteries from both the P1 PCA supply the nidus (PosThaP and PedP), and it is drained by MAPonMesV, PedV, and PComV, which then collect in the BVR.

The Posterior Midbrain AVM

The posterior midbrain AVM sits on the tectum/quadrigeminal plate, below the pineal gland and above the superior cerebellar peduncles, often intimate with the trochlear nerves (**Fig. 16.8**). Portions of the AVM reside in the quadrigeminal cistern. These AVMs are fed by the long circumflex perforator (CirP) from the P1 and P2 PCA segments, as well as branches from the s3 SCA, typically bilaterally. Venous drainage into the tectal vein and the vein of the cerebellomesen-

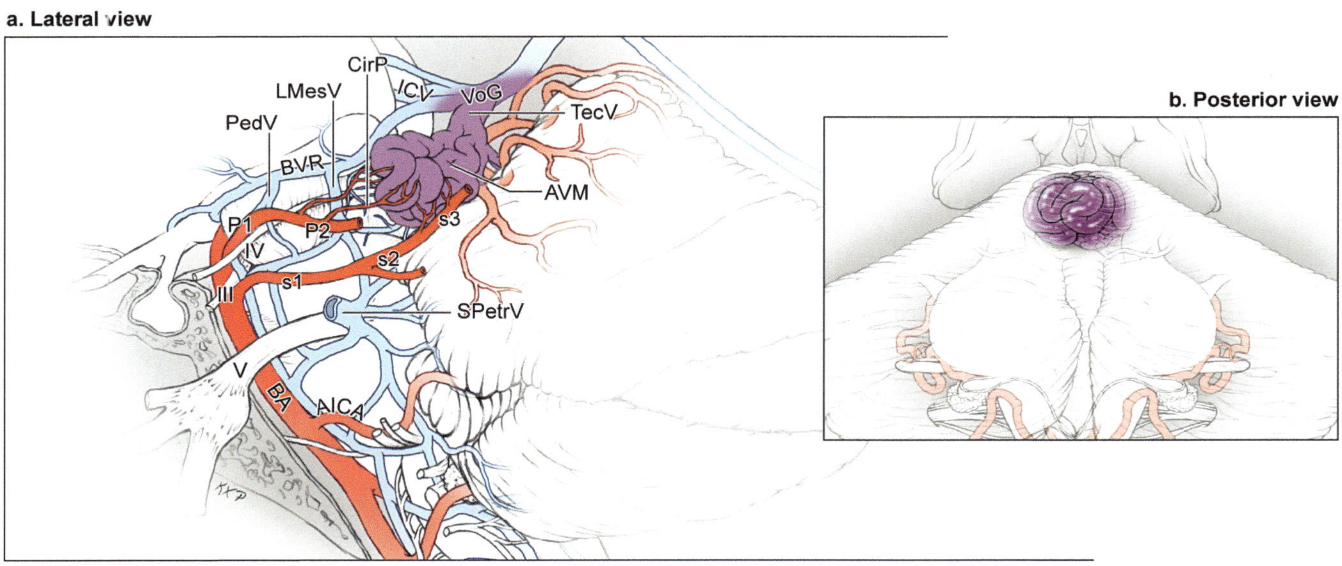

Fig. 16.8 The posterior midbrain AVM: (**a**) lateral and (**b**) posterior views. This AVM is located on the posterior midbrain surface on or adjacent to the quadrigeminal plate. It is supplied bilaterally by the PCA (long circumflex perforators from P1 and P2 segments) and the SCA (s3 branches), and is drained by veins ascending to the vein of Galen (TecV and VCMesF).

cephalic fissure (VCMesF) collect in the VoG. Although the lateral surface of the midbrain is sizable, no lateral midbrain AVM was encountered.

The Anterior Pontine AVM

The anterior pontine AVM sits on the rectangular surface between the basilar sulcus medially and the CN5 root laterally, and between the pontomesencephalic sulcus superiorly and the pontomedullary sulcus inferiorly (**Fig. 16.9**). These exophytic AVMs protrude into the prepontine and cerebellopontine cisterns. Despite its anterior location, this AVM is unilateral and does not cross the midline. It is located between the s1 SCA superiorly and the a1 AICA inferiorly, and is supplied by both arteries. Enlarged perforating branches from the basilar trunk also feed this AVM directly. Interestingly, arteries from the meningohypophyseal trunk of the internal carotid artery (ICA) travel through Meckel's cave along CN5 and can contribute to these AVMs (three cases). Venous drainage collects medially in MAPonMesV or more commonly in SPetrV and SPS laterally. These AVMs are intimately associated with CN5, often entangled in nerve fibers.

The Lateral Pontine AVM

The lateral pontine AVM sits on the triangular surface between the CN5 root medially and the V-shaped cerebellopontine fissure laterally, as the pons transitions into the middle cerebellar peduncle (**Fig. 16.10**). The extent of pial invasion varies among these AVMs, with some lying on the pial surface and others penetrating deeply into the middle cerebellar peduncle. Surprisingly, this portion of the brachium pontis tolerates surgical transgression, making intraparenchymal lateral pontine AVMs resectable lesions. They are supplied by the AICA (a2 and a3 segments) and, unlike anterior pontine AVMs, do not receive input from the SCA. Venous drainage collects in SPetrV and SPS. Lateral pontine AVMs are located in the cerebellopontine angle and more medial than petrosal cerebellar AVMs, which are also in the cerebellopontine angle but based on the petrosal surface in the cerebellar lobules rather than in the middle cerebellar peduncle. Lateral pontine AVMs were the most common brainstem subtype (27%). No posterior pontine AVM was encountered.

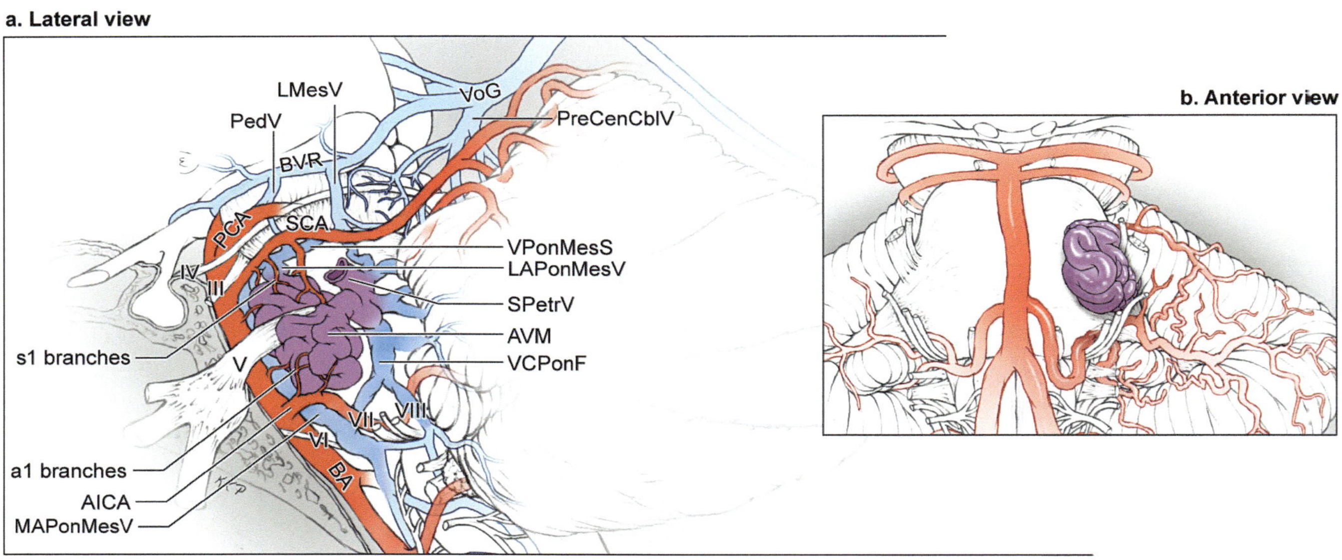

Fig. 16.9 The anterior pontine AVM: (**a**) lateral and (**b**) anterior views. This AVM is located on the rectangular surface between the basilar sulcus medially, the trigeminal root laterally, and the pontomesencephalic and pontomedullary sulci. It is supplied unilaterally by s1 SCA and a1 AICA branches, as well as direct branches from the basilar trunk, and drains to MAPonMesV medially or SPetrV laterally.

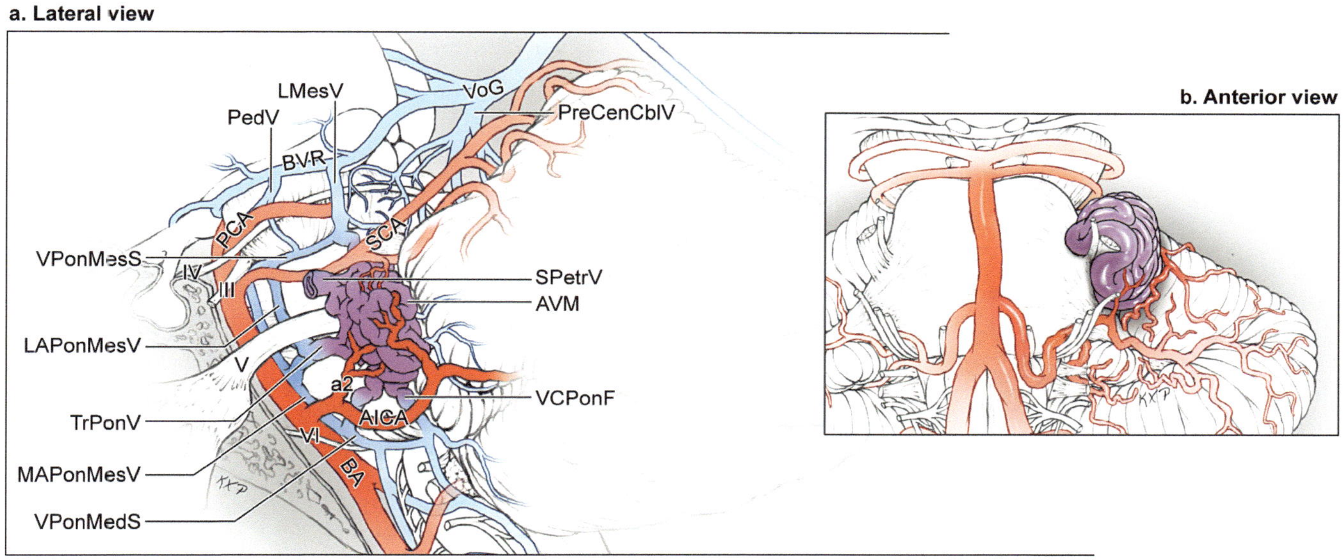

Fig. 16.10 The lateral pontine AVM: (**a**) lateral and (**b**) anterior views. This AVM is located on the triangular surface of the pons and brachium pontis between the CN5 root medially and the V-shaped cerebellopontine fissure laterally. It is supplied unilaterally by the a2 and a3 AICA branches and is drained by SPetrV.

The Anterior Medullary AVM

The anterior medullary AVM is located on the anterior surface below the pontomedullary sulcus, between the anterolateral sulci and anterior to the hypoglossal nerve rootlets (**Fig. 16.11**). Portions of the AVM reside in the premedullary cistern. This AVM sits posteroinferior to the vertebrobasilar junction (VBJ) in the midline and is supplied bilaterally by vertebral artery (VA) branches at the level of the anterior spinal artery origins (distal V4 segment). The PICA originates lateral to this area and does not contribute. Venous drainage is through MAMedV.

The Lateral Medullary AVM

The lateral medullary AVM is located below the pontomedullary sulcus, lateral to the anterolateral (preolivary) sulcus

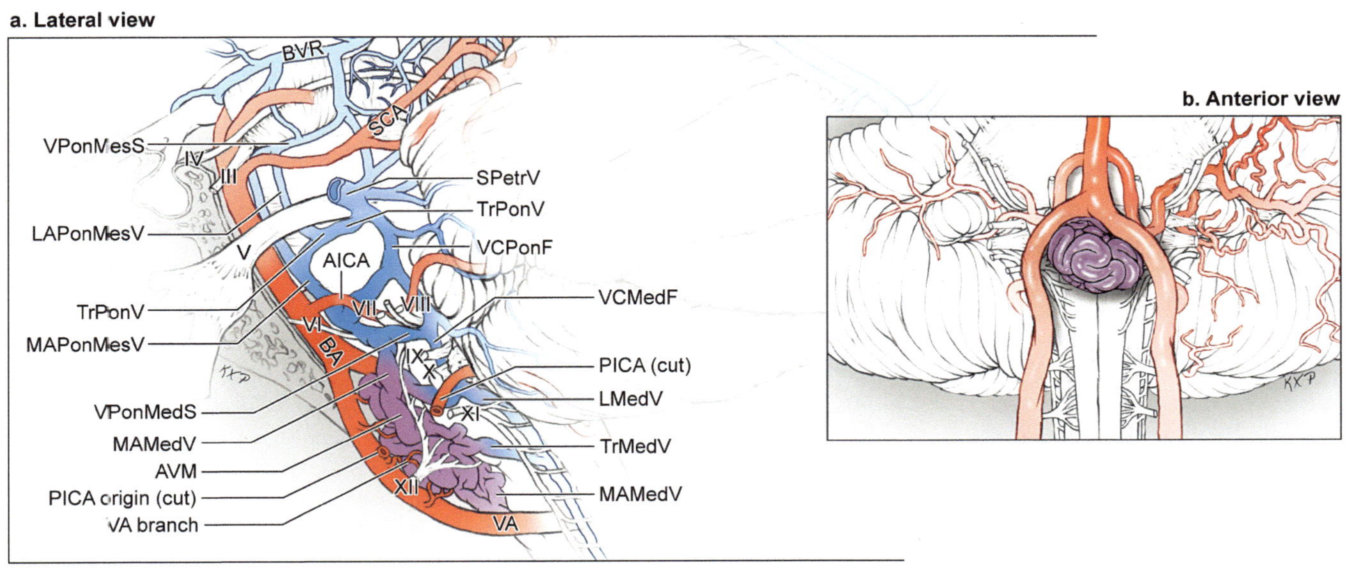

Fig. 16.11 The anterior medullary AVM: (**a**) lateral and (**b**) anterior views. This AVM is located below the pontomedullary sulcus, between the anterolateral sulci, and anterior to hypoglossal nerve rootlets. It is supplied by branches from the distal vertebral artery proximal to or at the vertebrobasilar junction and is drained in the midline by MAMedV and MAPonMesV.

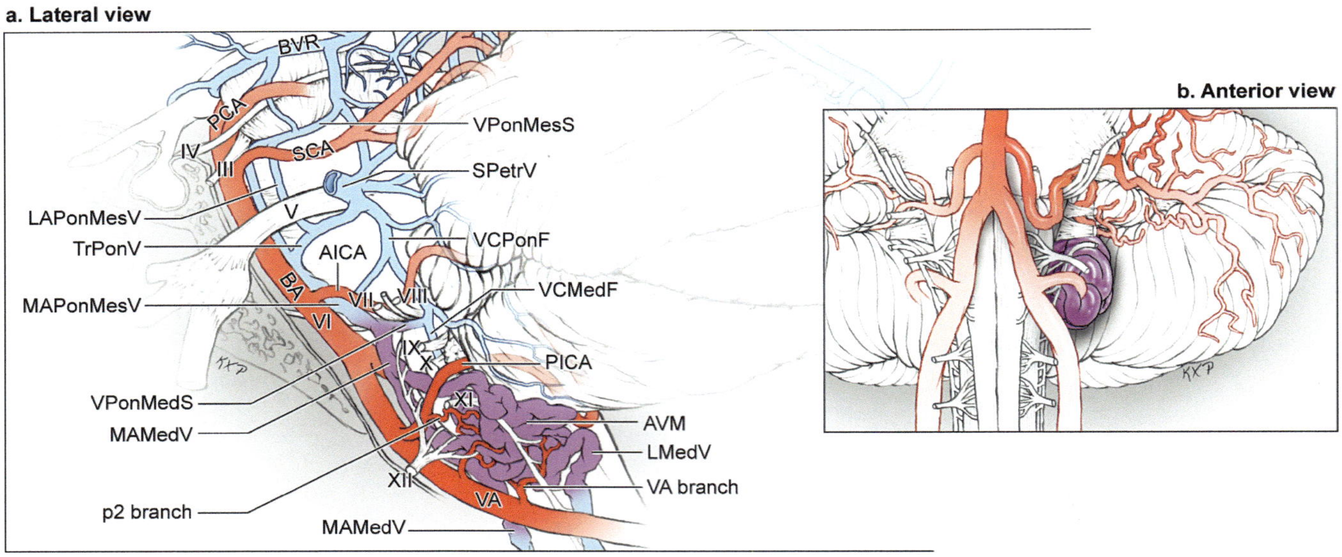

Fig. 16.12 The lateral medullary AVM: (**a**) lateral and (**b**) anterior views. This AVM is located below the pontomedullary sulcus, lateral to the anterolateral sulcus, and posterior to hypoglossal nerve rootlets. It is supplied by branches from the vertebral artery and PICA, and drains medially (MAMedV) and/or laterally (LMedV).

and posterior to the hypoglossal nerve rootlets (**Fig. 16.12**). This AVM is visible on the lateral medullary surface through a far lateral craniotomy in the location of the PICA's p2 segment. It tends to be small in size and respects the pia, with most of the AVM in the cerebellomedullary cistern. This AVM is unilateral and fed by small branches directly from the VA and PICA. It is drained by LMedV and MAMedV. Lateral medullary AVMs were more common than the anterior medullary AVM (19% vs. 4%, respectively). No posterior medullary AVMs were encountered.

Resection Strategies for Brainstem AVMs

Limited posterior fossa exposures and their unique location in or adjacent to vital structures make brainstem AVMs potentially dangerous to resect. They require a different surgical strategy that minimizes or avoids intraparenchymal dissection by completely occluding the AVM with circumferential pial dissection and does not transgress brainstem tissue. The occluded AVM is often left in situ rather than resected. Luckily, many brainstem AVMs are located on the pial layer and are small in size, allowing for this scaled back, simplified strategy of "occlusion in situ." The strategy still includes the optimal craniotomy (step 1), subarachnoid dissection to expose the AVM (step 2), and thorough appreciation of its venous (step 3) and arterial anatomy (step 4), but nidal dissection remains in the pia (step 5) without parenchymal invasion. Arteriovenous malformation dissection, even when confined to the pia, must still be circumferential and is depicted in the battle plan illustrations (step 6). The AVMs that do separate cleanly from the brainstem can be resected safely, requiring deep/ependymal dissection that is especially meticulous (step 7). However, when visualization is limited and brainstem perforators are at risk, I prefer this more cautious occlusion in situ. Complete circumdissection occludes the arterial input and darkens the draining vein, at which point the vein is divided and a lifeless nidus is left on the brainstem surface. Some neurosurgeons have alternatively described a "pial resection technique" with circumdissection that occludes arterial input at the pial margins and resects the portion of the nidus extending beyond the brainstem surface, leaving behind a deep portion that no longer poses the same threat of hemorrhage or may occlude on its own. In my experience, occlusion in situ is a safe and appropriate strategy for pial brainstem AVMs, particularly those that have never ruptured.

Ruptured brainstem AVMs are different because associated hematomas and neurologic deficits permit a more aggressive strategy beyond occlusion in situ. Hematomas create nonanatomic corridors to the nidus and enable transgression into brainstem parenchyma, facilitating the resection of these AVMs. Whether the surgical strategy is occlusion in situ or resection, brainstem AVMs demand the absolute preservation of normal perforating arteries. Uninvolved perforators are small in caliber, difficult to visualize, immediately adjacent to the nidus, and often indistinguishable from AVM feeders. The loss of even one perforator can devastate the patient, thus calling for delicate, deliberative, and cautious handling of each and every artery around a brainstem AVM.

Anterior Midbrain AVM Resection

The anterior midbrain AVM is approached with an orbitozygomatic-pterional craniotomy and transsylvian approach, as for a basilar bifurcation aneurysm or a medial temporal AVM (**Fig. 16.13**). With the full orbitozygomatic craniotomy (step 1), zygoma removal facilitates retraction of the temporal lobe and orbital removal expands the sylvian corridor. Subarachnoid dissection includes splitting of the sylvian fissure, opening carotid cistern, following the anterior choroidal artery (AChA) through the crural cistern, mobilizing the temporal pole, and entering the interpeduncular cistern

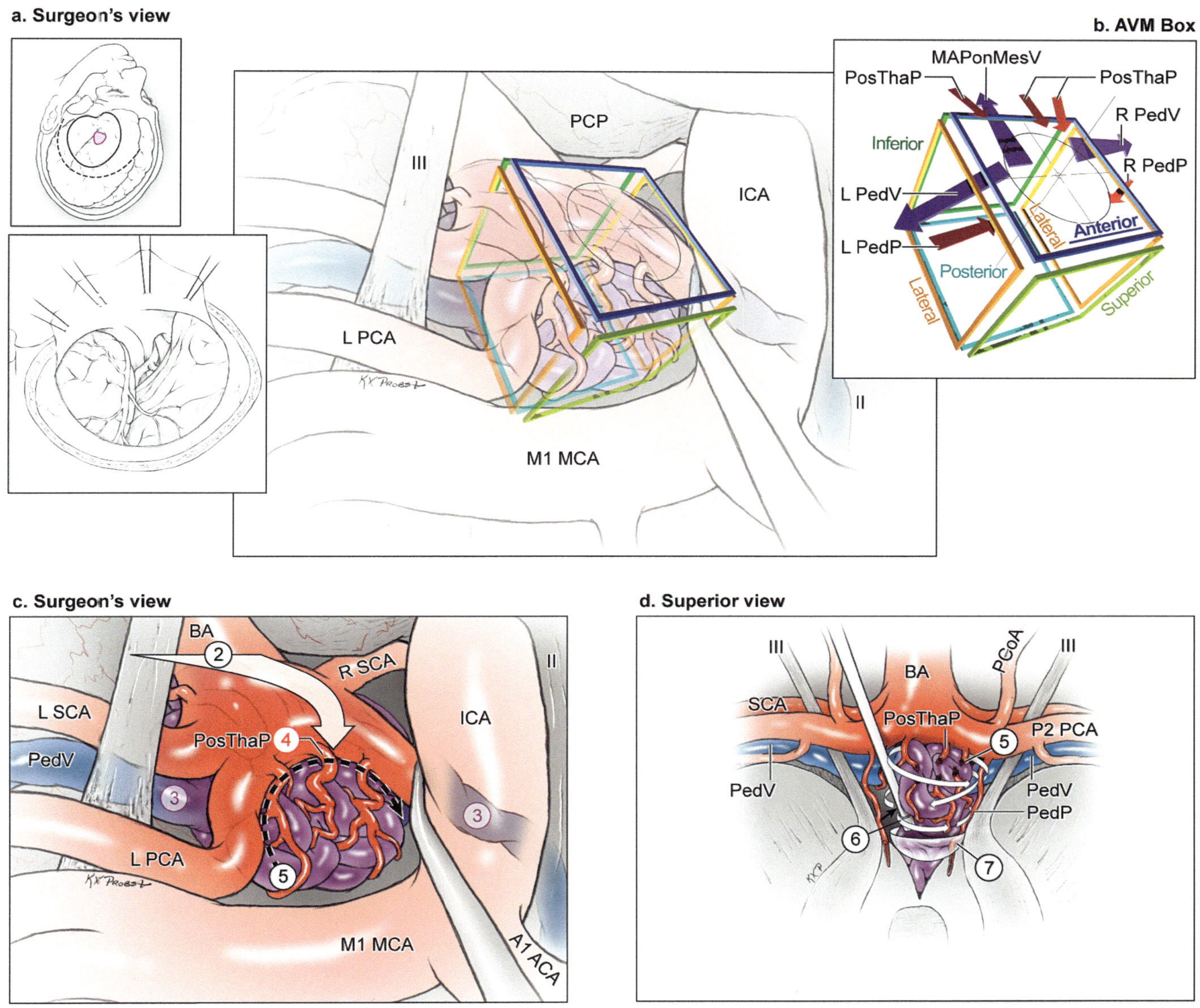

Fig. 16.13 Resection strategy for anterior midbrain AVMs. (**a**) Step 1, exposing the AVM with an orbitozygomatic-pterional craniotomy and transsylvian approach [surgeon's view, with scalp incision (*dashed line*), craniotomy (*solid line*), and AVM (*purple circle*) shown on *upper inset*, and the dural opening and transsylvian corridor shown on *lower inset*]. (**b**) AVM box showing arterial inputs from PCA branches (red inflow arrows), venous drainage to BVR bilaterally (blue outflow arrows), and proximity to oculomotor nerves and cerebral peduncles. (**c**) Step 2, approaching the AVM through the carotid-oculomotor triangle by splitting the sylvian fissure, opening the carotid cistern, following the AChA through the crural cistern, mobilizing the temporal pole, and entering the interpeduncular cistern through Liliequist's membrane (broad white arrow); step 3, identifying venous drainage laterally on both sides; step 4, locating feeding arteries from the P1 PCA; and step 5, interrupting the anterior front of feeders in the interpeduncular cistern (dashed black arrow, surgeon's view). (**d**) Step 6, circumdissecting in the interpeduncular fossa (*encircling arrows*); and step 7, mobilizing the AVM into the interpeduncular cistern (spherical scoop) to divide deep peduncular perforators.

through Liliequist's membrane (step 2). The carotid-oculomotor triangle provides access to the AVM, which can be augmented by working through the carotid-optic triangle, supracarotid triangle, and the lateral triangle between CN3 and the tentorium. The PCA, from the basilar bifurcation to the tentorial incisura, occupies the center of the surgical field, and normal perforators on the P1 and proximal P2 segments can be visualized. The AVM dissection progresses deep to PosThaP and PedP into interpeduncular fossa. Drainage to PedV and BVR is identified laterally in the crural cistern (step 3). The PCA feeders are differentiated from normal perforators at the AVM margins (step 4). Additional feeders might be found at the basilar bifurcation and distal basilar trunk. Feeding arteries are occluded along the anterior AVM margin until the draining vein darkens (step 5). The AVM is circumdissected within the pial confines of the interpeduncular fossa, taking care to protect the cerebral peduncles and oculomotor nerves (step 6). The AVM is either separated from the midbrain (step 7) and resected, or occluded in situ, with indocyanine green (ICG) videoangiography confirming the absence of arteriovenous shunting. Before permanently occluding the draining vein, test occlusion with a forceps or temporary clips also assesses the completeness of the arterial occlusion, watching for nidal expansion or changes in turgor (**Fig. 16.14**).

a 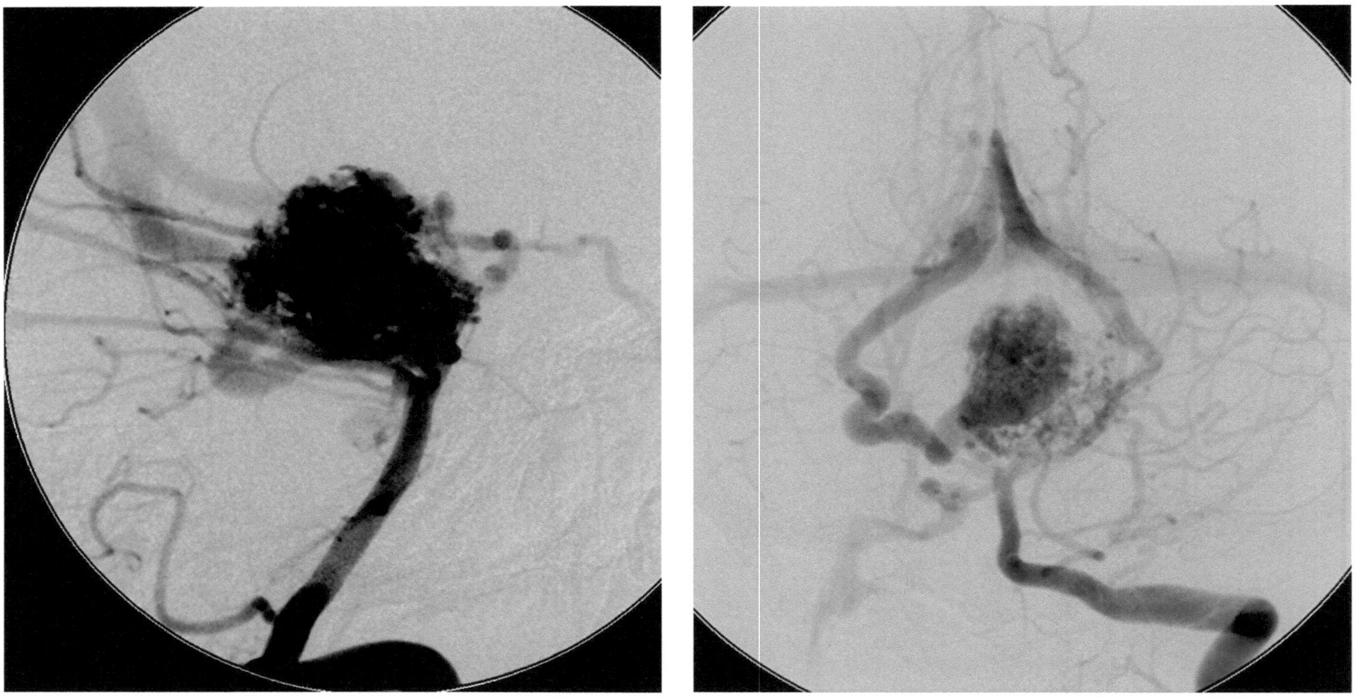 b

Fig. 16.14 This 19-year-old girl presented in a coma with a hemorrhage from this anterior midbrain AVM (supplemented Spetzler-Martin grade 4: S1V1E1/A1B0C0), supplied by left CirP, PedP, and ThGenP and drained by PedV and BVR bilaterally [left VA angiogram, (**a**) lateral and (**b**) anteroposterior views]. She recovered significantly with persistent hemiplegia on the right side from the hemorrhage, and underwent Gamma Knife radiosurgery with significant volume reduction.

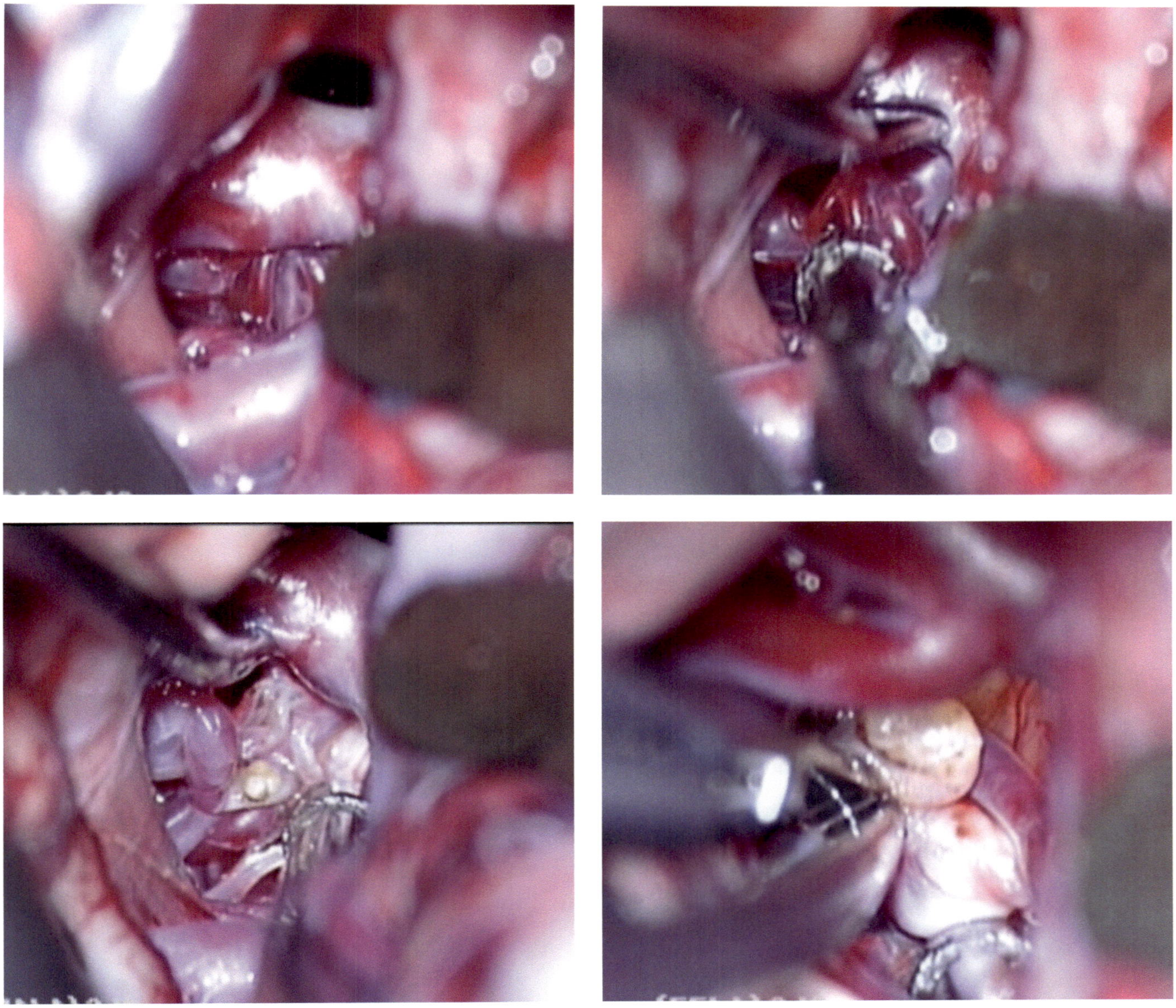

c d e f

Fig. 16.14 (*continued*) (**c**) The residual AVM was resected through a left orbitozygomatic-pterional craniotomy and transsylvian approach to the interpeduncular cistern. The carotid-oculomotor triangle was the workir g window, as with basilar bifurcation aneurysms. (**d**) Feeding arteries were visualized behind the basilar apex in the axilla of the P1 PCA and over the shoulder of the s1 SCA, medial to CN3. (**e**) Feeding arteries were cauterized as they intersected the AVM. (**f**) The nidus was separated from the gliotic walls of the previous hemorrhage cavity with preservation of normal perforating arteries.

Posterior Midbrain AVM Resection

Posterior midbrain AVMs are exposed through a torcular craniotomy and supracerebellar-infratentorial approach, with or without gravity retraction (**Fig. 16.15**). Gravity retraction requires the patient to be in the sitting position with the operating table flexed maximally to bring the back vertical and the head flexed forward to flatten the angle of the tentorium. A linear midline incision and a torcular craniotomy expose the torcular (step 1). A dural flap based superiorly on the transverse sinus (TrvS) and tented with sutures elevates the sinuses and provides entrée to the supracerebellar-infratentorial plane. Cerebellar sag widens the natural corridor to the quadrigeminal cistern. Placing the patient in the sitting position can make the surgery awkward for the neurosurgeon, who then has to hold his or her hands high to reach the surgical field. I sit on a rolling stool and support my elbows on a free-standing arm brace raised to shoulder level. The hands remain relaxed and stabilized in this position, but they fatigue more quickly. Still, I have not found this setup to be uncomfortable or problematic. Younger patients, those without a patent foramen ovale (as assessed by preoperative echocardiogram with the bubble test), and patients with smaller AVMs and short resection times are ideal for the sitting position. Patients with large AVMs that require prolonged resection time or have increased bleeding risk might be better positioned prone with the neck flexed. Air embolism is a major concern with a craniotomy that crosses three major venous sinuses, making the prone position a better choice for older patients with adherent dura and a greater likelihood of dural tears.

Cerebrospinal fluid (CSF) is released early from the cisterna magna to relax the cerebellum (step 2) and obviates the need for lumbar drains. The cerebellum is de-tethered by releasing the arachnoid adhesions bridging from the posterior edge of the superior cerebellum to the outer edge of the tentorium. Bridging veins to the tentorium are divided to open the corridor to the free edge of the tentorium. The arachnoid of the posterior incisural space is incised to drain the quadrigeminal cistern and expose the posterior midbrain. The supracerebellar-infratentorial approach in the sitting position opens an anatomic plane so widely that dissection is dramatically easier. Any discomfort from operating with raised hands is more than offset by the retractor-less panorama and a surgical field cleared by gravity.

The TecV and VCMesF drain the AVM and hang superficially in the field above the nidus (step 3). The long CirP and SCA branches supplying the AVM bilaterally can be found laterally in the posterior part of QuadC between the rising edge of the tentorium and tectum (step 4). These feeders form lateral fronts on both sides of the nidus that are occluded proximally (step 5). Circumdissection within the quadrigeminal cistern de-arterializes the AVM (step 6), and upward mobilization accesses the deep anterior plane (step 7). After the draining vein darkens, the nidus is either occluded in situ or resected, depending on how cleanly the anterior pial margin separates from the posterior midbrain (**Figs. 16.16** and **16.17**).

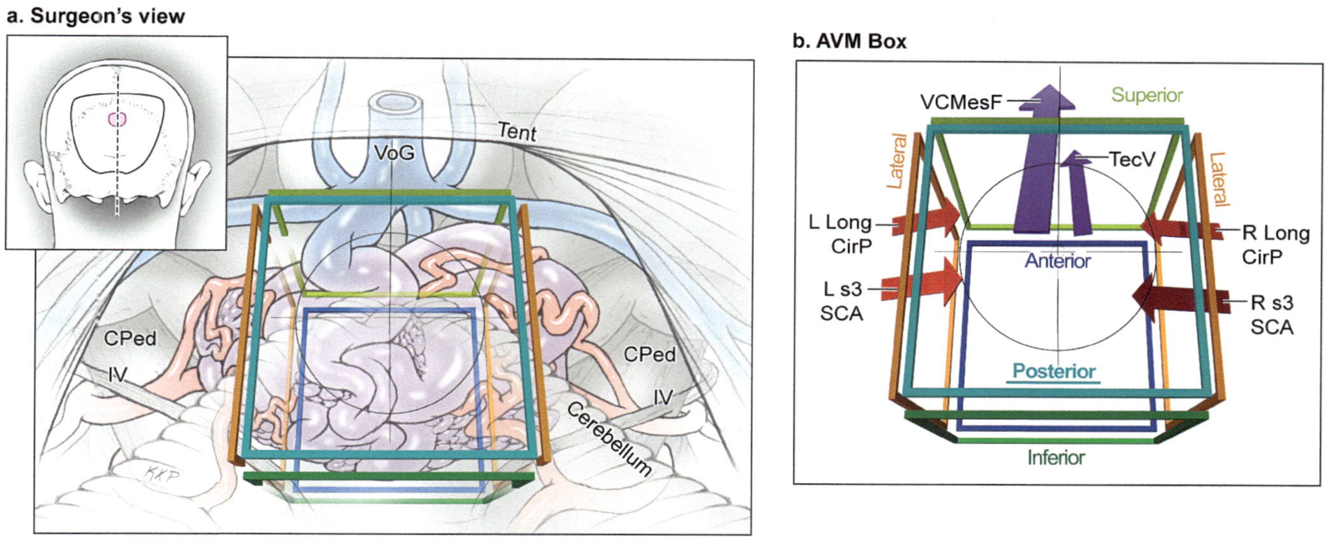

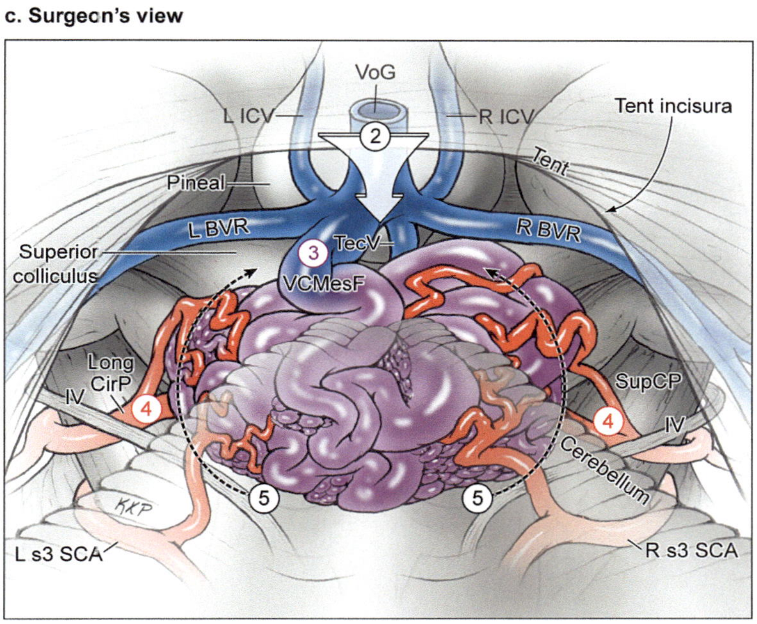

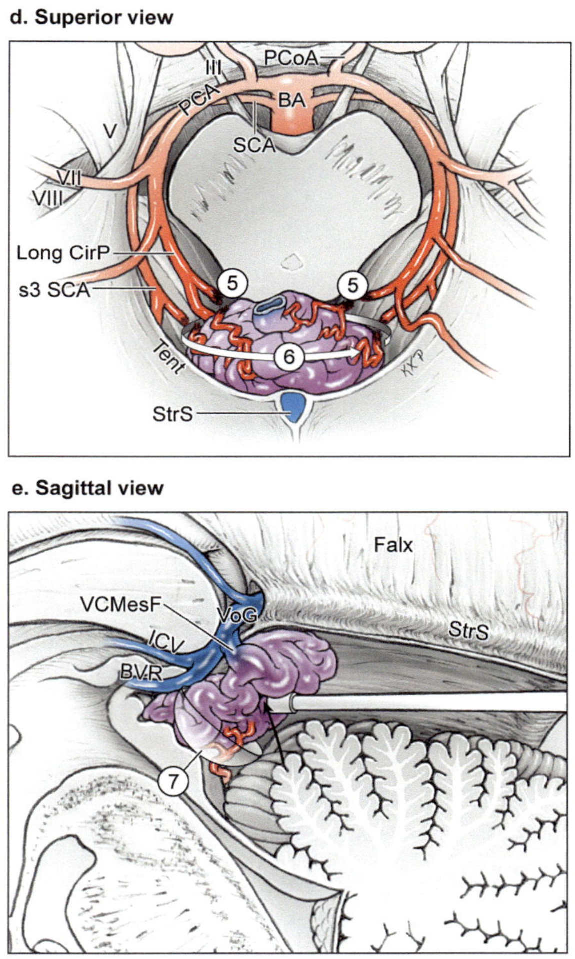

Fig. 16.15 Resection strategy for posterior midbrain AVMs. (**a**) Step 1, exposing the AVM with a torcular craniotomy and supracerebellar-infratentorial approach [surgeon's view, with scalp incision (*dashed line*), craniotomy (*solid line*), and AVM (*purple circle*) shown on *inset*]. (**b**) AVM box showing arterial inputs from long circumflex perforators and SCA branches, ascending drainage to the vein of Galen, and proximity to the trochlear nerves and quadrigeminal plate. (**c**) Step 2, approaching the AVM through the supracerebellar-infratentorial plane and quadrigeminal cistern; step 3, identifying the ascending veins superiorly (TecV and VCMesF); step 4, locating the feeding arteries laterally in the quadrigeminal cistern (Long CirP and s3 SCA branches); and step 5, interrupting the two lateral fronts (surgeon's view). (**d**) Step 6, circumdissecting in the quadrigeminal cistern (superior view of the midbrain and tentorium with both cerebral hemispheres removed). (**e**) Step 7, mobilizing the AVM upward to divide anterior feeders and connections to the tectal vein (sagittal cross-sectional view).

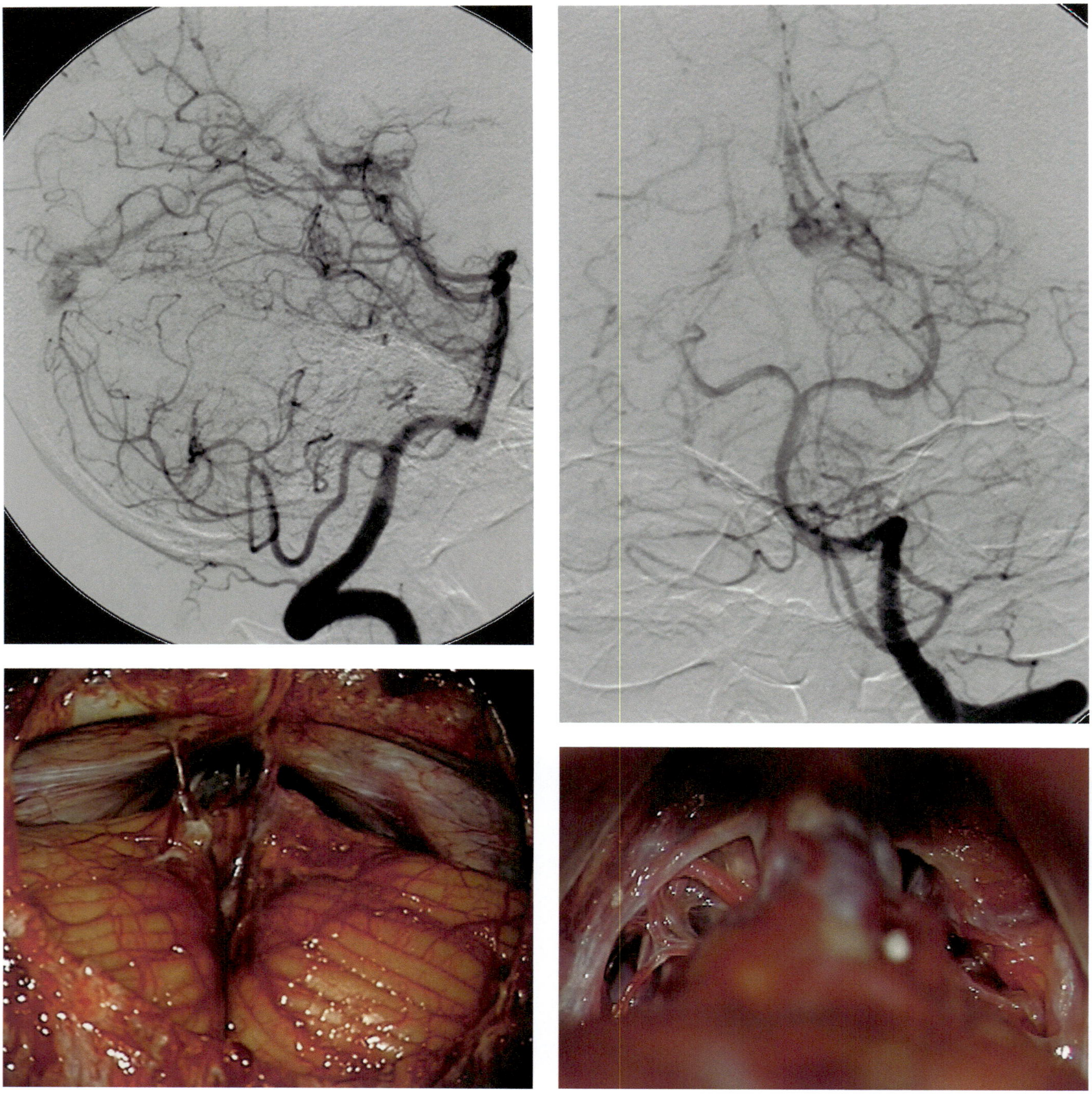

a b c d

Fig. 16.16 This 63-year-old woman presented with a midbrain hemorrhage beneath the tectum. A posterior midbrain AVM was found (supplemented Spetzler-Martin grade 6: S1V1E1/A3B0C0), supplied by CirP and drained by TecV [left VA angiogram, (**a**) lateral and (**b**) anteroposterior views]. (**c**) The AVM was exposed through a torcular craniotomy with the patient in the sitting position, with gravity retracting the cerebellum and opening the supracerebellar-infratentorial plane. The dural flap elevated the torcular superiorly, and dividing the superior hemispheric veins bridging to the tentorium de-tethered the cerebellum for even wider exposure. (**d**) The supracerebellar-infratentorial approach accessed the quadrigeminal cistern between the tentorial leaflets, with the ascending cerebellar veins (SVerV and PreCenCblV) in the center of the field.

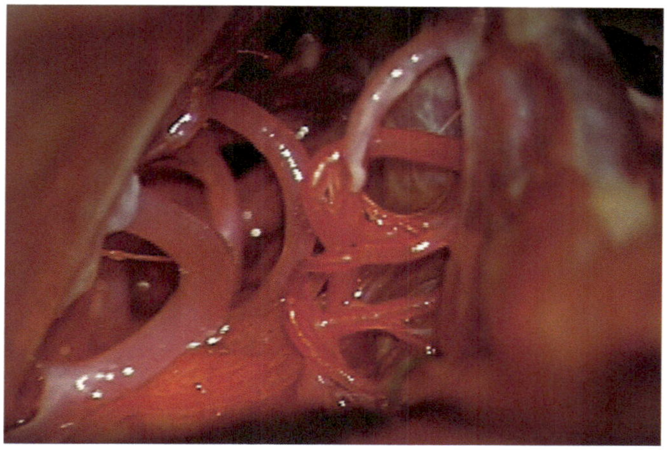
e

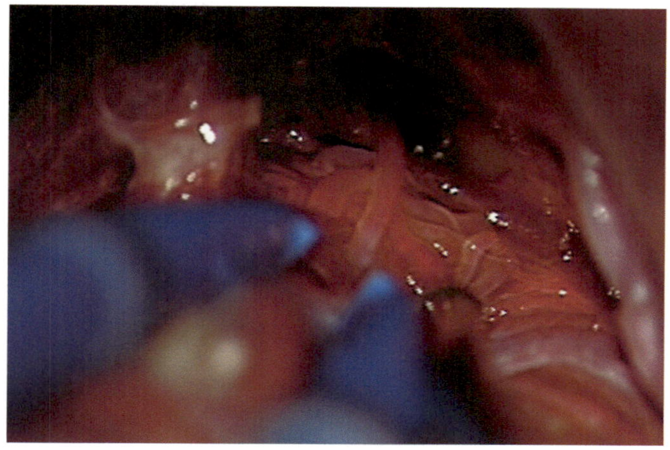
f

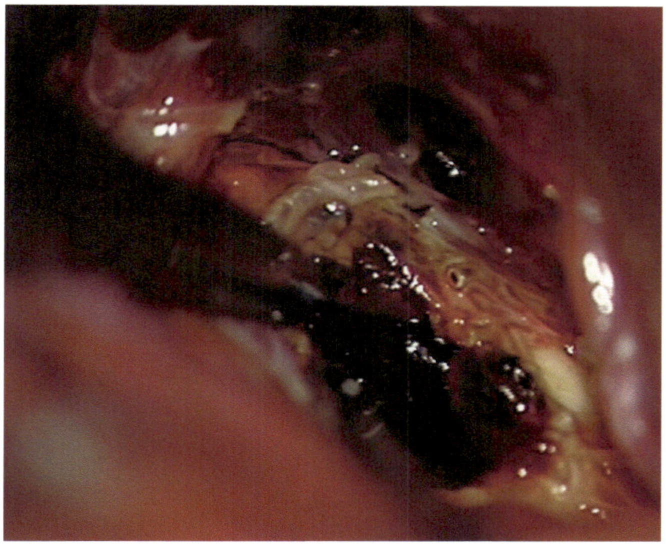
g

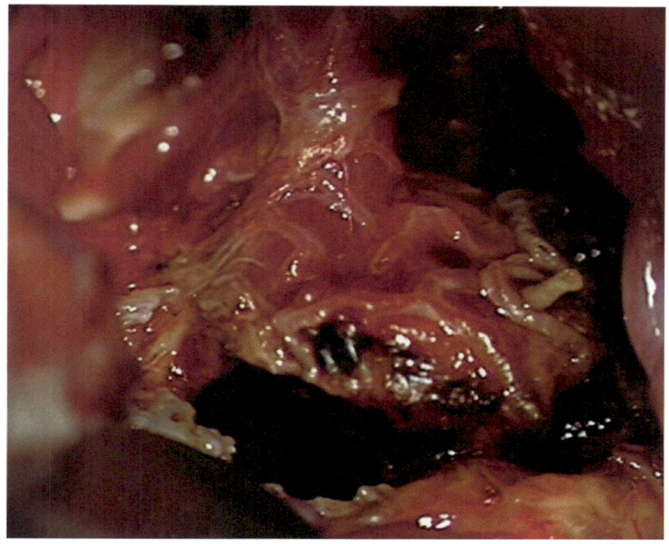
h

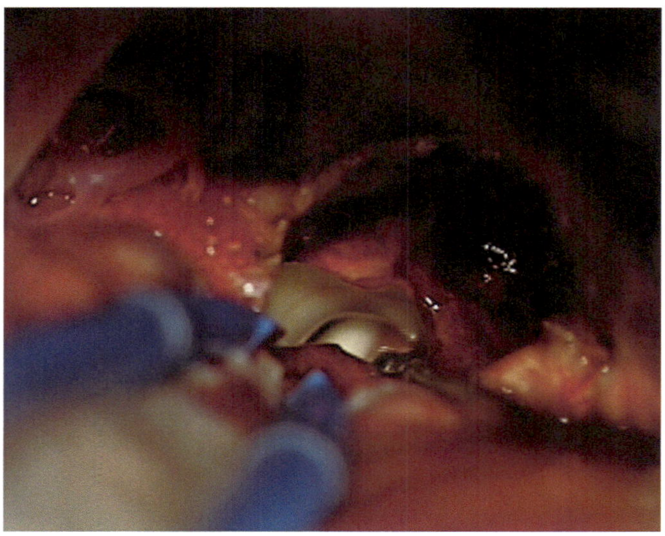
i

Fig. 16.16 (*continued*) (**e**) The left incisura had many arteries in transit, including PCA branches (CalcA, ParOccA) that continued supratentorially, SCA branches that emerged from the cerebellomesencephalic fissure, mPChA that ascended to the roof of the third ventricle, normal long CirP from the PCA that supplied the tectum, and abnormal AVM feeders. (**f**) Feeders on the right side were identified at the AVM margin, (**g**) cauterized, and incised to enter the underlying hematoma. (**h**) The nidus was dissected circumferentially around the draining TecV, with the hematoma separating the AVM's deep plane from the central midbrain. (**i**) After AVM resection, the view extended anteriorly through the hematoma cavity, up the aqueduct, and into the third ventricle (at the sucker tip).

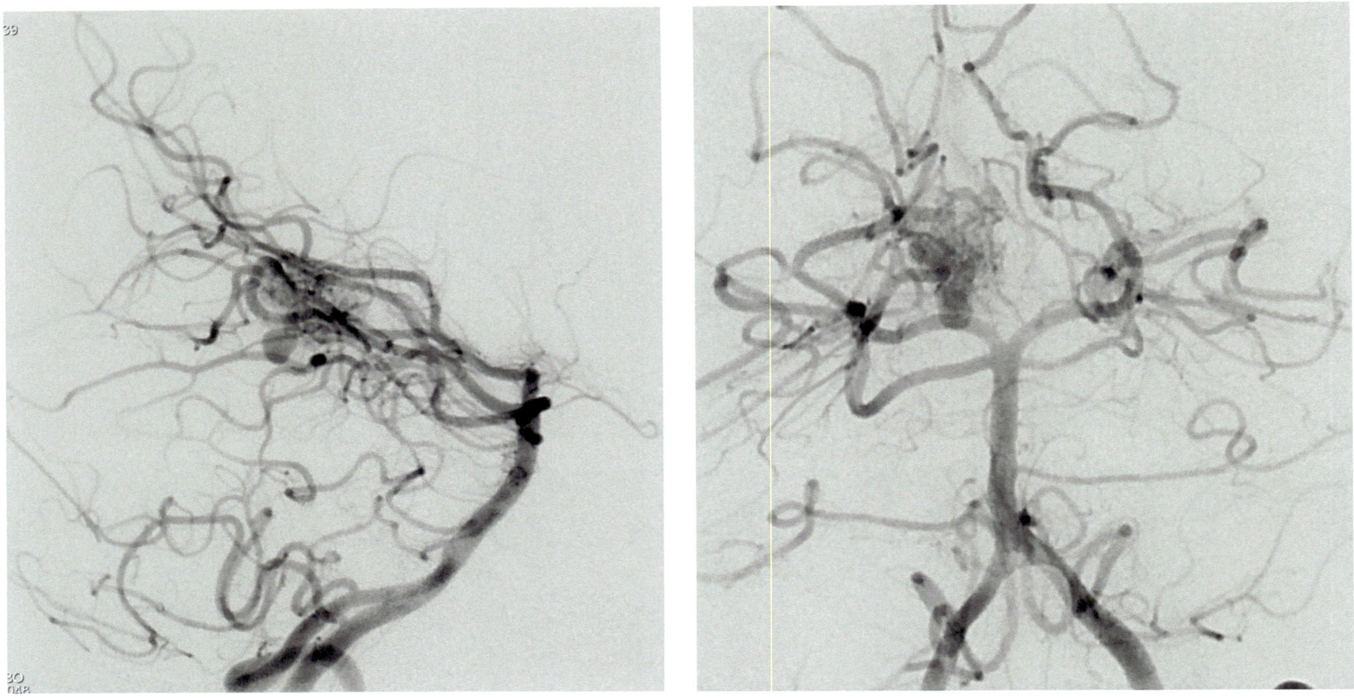

a b

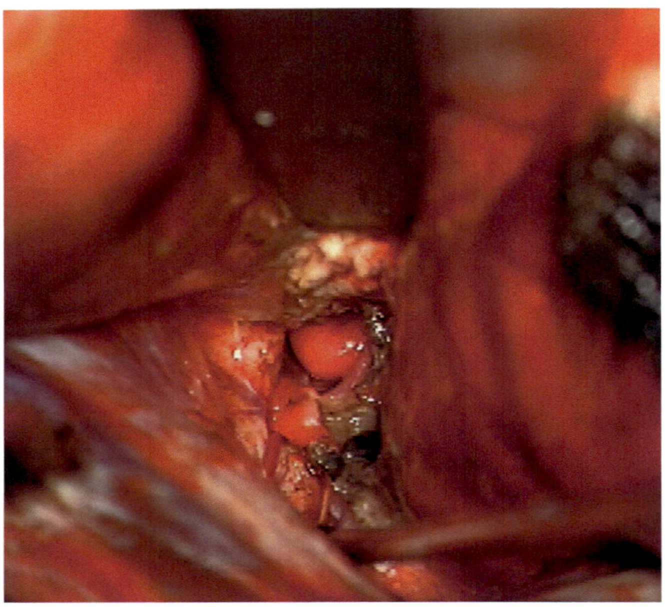

c

Fig. 16.17 This 30-year-old woman presented with a ruptured posterior midbrain AVM (supplemented Spetzler-Martin grade 5: S1V1E1/A2B0C0), supplied by right CirP and SCA branches and drained by TecV [right VA angiogram, (**a**) lateral and (**b**) anteroposterior views]. Preoperative echocardiogram demonstrated a patent foramen ovale that precluded placing the patient in the sitting position. (**c**) The AVM was exposed though a torcular craniotomy and a supracerebellar-infratentorial approach with the patient in the prone position. Cerebellar swelling from the hemorrhage and the absence of gravity retraction necessitated some resection of the vermis and fixed retraction.

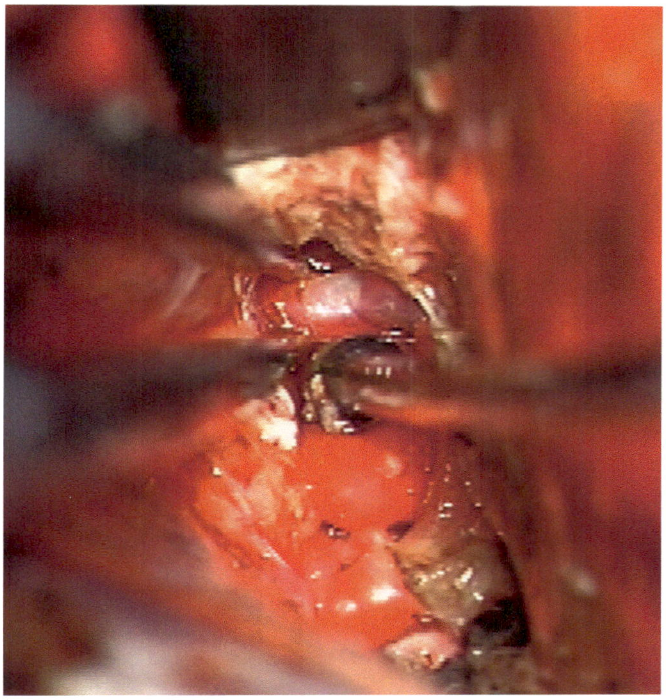

d

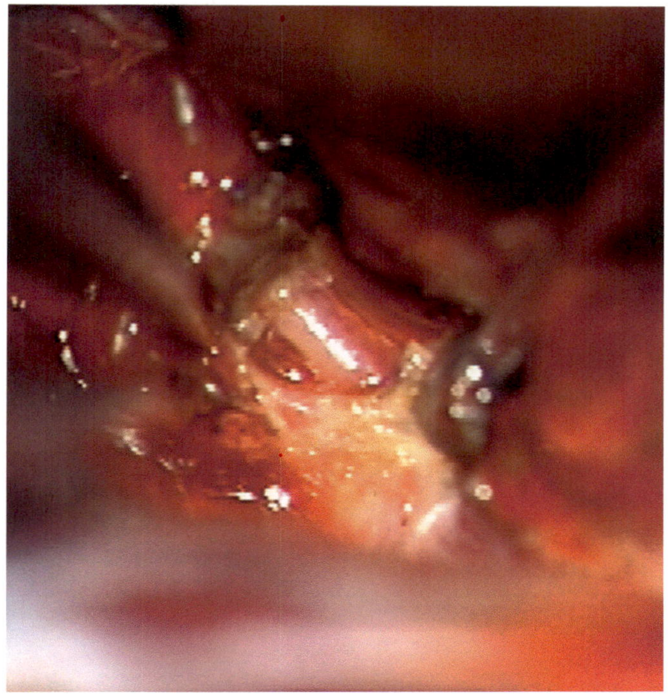

e

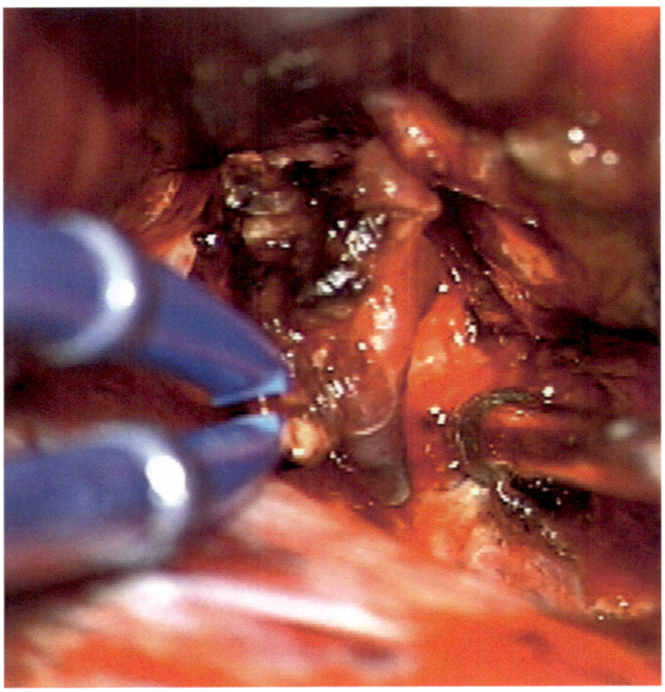

f

Fig. 16.17 (*continued*) **d**) AVM feeders from the right SCA were coagulated inferiorly (**e**) and superiorly. (**f**) The nidus was disconnected and resected completely.

Anterior Pontine AVM Resection

Anterior pontine AVMs are resected through an extended retrosigmoid craniotomy using a limited mastoidectomy and skeletonization of SigmS to increase the exposure of a traditional retrosigmoid approach (**Fig. 16.18,** step 1). A C-shaped skin incision is made behind the ear and, using a cutting burr on the drill, the mastoid air cells are entered through a vertical cut that is one fingerbreadth behind the external auditory canal (EAC). A posterior mastoidectomy exposes SigmS, which is skeletonized with a diamond drill bit from the transverse-sigmoid junction to the jugular bulb. After elevating a posterior craniotomy, the dural flap based on SigmS mobilizes the sinus anteriorly and enhances exposure of the cerebellopontine angle.

The cisterna magna (MagnC) is opened inferiorly to release CSF and relax the cerebellum, which can herniate as the dura is opened (step 2). Consequently, the dura is opened under the microscope for quick access to MagnC. The cerebellopontine cistern (CbPonC) is opened laterally, and adhesions between the flocculus and CN7/8 and CN9/10/11 are released to mobilize the cerebellum posteriorly. The arachnoid is preserved over the nerves for protection, and the labyrinthine and subarcuate arteries that supply the inner ear are also preserved. Anterior pontine AVMs are located on the anterior patch of the pons medial to the trigeminal nerve, and therefore access is limited to two windows: one above the trigeminal nerve between CN5 and the tentorium (the supratrigeminal triangle); and one below the trigeminal nerve between CN5 and CN7/8 (the infratrigeminal triangle). The supratrigeminal triangle is small but accesses the upper pontine surface and descending feeders from the SCA to the superior margin. The infratrigeminal triangle is larger and accesses the lower pontine surface and ascending feeders from the AICA to the inferior margin. Therefore, the approach is centered on the trigeminal nerve. The window between CN7/8 and CN9/10/11 is directed at the medulla and does not access anterior pontine AVMs, but

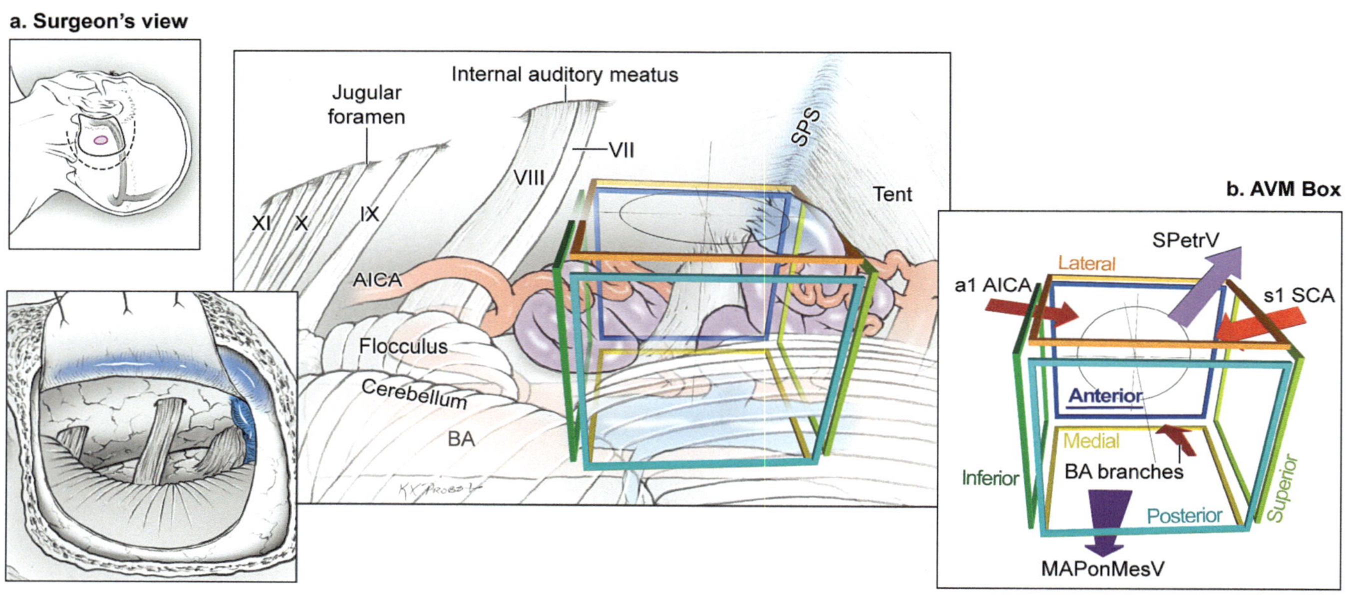

Fig. 16.18 Resection strategy for anterior pontine AVMs. (**a**) Step 1, exposing the AVM with an extended retrosigmoid approach that includes limited mastoidectomy and skeletonization of sigmoid sinus [surgeon's view, with scalp incision (*dashed line*), craniotomy (*solid line*), and AVM (*purple circle*) shown on *upper inset*, and dural flap mobilizing the skeletonized SigmS anteriorly shown on *lower inset*]. (**b**) AVM box showing arterial supply from s1 SCA, a1 AICA, and direct branches from the basilar trunk, venous drainage medially and laterally, and proximity to the trigeminal, facial, and vestibulocochlear nerves.

c. Surgeon's view **d. Superior view**

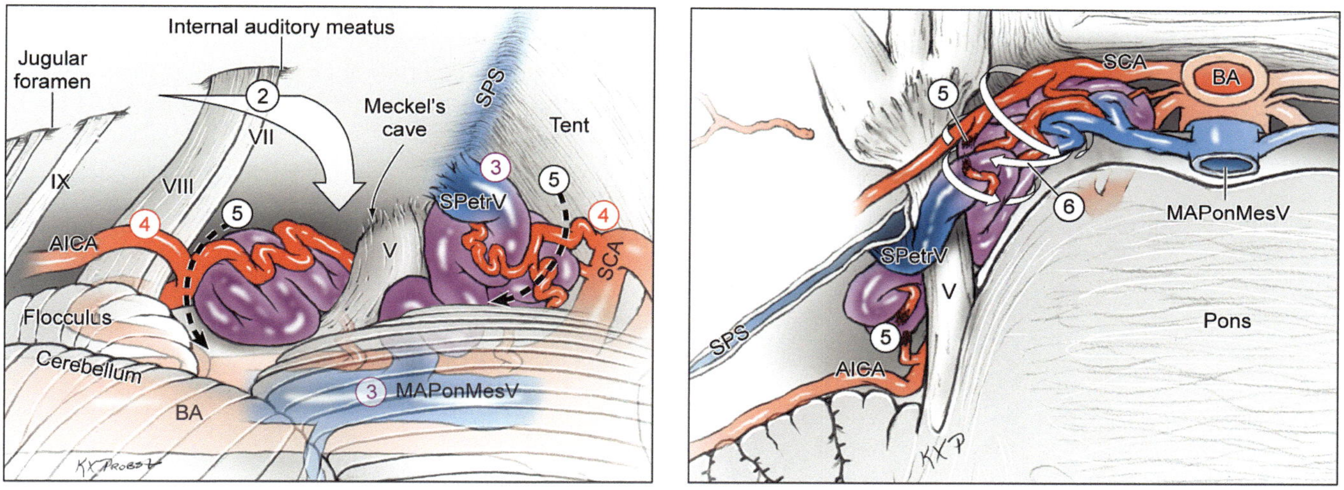

e. Superior view

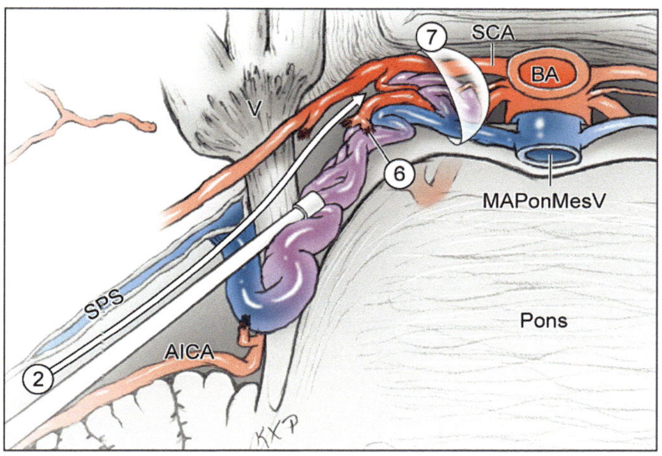

Fig. 16.18 *(continued)* (**c**) Step 2, approaching the AVM through the cerebellopontine and prepontine cisterns, and opening windows of access above and below the trigeminal nerve (supra- and infratrigeminal triangles, respectively); step 3, identifying ascending drainage laterally (SPetrV); step 4, locating SCA feeders in the supratrigeminal triangle and AICA feeders in the infratrigeminal triangle; and step 5, interrupting the superior front below the tentorium and the inferior front above CN7/8 (surgeon's view). (**d**) Step 6, circumdissecting in the prepontine cistern (superior view of pons and posterior fossa). (**e**) Step 7, mobilizing the AVM posteriorly to interrupt the medial front of basilar artery feeders and the medial drainage through MAPonMesV (superior view of pons and posterior fossa).

it may augment the view of AICA feeders traveling up to the nidus.

A dilated SPetrV may be another obstacle in the field, especially in the supratrigeminal triangle (step 3). Lateral bridging veins are not arterialized with midline drainage to MAPonMesV and may be taken to open the corridor. Descending SCA feeders in the supratrigeminal triangle and ascending AICA feeders in the infratrigeminal triangle (step 4) are occluded along the superior and inferior fronts, respectively (step 5). Although superficial in the field, the lateral border is covered by the trigeminal nerve and may be arterialized by the feeders from the meningohypophyseal trunk coursing along the nerve. The nidus must be circumdissected (step 6) and mobilized posteriorly toward the pons to visualize the medial front, which is arterialized by feeders directly from the basilar trunk (step 7). Venous connections to MAPonMesV are also visualized with this maneuver. The windows are long and narrow, the view is tangential, and there are blind spots deep to the trigeminal nerve, lateral draining veins, and the nidus. With these limitations, any angiographic anatomy such as arterial curves, dilatations, aneurysms, and embolic material that can be translated onto the field helps orient the dissection. These AVMs typically have three to five feeders, and their correct identification and interruption can normalize flow in the draining vein for occlusion in situ. The eloquence of the anterior pons and the limitations in exposure often make resection too dangerous here (**Figs. 16.19, 16.20, 16.21**).

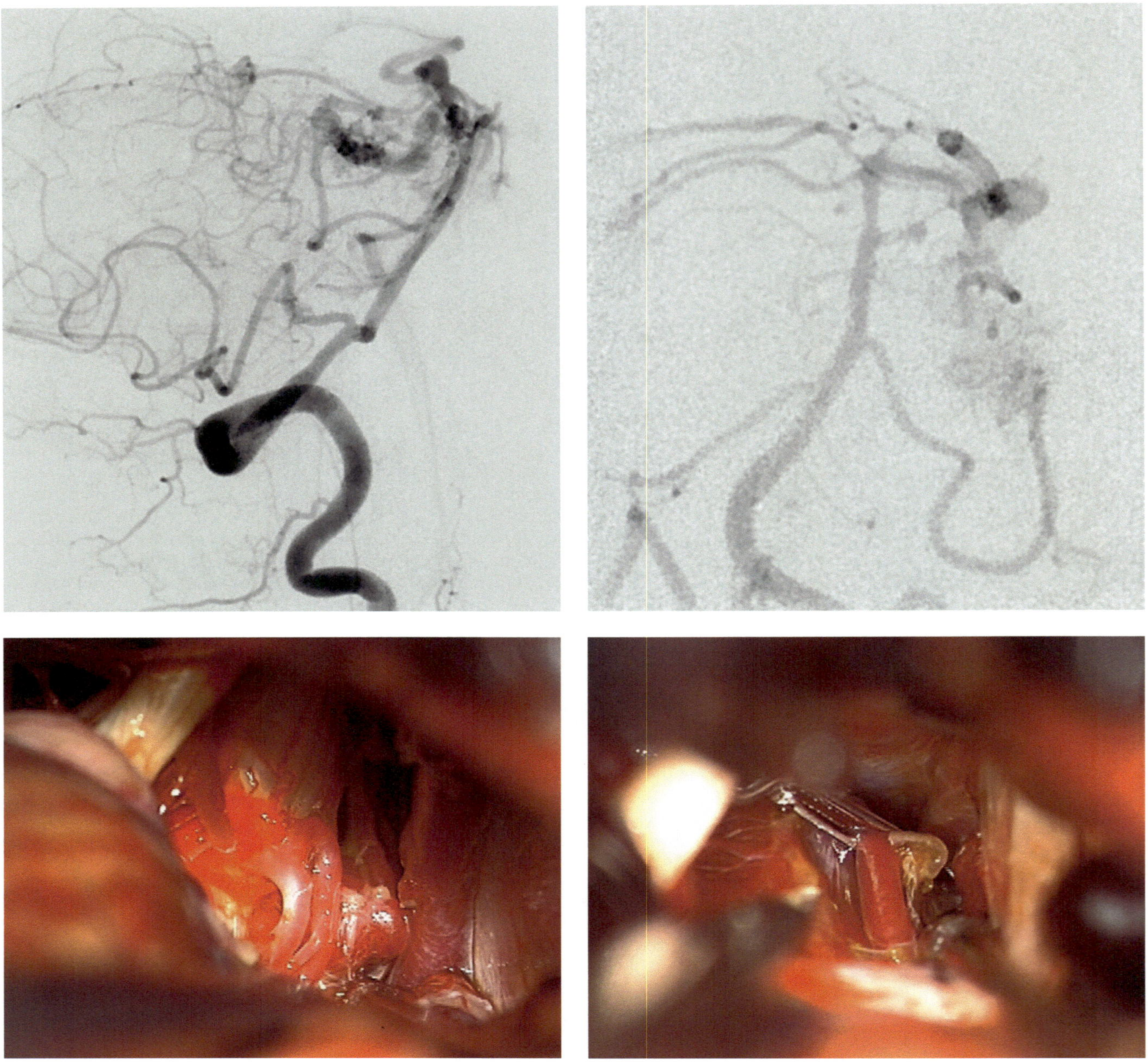

a b c d

Fig. 16.19 This 58-year-old man presented with a posterior fossa subarachnoid hemorrhage, and a left anterior pontine AVM was found (supplemented Spetzler-Martin grade 6: S1V1E1/A3B0C0). The AVM was supplied by the AICA, branches from the basilar trunk, and the SCA, which also had a feeding artery aneurysm [left VA angiogram, (**a**) lateral and (**b**) anteroposterior views]. (**c**) The AVM was exposed through a left extended retrosigmoid craniotomy, bringing the CN7-8 complex (*left*), CN5 (*center*), and tentorium (*right*) into view. The AICA feeder coursed medial to CN7-8 and lateral to CN5 to reach the AVM. (**d**) A feeder from the basilar trunk was clip occluded in the axilla of CN5 as it joined the nidus (infratrigeminal triangle).

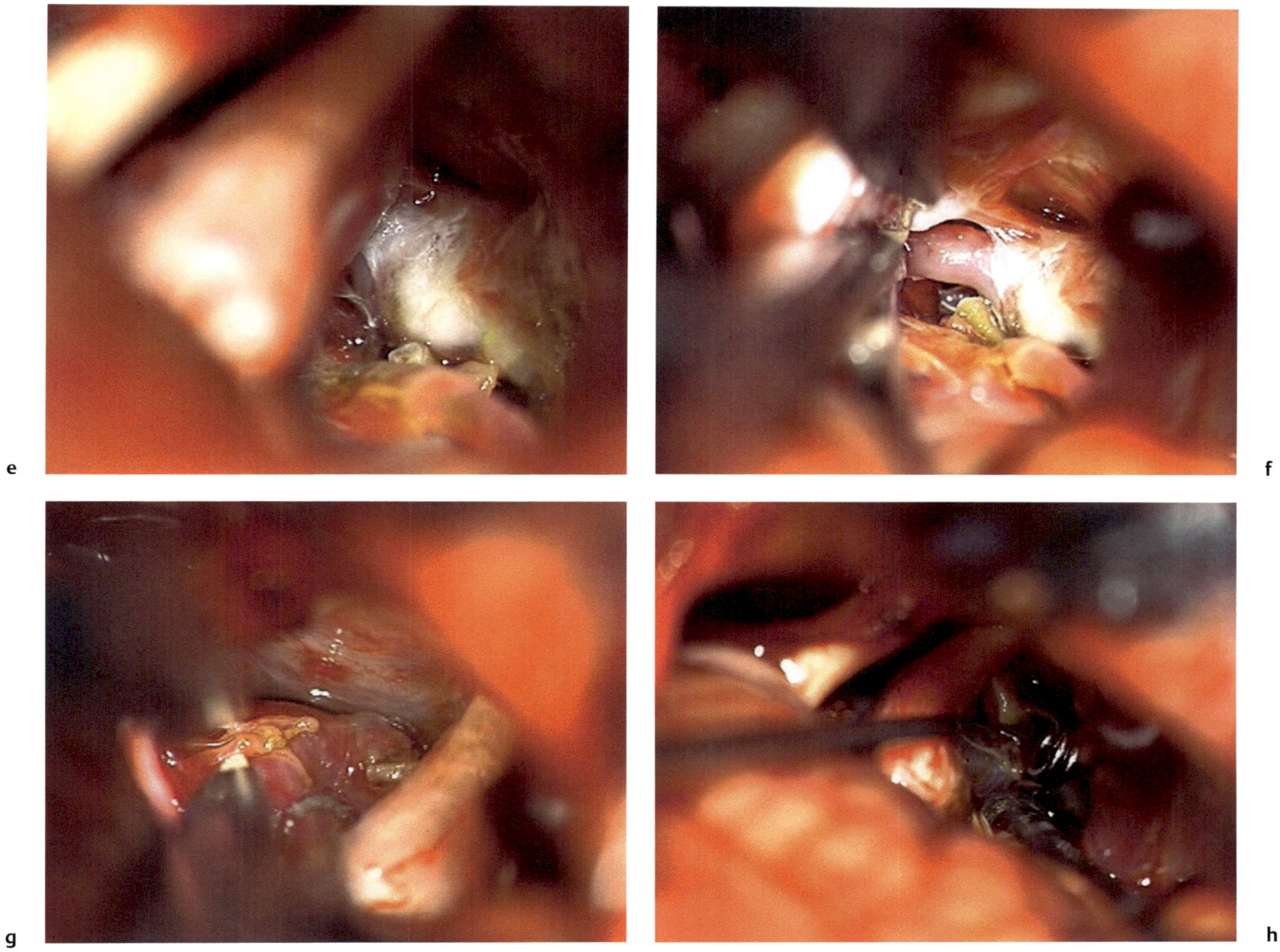

Fig. 16.19 (*continued*) (**e**) The feeding artery aneurysm on the SCA was located above CN5 (supratrigeminal triangle) in the angle between the tentorium and the petrous bone. (**f**) Proximal dissection exposed the afferent artery, which was clip occluded. (**g**) The draining vein was still red, but coagulation of several small feeders medially in the infratrigeminal triangle resulted in (**h**) darkening of the vein, seen coursing superiorly above CN5. The AVM was occluded in situ and a postoperative angiogram confirmed complete occlusion.

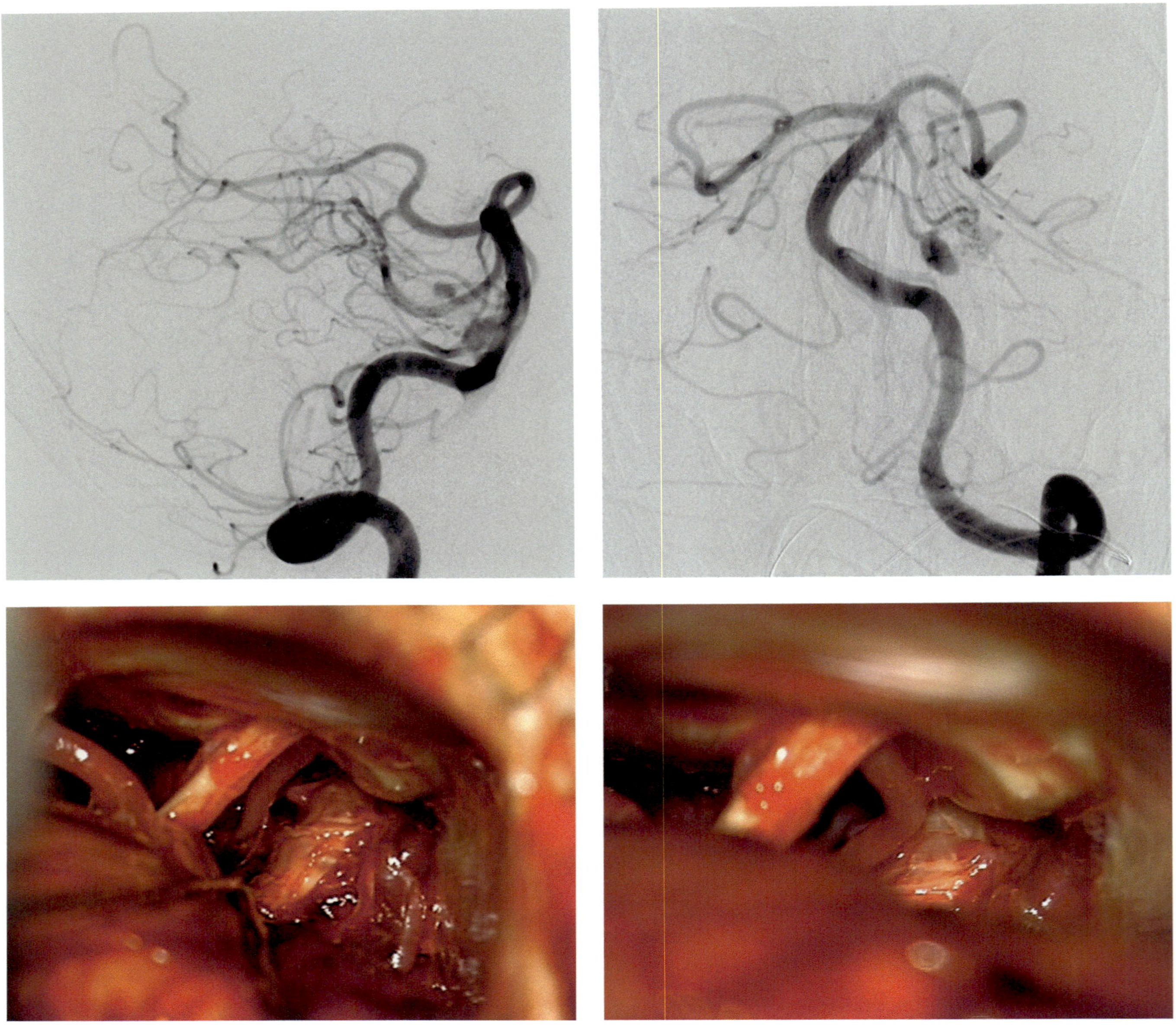

a b c d

Fig. 16.20 This 77-year-old man presented with a posterior fossa subarachnoid hemorrhage and a left anterior pontine AVM, similar to the previous case (supplemented Spetzler-Martin grade 6: S1V1E1/A3B0C0). The AVM was supplied by the SCA, a branch from the basilar trunk, and small distal AICA branches [left VA angiogram, (**a**) lateral and (**b**) anteroposterior views]. There was a feeding artery aneurysm on the basilar branch. (**c**) The AVM was exposed through a left extended retrosigmoid craniotomy. (**d**) The basilar branch coursed above CN7-8 through the infratrigeminal triangle and was divided.

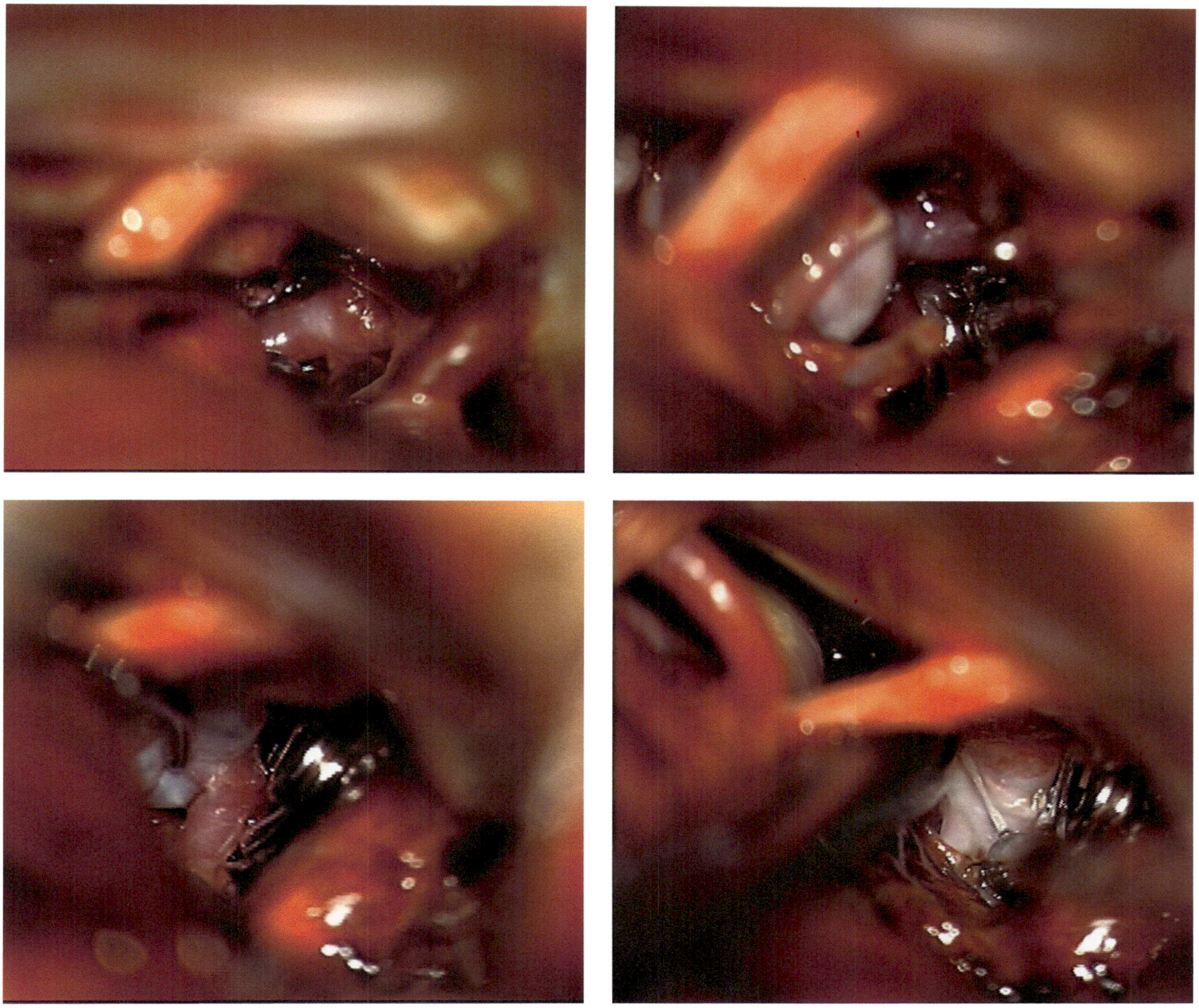

Fig. 16.20 (*continued*) (**e**) The SCA feeder coursed along the tentorium through the supratrigeminal triangle and was divided. (**f**) The feeding artery aneurysm was located medial to CN7-8 and (**g**) its afferent artery was occluded with a clip. (**h**) SPetrV was no longer arterialized (between microscissors and aneurysm clip) and the AVM was occluded in situ.

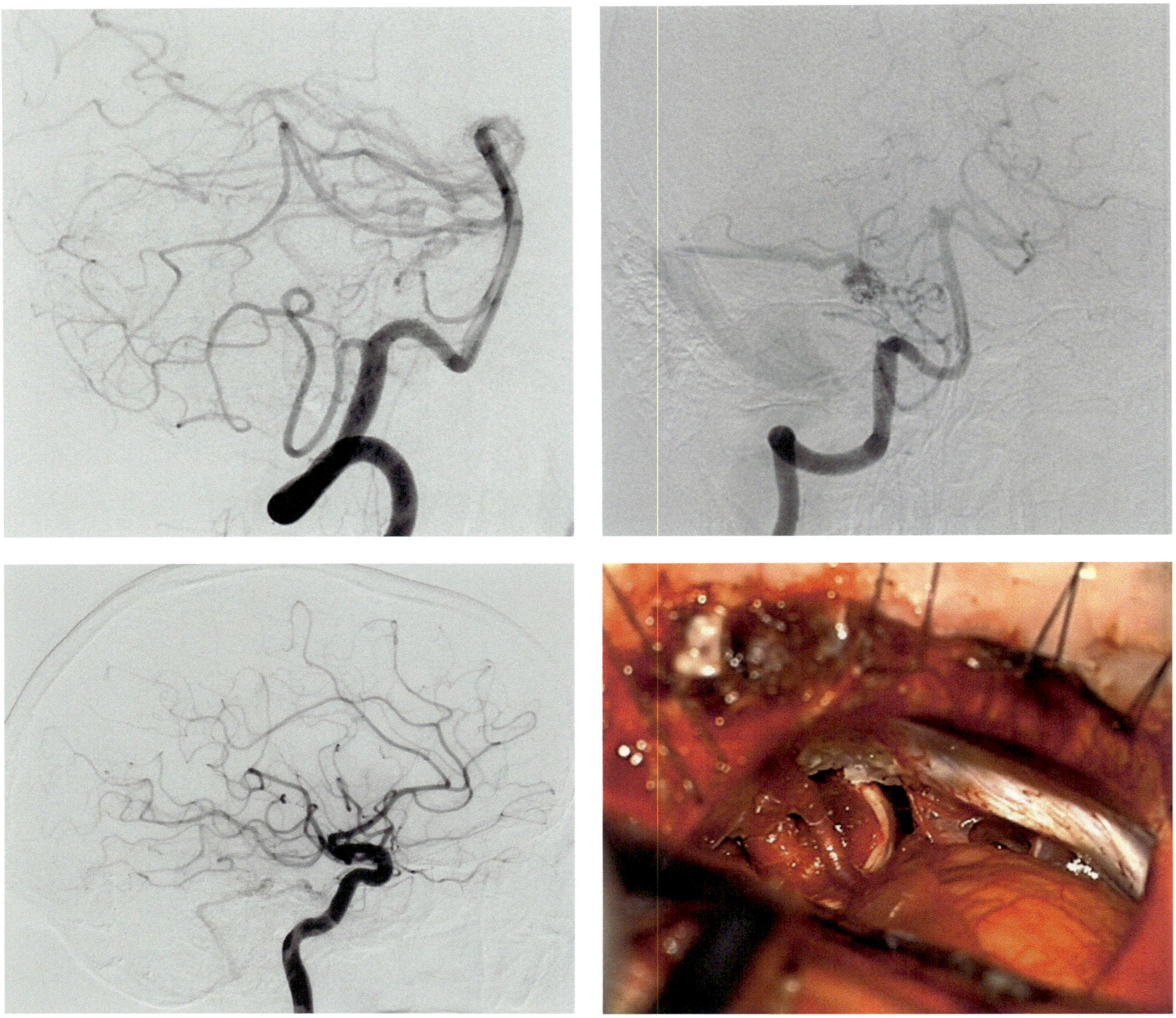

a b c d

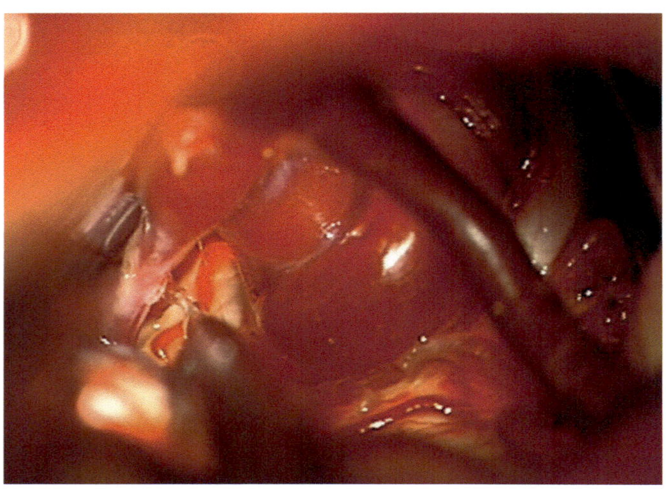

e

Fig. 16.21 This 58-year-old man presented with a left anterior pontine AVM located medial to the trigeminal nerve root (supplemented Spetzler-Martin grade 6: S1V1E1/A3B0C0), supplied not only by the AICA and branches from the basilar trunk [right VA angiogram, (**a**) lateral and (**b**) anteroposterior views], but also by dural arteries from the meningohypophyseal trunk [(**c**) right ICA angiogram, lateral view]. (**d**) The cerebellopontine angle was accessed through a right extended retrosigmoid approach and (**e**) an arterialized SPetrV was exposed.

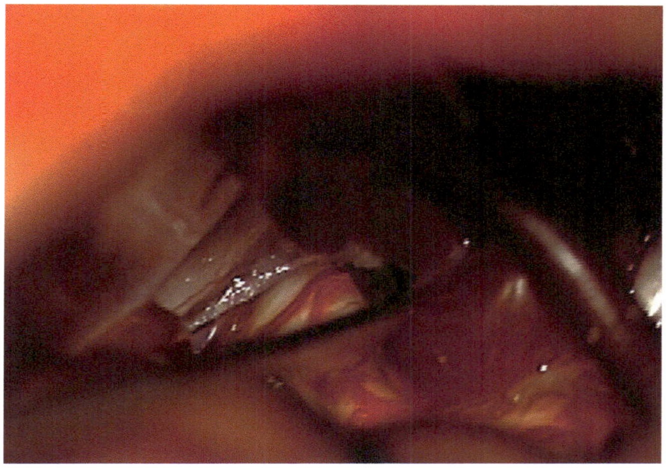

f

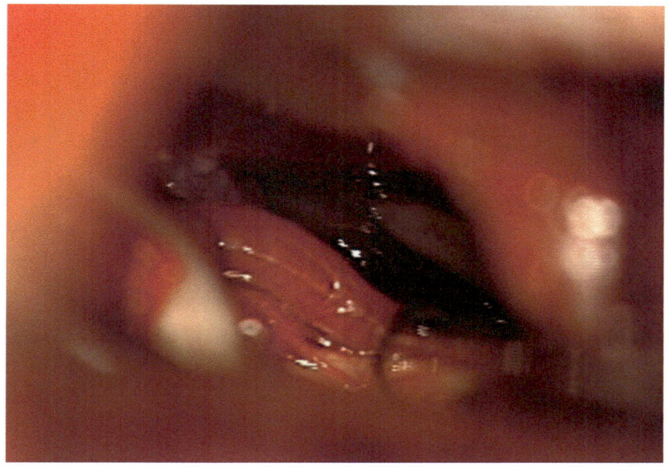

g

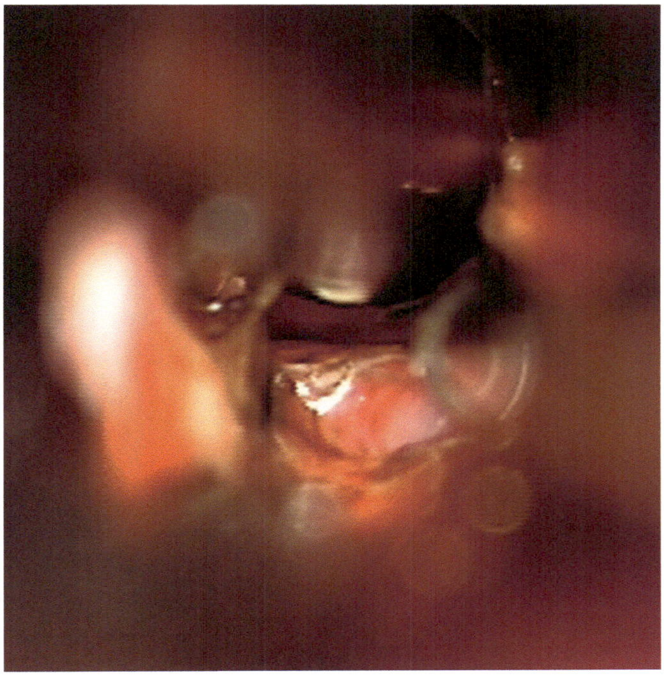

h

Fig. 16.21 (*continued*) (**f**) The trochlear nerve was identified along the tentorial incisura medial to the draining vein. (**g**) Feeders from the AICA were accessed in the infratrigeminal triangle and divided. The abducens nerve entered Dorello's canal medial to this feeder (above the sucker tip). (**h**) Although two additional feeders were occluded through the infratrigeminal triangle, the AVM was still supplied by dural arteries that could not be interrupted without injuring the trigeminal nerve. The AVM was incompletely occluded and treated subsequently with radiosurgery.

Lateral Pontine AVM Resection

Lateral pontine AVMs are also resected through an extended retrosigmoid craniotomy (**Fig. 16.22,** step 1) and initial subarachnoid dissection releases CSF from the cisterna magna, opens the cerebellopontine cistern, and frees the flocculus from the lower cranial nerves (step 2). Lateral pontine AVMs sit lateral to CN5 and do not need to be accessed through the supra- and infratrigeminal triangles. Surgical access is the wide open space of the cerebellopontine angle above CN7/8. Drainage through SupPetrV is not obstructive (step 3) and AICA supply is visualized in the infratrigeminal triangle proximally (step 4). This AICA input may extend anteriorly to the AVM's free surface but is controlled on the medial AVM margin, between the trigeminal and vestibulocochlear nerves (step 5). This AVM is based medially on the belly of the pons and posteriorly on or in the middle cerebellar peduncle, which comprise its eloquent borders. However, its superior, inferior, and lateral borders abut non-eloquent cerebellum, which is unusual for a brainstem AVM. These non-eloquent borders enable "back door" access to the AVM's deep borders, meaning that lateral half of the nidus can be mobilized with parenchymal circumdissection that closes feeders to these planes and rolls the nidus into the cerebellopontine angle (step 6). The plane involving the middle cerebellar peduncle is dissected posteriorly, and the plane

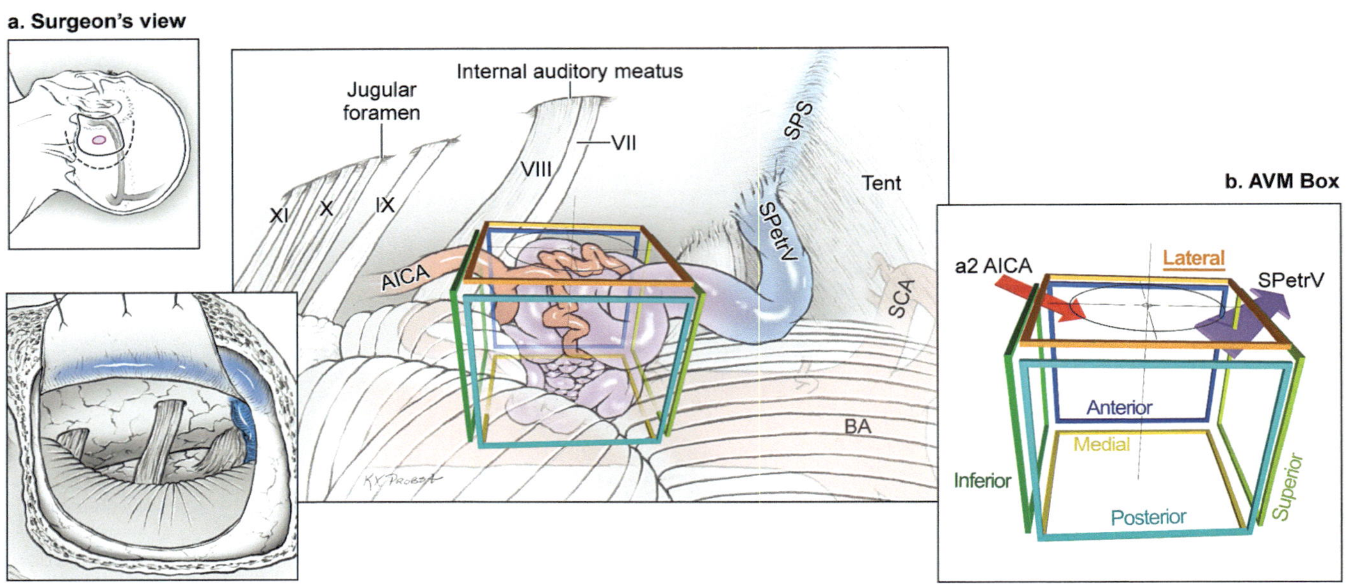

Fig. 16.22 Resection strategy for lateral pontine AVMs. (**a**) Step 1, exposing the AVM with an extended retrosigmoid approach that includes a limited mastoidectomy and skeletonization of the sigmoid sinus [surgeon's view, with scalp incision (*dashed line*), craniotomy (*solid line*), and AVM (*purple circle*) shown on *upper inset*, and dural flap mobilizing the skeletonized SigmS anteriorly shown on *lower inset*]. (**b**) AVM box showing arterial supply from the a2 and a3 AICA branches, venous drainage to SPetrV, and proximity to the trigeminal, facial, and vestibulocochlear nerves.

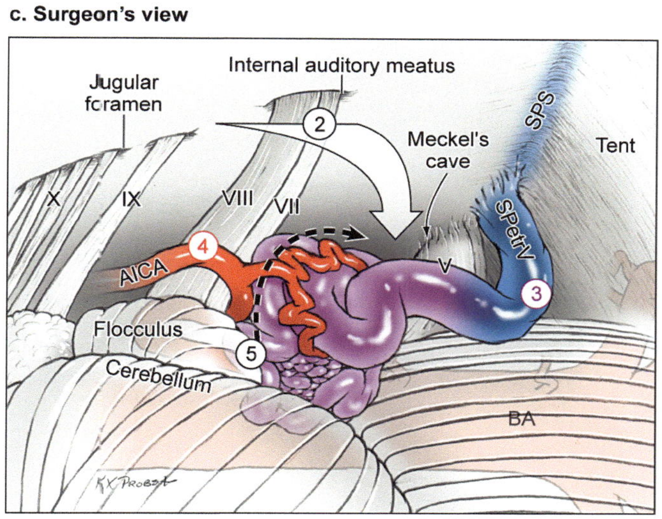

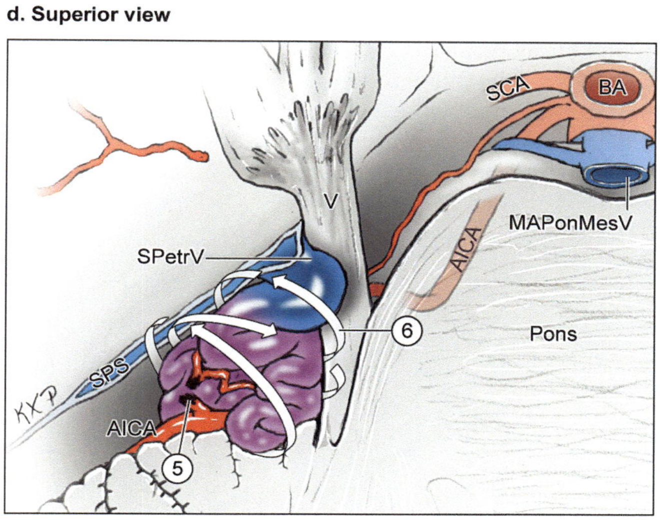

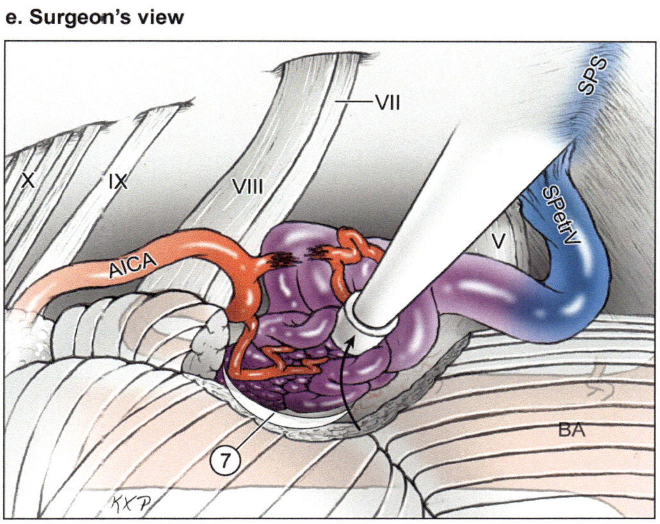

Fig. 16.22 (*continued*) (**c**) Step 2, approaching the AVM through the cerebellopontine cistern; step 3, identifying ascending drainage laterally (SPetrV); step 4, locating AICA feeders in the infratrigeminal triangle; and step 5, interrupting the medial front between the trigeminal and vestibulocochlear nerves (surgeon's view). (**d**) Step 6, circumdissecting the lateral, superior, and inferior margins in the cerebellum ("back door" technique, superior view of pons and posterior fossa). (**e**) Step 7, mobilizing the AVM anteriorly to dissect the posterior plane along the brachium pontis and the medial plane along the pons (surgeon's view).

involving the lateral pons is dissected medially. The remaining feeders along these deep margins are visualized increasingly as the AVM mobilizes forward out of its resection bed (step 7). This "back door" technique makes the lateral pontine AVM the easiest brainstem AVM to resect. Occlusions in situ are not performed with these AVMs, and all were resected completely. The middle cerebellar peduncle tolerates parenchymal dissection without neurologic consequences, and these patients had the best surgical outcomes of all brainstem AVM patients. Preserving the arachnoid over CN5 and CN7-8 adjacent to these AVMs helps protect the nerves (**Fig. 16.23**).

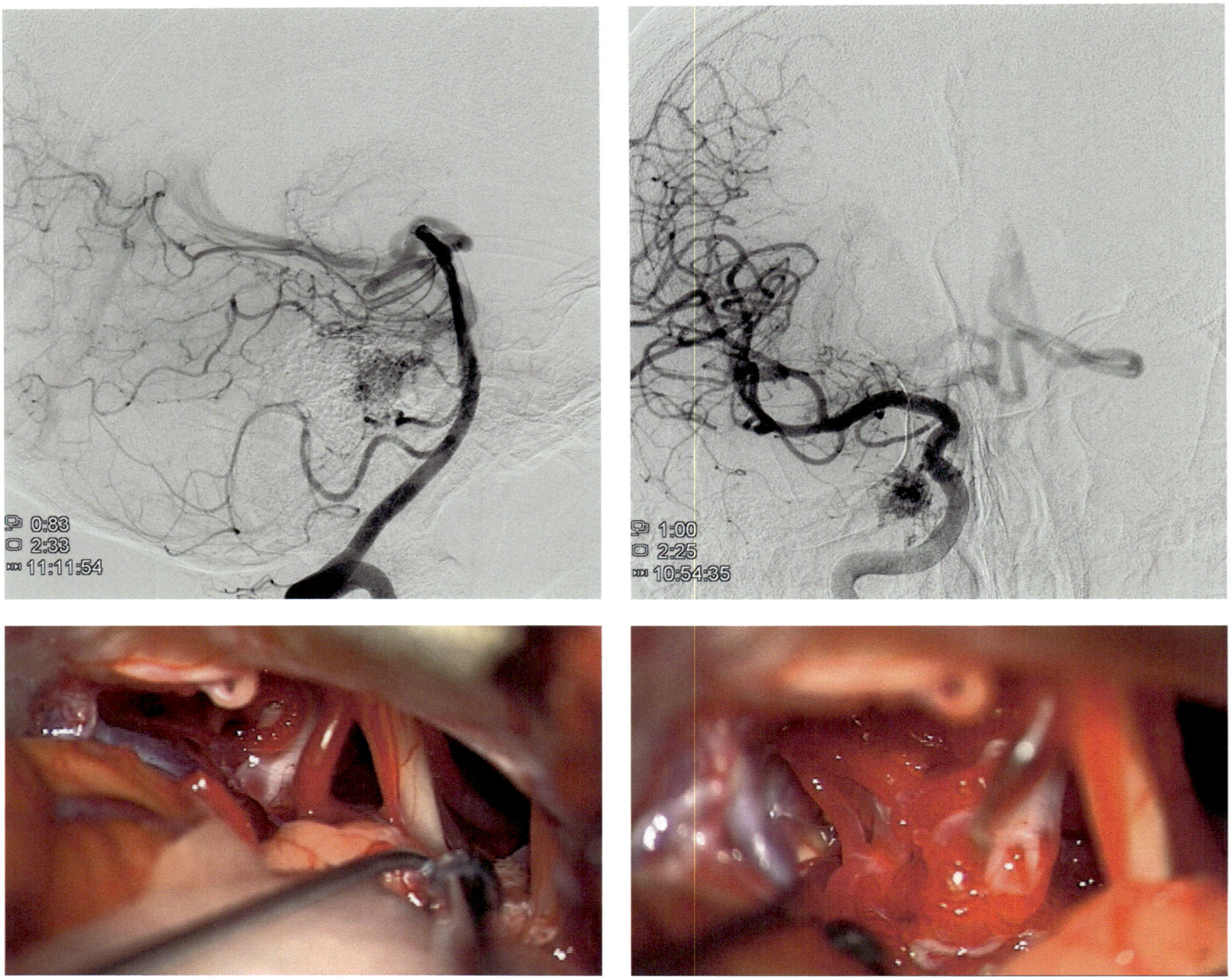

Fig. 16.23 This 75-year-old man presented with a remote hemorrhage from this right lateral pontine AVM (supplemented Spetzler-Martin grade 6: S1V1E1/A3B0C0), supplied as in the last case by the AICA [(**a**) right VA angiogram, lateral view] and dural arteries from meningohypophyseal trunk [(**b**) right ICA angiogram, anteroposterior view]. (**c**) The AVM was approached through a right extended retrosigmoid craniotomy, which exposed CN5, CN7-8 (at tips the sucker and Rhoton No. 6, respectively), and CN9 (right of sucker tip). (**d**) The AVM infiltrated the trigeminal nerve root but was mostly lateral to it.

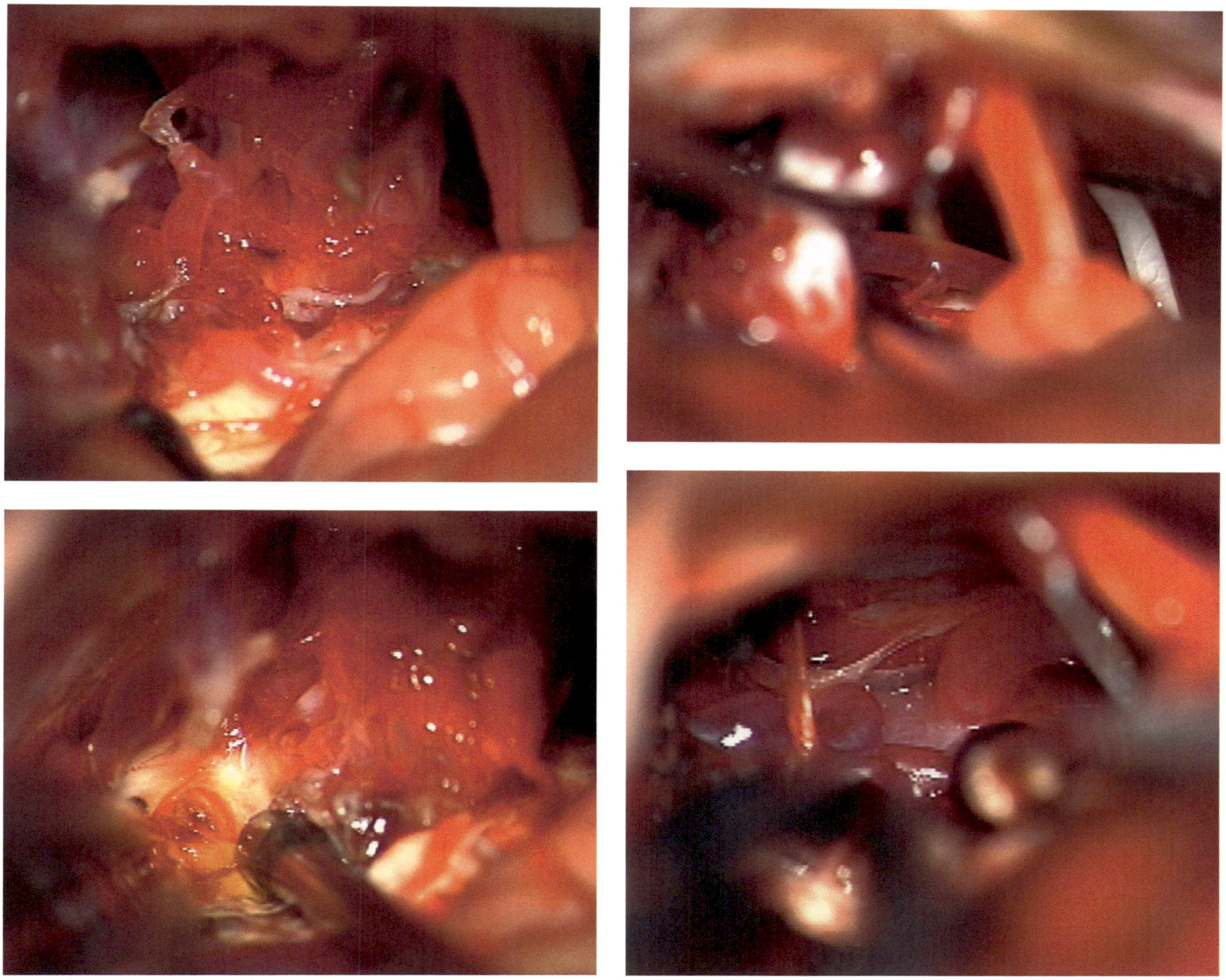

e f g h

Fig. 16.23 (*continued*) (**e**) Pial dissection along the AVM's lateral border interrupted small feeders, and (**f**) a large AICA feeder was interrupted through the infratrigeminal triangle. Note CN6 entering Dorello's canal below (to the right) of CN7-8. (**g**) Parenchymal dissection laterally entered a small hematoma cavity from the patient's prior bleed and defined the superior margin. (**h**) After resecting the AVM, the basilar trunk and AICA origin were visualized through the infratrigeminal triangle.

Anterior Medullary AVM Resection

Anterior medullary AVMs are resectable only when ruptured and with a hematoma that opens a posterior route of access through the fourth ventricle. Otherwise, the anterior medullary surface is difficult to access. A sizable hematoma in this location may devastate the patient and contraindicate surgery, and there was only one surgical patient in my experience. This AVM is exposed with a suboccipital craniotomy or a suboccipital–far lateral combined craniotomy (**Fig. 16.24,** step 1). For the simple suboccipital craniotomy, the patient is prone with the neck flexed to tuck the chin two fingerbreadths from the manubrium and open the occipital-cervical angle. Soft tissue dissection consists of a midline linear scalp incision, a Y-shaped incision in the cervical fascia to create three leaflets for water-tight closure, and a T-shaped incision in the muscle to mobilize paraspinous muscles inferolaterally. A suboccipital craniotomy with C1 laminectomy exposes the posterior cerebellum, tonsils, and cisterna magna. The MagnC is drained, the cerebellomedullary fissures are opened, the tonsils are mobilized laterally, and the fourth ventricle is entered (step 2). Hematoma is evacuated through the ventricular floor and the anterior medulla is reached. The MAMedV drains the AVM at the depths of the cavity in the midline and may be on the anterior side of the nidus, invisible until later in the dissection (step 3). Bilateral branches from the VA originate from the posteromedial aspect of the artery and supply the AVM along its anterolateral margins (step 4). The AVM is attacked with the feeding arteries and draining veins anteriorly on the opposite side of the AVM, which is a recipe for intraoperative bleeding. Furthermore, hematoma evacuation can stir up bleeding as the AVM is approached. Although the angle of attack is parallel, visualization and control of AVM anatomy is poor. The nidus is circumdissected from within the hematoma cavity, with attention to the inputs on the lateral margins (step 5). Circumdissection extends anteriorly in the premedullary cistern (step 6). The AVM is mobilized inferiorly

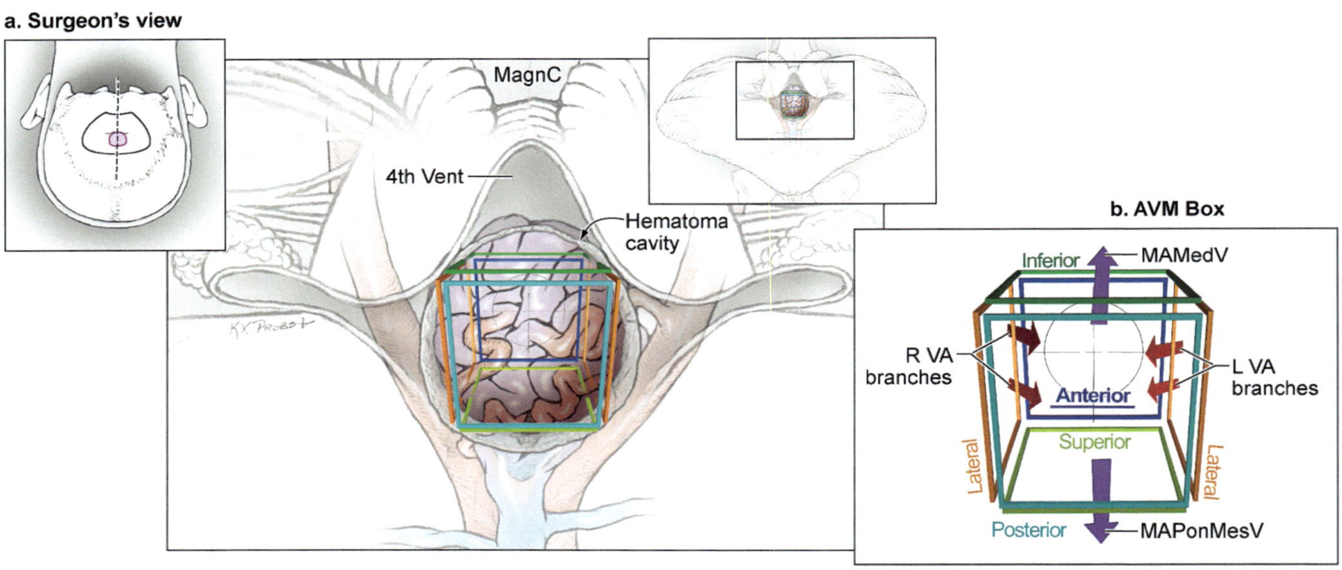

Fig. 16.24 Resection strategy for anterior medullary AVMs. (**a**) Step 1, exposing the AVM with a suboccipital craniotomy and transventricular approach [surgeon's view, with the patient prone and the scalp incision (*dashed line*), craniotomy (*solid line*), and AVM (*purple circle*) shown on the left inset]. (**b**) AVM box showing arterial supply from the distal vertebral artery and vertebrobasilar junction and venous drainage to the midline (MAMedV and MAPonMesV).

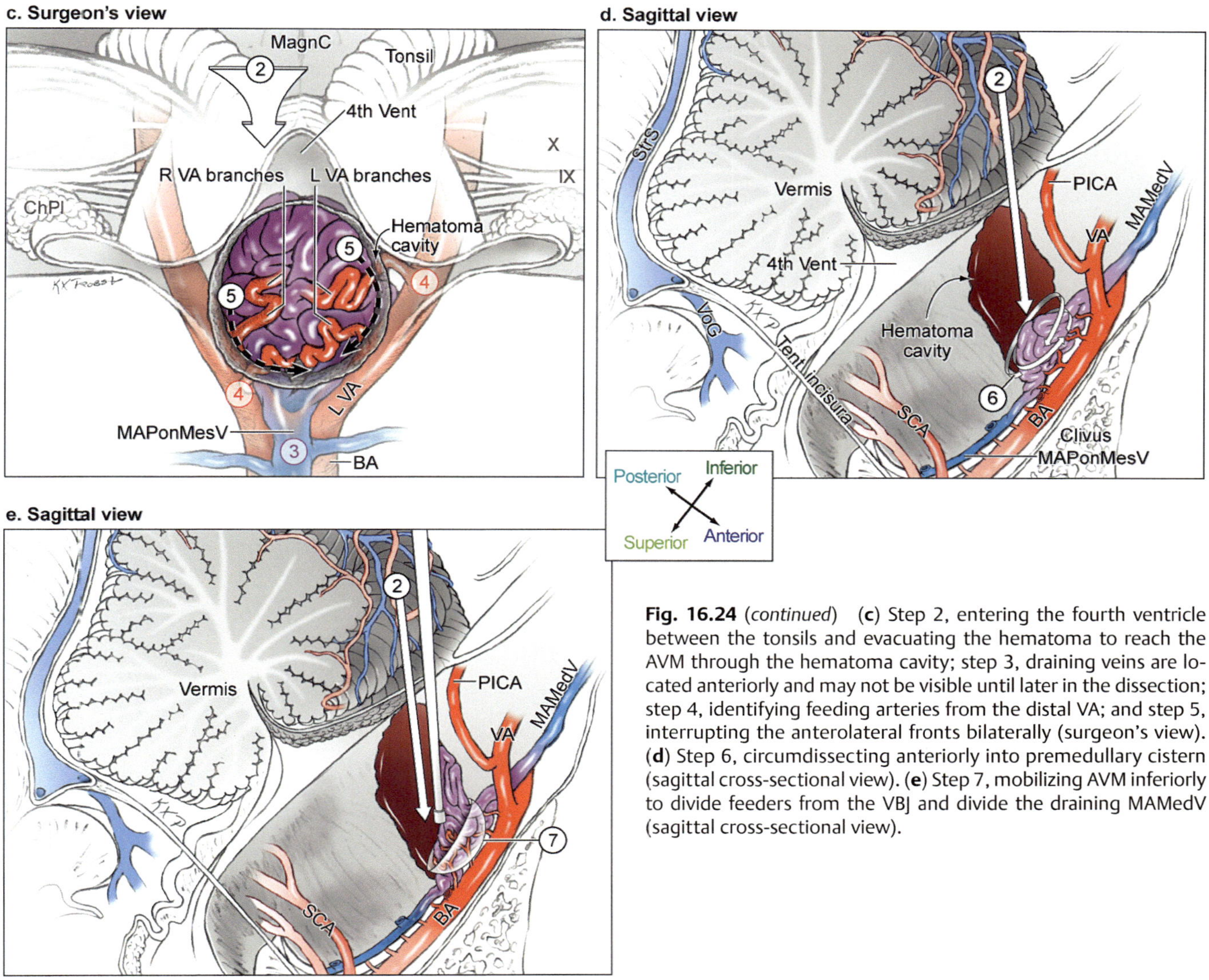

Fig. 16.24 *(continued)* (**c**) Step 2, entering the fourth ventricle between the tonsils and evacuating the hematoma to reach the AVM through the hematoma cavity; step 3, draining veins are located anteriorly and may not be visible until later in the dissection; step 4, identifying feeding arteries from the distal VA; and step 5, interrupting the anterolateral fronts bilaterally (surgeon's view). (**d**) Step 6, circumdissecting anteriorly into premedullary cistern (sagittal cross-sectional view). (**e**) Step 7, mobilizing AVM inferiorly to divide feeders from the VBJ and divide the draining MAMedV (sagittal cross-sectional view).

to dissect across the arterial connections to the vertebrobasilar junction on the deep anterior margin (step 7). My one anterior medullary AVM resection was memorable for its brisk bleeding. Fortunately, the initial hemorrhage already separated the AVM from its medullary attachments and pushed the pyramidal tracts and paramedian cranial nerve nuclei to the sides. The patient made a surprisingly good recovery (**Fig. 16.25**).

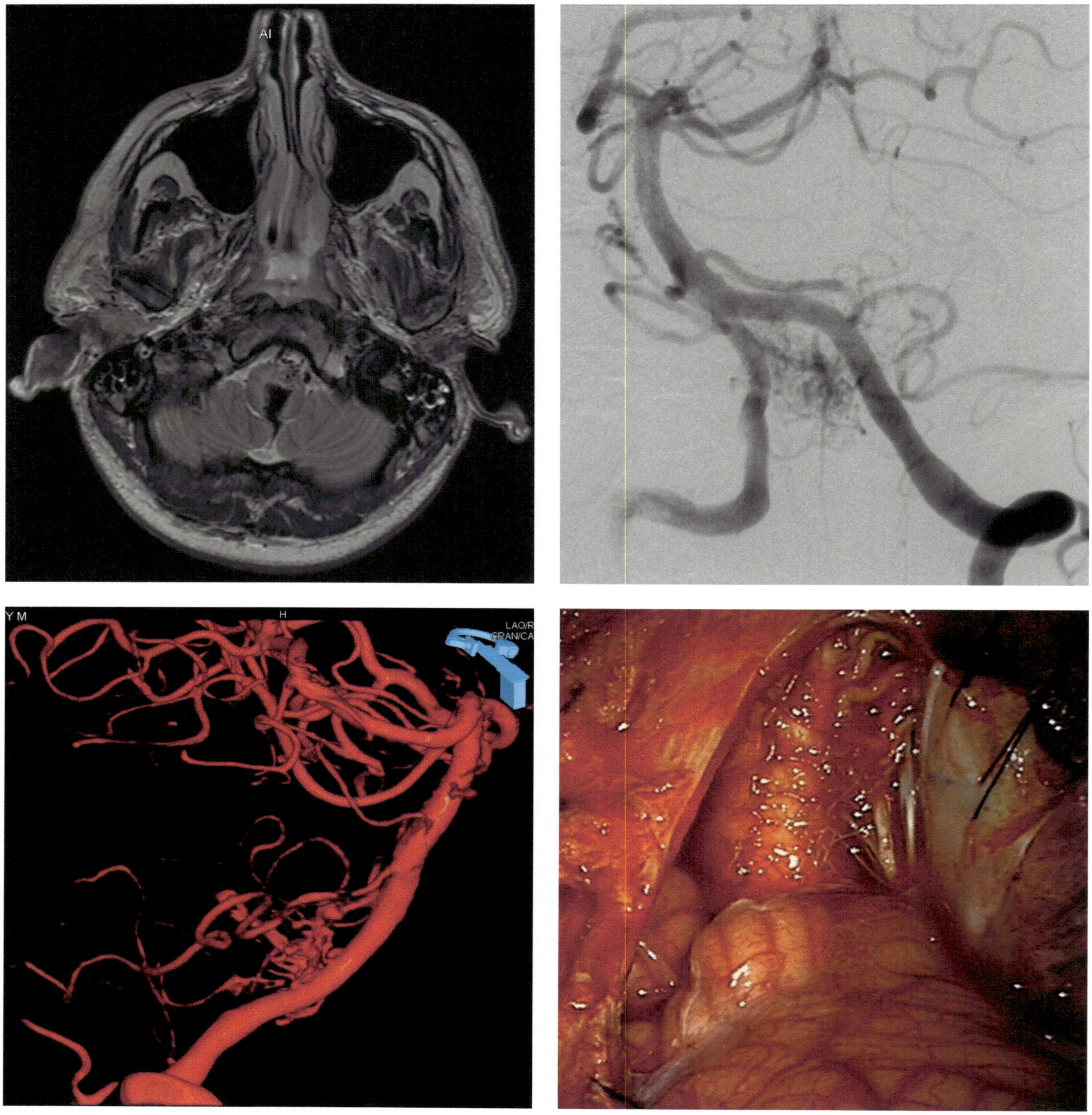

a b c d

Fig. 16.25 This 45-year-old man presented with an anterior medullary AVM (supplemented Spetzler-Martin grade 6: S1V1E1/A3B0C0) and an intramedullary hemorrhage that extended posteriorly into the fourth ventricle [(**a**) T2-weighted MRI, axial view]. The AVM was supplied by branches from the VA bilaterally (left more than right) that could not be embolized, and drained by MAMedV [(**b**) left VA angiogram, anterior oblique view and (**c**) 3D rotational angiogram, lateral view]. (**d**) A left suboccipital–far lateral craniotomy accessed both the left VA and the fourth ventricle.

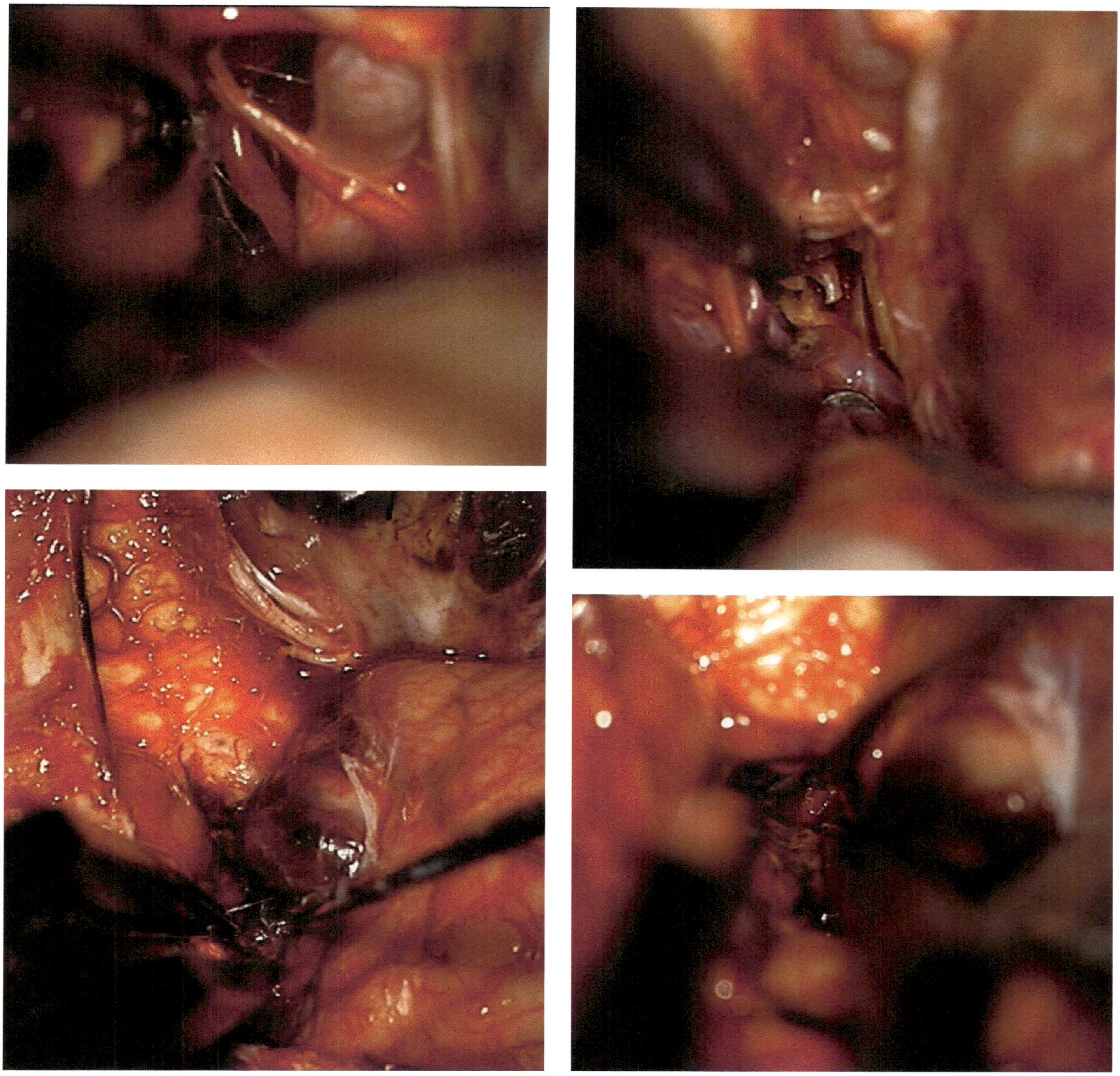

e f g h

Fig. 16.25 (*continued*) (**e,f**) The VA was followed anteriorly around the medulla where feeding arteries were identified and coagulated. (**g**) After interrupting this lateral front of arterial supply, the hematoma was entered through the fourth ventricular floor, evacuated, and (**h**) the AVM was dissected circumferentially. The AVM was resected completely and the patient improved dramatically.

Lateral Medullary AVM Resection

Lateral medullary AVMs are exposed through a far lateral craniotomy (**Fig. 16.26,** step 1) with the patient in the three-quarter prone ("park bench") position and the head flexed to tuck the chin to the manubrium, rotated 45 degrees away from the lesion to bring the nose toward the floor, and laterally flexed downward. A "hockey stick" scalp incision is used, and incisions in the midline nuchal ligament and below the superior nuchal line release the paraspinous muscles inferolaterally. Bone removal consists of a C1 laminectomy, lateral occipital craniotomy, and condylectomy. Thorough condylectomy reduces its size and enables the dura flapped against the condyle to be completely flat, opening an unobstructed surgical corridor down the axis of the VA. Subarachnoid dissection releases CSF from the MagnC, opens the CbMedC, identifies the VA where it pierces the dura, incises the overlying dentate ligament, opens the cerebellomedullary fissure,

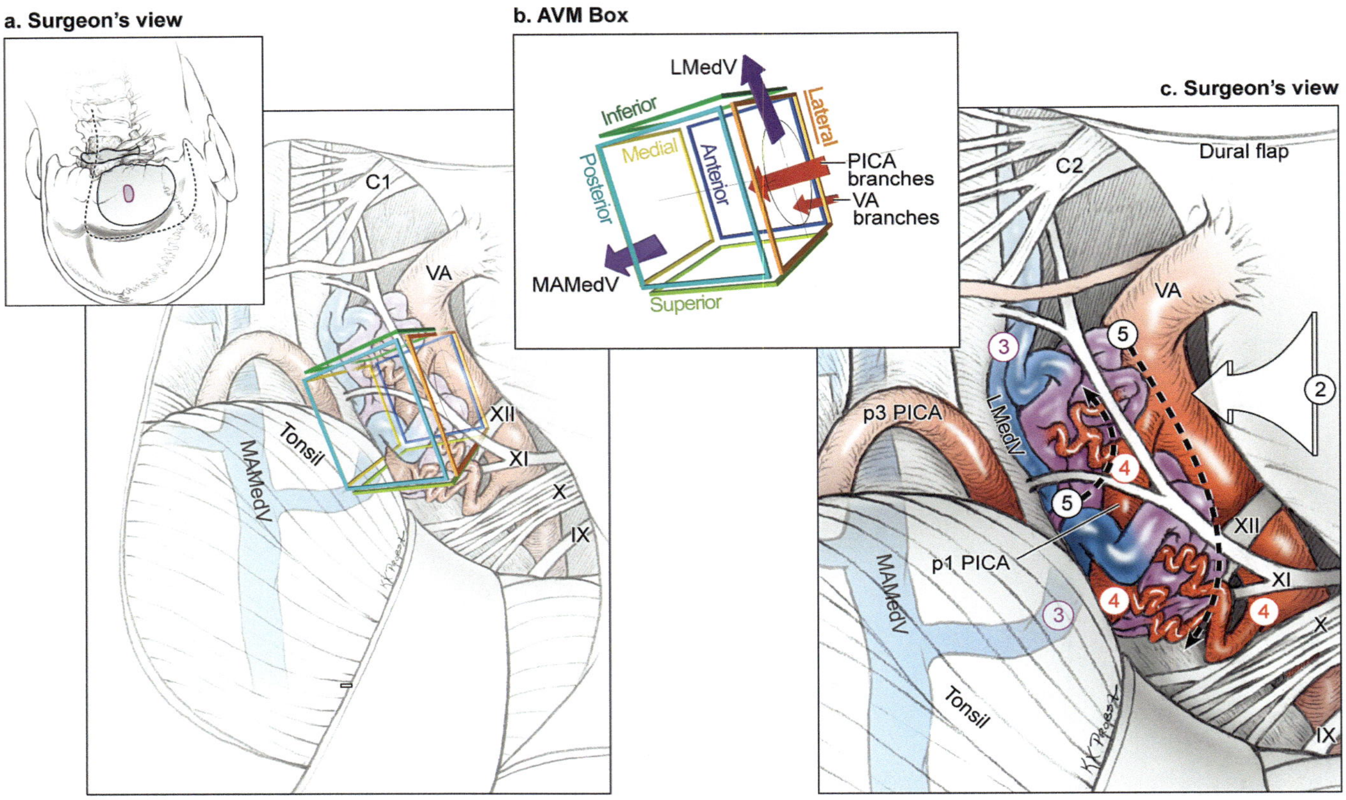

Fig. 16.26 Resection strategy for lateral medullary AVMs. (**a**) Step 1, exposing the AVM with a far lateral craniotomy [surgeon's view, with the patient in the park bench position and the scalp incision (*dashed line*), craniotomy (*solid line*), and AVM (*purple circle*) shown on *the inset*]. (**b**) AVM box showing arterial supply from the proximal vertebral artery and PICA, venous drainage medially and/or laterally, and proximity to the lower cranial nerves. (**c**) Step 2, opening the cisterna magna and dissecting the vagoaccessory, suprahypoglossal, and infrahypoglossal triangles; step 3, identifying the lateral draining vein (LMedV); step 4, locating the feeding arteries from the VA and PICA; and step 5, skeletonizing the VA and PICA to interrupt the lateral front while preserving distal flow (surgeon's view).

d. Axial section

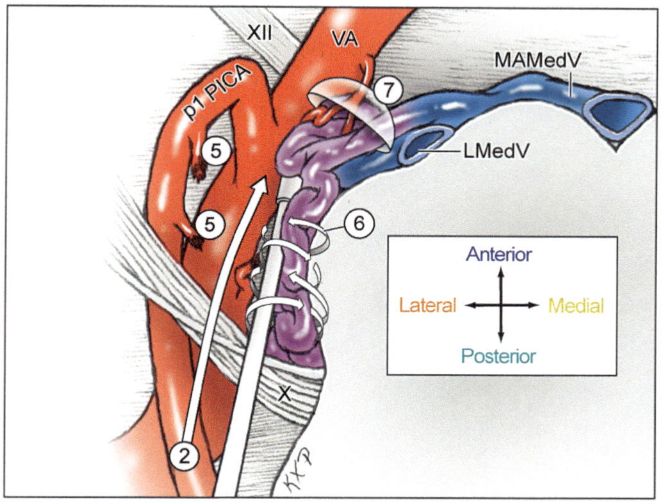

Fig. 16.26 (*continued*) (**d**) Step 6, circumdissecting in the cerebellomedullary cistern and along the pial margin; and step 7, mobilizing AVM medially away from the VA to interrupt deep arterial connections and visualize anterior drainage to MAMedV (axial cross-sectional view).

and elevates the tonsil (step 2). The vagoaccessory triangle is opened to clarify the course of CN9/10/11, and hypoglossal nerve roots are identified inside this triangle to define the supra- and infrahypoglossal triangles. The lateral medullary AVM sits on the lateral surface intermingled with the lower cranial nerves. Lateral drainage through LMedV is identified to monitor AVM occlusion, but medial drainage through MAMedV may not be visible until later (step 3). Feeding arteries originate from the posterolateral aspect of the VA between its point of dural entry and the VBJ (V4 segment), and from the proximal PICA branches (p1 and p2 segments, step 4). Feeding arteries are occluded at the lateral AVM margin, skeletonizing the VA so that it can continue to nourish medullary perforators and contribute to the basilar circulation (step 5). All of the lateral medullary AVMs in my surgical experience were pial and were circumdissected without parenchymal transgression (step 6). Mobilization of the AVM medially toward the medulla and away from the VA helps to visualize any remaining inputs from the VA more distally as well as the anterior venous drainage to MAMedV (step 7). Two-thirds of these AVMs separated cleanly from the medulla and lower cranial nerves and were resected; the remaining one-third were occluded in situ, as seen on ICG videoangiography, which demonstrated cessation of arteriovenous shunting before coagulating the dark draining vein (**Figs. 16.27** and **16.28**).

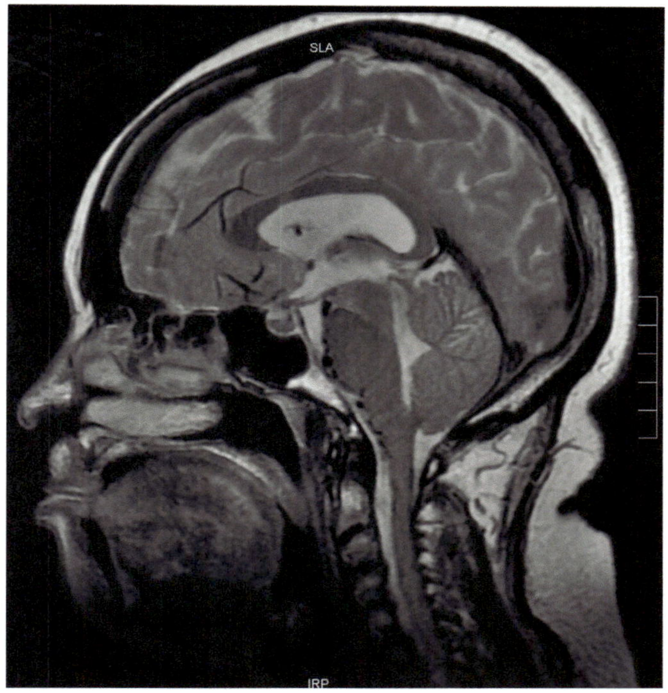

a

Fig. 16.27 This 55-year-old woman presented with an intraventricular hemorrhage from a right lateral medullary AVM (supplemented Spetzler-Martin grade 6: S1V1E1/A3B0C0), located on the pial surface of the medulla with dilated draining veins anteriorly [(**a**) sagittal T2-weighted MRI]. (*continued on next page*)

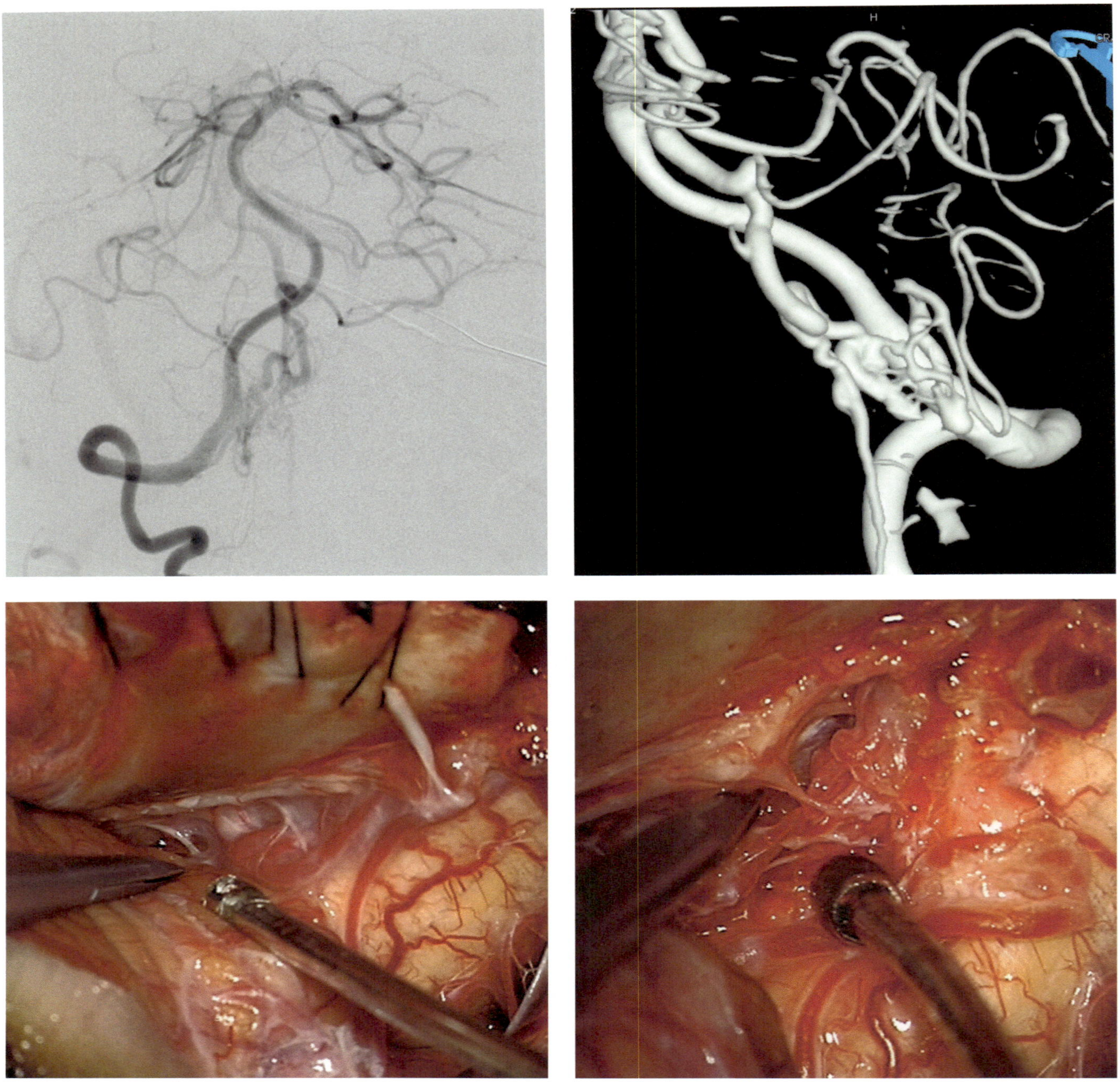

b c d e

Fig. 16.27 (*continued*) The AVM was supplied by PICA branches and AntSpA, and drained by MAMedV [(**b**) right VA angiogram, anteroposterior view and (**c**) 3D rotational angiogram, lateral view]. (**d**) A right far lateral craniotomy with aggressive condylectomy exposed the cerebellomedullary fissure and lateral medulla. (**e**) The AVM was on the pial surface of the lateral medulla.

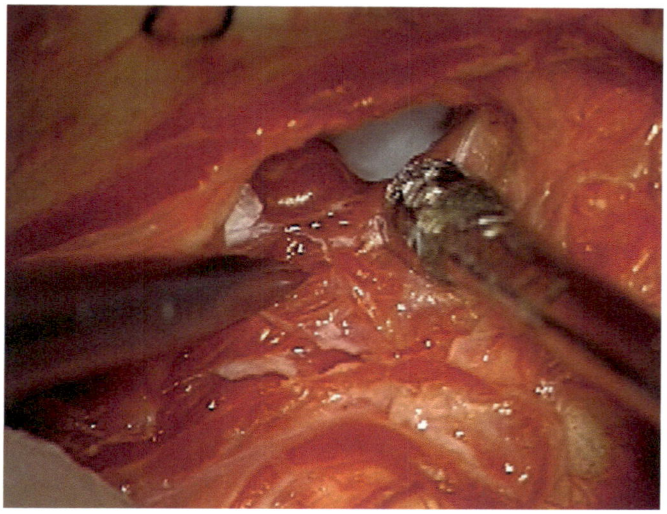
f

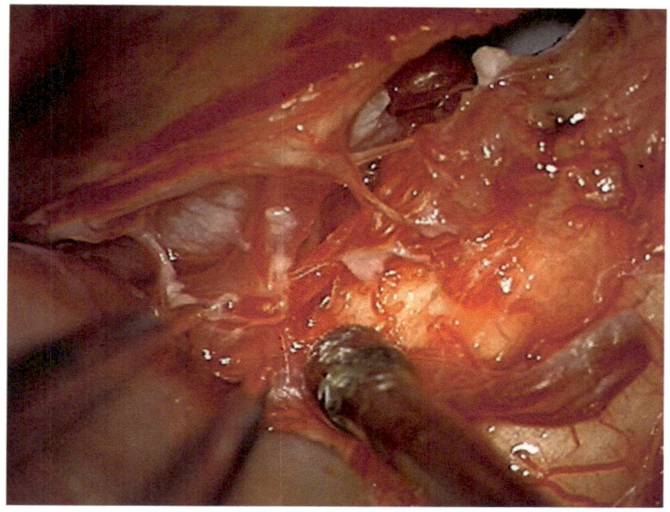
g

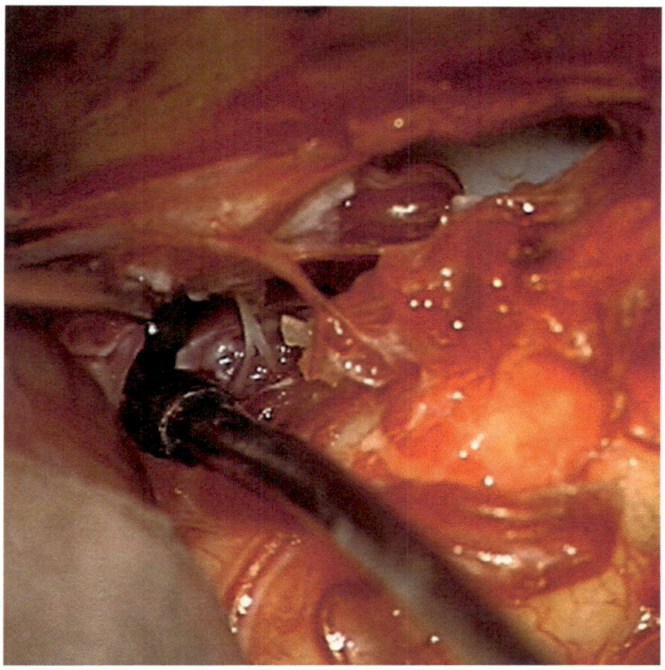
h

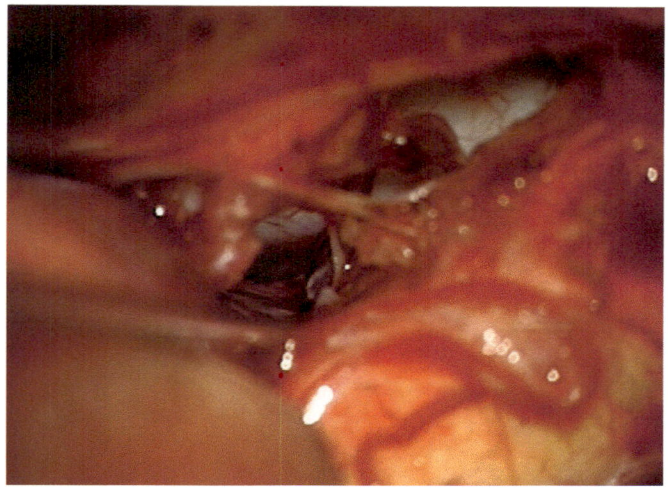
i

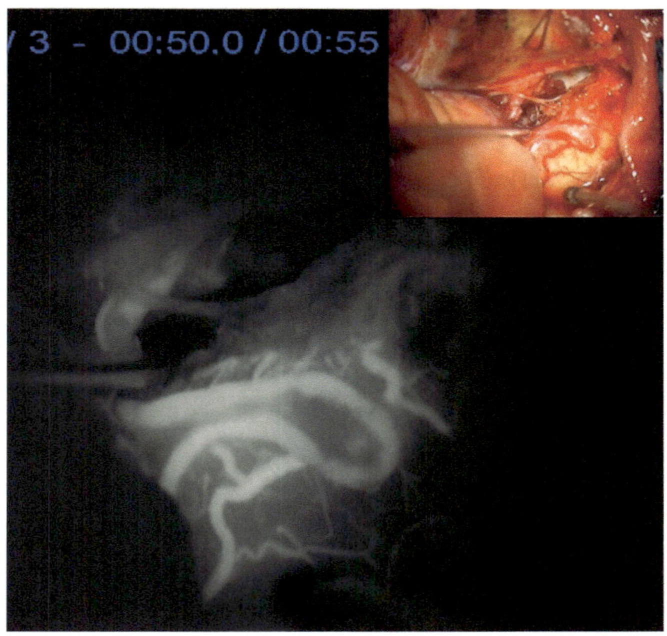

j

Fig. 16.27 (*continued*) (**f**) The AVM extended inferiorly to the cervical spinal cord. (**g**) The PICA originated proximally from the right VA, seen under CN11, and sent branches to the AVM. (**h**) As these branches were interrupted, the PICA separated from the AVM and was swept laterally by the Rhoton No. 6 dissector. (**i**) The MAMedV, seen on the anterior medullary surface, darkened and (**j**) indocyanine green videoangiography confirmed the absence of arteriovenous shunting. The AVM was occluded in situ and angiography confirmed complete occlusion.

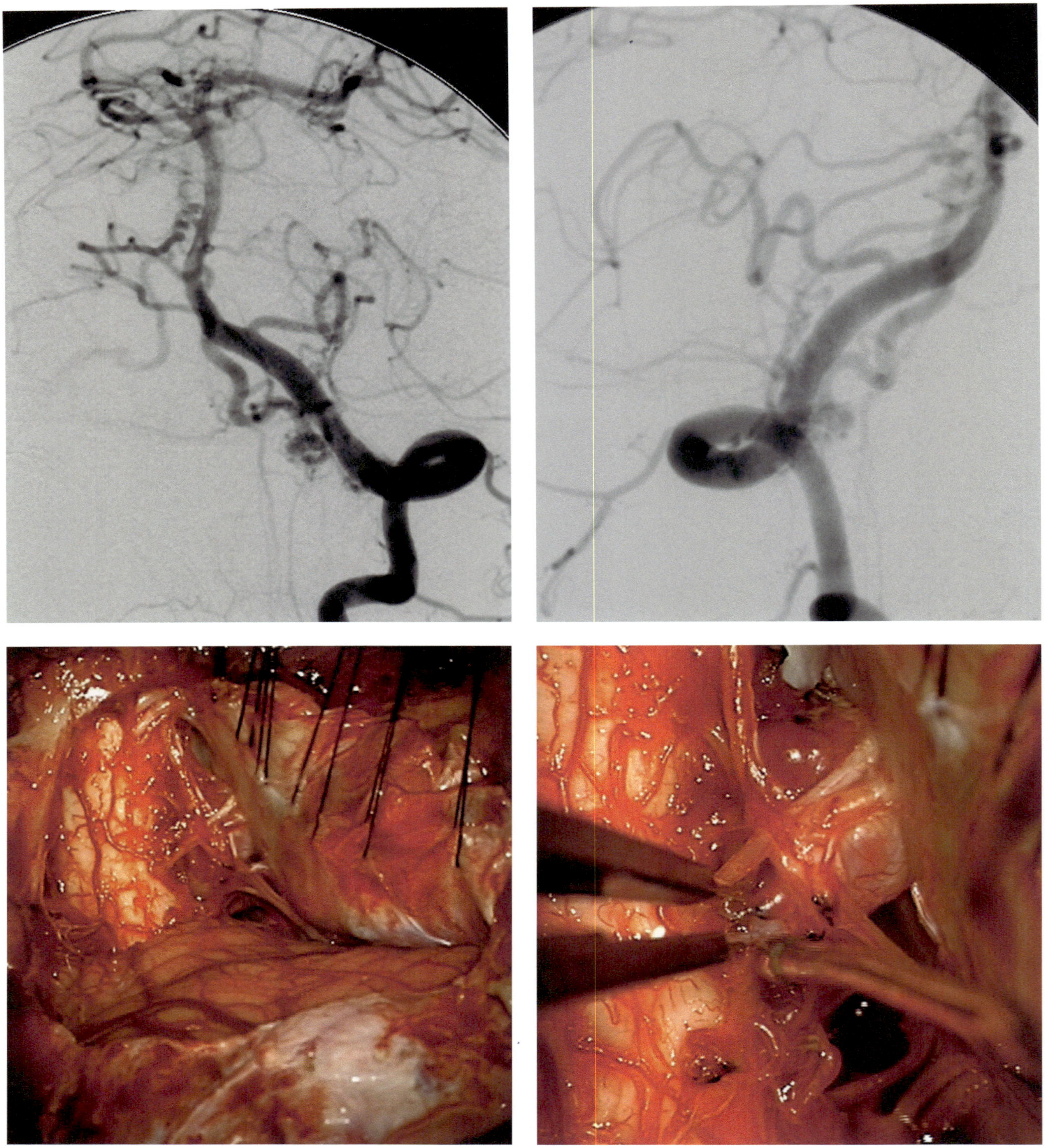

a b c d

Fig. 16.28 This 55-year-old man presented with subarachnoid hemorrhage from a left lateral medullary AVM (supplemented Spetzler-Martin grade 6: S1V1E1/A3B0C0), supplied by VA branches and drained by MAMedV [left VA angiogram, (**a**) anteroposterior and (**b**) lateral views]. Unlike the previous case, he had an AICA-PICA that did not contribute to the AVM. (**c**) The AVM was exposed through a left far lateral craniotomy and (**d**) direct arterial feeders from the VA were coagulated.

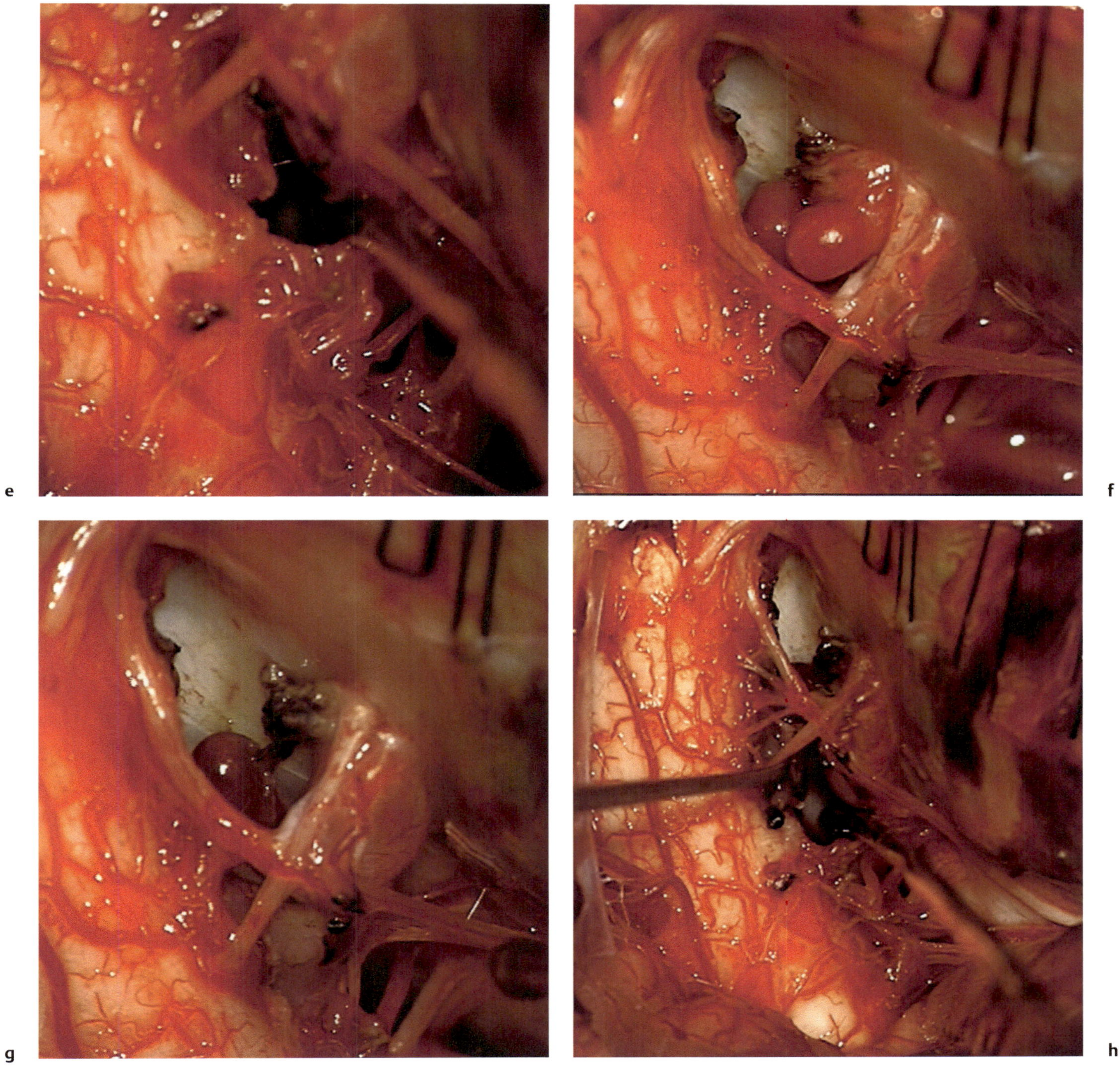

Fig. 16.28 (*continued*) (**e**) The VA was mobilized away from the AVM. (**f**) The major feeder originated from the VA as it pierced the dura, inferior to the C1 nerve rootlet and lateral to CN11. (**g**) After coagulating and (**h**) dividing this artery, MAMedV darkened and the nidus was occluded in situ, with confirmation by both ICG videoangiography intraoperatively and conventional angiography postoperatively.

Conclusion

Brainstem AVMs, like deep AVMs, are intimidating and lead many neurosurgeons to consider them inoperable. However, brainstem AVMs have a hemorrhage rate that is higher than that of supratentorial AVMs (estimated to be as high as 15% per year), making them difficult to observe. Furthermore, they are not as amenable to radiosurgery as other AVMs because of the brainstem's sensitivity to radiation. Surgical options are not ideal, particularly when the skull base makes anterior brainstem AVMs so inaccessible. However, lateral brainstem AVMs, specifically the lateral pontine and lateral medullary subtypes, can be exposed adequately with extended retrosigmoid and far lateral approaches, and results in these patients have been good. The lateral pontine AVM is a resectable AVM, and occlusion in situ offers a safe alternative for other AVMs that prove too risky to resect. Complete occlusion rates are lower with occlusions in situ, but this approach represents a conservative option that still may be better than observation or radiosurgery alone. Brainstem AVMs that are incompletely occluded in situ are typically smaller targets and are treated with radiosurgery, usually with smaller doses than would have been required without surgery, to achieve complete obliteration.

17 Cerebellar Arteriovenous Malformations

Microsurgical Anatomy

Brain

The cerebellum is composed of two hemispheres joined in the midline by the vermis (**Fig. 17.1**). The cerebellum has three surfaces: suboccipital, tentorial, and petrosal. Each of the surfaces is divided by a major fissure named according to its surface: suboccipital, tentorial, and petrosal fissures. The hemispheric part of the tentorial surface in composed of the quadrangular, simple, and superior semilunar lobules. The tentorial surface is divided into anterior and posterior parts by its major fissure, the tentorial (primary) fissure. This fissure separates the quadrangular and simple lobules on the hemisphere, and the culmen and declive on the vermis. The postclival fissure separates the simple and superior semilunar lobules.

The hemispheric portion of the suboccipital surface is composed of the superior semilunar lobule, inferior semilunar lobule, biventral lobule, and tonsil. The suboccipital surface is divided into superior and inferior parts by its major fissure, the suboccipital fissure. The vermian part of this fissure is called the prepyramidal fissure, and the hemispheric part of this fissure is called the prebiventral fissure. Minor fissures on the suboccipital surface include the petrosal (horizontal) fissure between the superior and inferior semilunar lobules, which is an extension of the major fissure on the petrosal surface, and the tonsillobiventral fissure.

The inferior vermis lies in a deep vertical depression in the suboccipital surface called the posterior cerebellar incisura, which also contains the falx cerebelli. The inferior vermis forms the posterior cortical surface in the midline within this incisura. In contrast, the superior vermis is the highest point on the cerebellum, occupying the space under the straight sinus where the tentorial leaflets intersect with the falx cerebri. The superior vermis slopes downward from its apex anteriorly to the posterior cerebellar incisura. The tentorial part of the vermian surface includes (from anterior

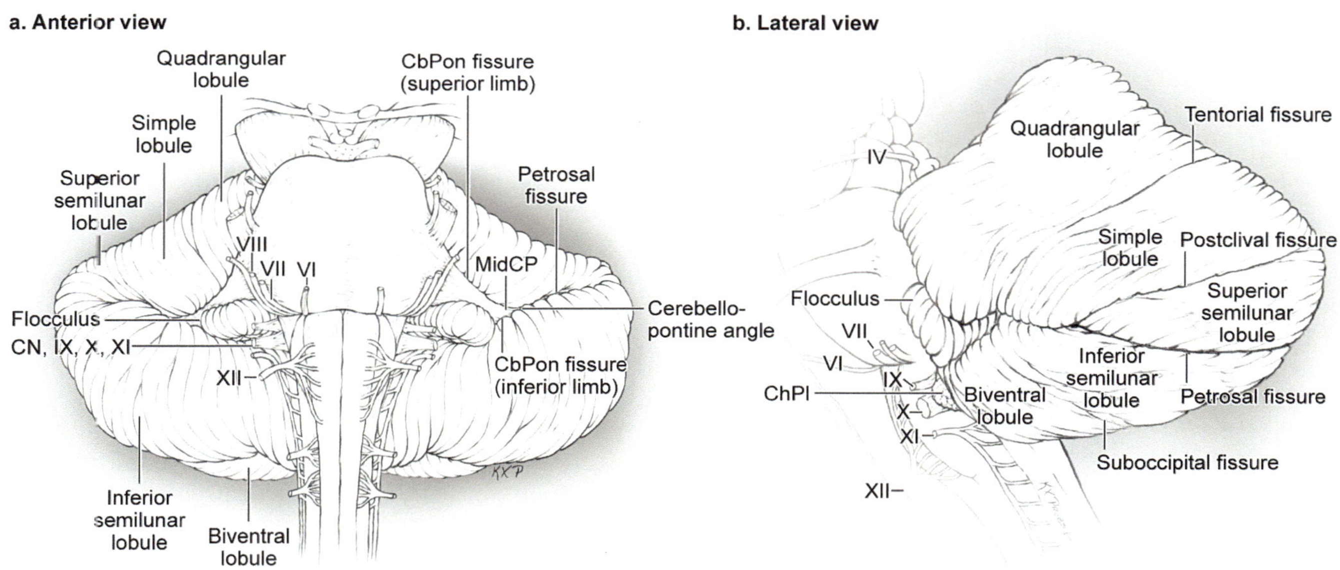

Fig. 17.1 Microsurgical anatomy of the cerebellum. The cerebellum is composed of two hemispheres joined in the midline by the vermis and has three surfaces (suboccipital, tentorial, and petrosal), each divided by a major fissure named according to its surface (suboccipital, tentorial, and petrosal fissures). (**a**) Anterior view (petrosal surface). (**b**) Lateral view (tentorial, suboccipital, and petrosal surfaces). (*continued on next page*)

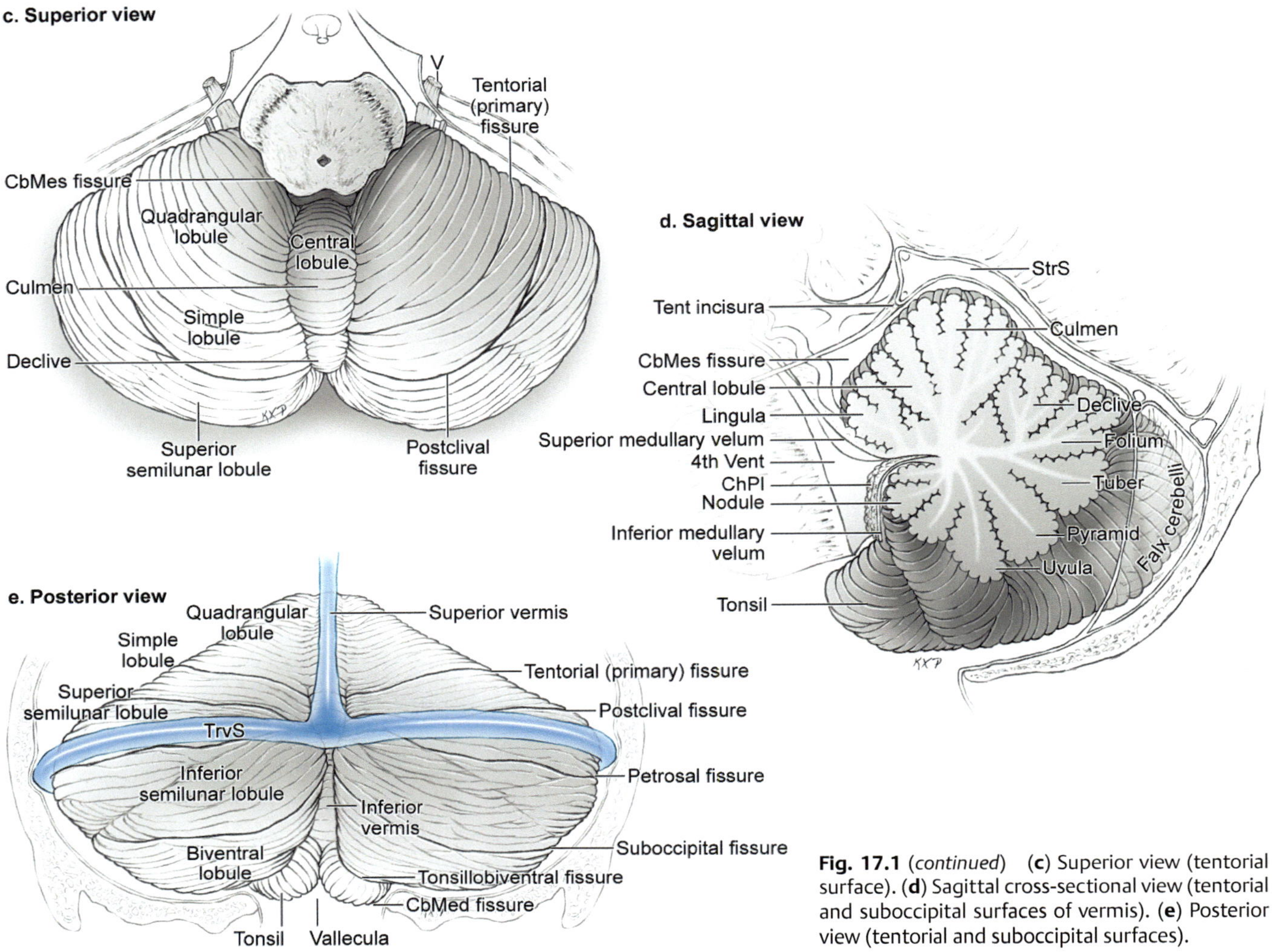

Fig. 17.1 *(continued)* (**c**) Superior view (tentorial surface). (**d**) Sagittal cross-sectional view (tentorial and suboccipital surfaces of vermis). (**e**) Posterior view (tentorial and suboccipital surfaces).

to posterior) the culmen, declive, and folium. The suboccipital part of the vermian surface includes (from superior to inferior) the tuber, pyramid, uvula, and nodule. The nodule is hidden deep to the uvula.

The tonsils are ovoid structures on the inferomedial aspect of the cerebellar hemispheres that attach to the cerebellum superolaterally through the tonsillar peduncles. The other tonsillar surfaces are free, with the inferior pole and posterior surfaces in the cisterna magna. The anterior tonsil faces the posterior medulla and is separated by the cerebellomedullary fissure. The medial tonsils face each other and are separated by the vallecula, a cleft that leads into the fourth ventricle. The ventral aspect of the superior tonsil faces the lower half of the roof of the fourth ventricle, which is formed by the tela choroidea, inferior medullary velum, and nodule. The lateral tonsil is separated from the hemisphere by the tonsillobiventral fissure.

The petrosal surface of the cerebellum faces the posterior petrous bone and is divided into superior and inferior parts by the petrosal (horizontal) fissure, which extends onto the suboccipital surface between the superior and inferior semilunar lobules. The cerebellopontine angle is the V-shaped intersection of the petrosal and cerebellopontine fissures, the latter one formed where the hemispheric lobules wrap around the pons and middle cerebellar peduncle. The superior and inferior limbs of the cerebellopontine fissure meet laterally at the apex of the cerebellopontine angle, at the anterior end of the petrosal fissure. The petrosal surface is formed by the anterior surfaces of the quadrangular, simple, semilunar, and biventral lobules, and the flocculi. The two halves of the petrosal surface are not connected by a continuous strip of vermis like the other two surfaces, because of the interposition of the fourth ventricle. Anterior vermis above the fourth ventricle are the lingula, central lobule, and culmen, and below are the nodule and uvula.

Arteries

The arteries that supply cerebellar arteriovenous malformations (AVMs) are the cortical segments of the cerebellar arteries discussed with brainstem AVMs: the s4 superior cerebellar artery (SCA), a4 anterior inferior cerebellar artery (AICA), and the p4 and p5 posterior inferior cerebellar artery (PICA) (**Fig. 17.2**). The s3 segment of the SCA climbs up from the cerebellomesencephalic fissure to reach the anterior edge of the tentorial cerebellar surface, by which time it bifurcates into rostral and caudal trunks. The rostral trunk supplies the superior vermis and the caudal trunk supplies the hemispheric surface. Before exiting the cerebellomesencephalic fissure and becoming cortical segments, these trunks (particularly the rostral trunk) give rise to as many as eight precerebellar arteries that supply the dentate and deep cerebellar nuclei, and become the deep perforating artery supply to large cerebellar AVMs, or the equivalent of the "red devils" in the cerebellum that can be difficult to coagulate along the deep plane. The cortical branches divide into the hemispheric (medial, intermediate, and lateral) and vermian (medial and paramedian) segments.

The AICA courses through the cerebellopontine angle near cranial nerves (CN) 7/8 and, after sending branches to the nerves entering the acoustic meatus and to the choroid plexus protruding from the foramen of Luschka, it supplies the petrosal surface of the cerebellum. The AICA typically bifurcates near the nerve complex into rostral and caudal trunks, the former supplying the middle cerebellar peduncle and superior lip of the cerebellopontine fissure, and the latter supplying the inferior lip of the cerebellopontine fissure, flocculus, and choroid plexus. Important AICA branches include brainstem perforators, labyrinthine, recurrent perforating, and subarcuate arteries.

The PICA is intimate with the cerebellomedullary fissure, lower half of the ventricular roof, inferior cerebellar peduncle, and suboccipital surface. After exiting the cerebellomedullary fissure, the PICA typically bifurcates along its p4 telovelotonsillar segment into a smaller medial trunk that sends branches to the inferior vermis and adjacent hemisphere (median and paramedian vermian arteries), and a larger lateral trunk that sends branches to the suboccipital surface and tonsils (medial, intermediate, and lateral hemispheric arteries; tonsillar arteries). Cortical branches emerge from the telovelotonsillar or tonsillobiventral fissure and radiate outward from the superior and lateral borders of the tonsil. Cortical branches arising near the superior tonsil send branches to the dentate nucleus and can also be a source of deep perforating artery supply to large AVMs.

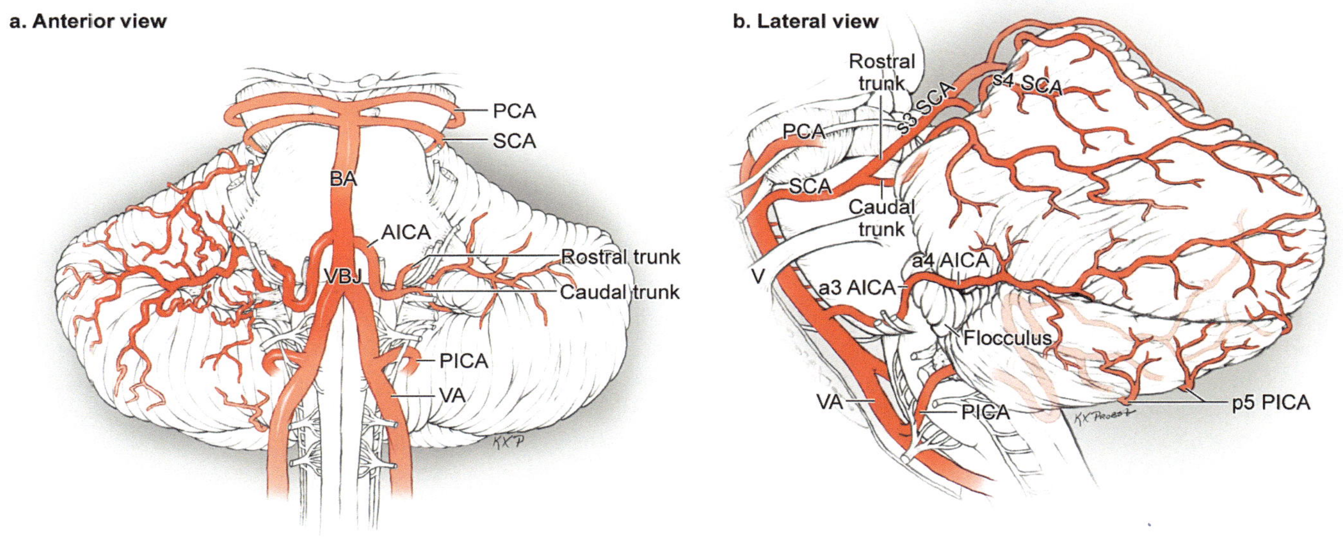

Fig. 17.2 Microsurgical anatomy of the cerebellar arteries. (**a**) The petrosal surface of cerebellum is supplied by the cortical branches of the AICA (anterior view). (**b**) The lateral hemisphere is supplied by all three cerebellar arteries (lateral view). (*continued on next page*)

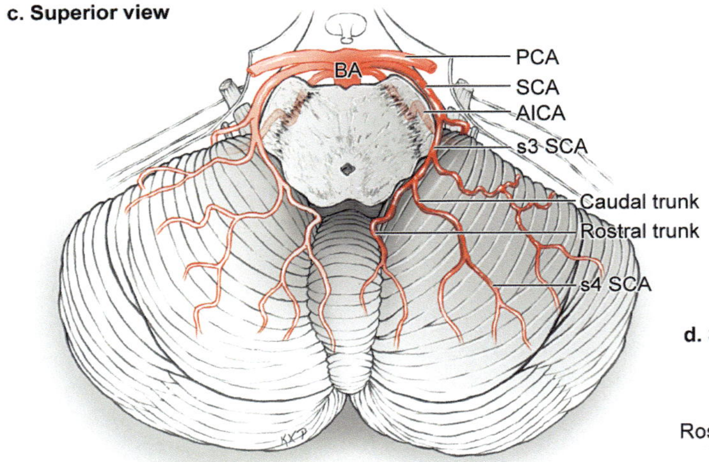

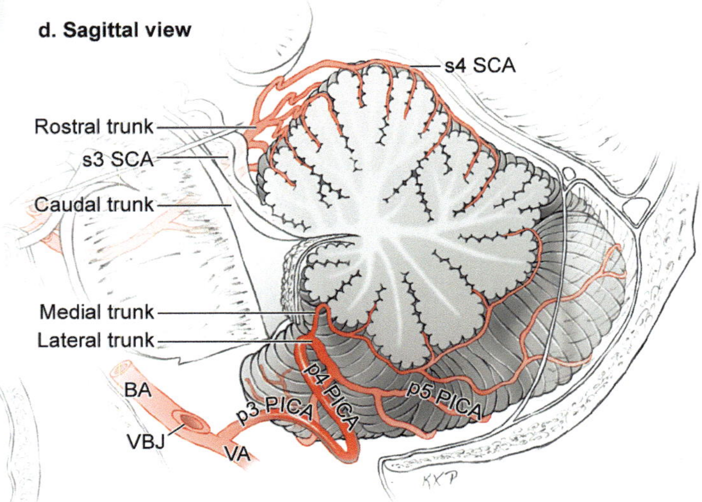

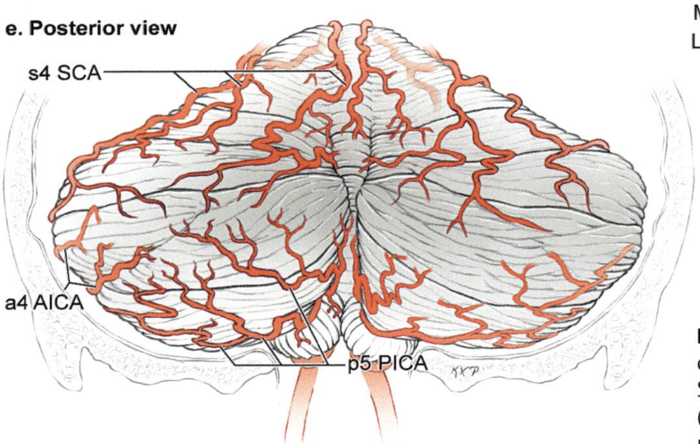

Fig. 17.2 (*continued*) (**c**) The tentorial surface is supplied by cortical branches of the SCA (superior view). (**d**) Vermis is supplied by the SCA superiorly and the PICA inferiorly (sagittal cross-sectional view). (**e**) The posterior cerebellar hemispheres are supplied by the SCA superiorly, AICA laterally, and PICA inferiorly (posterior view).

Veins

Superficial veins draining the tentorial surface include the superior hemispheric vein (SHemV) and superior vermian vein (SVerV) (**Fig. 17.3**). The suboccipital surface is drained by inferior hemispheric veins (IHemV) and inferior vermian veins (IVerV). The tonsils are drained by medial and lateral tonsillar veins (TonsV) and retrotonsillar veins (ReTonsV). The petrosal surface is drained by anterior hemispheric veins (AHemV). Deep veins course through the main fissures of the cerebellum and brainstem, including the vein of the cerebellomesencephalic fissure (VCMesF) related to the superior half of the fourth ventricular roof, the vein of the cerebellomedullary fissure (VCMedF) related to the inferior half of the fourth ventricular roof, and the vein of the cerebellopontine fissure (VCPonF) related to the lateral recess. Bridging veins from the three cerebellar surfaces include the Galenic group from superior surfaces to the vein of Galen (VoG); the tentorial group from the tentorial surface to the torcula (Torc) or tentorial sinus (TentS); and the petrosal group from the petrosal surface to the superior petrosal sinus (SPS) and inferior petrosal sinus (IPS).

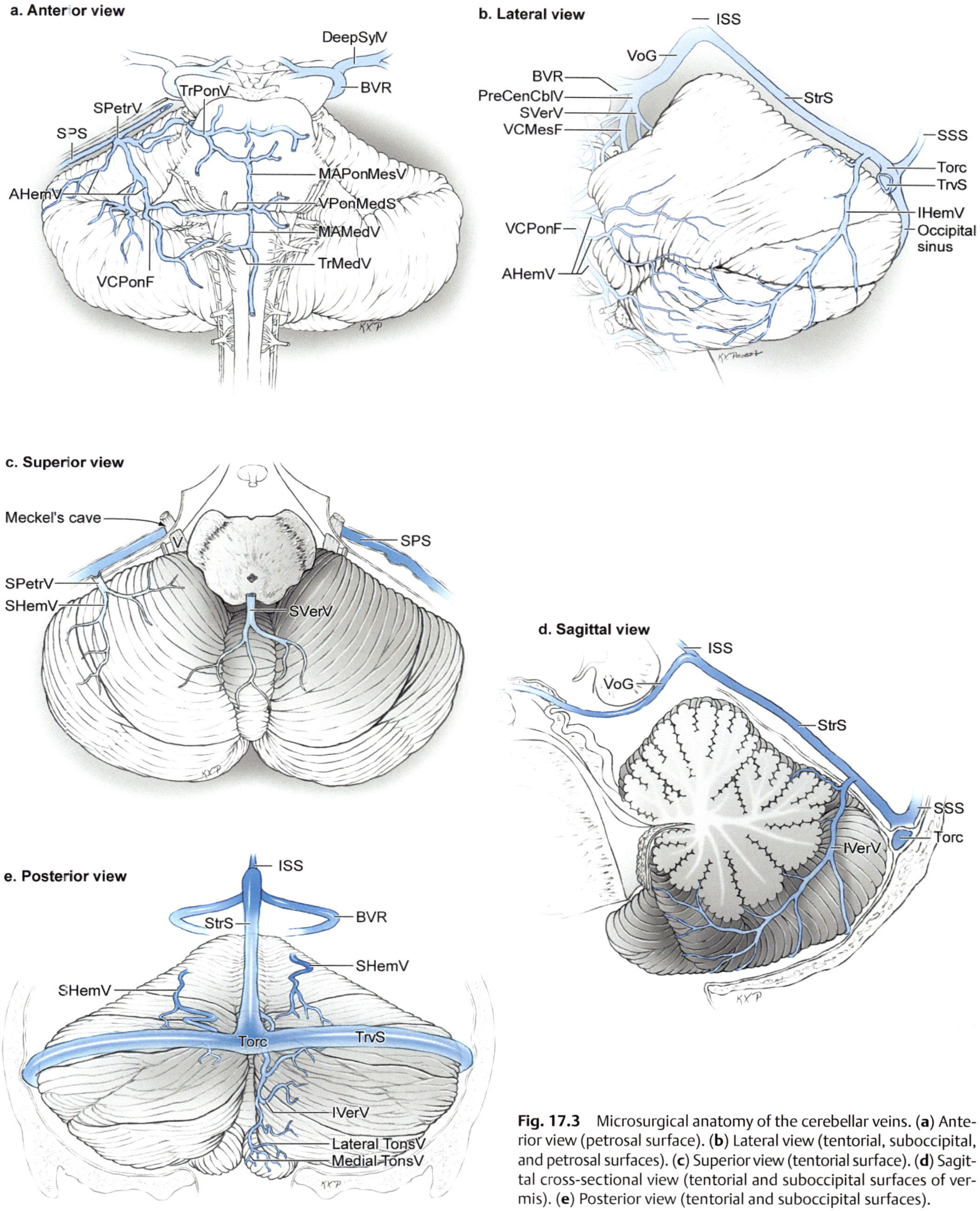

Fig. 17.3 Microsurgical anatomy of the cerebellar veins. (**a**) Anterior view (petrosal surface). (**b**) Lateral view (tentorial, suboccipital, and petrosal surfaces). (**c**) Superior view (tentorial surface). (**d**) Sagittal cross-sectional view (tentorial and suboccipital surfaces of vermis). (**e**) Posterior view (tentorial and suboccipital surfaces).

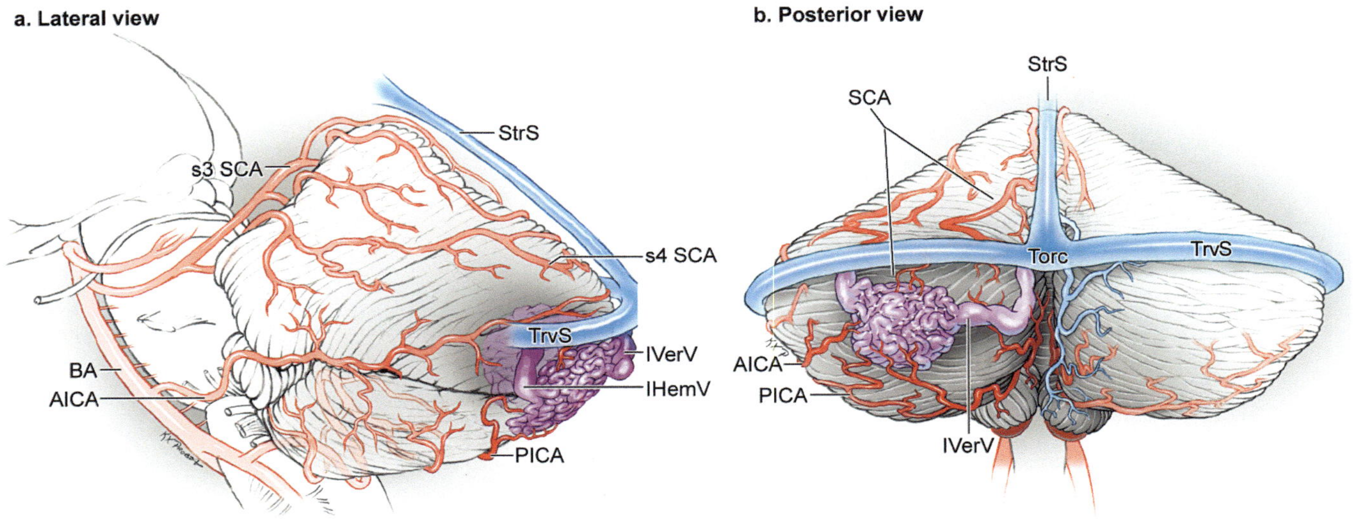

Fig. 17.4 The suboccipital cerebellar AVM: (**a**) lateral and (**b**) posterior views. This AVM is based unilaterally on the suboccipital surface, can be supplied by all three cerebellar arteries, and has superficial, ascending venous drainage to the torcula and transverse sinuses.

Five Cerebellar AVM Subtypes

The Suboccipital Cerebellar AVM

Suboccipital AVMs are based on the suboccipital cerebellar surface facing the occipital bone in the superior semilunar, inferior semilunar, and biventral lobules, below and between the transverse (TrvS) and the sigmoid sinuses (SigmS) (**Fig. 17.4**). They are the second most common cerebellar AVMs, accounting for one fifth of all cerebellar AVMs. They are unilateral and their location varies in the medial-lateral and superior-inferior directions. Suboccipital cerebellar AVMs receive supply from the cortical branches of all three cerebellar arteries because of collateral connections on this surface, with increased participation from the SCA, AICA, and PICA with AVMs located more superiorly, laterally, and inferiorly, respectively. Venous drainage is superficial through IHemV and/or IVerV, which a bridge to Torc and TrvS. Suboccipital AVMs are eloquent only when they extend to deep cerebellar nuclei. Midline AVMs based in the inferior vermis differ from lateral suboccipital AVMs and are categorized instead as vermian cerebellar AVMs.

The Tentorial Cerebellar AVM

Tentorial AVMs are based on the tentorial surface in the quadrangular, simple, and superior semilunar lobules (**Fig. 17.5**). These AVMs also accounted for one fifth of all cerebellar AVMs and are unilateral. Their arterial supply is from hemispheric branches of the SCA that intersect the anterior and medial margins of the nidus. Venous drainage is through SHemV that can bridge anteriorly to the VoG, posteriorly to Torc, or superiorly to TentS or StrS. Tentorial AVMs typically do not extend to the deep cerebellar nuclei and are non-eloquent. Midline AVMs based in the superior vermis differ from tentorial AVMs and are categorized instead as vermian AVMs.

The Vermian Cerebellar AVM

Vermian AVMs are the most common cerebellar AVM (30%) and sit in the midline in the superior vermis (tentorial surface, **Fig. 17.6**) or the inferior vermis (suboccipital surface), with the superior vermian being more common (90% vs. 10%, respectively). Superior vermian AVMs are located in the lingula, central lobule, culmen, and/or declive, whereas inferior vermian AVMs are located in the folium, tuber, pyramid, uvula, and/or nodule. Arterial supply is bilateral and depends on location, with superior vermian AVMs fed by the SCAs and inferior vermian AVMs fed by PICAs. Superior vermian AVMs drain deep to SVerV and VoG, whereas inferior vermian AVMs drain superficially to IVerV and Torc. Most vermian AVMs are non-eloquent.

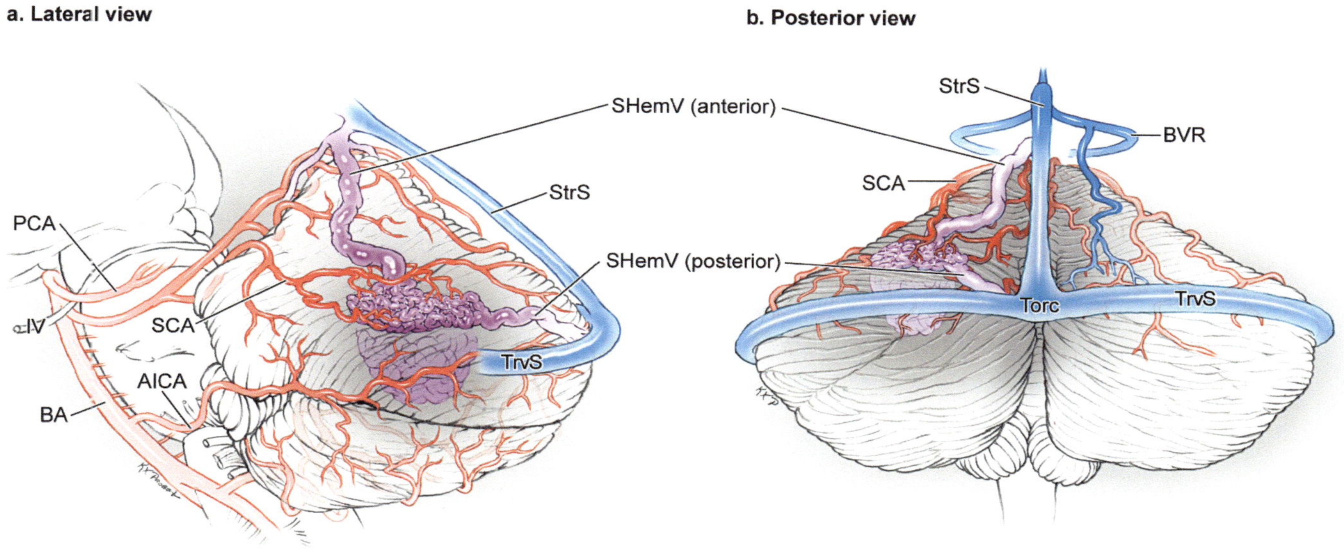

Fig. 17.5 The tentorial cerebellar AVM: (**a**) lateral and (**b**) posterior views. This AVM is based unilaterally on the tentorial surface, is supplied by hemispheric branches of the SCA, and drains to the superior hemispheric veins that may course deeply to the VoG (anterior SHemV) or superficially to the torcula or transverse sinus (posterior SHemV).

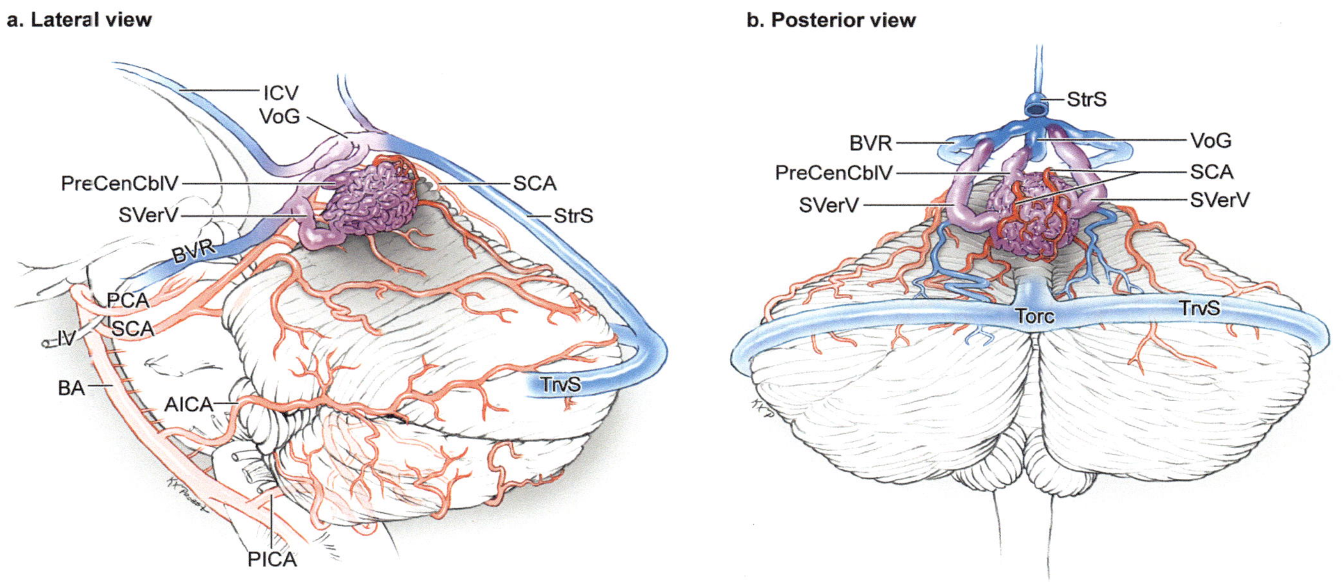

Fig. 17.6 The vermian cerebellar AVM: (**a**) lateral and (**b**) posterior views. This AVM is based in the midline either on the superior vermis (tentorial surface, as shown) or on the inferior vermis (suboccipital surface, not shown). This AVM is supplied bilaterally by the SCA in the superior vermis and by the PICA in the inferior vermis. Superior vermian AVMs drain deeply to the VoG via SVerV and inferior vermian AVMs drain superficially to the torcula via IVerV.

The Tonsillar Cerebellar AVM

Tonsillar AVMs lie in the cerebellar tonsils at the lower edge of the suboccipital surface (**Fig. 17.7**) and were the least common cerebellar AVM (8%). These are unilateral AVMs fed by the ipsilateral PICA, and have superficial drainage to medial and lateral TonsV as well as ReTonsV. Tonsillar AVMs are small in size and non-eloquent.

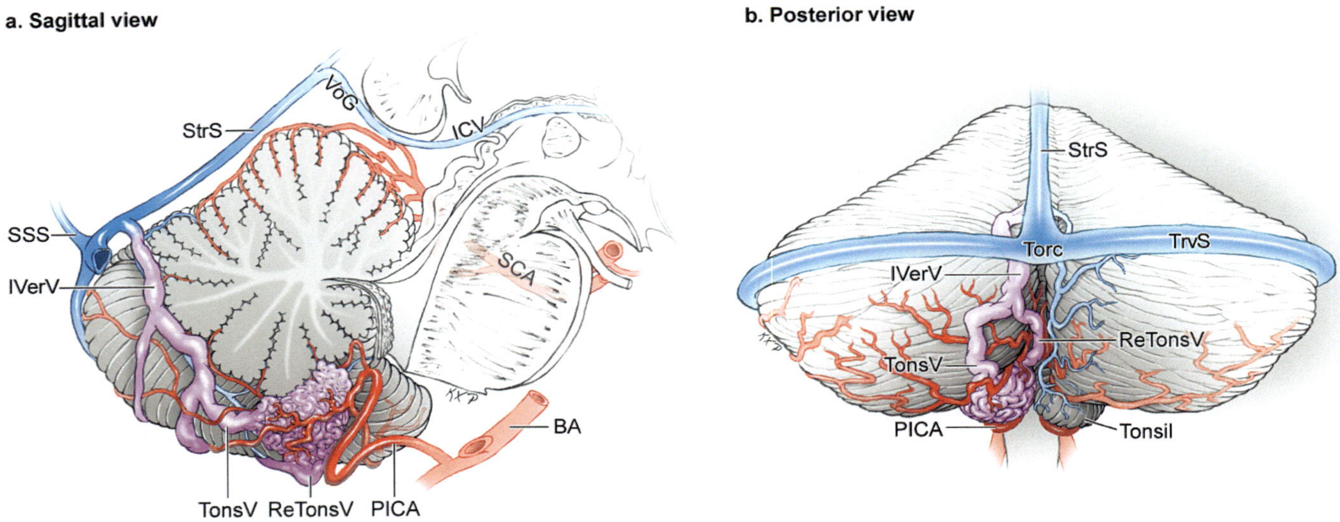

Fig. 17.7 The tonsillar cerebellar AVM: (**a**) sagittal cross-sectional and (**b**) posterior views. This AVM is based in the cerebellar tonsil unilaterally, supplied by the ipsilateral PICA, and drained by the tonsillar veins.

The Petrosal Cerebellar AVM

Petrosal AVMs are based on the petrosal surface, which is the anterior cerebellum that faces the posterior petrous bone (**Fig. 17.8**). These AVMs are located in the parts of the cerebellar lobules that wrap around to the anterior surface: the quadrangular, simple, superior semilunar, inferior semilunar, and biventral lobules. They are distinct from lateral pontine AVMs that are based in the lateral pons and middle cerebellar peduncle. These AVMs are unilateral and supplied by cortical branches of the AICA. They drain to AHemV and VCPonF, which then course to SPetrV and SPS. These AVMs are non-eloquent, but not far from CN5, CN7/8, and pons.

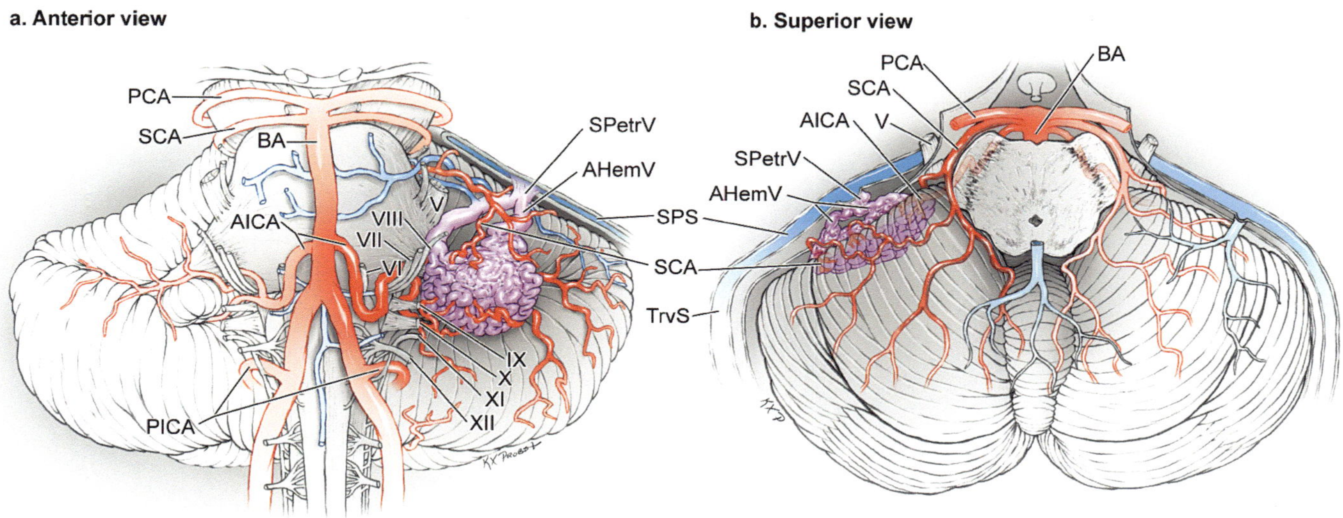

Fig. 17.8 The petrosal cerebellar AVM: (**a**) superior and (**b**) anterior views. This AVM is based on the petrosal surface lateral to the brachium pontis. It s supplied by cortical branches of the AICA and is drained by the anterior hemispheric veins and petrosal vein.

Resection Strategies for Cerebellar AVMs

Suboccipital Cerebellar AVM Resection

Suboccipital AVMs are exposed with a lateral suboccipital craniotomy (**Fig. 17.9**, step 1). Combination approaches are used for larger AVMs at the margins of the suboccipital surface, with the far lateral craniotomy adding an inferolateral exposure, the extended retrosigmoid craniotomy adding a superolateral exposure, and the torcular craniotomy adding a superior exposure. The patient is positioned prone with the head flexed to open the cranial-cervical angle. The skin incision is typically a linear midline incision for more medial craniotomies and a "hockey stick" or lateral horseshoe incision for more lateral or combination craniotomies. The suboccipital surface is the largest and most accessible of the cerebellar surfaces, and suboccipital AVMs are on the convexity requiring minimal subarachnoid dissection to expose their borders medially, laterally, superiorly, and inferi-

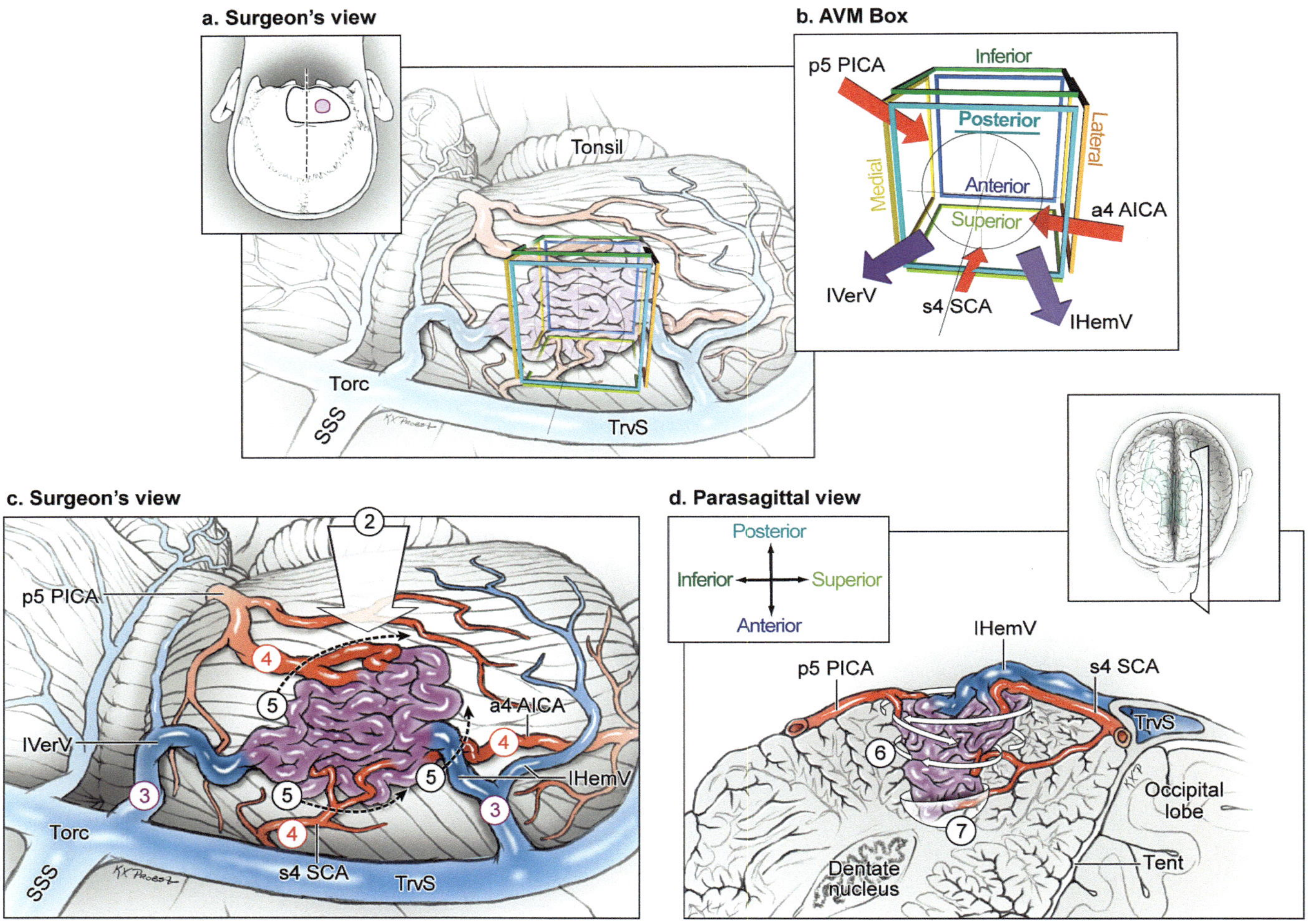

Fig. 17.9 Resection strategy for suboccipital cerebellar AVMs. (**a**) Step 1, exposing the AVM with a lateral suboccipital craniotomy that may be enlarged medially, laterally, or superiorly depending on AVM size [surgeon's view, with the patient in the prone position; scalp incision (*dashed line*), craniotomy (*solid line*), and AVM (*purple circle*) are shown on *inset*]. (**b**) AVM box showing arterial inputs from all three cerebellar arteries and superficial venous drainage through the inferior hemispheric and inferior vermian veins. Note that the AVM's cortical surface is depicted with a circle on its base side and that side's label is underlined. The AVM's axis is depicted with a line through the box. Arterial and venous anatomy is superimposed on the box with red inflow arrows and blue outflow arrows, respectively. (**c**) Step 2, dissecting margins on the suboccipital cerebellar surface (broad white arrow); step 3, identifying ascending veins; step 4, locating feeders from the SCA, AICA, and PICA; and step 5, interrupting the superior, lateral, and inferior fronts near the superior semilunar, inferior semilunar, and biventral lobules, respectively (dashed black arrow, surgeon's view). (**d**) Step 6, circumdissecting into the cerebellar parenchyma (*encircling arrows*); and step 7, mobilizing the AVM to interrupt deep feeders from the SCA and PICA (parasagittal cross-sectional view).

orly (step 2). The cisterna magna (MagnC) is opened to drain cerebrospinal fluid (CSF) and relax the cerebellum. Venous drainage to IHemV and IVerV courses superficially to Torc and TrvS (step 3). Arterial supply through the distal cortical branches from the s4 SCA superiorly, p5 PICA inferiorly, and a4 AICA laterally depends on AVM size and location in the hemisphere (step 4). The SCA feeders are identified as a superior front as they course inferiorly over the superior semilunar lobule (step 5). The PICA feeders are identified as an inferior front as they emerge from the tonsillobiventral fissure and course superiorly over the biventral lobule. The AICA feeders are identified as a lateral front as they course medially over the superior and inferior semilunar lobules. These convexity AVMs have a parallel attack angle with circumferential access to all sides of the nidus and no associated cranial nerves or eloquence, unless they extend to deep cerebellar nuclei (step 6). Deep perforating arteries from the PICA and SCA are encountered along the deep plane of the nidus and may require microclips due to their poor coagulability (step 7) (**Figs. 17.10** and **17.11**).

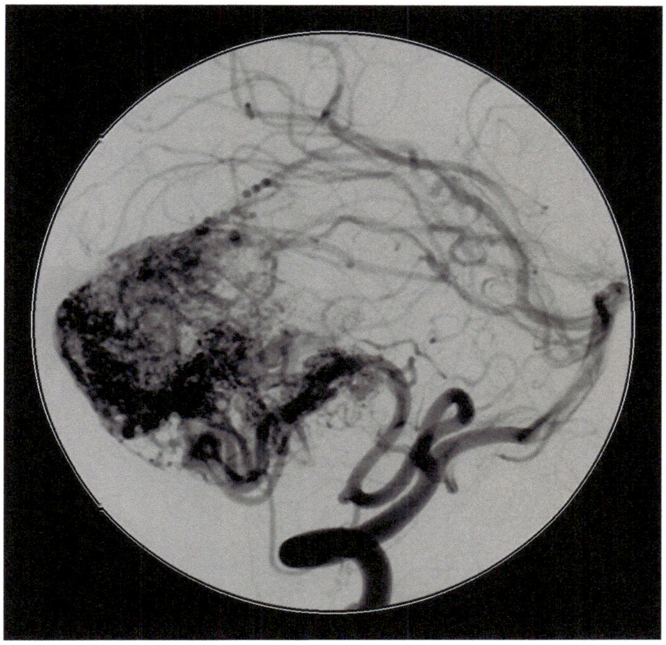

a

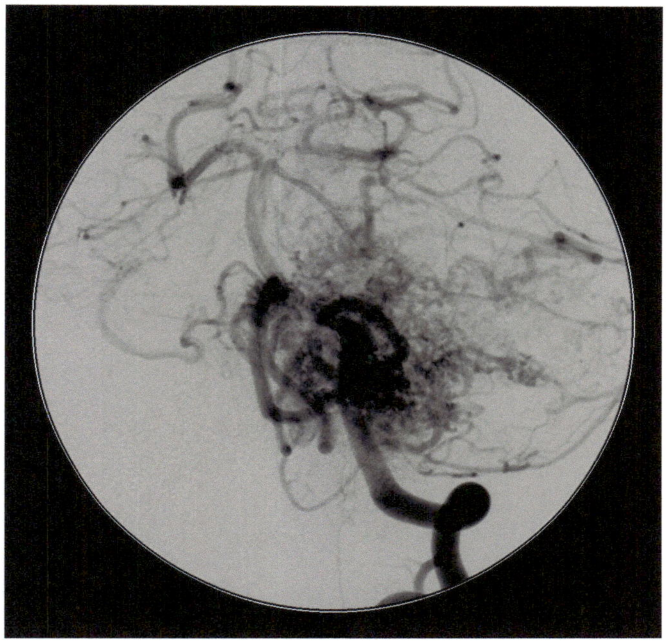

b

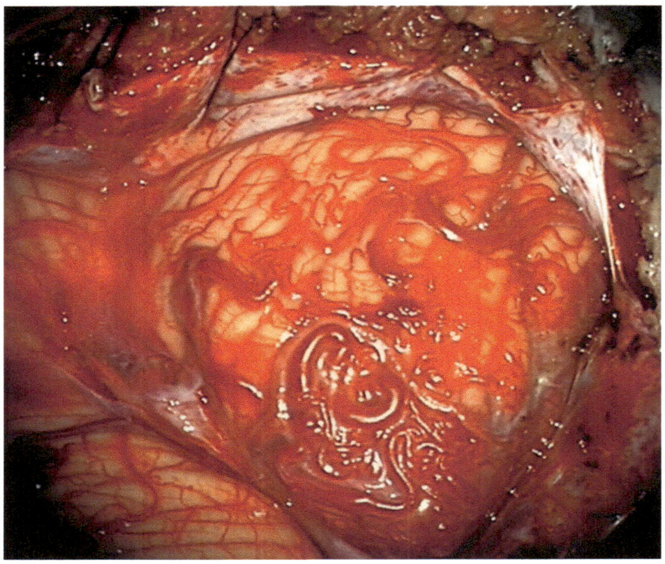

c

Fig. 17.10 This 6-year-old boy presented with a cerebellar hemorrhage from a left suboccipital cerebellar AVM (supplemented Spetzler-Martin grade 6: S2V1E1/A1B0C1), supplied by a large left PICA and smaller SCA branches [left VA angiogram, (**a**) lateral and (**b**) anteroposterior views]. (**c**) The left suboccipital surface was exposed with a torcular craniotomy extending to the foramen magnum, accessing the PICA feeders inferiorly and SCA feeders superiorly (prone position, with vertex at bottom right). (*continued on next page*)

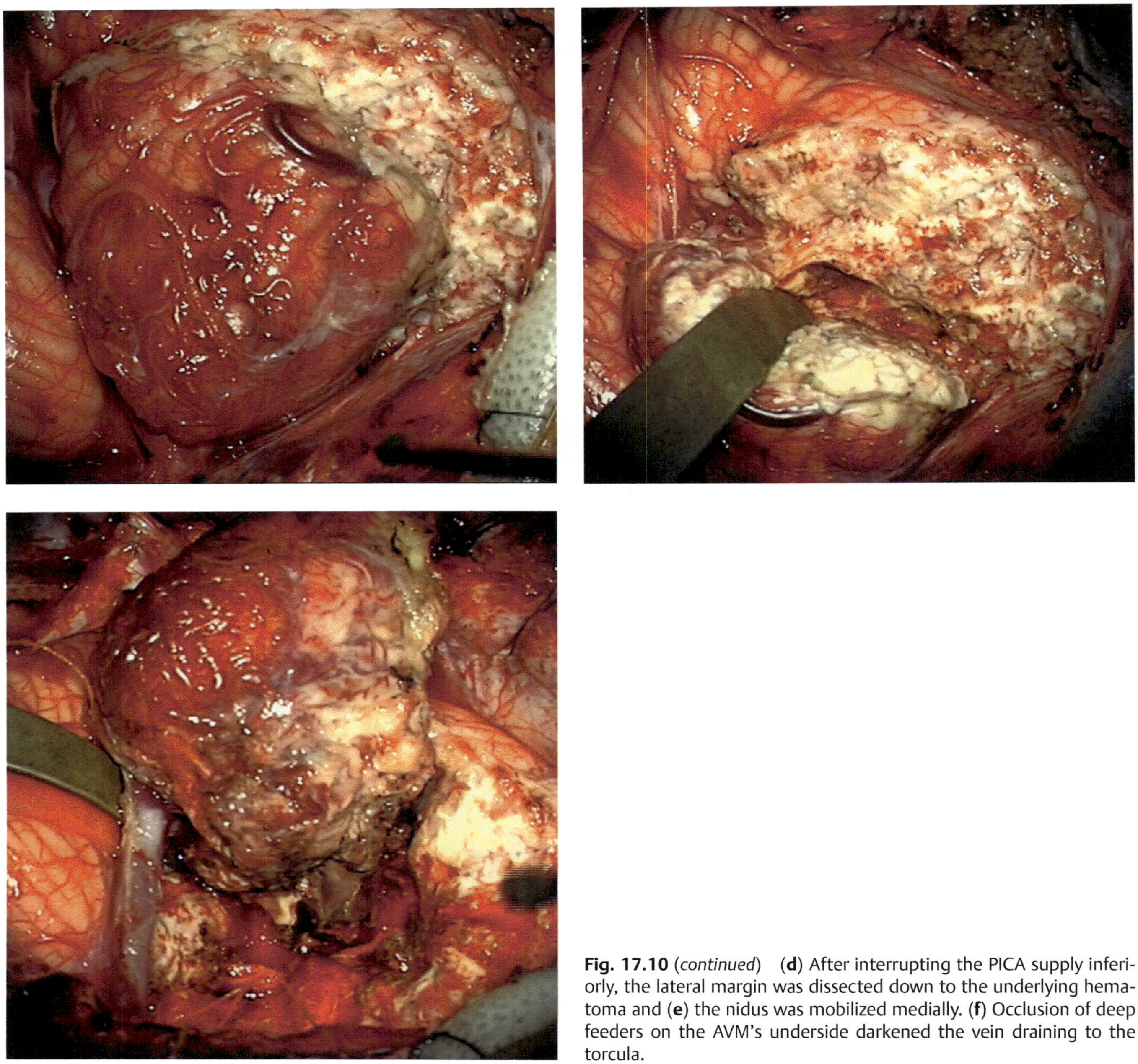

d e f

Fig. 17.10 (*continued*) (**d**) After interrupting the PICA supply inferiorly, the lateral margin was dissected down to the underlying hematoma and (**e**) the nidus was mobilized medially. (**f**) Occlusion of deep feeders on the AVM's underside darkened the vein draining to the torcula.

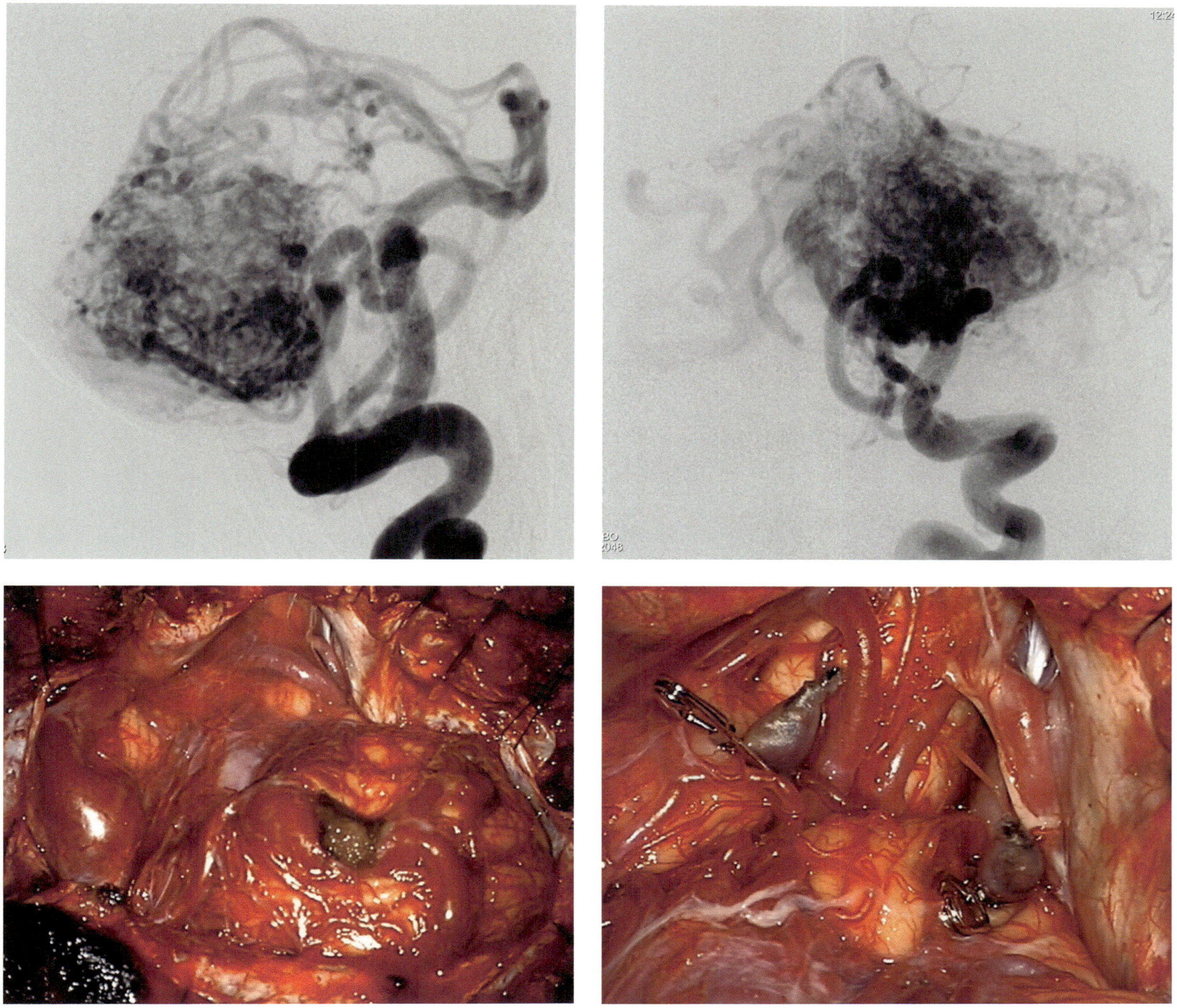

a b c d

Fig. 17.11 This 34-year-old man presented with a left suboccipital cerebellar AVM (supplemented Spetzler-Martin grade 7: S2V1E1/A2B1C0), supplied by the SCA, AICA, and PICA [left VA angiogram, (**a**) lateral and (**b**) anteroposterior views]. (**c**) An extended torcular craniotomy exposed the entire suboccipital surface, and the complex of draining varices was seen over both cerebellar hemispheres. (**d**) A large PICA trunk was occluded with clips and divided in the cisterna magna. (*continued on next page*)

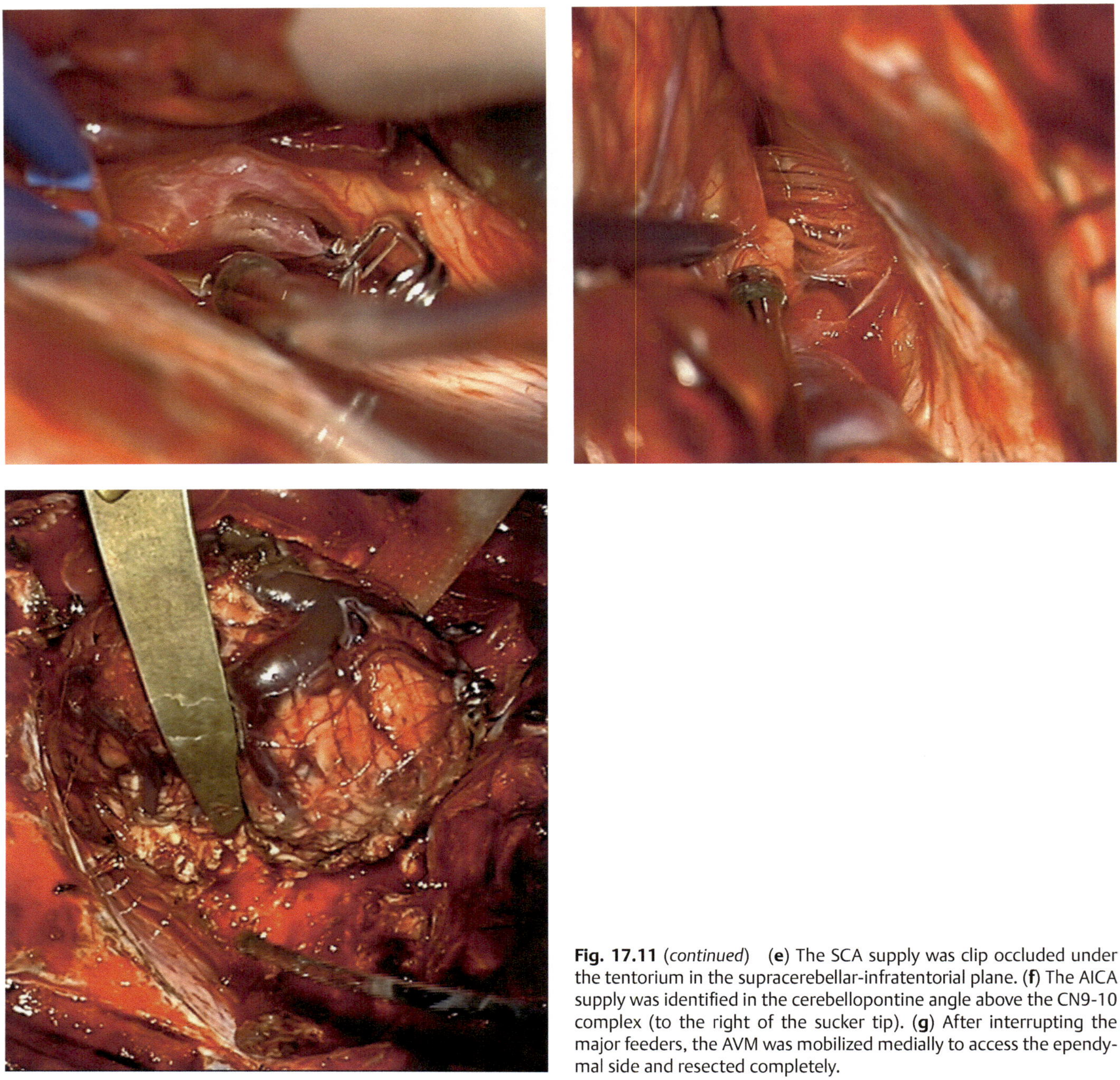

e f g

Fig. 17.11 (*continued*) (**e**) The SCA supply was clip occluded under the tentorium in the supracerebellar-infratentorial plane. (**f**) The AICA supply was identified in the cerebellopontine angle above the CN9-10 complex (to the right of the sucker tip). (**g**) After interrupting the major feeders, the AVM was mobilized medially to access the ependymal side and resected completely.

Tentorial Cerebellar AVM Resection

Tentorial AVMs are resected through torcular craniotomies, which improve access to the tentorial surface, relative to the standard suboccipital craniotomy, by removing the ledge of overhanging bone and lifting the TrvS with tacking sutures on the dural flap (**Fig. 17.12,** step 1). After this craniotomy, the dural flap elevates the sinuses and widens this supracerebellar-infratentorial plane. The AVMs that reach the lateral tentorial surface may require the additional exposure of a retrosigmoid craniotomy, as with a lateral supracerebellar-infratentorial approach. Patient position is prone with the chin tucked as described for suboccipital AVMs. The skin incision is linear, the fascial incision is Y-shaped to create three leaflets for a watertight closure, and the paraspinous muscle incision is T-shaped, as described for anterior medullary AVMs. Release of dense arachnoid adhesions between the posterior border of the tentorial surface and the tentorium

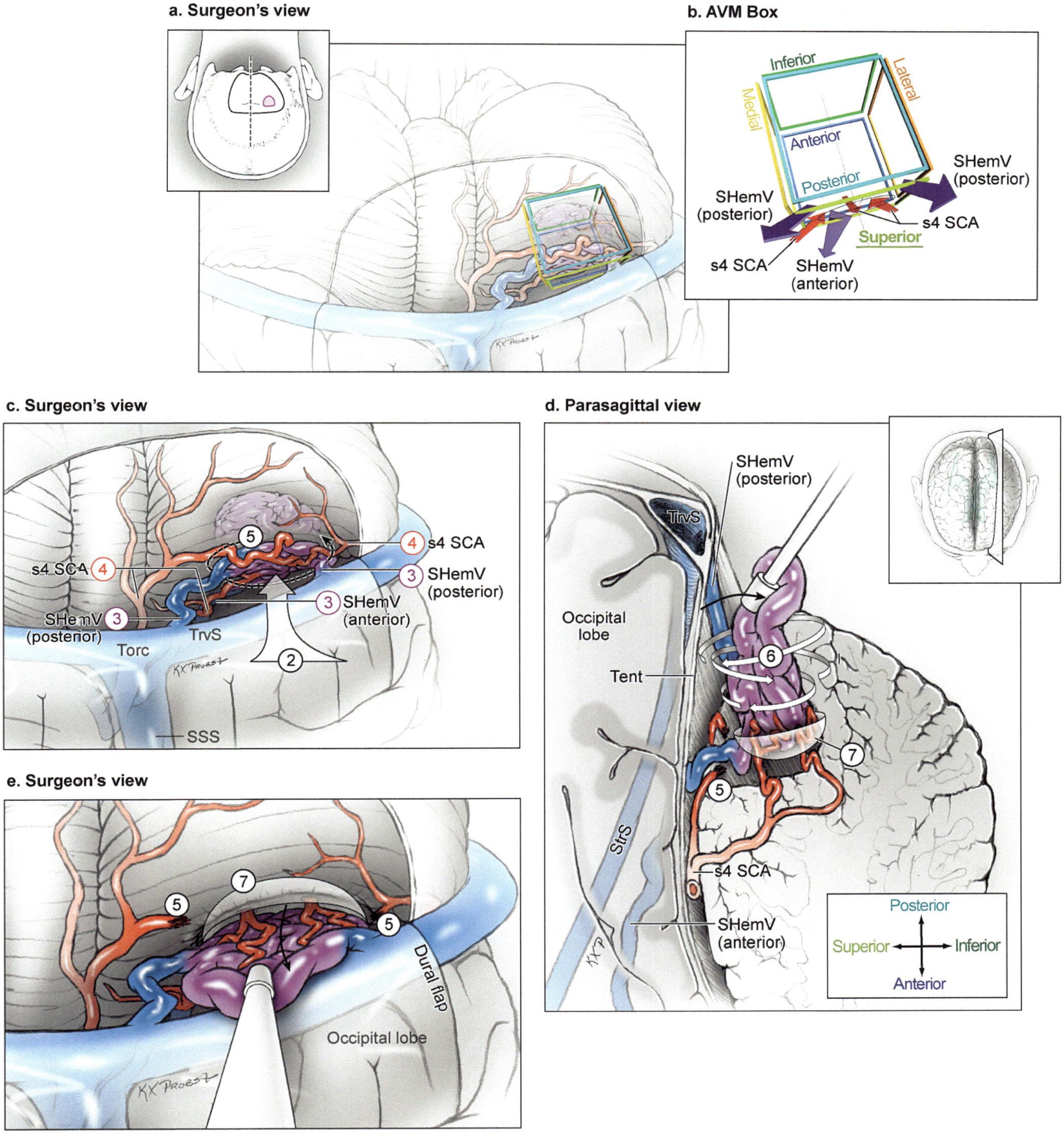

Fig. 17.12 Resection strategy for tentorial cerebellar AVMs. (**a**) Step 1, exposing the AVM with a torcular craniotomy and lateral supracerebellar-infratentorial approach [surgeon's view, with the patient in the prone position; scalp incision (*dashed line*), craniotomy (*solid line*), and AVM (*purple circle*) are shown on *inset*]. (**b**) AVM box showing arterial inputs from the hemispheric branches of the SCA and venous outflow to the superior hemispheric veins. (**c**) Step 2, approaching the AVM in the lateral supracerebellar-infratenorial plane; step 3, identifying the superficial veins (posterior SHemV); step 4, locating the SCA feeders; and step 5, interrupting the anterior front along the quadrangular lobule (surgeon's view). (**d**) Step 6, circumdissecting inferiorly into the cerebellar parenchyma (parasagittal cross-sectional view). (**e**) Step 7, mobilizing the AVM superiorly to visualize deep SCA feeders and anterior superior hemispheric veins (surgeon's view).

begins the dissection over the cerebellum (step 2). The MagnC is opened to drain CSF and relax the cerebellum. Bridging veins to the tentorium can be sacrificed if they do not drain the AVM. Dissection deepens to the AVM, which can be superficial in the superior semilunar lobule or deeper in the quadrangular lobule. The draining SHemV is easily visualized on the tentorial surface when it courses superficially to Torc, StrS, or TentS (posterior SHemV), but may be more difficult to visualize when it courses deep to the VoG (anterior SHemV) (step 3). Tentorial AVMs are fed unilaterally by distal cortical SCA branches (step 4) that can be interrupted early in the supracerebellar-infratentorial dissection anteri-

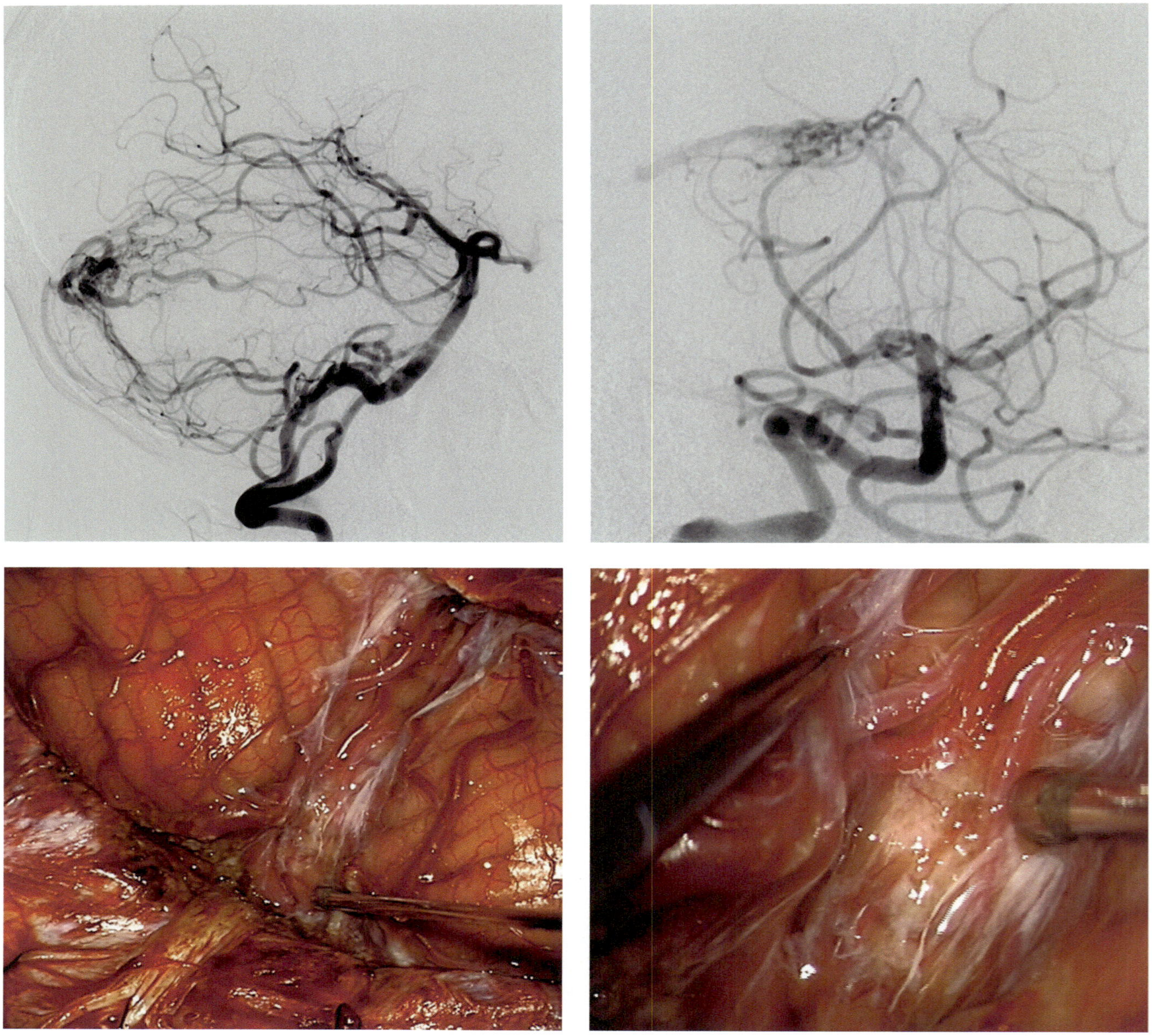

a b c d

Fig. 17.13 This 77-year-old woman presented with a cerebellar hemorrhage from a right tentorial cerebellar AVM (supplemented Spetzler-Martin grade 5: S1V1E0/A3B0C0), supplied bidirectionally by the PICA and SCA [right VA angiogram, (**a**) lateral and (**b**) anteroposterior views]. (**c**) The tentorial surface of the cerebellum was accessed through a torcular craniotomy (patient prone, with the vertex at bottom), with only the AVM's arterialized draining vein apparent on the suboccipital surface. (**d**) The PICA feeders ascended along the inferior vermis to reach the nidus.

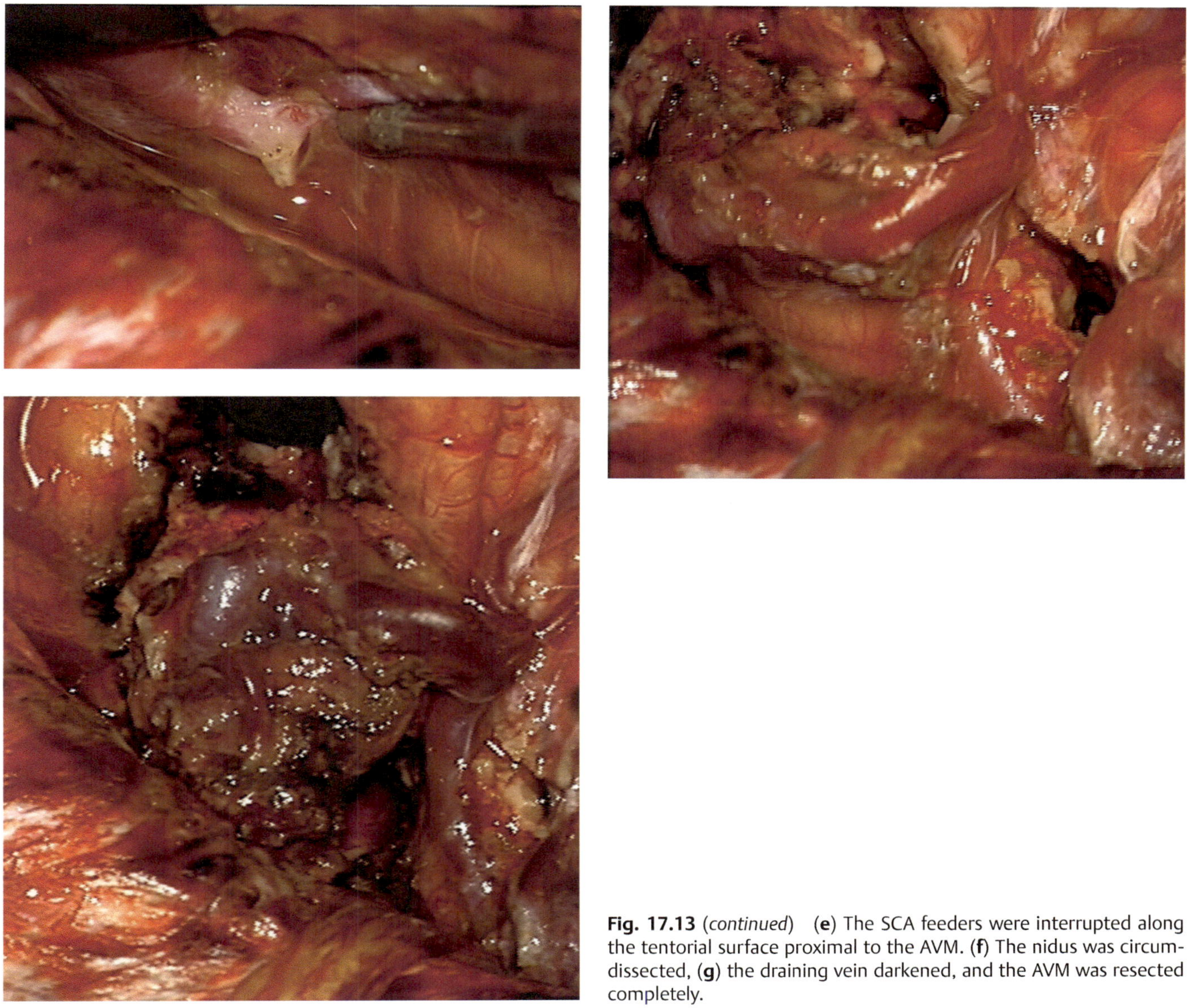

e

f

g

Fig. 17.13 (*continued*) (**e**) The SCA feeders were interrupted along the tentorial surface proximal to the AVM. (**f**) The nidus was circumdissected, (**g**) the draining vein darkened, and the AVM was resected completely.

orly along the quadrangular lobule (step 5). The draining vein may be centered in the surgical field and the parenchymal dissection deepens around it (step 6). This perpendicular approach may require a cortical incision into the cerebellum that helps visualize the posterior and inferior margins. Evacuation of associated hemispheric hematomas facilitates this perpendicular dissection. The AVM is mobilized upward out of the hemisphere toward the tentorium to visualize the deep plane and its connections to SCA feeders and the anterior SHemV (step 7). Tentorial AVMs are non-eloquent, but may extend anteriorly near the midbrain and CN4 (**Figs. 17.13** and **17.14**).

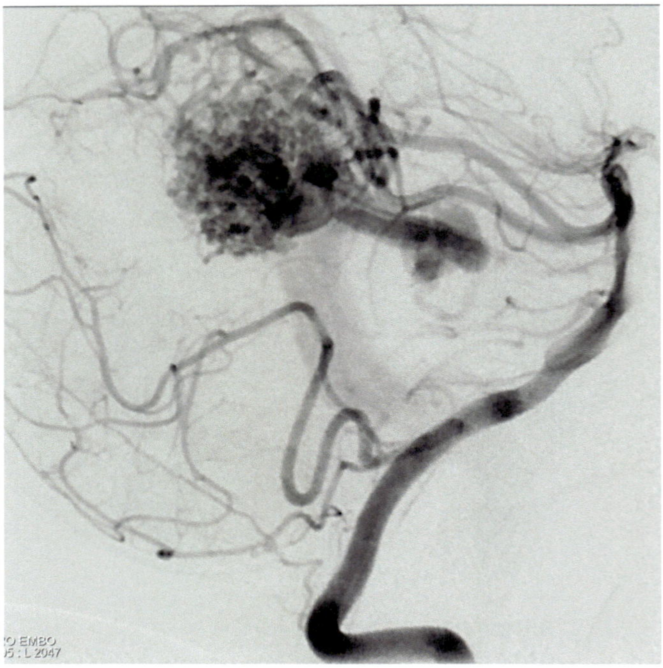

a

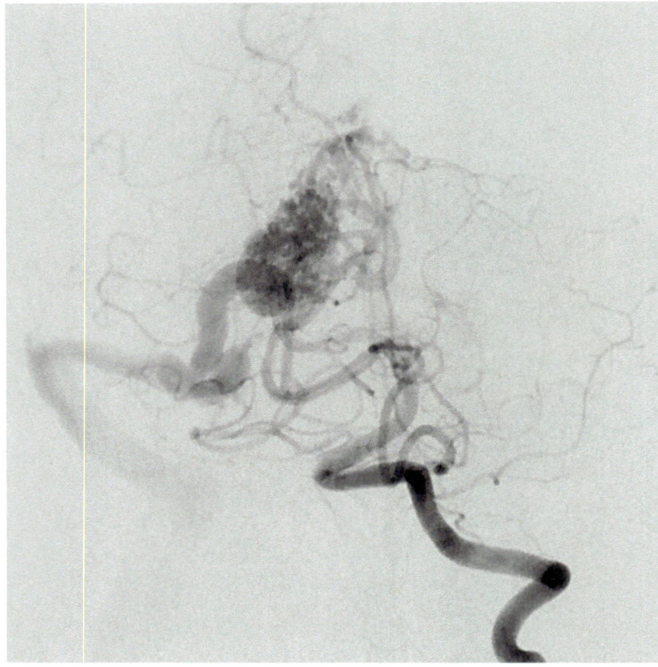

b

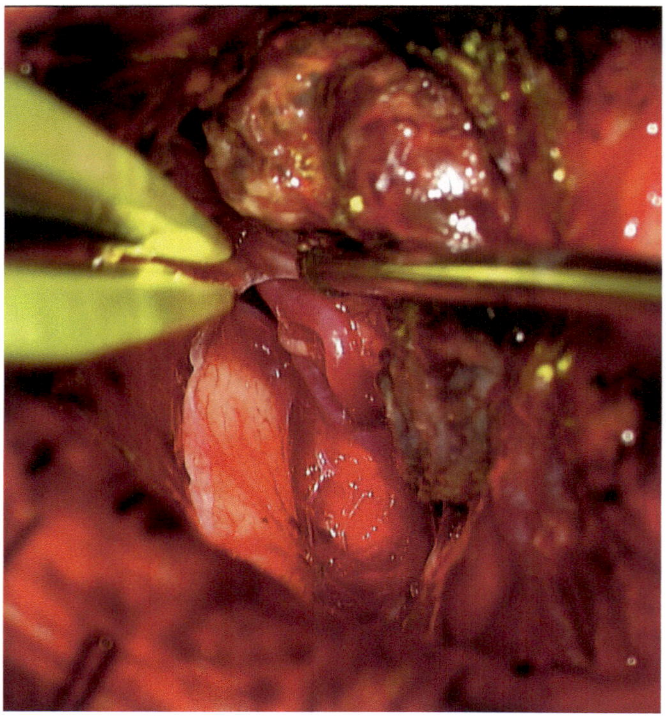

c

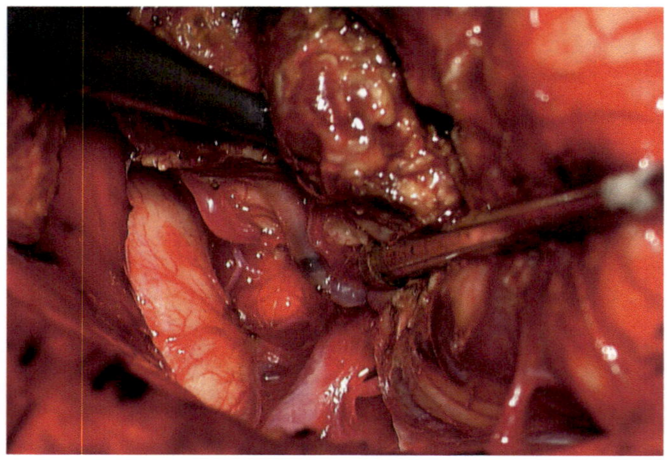

d

Fig. 17.14 This 51-year-old woman presented with a right tentorial cerebellar AVM (supplemented Spetzler-Martin grade 6: S1V1E0/A3B1C0), situated anteriorly on the tentorial surface and supplied only by the right SCA (no PICA supply) [right VA angiogram, (**a**) lateral and (**b**) anteroposterior views]. (**c**) After resecting some cerebellum to reach the inferior margin of the AVM, the arachnoid over the cerebellomesencephalic fissure was opened to identify the SCA feeders emerging from this fissure. (**d**) These lateral SCA feeders were cauterized and divided.

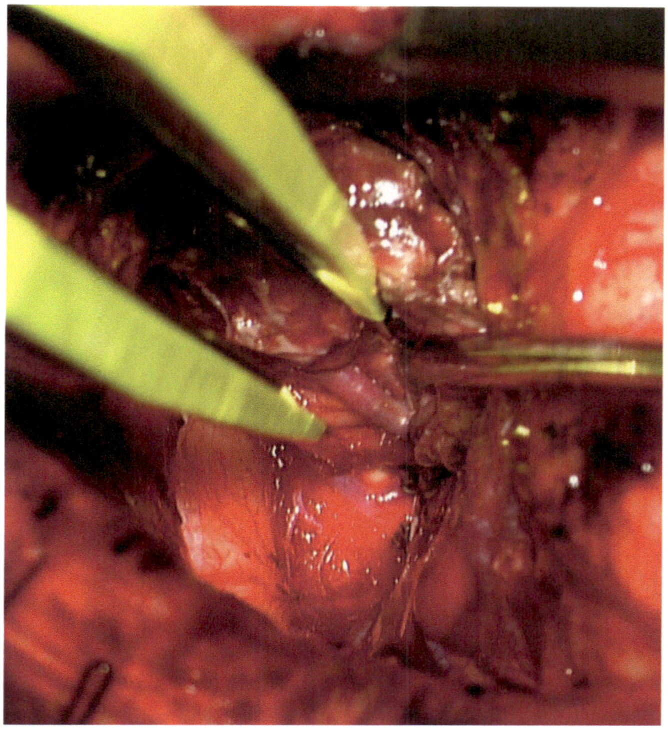
e

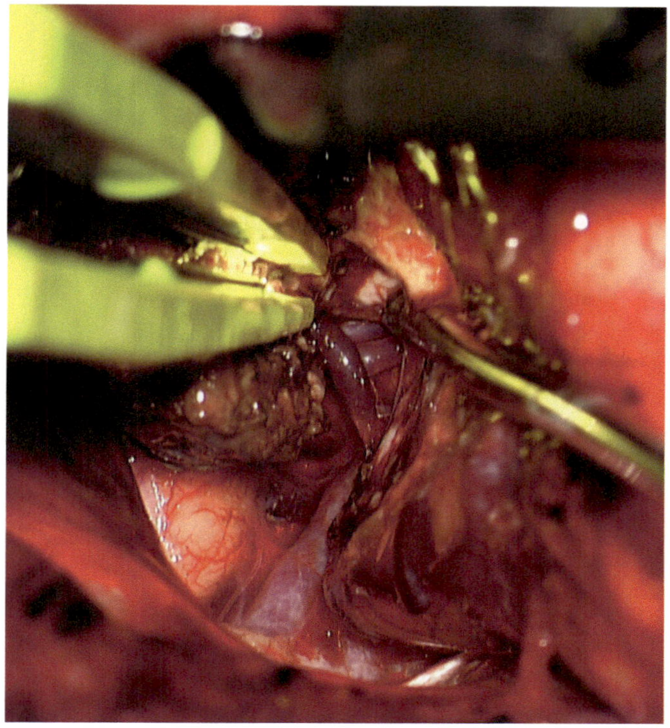
f

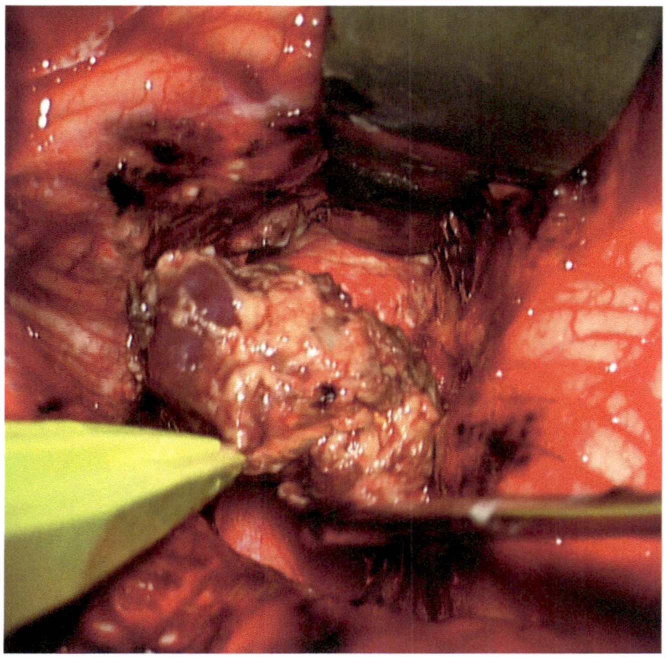
g

Fig. 17.14 (*continued*) (**e,f**) The medial SCA feeders from the cerebellomesencephalic fissure were also identified and interrupted, (**g**) freeing the AVM for resection.

Vermian Cerebellar AVM Resection

Vermian AVMs are also resected through torcular craniotomies (**Fig. 17.15,** step 1), which gain access to both the suboccipital and tentorial surfaces in the midline. The suboccipital part of the vermis (tuber, pyramid, uvula, and nodule) is superficial and easily accessed as a convexity lesion, but the tentorial part (culmen, declive, and folium) is deep and requires subarachnoid dissection in the midline supracerebellar-infratentorial plane (step 2). The ascending slope of the tentorial part of the vermis requires significant neck flexion when positioning the head, tucking the chin two fingerbreadths from the manubrium with the patient in the prone position to align the tentorium vertically. Alterna-

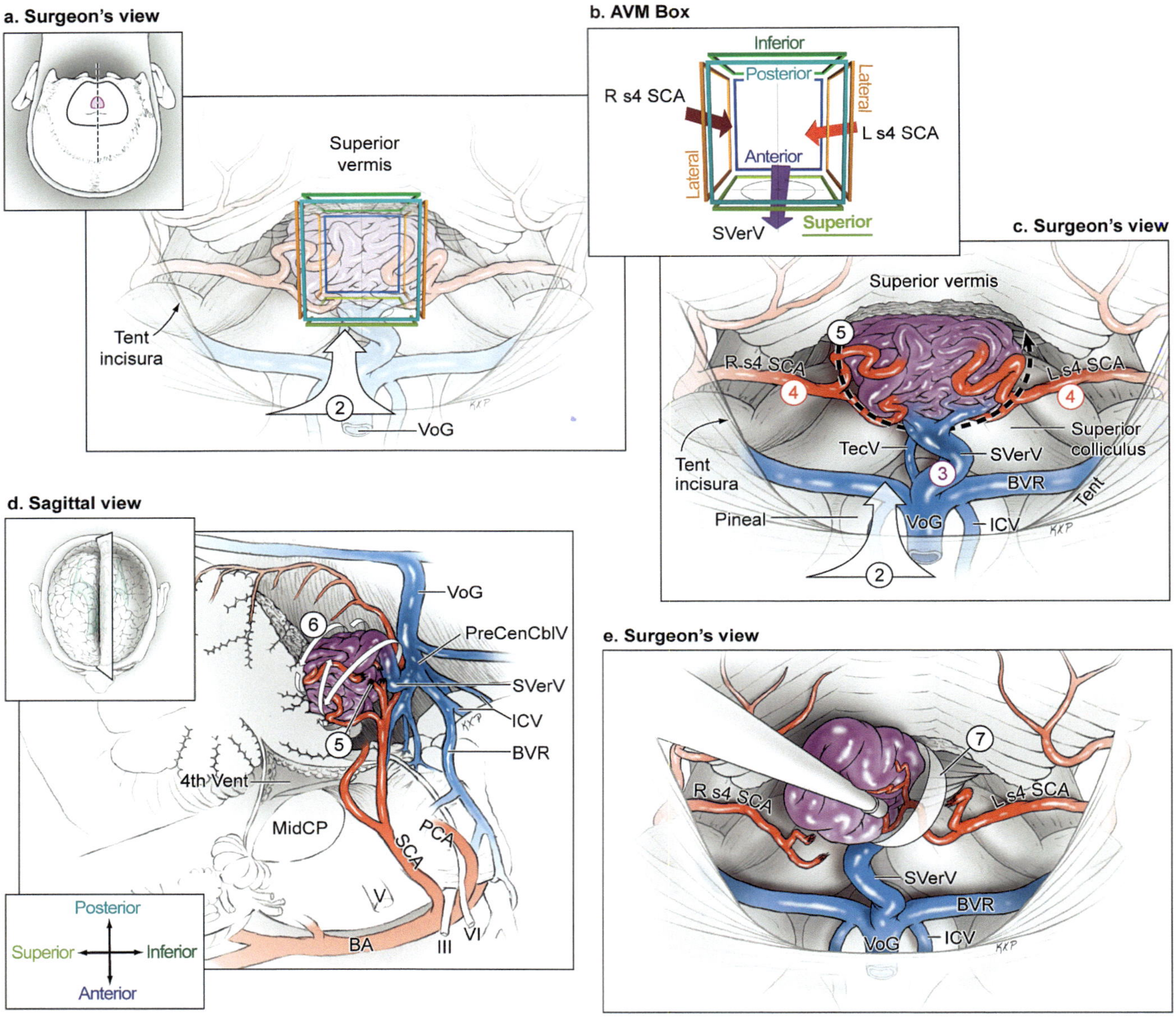

Fig. 17.15 Resection strategy for vermian cerebellar AVMs. (**a**) Step 1, exposing the AVM with a torcular craniotomy and midline supracerebellar-infratentorial approach [surgeon's view, with the patient in the prone position; scalp incision (*dashed line*), craniotomy (*solid line*), and AVM (*purple circle*) are shown on *inset*]. (**b**) AVM box showing arterial inputs bilaterally from the SCA and deep venous drainage to SVerV. (**c**) Step 2, approaching the AVM in the midline supracerebellar-infratentorial plane; step 3, identifying the ascending drainage to the VoG; step 4, locating the SCA feeders bilaterally; and step 5, interrupting the anterior front along the anterolateral margins of the superior vermis (surgeon's view). (**d**) Step 6, circumdissecting inferiorly into vermian parenchyma (parasagittal cross-sectional view). (**e**) Step 7, mobilizing the AVM laterally to enter the cerebellomesencephalic fissure and divide the anterior SCA feeders (surgeon's view).

tively, small AVMs at the apex of the vermis or anteriorly next to the quadrigeminal cistern can be approached with the patient in the sitting position, which facilitates subarachnoid dissection with gravity retraction of the cerebellum and a wide-open supracerebellar-infratentorial plane. Subarachnoid dissection of superior vermian AVMs extends to the posterior arachnoid of the quadrigeminal cistern (QuadC) on both sides of the vermian apex and to the cerebellomesencephalic fissure where the cortical the s4 SCA branches emerge. Cerebrospinal fluid drainage from these cisterns relaxes the cerebellum and opens the infratentorial plane. Superior vermian AVMs drain deep to SVerV and VoG, which are easily avoided, whereas inferior vermian AVMs drain superficially to IVerV and Torc, which are centered in the surgical corridor (step 3). Vermian AVMs attract a bilateral feeding artery supply from the SCA in the superior vermis and the PICA in the inferior vermis (step 4). The SCA feeders form an anterior front that is interrupted along the anterolateral AVM margins in the superior vermis, preserving more proximal branches to the tectum and posterior midbrain (step 5). The PICA feeders form an inferior front that is interrupted along the inferolateral AVM margins in the inferior vermis. The attack angle is parallel with inferior vermian AVMs but perpendicular with superior vermian AVMs, requiring some transgression of the posterior vermis to access their inferior margin (step 6). Vermian AVMs are not considered eloquent unless they extend to the cerebellar nuclei; however, division of the vermis can cause cerebellar mutism. With the AVM tethered to its ascending draining vein, accessing the deep anterior plane requires mobilization of the nidus from side to side (step 7). Deep dissection can extend into the cerebellomesencephalic fissure, where CN4, tectum, and midbrain perforators are protected (**Figs. 17.16** and **17.17**).

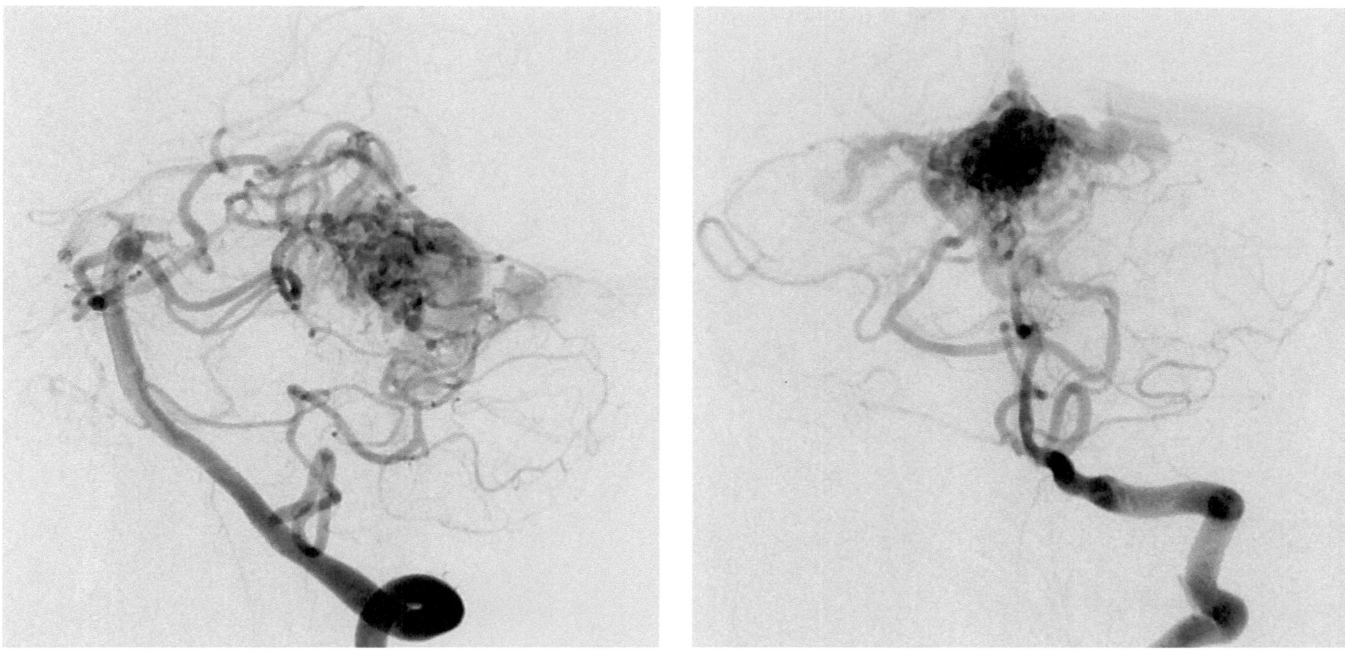

a b

Fig. 17.16 This 61-year-old man presented with the vermian cerebellar AVM (supplemented Spetzler-Martin grade 7: S2V1E0/A3B1C0), situated on the posterior downslope of the superior vermis and supplied by both the SCA and PICA bilaterally [left VA angiogram, (**a**) lateral and (**b**) anteroposterior views]. (*continued on next page*)

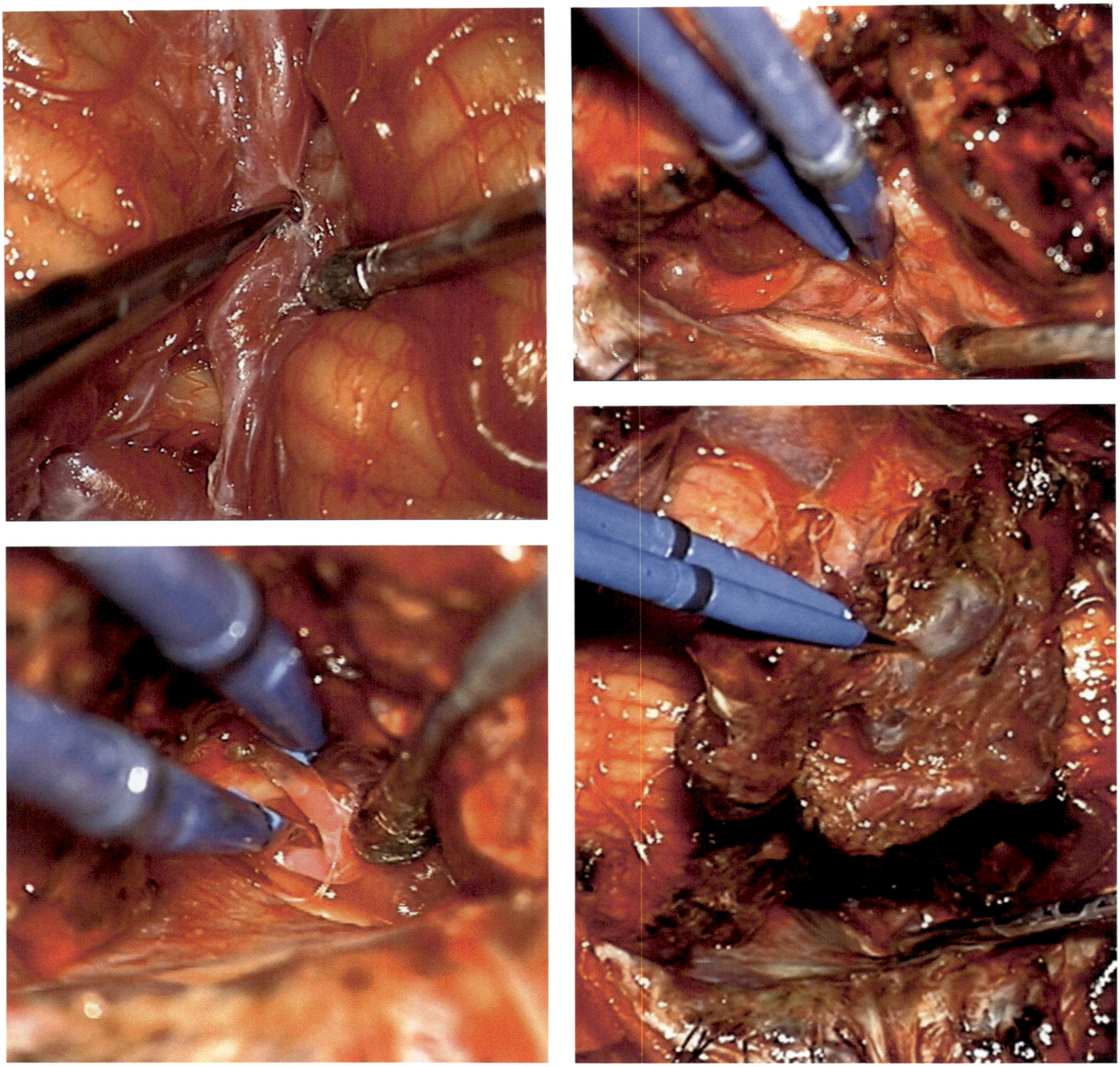

c d e f

Fig. 17.16 (*continued*) (**c**) The PICA feeders ascended in the posterior cerebellar incisura and were coagulated at the AVM margin inferiorly. (**d**) The supracerebellar-infratentorial plane was opened and (**e**) the SCA feeders were interrupted at the AVM margin anteriorly. **(f)** The AVM was resected completely.

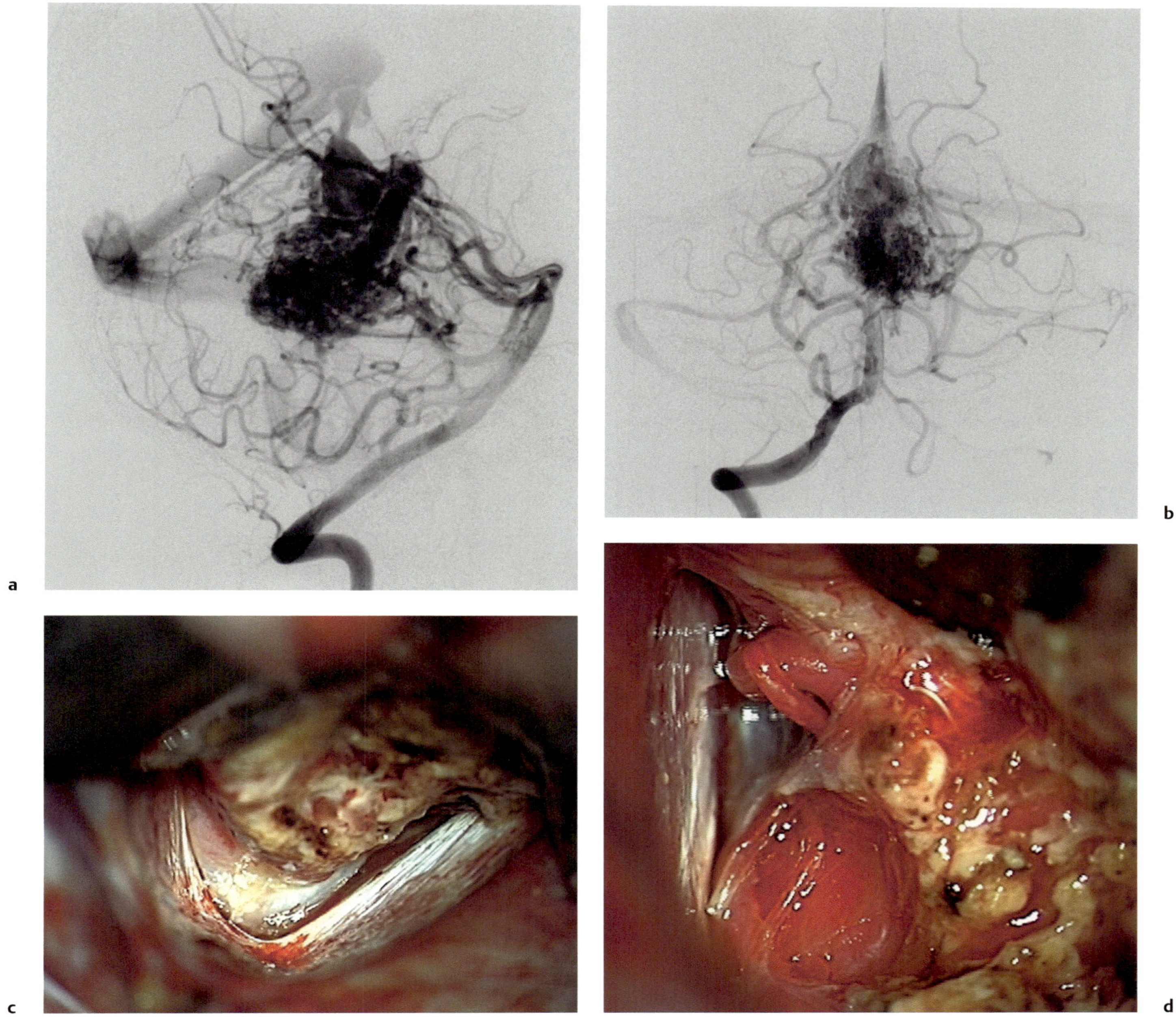

Fig. 17.17 This 28-year-old woman presented with an intraventricular hemorrhage from a vermian cerebellar AVM (supplemented Spetzler-Martin grade 5: S2V1E0/A2B0C0), situated on the anterior downslope of superior vermis, supplied by the SCA bilaterally and drained by PreCenCblV [right VA angiogram, (**a**) lateral and (**b**) anteroposterior views]. (**c**) A torcular craniotomy and supracerebellar-infratentorial approach (prone position, the vertex at bottom) opened a surgical corridor along the triangular roof of the tentorium to the quadrigeminal cistern. (**d**) Dissection into the vermis to the right of the midline exposed the arterialized draining vein and an SCA feeding artery. *(continued on next page)*

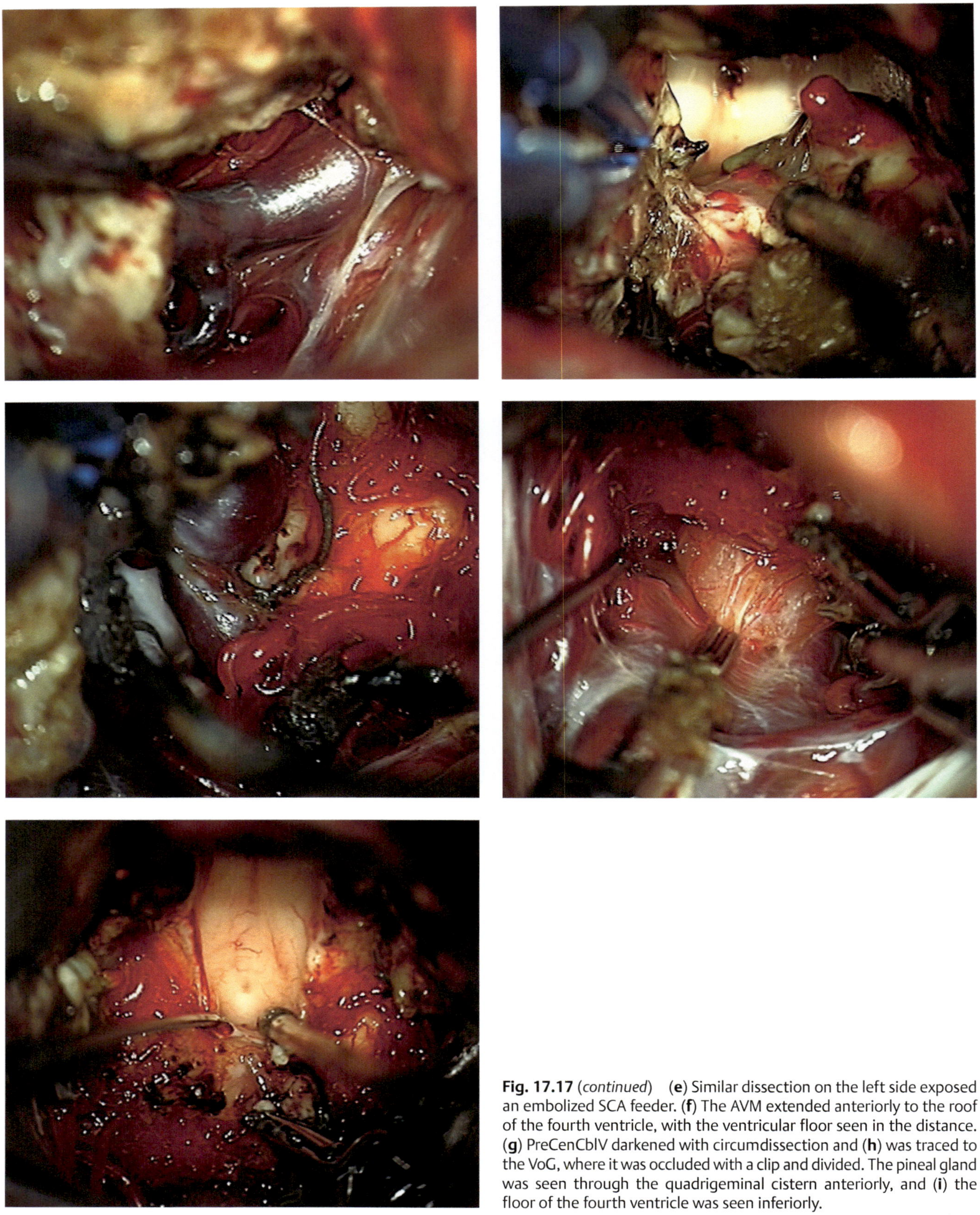

Fig. 17.17 (*continued*) (**e**) Similar dissection on the left side exposed an embolized SCA feeder. (**f**) The AVM extended anteriorly to the roof of the fourth ventricle, with the ventricular floor seen in the distance. (**g**) PreCenCblV darkened with circumdissection and (**h**) was traced to the VoG, where it was occluded with a clip and divided. The pineal gland was seen through the quadrigeminal cistern anteriorly, and (**i**) the floor of the fourth ventricle was seen inferiorly.

Tonsillar Cerebellar AVM Resection

Tonsillar AVMs are paramedian and small, and they are exposed with a standard suboccipital craniotomy (**Fig. 17.18**, step 1). Subarachnoid dissection includes opening the MagnC, widening the vallecula to separate the tonsils, opening the cerebellomedullary fissure, and splitting the tonsillobiventral fissure (step 2). These maneuvers circumferentially mobilize the tonsil and gain control of the PICA as it courses around the medulla. Drainage courses through the tonsillar veins: the medial and lateral TonsV drain to the superior and inferior ReTonsV, which collect in IVerV en route to Torc and TrvS (step 3). Upward retraction on the inferior pole of the tonsillar AVM exposes the PICA proximally for early in-

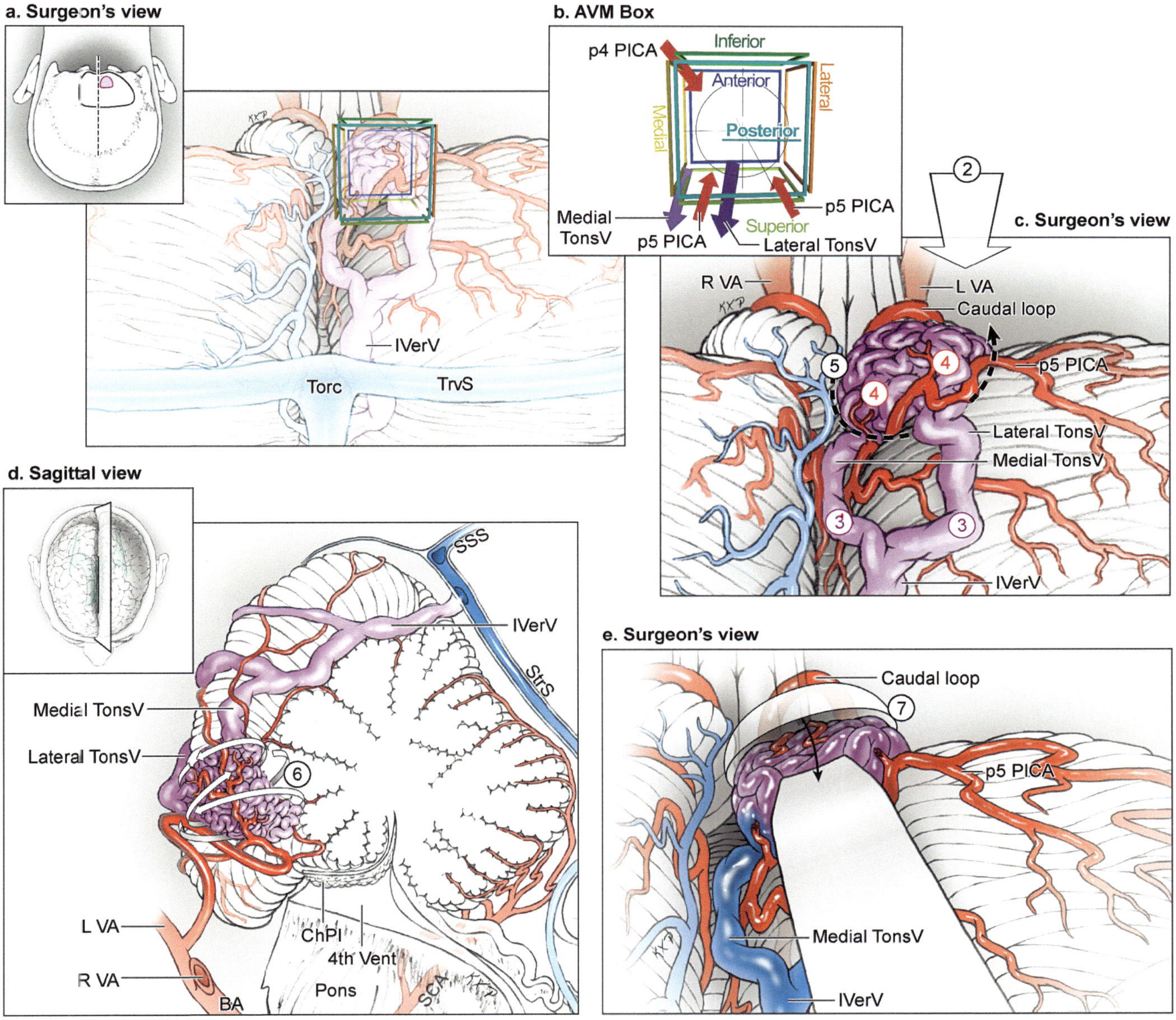

Fig. 17.18 Resection strategy for tonsillar cerebellar AVMs. (**a**) Step 1, exposing the AVM with a suboccipital craniotomy [surgeon's view, with the patient in the prone position; scalp incision (*dashed line*), craniotomy (*solid line*), and AVM (*purple circle*) are shown on *inset*]. (**b**) AVM box showing arterial inputs from the ipsilateral PICA and drainage through the tonsillar veins. (**c**) Step 2, opening the cerebellomedullary fissure, tonsillobiventral fissure, and vallecula to free the tonsillar borders; step 3, identifying the draining tonsillar veins; step 4, locating the PICA and its tonsillar branches feeding the AVM; and step 5, skeletonizing the PICA to interrupt the superior front (surgeon's view). (**d**) Step 6, circumdissecting superolaterally across the tonsillar peduncle (sagittal cross-sectional view). (**e**) Step 7, mobilizing the AVM superiorly to disconnect the AVM anteriorly (surgeon's view).

terruption of the tonsillar arteries feeding the AVM (step 4). The cranial loop of the PICA courses over the superior pole of the tonsil with feeding arteries originating from the p4 and p5 PICA segments and forming a superior front of arteries (step 5). The PICA frequently terminates in the AVM, but distal en passage arteries are preserved when present. Tonsillar surfaces are free except for the attachment to the cerebellum superolaterally through the tonsillar peduncle, keeping parenchymal dissection to a minimum (step 6). Tonsillar AVMs are non-eloquent, but deep dissection is adjacent to the medulla and CN9/10/11 (step 7) (**Fig. 17.19**).

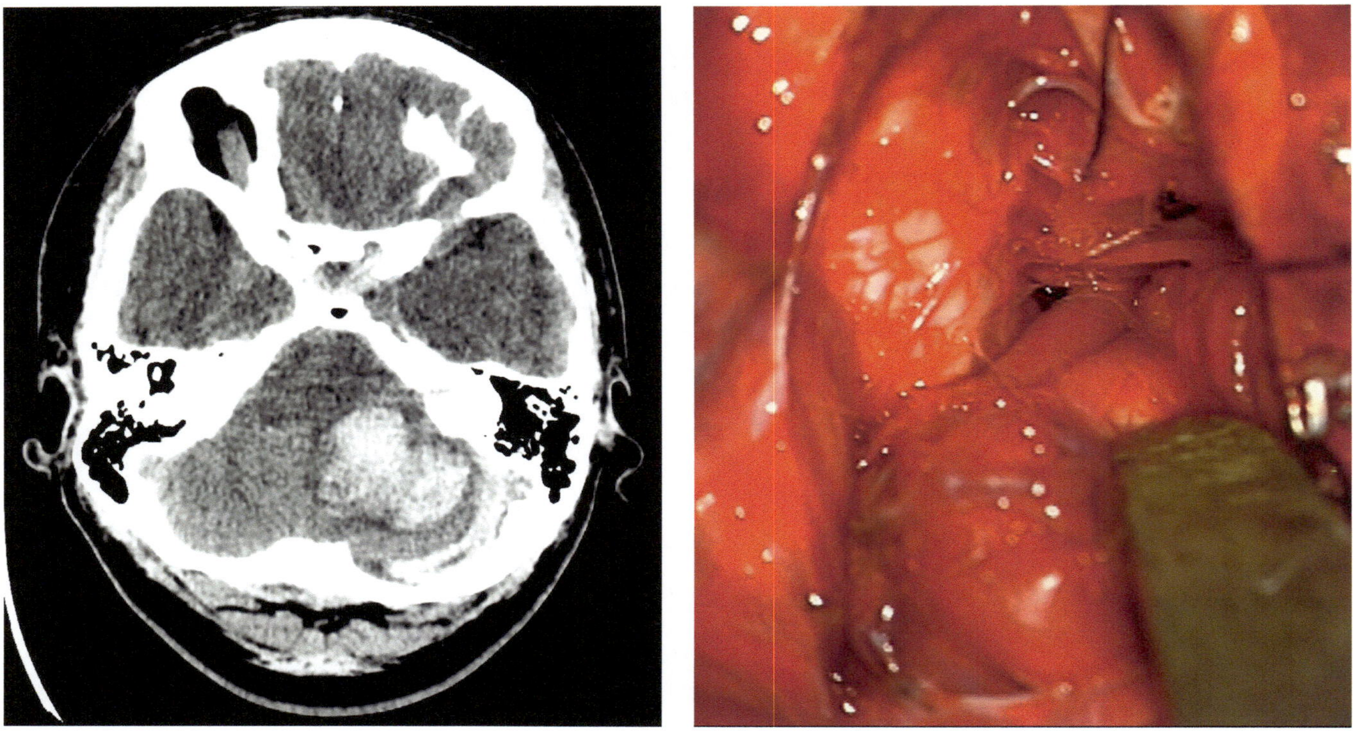

a b

Fig. 17.19 This 31-year-old woman presented with headache and acutely decompensated in the emergency room, from speaking normally to flexor posturing. (**a**) Axial computed tomography (CT) scan demonstrated a large left cerebellar hemorrhage and she was taken to the operating room directly. (**b**) After exposing the cerebellum through a suboccipital craniotomy, an AVM was found in the left tonsil supplied by an enlarged left PICA seen in the cerebellomedullary fissure (supplemented Spetzler-Martin grade 4: S1V1E0/A2B0C0).

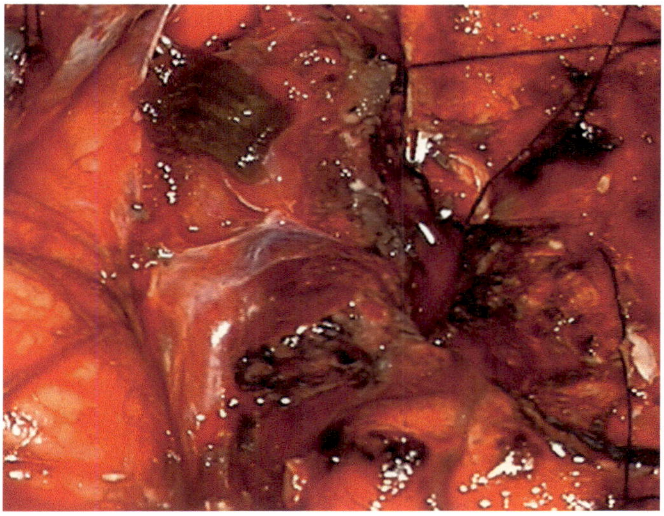
c

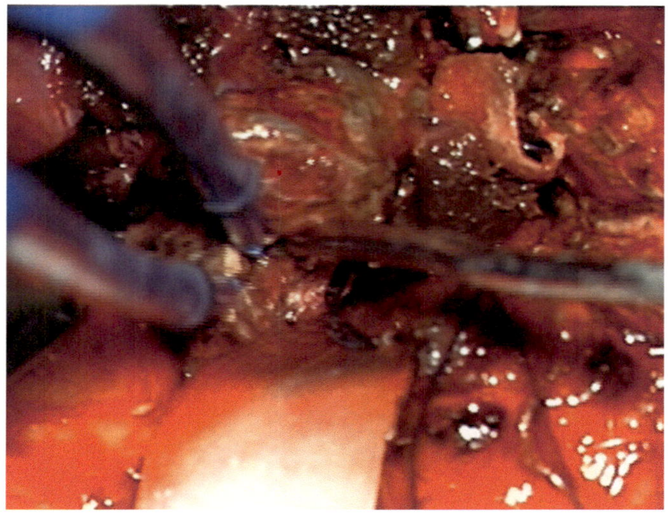
d

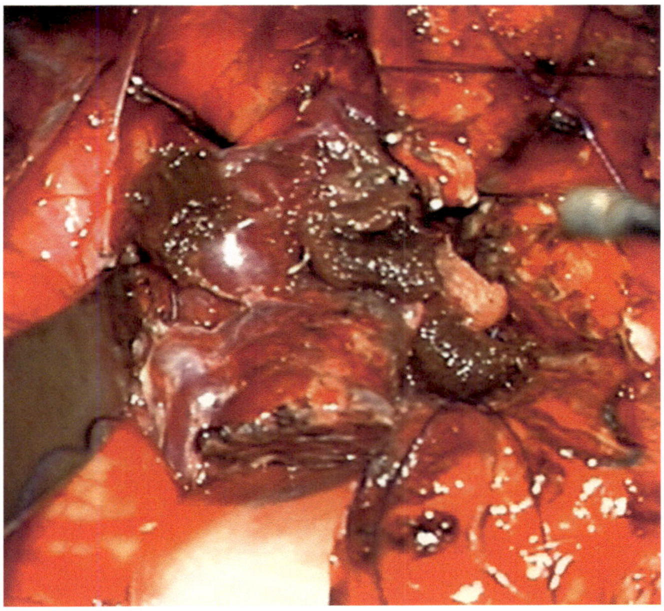
e

Fig. 17.19 (*continued*) (**c**) The PICA feeder was divided and the hematoma was evacuated laterally. (**d**) The AVM was dissected circumferentially, after which the draining tonsillar vein was divided superiorly and (**e**) the AVM was removed.

Petrosal Cerebellar AVM Resection

Petrosal AVMs are accessed through an extended retrosigmoid approach that skeletonizes SigmS from the transverse-sigmoid junction to the jugular bulb, allowing the dural flap to pull the sinus anteriorly and maximize the opening into the cerebellopontine angle (**Fig. 17.20,** step 1). This craniotomy minimizes the need for fixed retraction. Subarachnoid dissection opens the arachnoid of the brainstem cisterns, including CbPonC, PonC, CbMedC, and MedC (step 2). Dissection is centered around CN7/8 and the AICA, but extends superiorly to CN5 when the SCA contributes to the AVM and inferiorly to CN9/10/11 when the PICA contributes. Petrosal AVMs are cerebellar rather than pontine, and therefore reside lateral to CN7/8. The AVM drainage is deep via AHemV and VCPonF, which course to SPetrV (Dandy's vein) and SPS (step 3). The AICA feeders arise from the a3 and a4 segments (step 4) and are interrupted early by advancing medial to the nidus (step 5). However, many of these medial feeders cannot be visualized early in the resection, and their interruption must wait until the deep dissection. The approach trajectory is perpendicular rather than parallel, which means that the lateral and posterior AVM margins are accessed at the expense of some overlying cerebellum. An incision in the cerebellar cortex is made lateral to the AVM and some intervening lobule is resected to reach the lateral AVM margin and open a seam to the medial side. With ruptured AVMs, hemispheric hematomas may have already opened

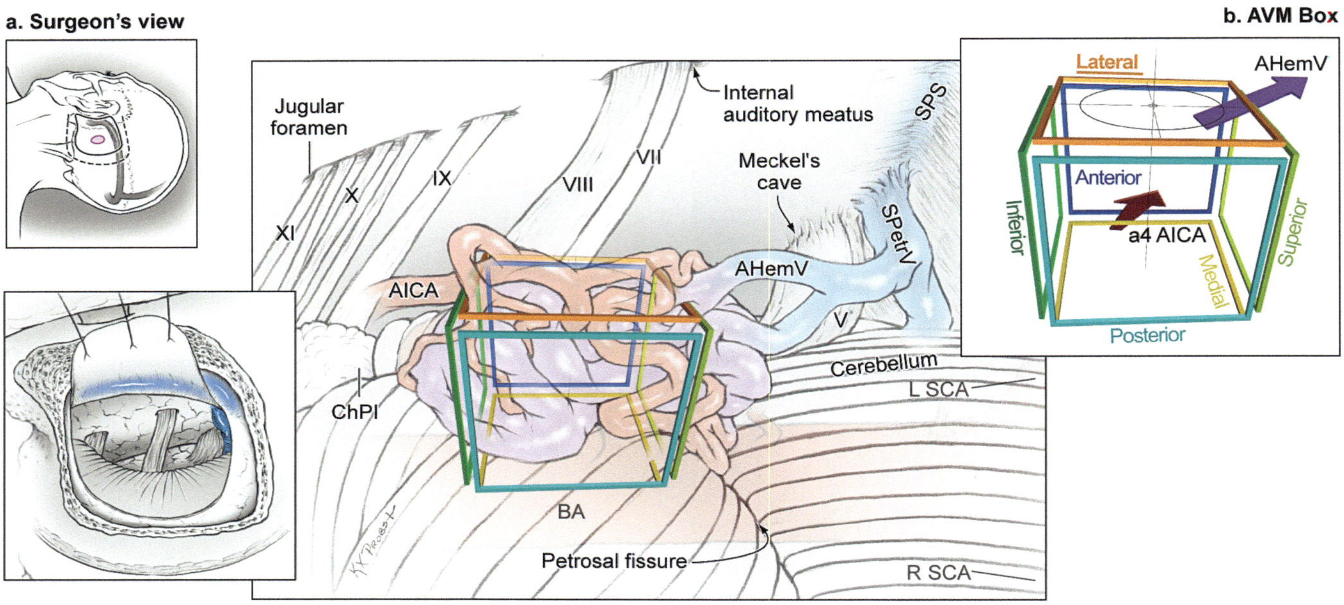

Fig. 17.20 Resection strategy for petrosal cerebellar AVMs. (**a**) Step 1, exposing the AVM with an extended retrosigmoid craniotomy that includes limited mastoidectomy and skeletonization of the sigmoid sinus [surgeon's view, with scalp incision (*dashed line*), craniotomy (*solid line*), and AVM (*purple circle*) shown on *upper inset,* and dural flap mobilizing the skeletonized SigmS anteriorly shown on *lower inset*). (**b**) AVM box showing arterial inputs from cortical branches of the AICA and drainage by anterior hemispheric veins, the vein of the cerebellopontine fissure, and the petrosal vein.

c. Surgeon's view

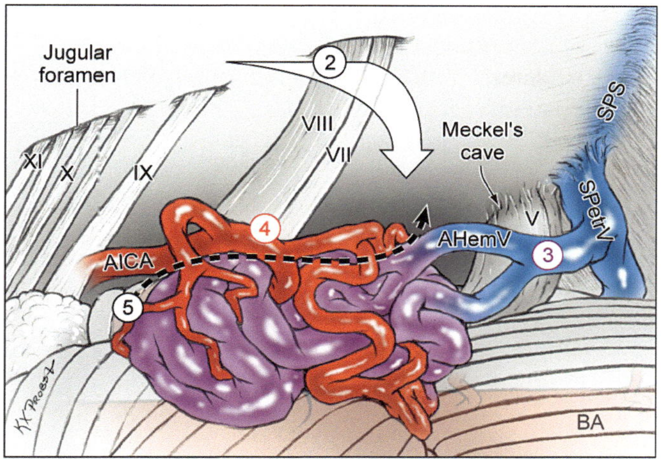

d. Superior view

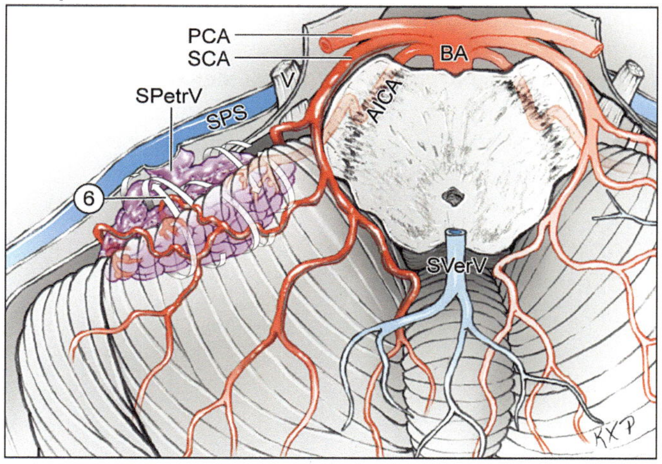

e. Surgeon's view

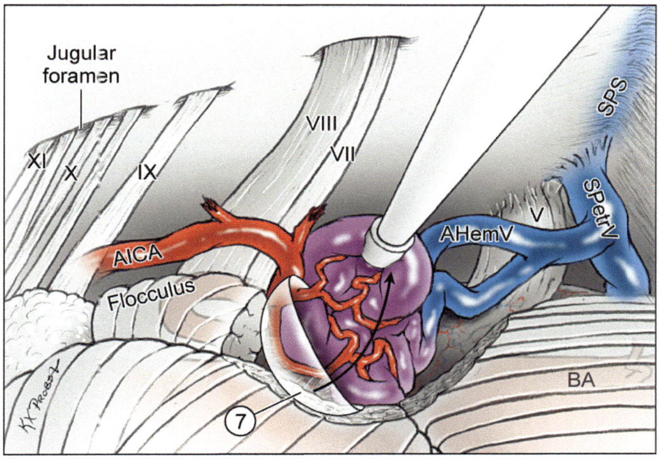

Fig. 17.20 (*continued*) (**c**) Step 2, approaching the AVM through the cerebellopontine cistern; step 3, identifying the draining veins ascending medially; step 4, locating the AICA feeders lateral to CN7/8; and step 5, interrupting the medial front near the flocculus (surgeon's view). (**d**) Step 6, circumdissecting the lateral, superior, and inferior margins in the cerebellum ("back door" technique, superior view of the cerebellum). (**e**) Step 7, mobilizing the AVM anteriorly to dissect the posterior and medial planes and divide the medial AICA feeders (surgeon's view).

this seam, and early evacuation accesses the medial side while also relaxing swollen cerebellum. The AVM is then circumscribed, dissecting around the back side and rolling it anteriorly away from the middle cerebellar peduncle and cranial nerves deep to the nidus (step 6). Scooping the AVM from behind leaves deep medial feeders until the end of the dissection and also preserves the attachment of the draining vein to SPS (step 7). Petrosal AVMs are non-eloquent but adjacent to pons, middle cerebellar peduncle, and CN7/8. The dissection lateral to the cranial nerves avoids entry into the brainstem (**Figs. 17.21** and **17.22**).

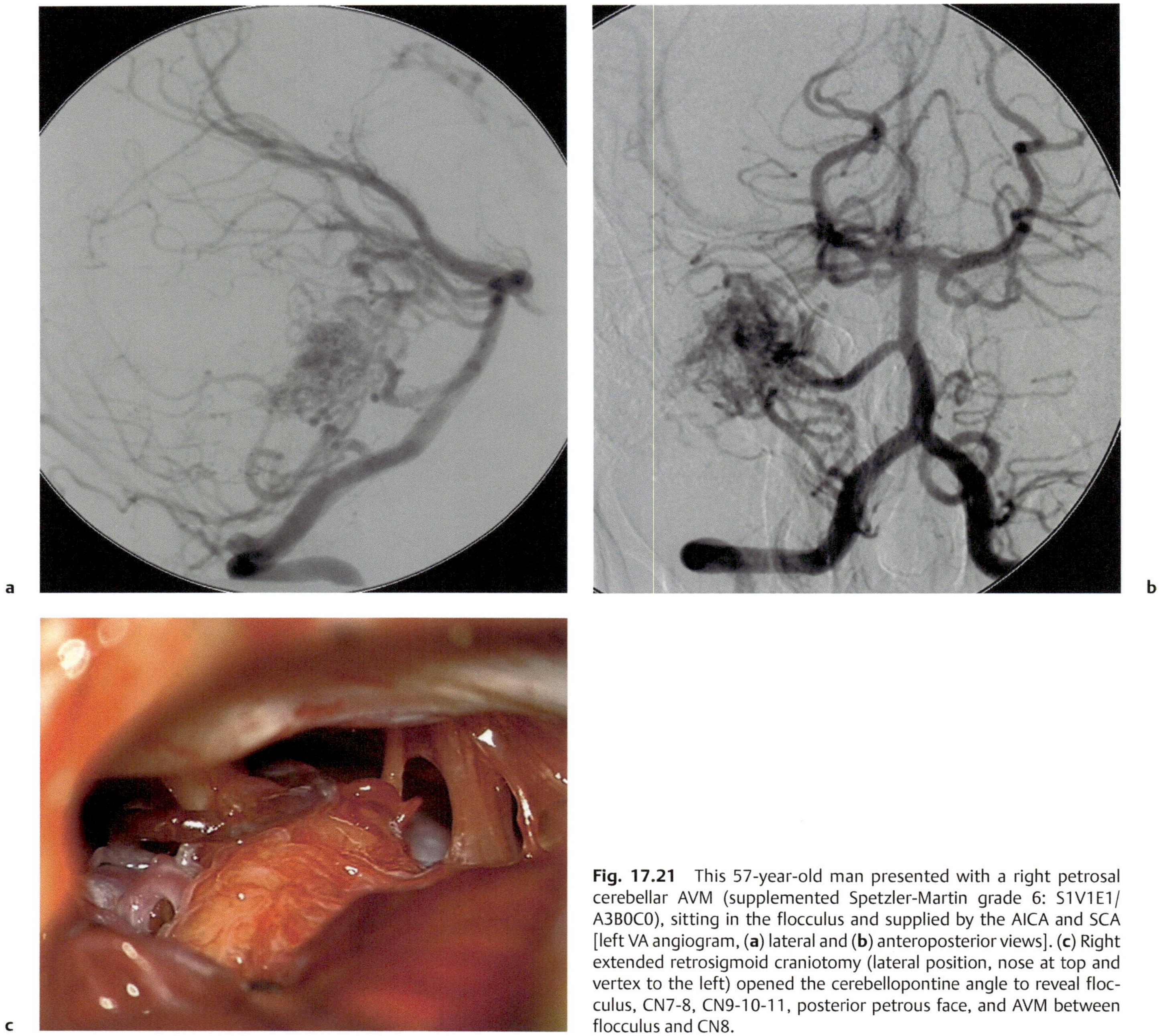

Fig. 17.21 This 57-year-old man presented with a right petrosal cerebellar AVM (supplemented Spetzler-Martin grade 6: S1V1E1/A3B0C0), sitting in the flocculus and supplied by the AICA and SCA [left VA angiogram, (**a**) lateral and (**b**) anteroposterior views]. (**c**) Right extended retrosigmoid craniotomy (lateral position, nose at top and vertex to the left) opened the cerebellopontine angle to reveal flocculus, CN7-8, CN9-10-11, posterior petrous face, and AVM between flocculus and CN8.

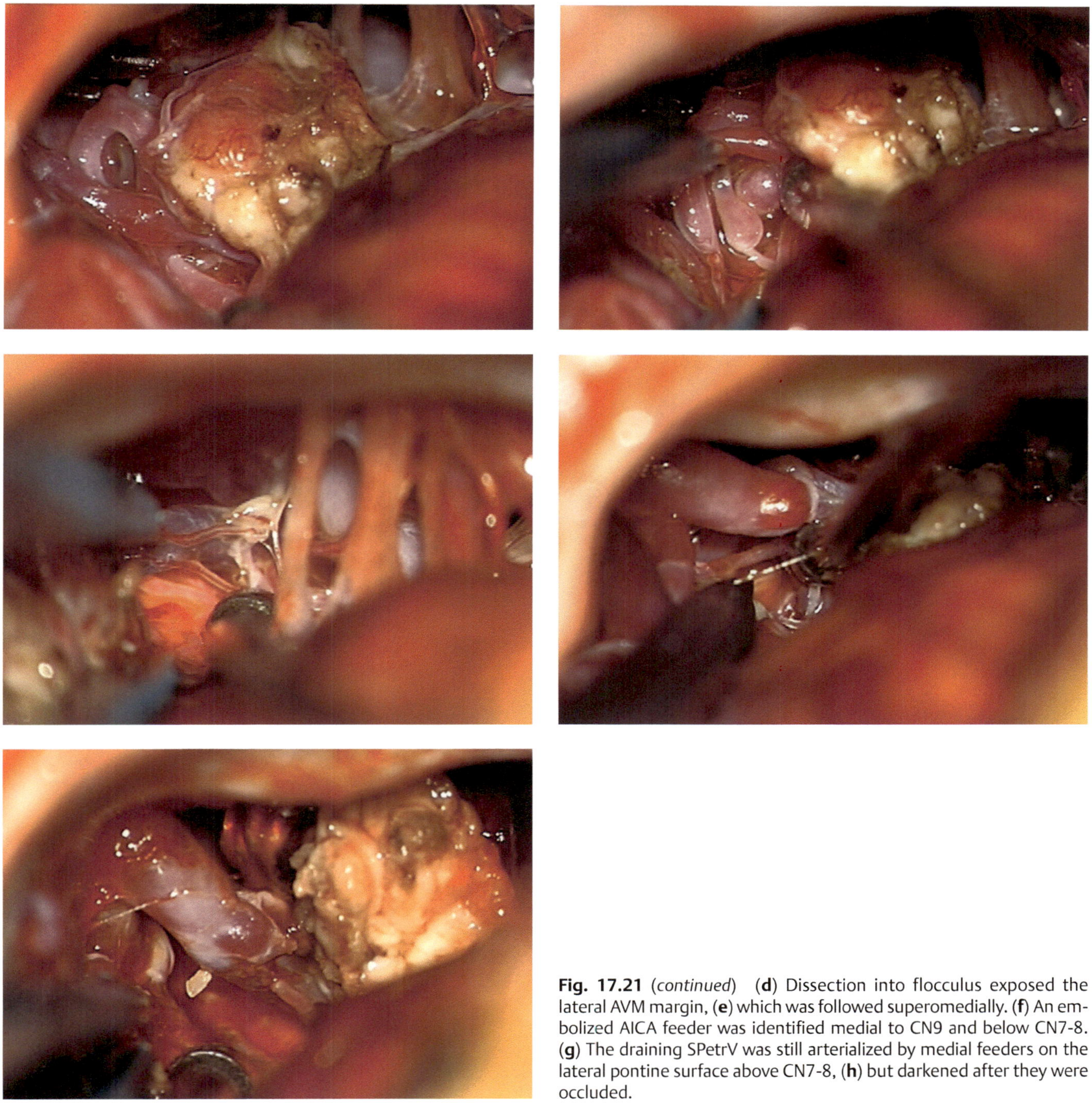

d

e

f

g

h

Fig. 17.21 (*continued*) (**d**) Dissection into flocculus exposed the lateral AVM margin, (**e**) which was followed superomedially. (**f**) An embolized AICA feeder was identified medial to CN9 and below CN7-8. (**g**) The draining SPetrV was still arterialized by medial feeders on the lateral pontine surface above CN7-8, (**h**) but darkened after they were occluded.

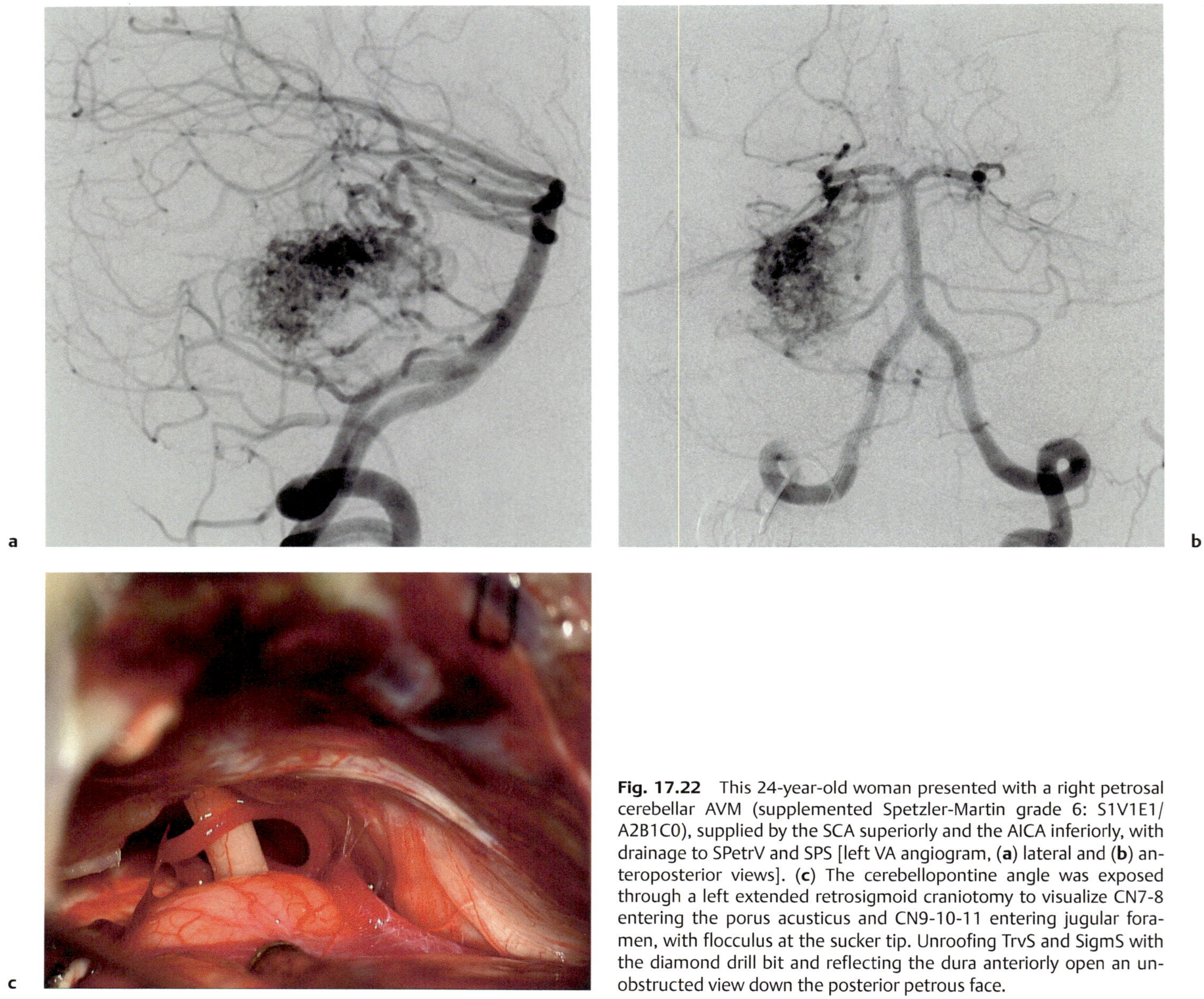

Fig. 17.22 This 24-year-old woman presented with a right petrosal cerebellar AVM (supplemented Spetzler-Martin grade 6: S1V1E1/A2B1C0), supplied by the SCA superiorly and the AICA inferiorly, with drainage to SPetrV and SPS [left VA angiogram, (**a**) lateral and (**b**) anteroposterior views]. (**c**) The cerebellopontine angle was exposed through a left extended retrosigmoid craniotomy to visualize CN7-8 entering the porus acusticus and CN9-10-11 entering jugular foramen, with flocculus at the sucker tip. Unroofing TrvS and SigmS with the diamond drill bit and reflecting the dura anteriorly open an unobstructed view down the posterior petrous face.

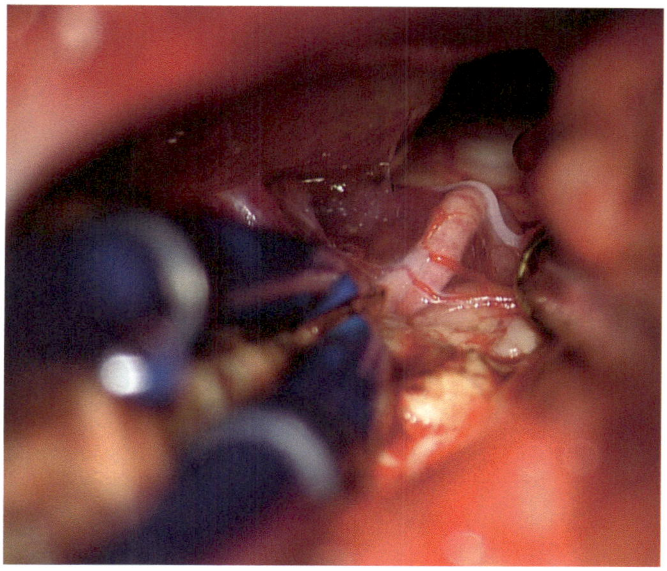

c

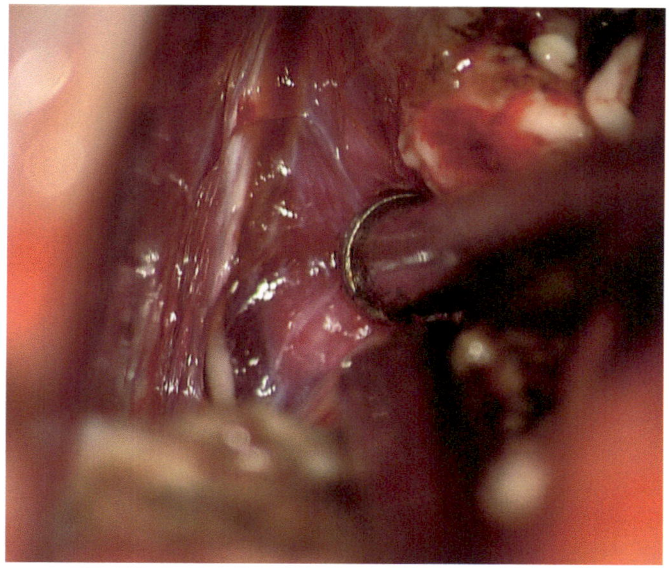

e

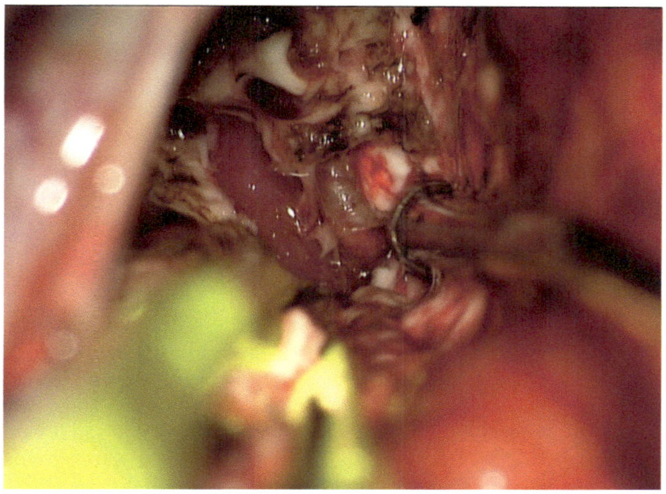

f

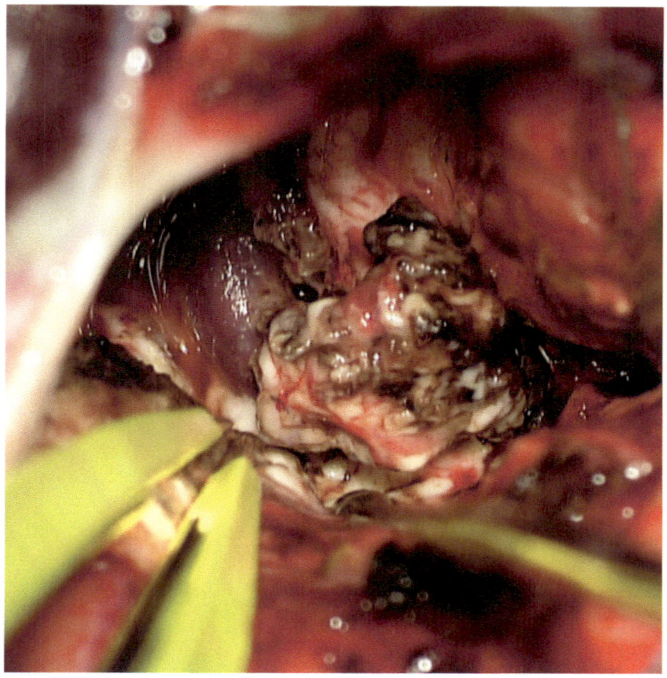

g

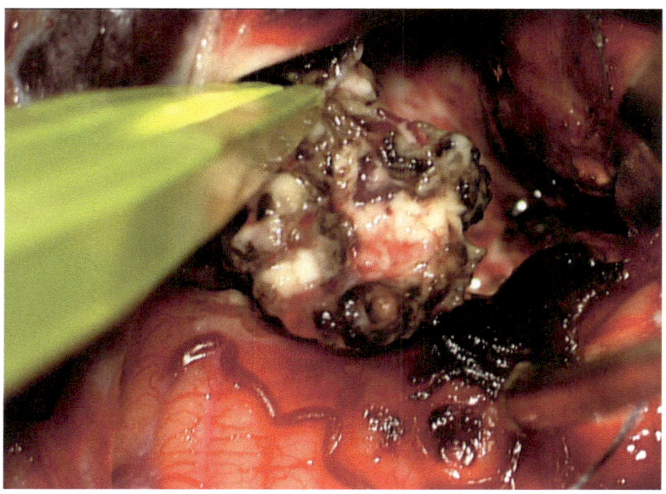

h

Fig. 17.22 (*continued*) (**d**) An embolized SCA feeder was followed into the cerebellopontine fissure. (**e**) Larger SCA feeders were identified under the tentorium at the lateral wall of the ambient cistern, where CN4 was seen through the arachnoid paralleling the free edge of the tentorium, then entering its dural canal. (**f**) Parenchymal dissection laterally exposed the draining vein and descending SCA feeders, which were coagulated. (**g**) SPetrV darkened as the AVM was dissected circumferentially, and (**h**) the AVM was removed.

■ Conclusion

Cerebellar AVMs comprise almost 15% of all brain AVMs. Patients with cerebellar AVMs are significantly more likely to present with hemorrhage than are patients with cerebral AVMs (three quarters vs. one half), and hemorrhagic presentation results in more neurologic deficits both preoperatively and at late follow-up. The explanation for increased bleeding from cerebellar AVMs is unclear. Deep venous drainage is associated with increased rupture risk and was significantly increased in our cerebellar AVMs. Small nidus size is also associated with increased rupture risk, but there were no differences in size between cerebellar and cerebral AVMs. Cerebellar AVMs have less eloquence and less deep perforator supply, but these factors are not associated with AVM rupture. The difference in hemorrhage rates between cerebellar and cerebral AVMs may simply be explained by the absence of seizures in patients with cerebellar AVMs. Overall, 23% of patients with cerebral AVMs presented with seizures, which approximated the difference in hemorrhagic presentation between patients with cerebellar and patients with cerebral AVMs.

Whatever the explanation, the increased rupture rate associated with cerebellar AVMs and its costly sequelae support an aggressive management posture. Surgery is recommended to most patients presenting with ruptured cerebellar AVMs, including 13% with high Spetzler-Martin grades. Treatment is recommended to many patients with unruptured cerebellar AVMs as well, selecting patients with low- and intermediate-grade AVMs for surgery and high-grade AVMs for radiosurgery. Even though they are infratentorial AVMs, cerebellar AVMs are not the same as brainstem AVMs. Cerebellar AVMs require the same complex approaches that work around major venous sinuses, skull base anatomy, and cranial nerves, but surgical exposures are more satisfactory, the risks are less, and results are more favorable with cerebellar AVMs than with brainstem AVMs.

III Selection Strategies

18 Patient Selection

Judicious patient selection is essential to avoid surgical complications and poor neurologic outcomes with microsurgical resection of brain arteriovenous malformations (AVMs); it is the secret to success. The wide variety of AVM anatomy, size, location, and clinical presentation makes patient selection for surgery a difficult process. Neurosurgeons have analyzed their surgical experiences to identify factors that determine the risks of surgery in order to assist them in this selection process. Numerous classification schemes have been developed each with its own emphasis, accuracy, advantages, and disadvantages. Some are complex and others simple, each striving to predict surgical risk and achieve bedside applicability. These classification schemes have value because they transform complex decisions into algorithms. This chapter describes my approach to patient selection.

Pre-Spetzler-Martin Grading Systems

The first major AVM grading scheme, developed by Luessenhop and Gennarelli, in 1977 formulated a grade from I to IV based on the number of feeding arteries, counting the number of tertiary arteries feeding the AVM from a single vascular territory [middle cerebral artery (MCA), anterior cerebral artery (ACA), or posterior cerebral artery (PCA)]. When the AVM was supplied by multiple territories, the grade was determined by the vascular territory with the largest number of feeders. No additional grade was assigned for large AVMs with more than four arteries, as these lesions were deemed inoperable. Surgical results in 49 patients demonstrated that grade I AVMs were associated with low risk, higher grade AVMs were associated with increasing risks, and grade IV AVMs were managed nonoperatively. Luessenhop and Rosa simplified this grading scheme in 1984 by considering only the angiographic size of the AVM, which was easier than counting arterial feeders. The new grades were assigned based on nidus diameter: grade I, < 2 cm; grade II, 2 to 4 cm; grade III, > 4 to 6 cm; and grade IV, > 6 cm. Surgical results in 90 patients demonstrated low morbidity and mortality with grades I and II AVMs, and surgical resection was recommended for these lesions, with minimal consideration of nidus location, patient age, or comorbidities. Conservative management was recommended for patients with high-grade lesions (grades III and IV).

Shi and Chen presented an alternative classification scheme in 1986 that considered AVM size, location and depth, arterial supply, and venous drainage. Each of these four aspects was divided into four grades. Specifically, size was graded as < 2.5 cm (grade I), 2.5 to 5 cm (grade II), > 5 to 7.5 cm (grade III), or > 7.5 cm (grade IV). Location and depth were graded as superficial/nonfunctional (grade I), superficial/functional (grade II), deep (grade III), and deep/vital (grade IV). Arterial supply was graded as single superficial branch of MCA or ACA (grade I), multiple superficial branches of MCA and/or ACA (grade II), PCA branches or deep MCA and/or ACA branches (grade III), and branches of all three cerebral arteries or vertebrobasilar artery (grade IV). Finally, venous drainage was graded as single superficial (grade I), multiple superficial (grade II), deep (grade III), and deep with variceal dilatation (grade IV). The final AVM grade was determined based on the highest of the grades. Excellent results were achieved in patients with low-grade AVMs, and morbidity/mortality increased with high-grade AVMs. This classification scheme demonstrated that complexity will ruin a grading scheme and prevent it from gaining acceptance.

Spetzler-Martin Grading System

In 1986, Spetzler and Martin published what has become the predominant classification scheme for brain AVMs. After considering a range of factors including size, number of feeding arteries, location, operative accessibility, shunt flow, vascular steal, location, and venous drainage, the authors settled on a simplified scheme utilizing only size, eloquence of surrounding brain parenchyma, and venous drainage pattern. Simplicity, applicability at the bedside, and accurate outcome prediction were the authors' principal objectives.

Each factor in the grading scale was scored independently. Size was divided into three categories, with small AVMs, < 3 cm, assigned 1 point; medium AVMs, 3 to 6 cm, assigned 2 points; and large AVMs, > 6 cm, assigned 3 points. Venous drainage was considered superficial if it drained into cortical veins and convexity sinuses and assigned 0 points, or deep if it drained into veins that coursed to the vein of Galen [i.e., internal cerebral vein (ICV), basal vein of Rosenthal (BVR), and precentral cerebellar vein (PreCenCblV)] and assigned 1 point. In the posterior fossa, only veins draining to the straight or transverse sinuses were considered superficial. Arteriovenous malformation eloquence was assessed anatomically based on the presumed function of surrounding brain tissue, with 1 point assigned to lesions located in sensorimotor cortex, language areas, visual cortex, hypothalamus, internal capsule, brainstem, cerebellar peduncles, or deep cerebellar nuclei. Arteriovenous malformations not in these regions were assigned 0 points for eloquence. The final AVM grade was the sum of points across the three domains, with a grade range from I to V. Arteriovenous malformations that are too complex for resection, such as intrinsic brainstem and holohemispheric AVMs, were deemed grade VI.

The Spetzler-Martin grading system was initially evaluated in 100 consecutive surgically resected AVMs. Outcomes were categorized as "no deficit," "minor deficit" (temporary worsening of neurologic function, mild ataxia, or mild increase in brainstem deficit), or "major deficit" (aphasia, hemianopsia, or hemiparesis). There were no major deficits and only one minor deficit in patients with low-grade AVMs (grades I and II). Patients with high-grade AVMs experienced much higher rates of both major (grade IV, 7%; grade V, 12%) and minor deficits (grade IV, 20%; grade V, 19%). Prospective analysis as well as independent analyses by other groups confirmed the accuracy of the grading system to predict operative morbidity and mortality.

This grading system has been widely accepted by neurosurgeons and other clinicians for its simplicity and practicality, quickly providing estimates of surgical risk. Furthermore, its easy applicability has made the grading system an integral part of the description and language of brain AVMs. Experience with this grading has demonstrated three distinct groups of patients. Low-grade AVMs (grades I and II) have low morbidity rates associated with their resection and are frequently treated surgically. High-grade AVMs (grades IV and V) have high morbidity rates associated with their resection and are frequently managed conservatively. Grade III AVMs have intermediate morbidity rates associated with their surgical resection, and treatment recommendations require an individualized approach with multimodality treatment.

A Modification to the Spetzler-Martin Grading System

One deficiency of the Spetzler-Martin grading system is its handling of grade III AVMs. A 2-cm thalamic AVM with deep drainage has the same score as a 7-cm right frontal pole AVM with superficial drainage, yet these two very different lesions have the same grade. Grade III AVMs are the most heterogeneous of the five grades, with four different combinations of size, venous drainage, and eloquence, and one third of all combinations of these elements of the grading scale. In addition, these AVMs are technically challenging, at the limit of what many neurosurgeons are willing to accept in terms of technical difficulty and potential morbidity. The Spetzler-Martin grading system lumps these diverse lesions together and fails to provide the clarity in management that it does for low- and high-grade AVMs.

In an analysis of a consecutive series of 76 of my grade III AVMs, neurologic outcomes varied according to the subtype of grade III AVM (**Table 18.1**). Small grade III AVMs, with 1 point assigned for size, deep venous drainage, and eloquence (S1V1E1), were the most common and had the lowest surgical risk (3% morbidity). In contrast, medium-sized/eloquent grade III AVMs (S2V0E1) had the highest surgical risk (15% morbidity). Medium-sized/deep grade III AVMs (S2V1E0) had an intermediate surgical risk (7%). Large grades III AVMs (S3V0E0) are exceedingly rare, with none in this surgical experience.

Based on these data, grade III AVMs should not be considered a homogeneous group with equivalent risks for all subtypes, as the Spetzler-Martin scheme suggests. Instead, grade III AVMs should be analyzed according to the four subtypes defined by the Spetzler-Martin scheme. A modification to the Spetzler-Martin scheme emphasizes these differences. Small grade III AVMs are designated grade III– because their surgical risk was less than the average grade III lesion,

Table 18.1 Surgical Risk, According to the Type of Spetzler-Martin Grade III AVM

Grade III AVM Type	Total Patients	Improved/ Unchanged		New Deficit/ Death		Modified Grade
	N	*N*	%	*N*	%	
S1V1E1	34	33	97.1	1	2.9	III–
S2V1E0	14	13	92.9	1	7.1	III
S2V0E1	27	23	85.2	4	14.8	III+
S3V0E0	0	0	0.0	0	0.0	III*
Overall	75	69	92.0	6	8.0	

more like a grade II lesion. Medium/eloquent grade III AVMs are designated grade III+ because their surgical risk was more than the average grade III lesion, more like a grade IV lesion. Medium/deep grade III AVMs are designated plain grade III because their surgical risk was the same as the average grade III lesion. Large grade III AVMs are designated grade III* because they are lesions fabricated by the grading system with an incidence so low that their surgical risk is unclear. Large, superficial AVMs in non-eloquent brain can only occur in the frontal or temporal poles; large AVMs in other locations are likely to have a deep draining vein or abut eloquent brain tissue.

This modification to the Spetzler-Martin system facilitates treatment recommendations. Grade III– and III AVMs are typically managed surgically, whereas grade III+ lesions are managed conservatively. This modification improves the Spetzler-Martin grading system's capacity for bedside decision-making.

New and Supplementary Grading Systems

Although the original Spetzler-Martin classification scheme has become an established part of the AVM literature, Spetzler himself recognized redundancy in the grading system, with low-grade AVMs managed similarly with surgery and high-grade AVMs managed conservatively. Therefore, Spetzler and Ponce condensed the original five-tier grading system into three tiers: grades I and II were combined into class A; grade III became class B; and grades IV and V became class C. In a compilation of 1,476 cases from the literature, the differences in surgical outcomes were smallest between grades I and II AVMs and again between grades IV and V AVMs. The predictive power for the three-tiered system was identical to that for the five-tiered system, supporting this condensed classification system.

Spetzler and Ponce made broad treatment recommendations based on AVM class. Class A lesions are managed surgically with a goal of complete resection; class B are managed with multimodality treatment that includes endovascular and radiosurgical intervention in addition to surgical resection; and class C lesions are largely deemed nonsurgical, with exceptions made for recurrent hemorrhage, progressive neurologic deficits, steal-related symptoms, and AVM-related aneurysm. Proponents of this simplification of the grading system emphasize that fewer classes lump together patients with a rare disorder and that the larger groups correspond more directly with treatment recommendations. Opponents of this simplification argue that it does not simplify the analysis of the AVM because the same scoring steps of the original Spetzler-Martin scale are required with an additional step to reclassify the AVM. Opponents also emphasize that the class-specific recommendations are vague and encumbered with exceptions. For example, the class system does nothing to shed light on the heterogeneous group of grade III lesions. Patient selection is a sophisticated process that requires more complexity, not less.

To counter this trend toward simplification, new and supplementary classification schemes have been proposed. Additional factors are important to patient selection but are not part of the Spetzler-Martin grading scale, including hemorrhagic presentation, patient age, deep perforating artery supply, and diffuseness. Presentation with hemorrhage not only indicates AVMs with high risk of rehemorrhage, but also facilitates surgery. Hematomas help separate AVMs from adjacent brain; evacuation of hematoma creates working space around the AVM that can minimize transgression of normal brain or access a deep nidus that might otherwise have been unreachable; and hemorrhage can obliterate some of the AVMs arterial supply to reduce its flow during resection. AVM hemorrhage and microsurgery can injure brain tissue, but young age and plasticity can enhance a patient's ability to recover neurologic function. Compact AVMs with tightly woven arteries and veins often have distinct borders that separate cleanly from the adjacent brain, whereas diffuse AVMs with ragged borders and intermixed brain force the neurosurgeon to establish dissection planes that can extend into normal brain. Deep perforating arteries are thin, fragile, and difficult to occlude with cautery. Bleeding during surgery can escape into deep white matter tracts and cause significant deficits. All of these factors—hemorrhagic presentation, young age, compactness, and absence of deep perforator supply–have been identified as predictors of good outcomes after microsurgical resection.

Alternative AVM classification schemes have been proposed since the introduction of the Spetzler-Martin grading system to incorporate these other factors and improve surgical risk prediction and patient selection. One alternative scheme incorporated a clinical variable, namely the Hunt and Hess grade, as a surrogate for hemorrhagic presentation. Another from the University of Toronto Brain AVM Study Group recognized nidus diffuseness as a critical predictor variable, but combined it with eloquence and deep venous drainage such that it competed with the Spetzler-Martin grading system, re-affiliating eloquence and venous drainage with the newer scale. My group, the University of California–San Francisco (UCSF) Brain AVM Study project, envisioned a grading system that would supplement rather than replace the already entrenched Spetzler-Martin grading system (**Table 18.2**). This supplementary grading system has its own unique variables separate from the Spetzler-Martin scale. Points were assigned for the ABC's of AVMs: patient age, bleeding or hemorrhagic presentation, and AVM compactness, analogous to the Spetzler-Martin scoring system. Pediatric patients (age < 20 years) were assigned 1 point; adults (age 20 to 40 years) were assigned 2 points; and older pa-

Table 18.2 Comparison of Spetzler-Martin and Supplementary Grading Systems

Spetzler-Martin Grading		Points	Supplementary Grading	
Size	< 3 cm	1	Age	< 20 years
	3 to 6 cm	2		20 to 40 years
	> 6 cm	3		> 40 years
Venous drainage	Superficial	0	Bleeding	Yes
	Deep	1		No
Eloquence	No	0	Compactness	Yes
	Yes	1		No
Total		5		

tients (> 40 years) were assigned 3 points. Patients presenting with unruptured AVMs were assigned 1 point and ruptured AVMs 0 points. Diffuse AVMs were assigned 1 point and compact AVMs 0 point. These points were added together for a supplementary AVM grade that ranged from 1 to 5. Simplicity is a critical aspect of a popular grading scale, and a supplementary grading scale was designed with this in mind. In addition, the two grading systems are analogous in their structure to make the supplementary grading scale memorable. In a consecutive surgical series of 300 patients, the supplementary grading system had higher predictive accuracy than the Spetzler-Martin system and stratified surgical risk more evenly (**Table 18.3**).

I use this supplementary grading system to improve and refine patient selection for AVM surgery. Clinical decisions begin with an analysis of nidus size, venous drainage, location, patient age, bleeding presentation, and compactness, generating Spetzler-Martin and supplementary grades. The Spetzler-Martin grade provides an initial risk estimate. The supplementary grade can be considered separately, with supplementary grades ≤ 3 having an acceptably low risk of AVM resection. It can also be added to the Spetzler-Martin grade, with combined grades ≤ 6 having an acceptably low surgical morbidity. An analysis of supplementary factors can impact a management decision by confirming the risk predicted by the Spetzler-Martin grade. For example, an AVM with a low Spetzler-Martin grade (grade I to III) may be favorable for microsurgical resection, and a low supplementary grade (grade I to III) may strengthen the recommendation for surgery. We found that 62% of patients had low-grade AVMs according to both grading systems, and 85% of these patients were improved or unchanged after surgery (**Table 18.4**). Conversely, an AVM with a high Spetzler-Martin grade (IV or V) may be unfavorable for microsurgical resection, and a high supplementary grade (IV or V) may strengthen the recommendation for nonoperative management. In these cases of matched Spetzler-Martin and supplementary grades, the supplementary grading system has a confirmatory role and may not alter management decisions.

However, in cases of mismatched Spetzler-Martin and supplementary grades, the supplementary grading system may alter management decisions and therefore has a more important role. We found that 28% of patients had low Spetzler-Martin grades and high supplementary grades, and 41% of these patients were neurologically worse after surgery (**Table 18.4**), which is a higher morbidity than that of Spetzler-Martin grade IV AVMs (31%). Insight provided by the supplementary grade might have discouraged the recommendation for surgery in some of these patients. Similarly, 7% of patients had high Spetzler-Martin grades and

Table 18.3 Application of Spetzler-Martin, Supplementary, and Supplemented Spetzler-Martin Grading Systems

	Total	Improved/ Unchanged		Worse/ Dead	
	N	*N*	%	*N*	%
Spetzler-Martin grade					
I	56	51	91	5	9
II	123	93	76	30	24
III	90	63	70	27	30
IV	29	20	69	9	31
V	2	0	0	2	100
Supplementary grade					
I	27	26	96	1	4
II	67	59	88	8	12
III	113	88	78	25	22
IV	79	47	59	32	41
V	14	7	50	7	50
Supplemented Spetzler-Martin grade					
1	0	0	0	0	0
2	7	7	100	0	0
3	21	21	100	0	0
4	55	50	91	5	9
5	90	71	79	19	21
6	70	51	73	19	27
7	44	20	45	24	55
8	8	4	50	4	50
9	5	3	60	2	40
10	0	0	0	0	0

Table 18.4 Matched and Mismatched Prediction of Surgical Risk

	Total		Improved/ Unchanged		Worse/ Dead	
	N	%	*N*	%	*N*	%
Matched risk prediction						
Low Spetzler-Martin and Supplementary grades	186	62	158	85	28	15
High Spetzler-Martin and Supplementary grades	10	3	5	50	5	50
Mismatched risk prediction						
Low Spetzler-Martin, high supplementary grades	83	28	49	59	34	41
High Spetzler-Martin, low supplementary grades	21	7	15	71	6	29
Total	300	100	227		73	

low supplementary grades, and 29% of these patients were neurologically worse after surgery (**Table 18.4**). This proportion of worsening was lower than the 35% morbidity for the overall group of Spetzler-Martin grade IV and V AVMs, and equivalent to the 30% morbidity seen for grade III AVMs. Again, insight provided by the supplementary grade might have encouraged the recommendation for surgery in some of these patients. Spetzler-Martin grade III AVMs have surgical risks that depend on the subtype, with small grade III– lesions associated with lower risk and medium/eloquent grade III+ lesions associated with higher risk. In addition to considering the grade III subtype, considering the supplementary grade may influence surgical decisions for AVM patients at the borderline between high and low risk. Our experience demonstrates that factors outside of the Spetzler-Martin grading system improve the prediction of neurologic outcome after AVM resection, and that a simple supplementary grading system can be easily applied at the bedside to refine patient selection for AVM surgery.

Natural History Risk Prediction

Neurosurgeons have focused on the prediction of surgical risk with classification schemes to help them recommend AVM resection. However, the natural alternative to AVM resection is observation, which is particularly important with high-grade AVMs associated with high surgical risks. Therefore, predicting the natural history risk of an AVM is as important in the clinical decision as predicting the surgical risk. An accurate understanding of the hemorrhagic behavior of untreated AVMs is essential when comparing conservative and surgical options.

Patients typically present between 20 and 40 years of age with hemorrhage, seizures, neurologic deficits, and/or headaches. In Ondra's cohort of 160 AVM patients managed nonoperatively and observed prospectively over a 33-year period in Finland, drawn from a population that included over 90% of AVM patients in that country, patients presented with hemorrhage (71%), seizures without evidence of hemorrhage (24%), or other symptoms including headaches, asymptomatic bruits, or other neurologic complaints (5%). The annual rate of AVM hemorrhage was 4%, regardless of presentation and constant over a mean follow-up of 24 years. The mortality rate was 1% annually and the combined major morbidity/mortality rate was 2.7% annually. The mean interval between presentation and subsequent hemorrhagic events was 7.7 years. To simplify the data for patients, I cite an annual hemorrhage rate of 1 to 4%, a rehemorrhage rate of 6 to 10% in the first year after hemorrhage, and thereafter an annual hemorrhage rate of 1 to 4%. The morbidity and mortality rates associated with AVM hemorrhage are between 25 and 50% and 10 and 20%, respectively.

Other reports estimate the annual risk of AVM hemorrhage to be 2 to 4%. The New York Islands AVM Hemorrhage Study, a prospective survey of a zip code–defined population of nearly 10 million inhabitants, found an AVM detection rate of 1.21/100,000 person-years, with incidence of hemorrhage being 0.42/100,000 person-years. The Northern Manhattan Stroke Study found the incidence of first-ever AVM hemorrhage to be 0.55/100,000 person-years. Similar estimates were obtained from studies in a defined population in Northern California. These studies offer insight into the clinical and anatomic factors that influence AVM natural history. Data from the Columbia AVM Databank showed that deep brain location, exclusively deep venous drainage, and presentation with AVM hemorrhage were all associated with increased risk of new hemorrhage. The hemorrhage risks associated with these factors were additive, with an average annual rupture rate that ranged from 0.9% with no risk factors to 34.4% with all three. In addition, associated arterial aneurysms increased the risk of hemorrhage, with a relative risk of 2.28 for patients with intranidal aneurysms and 1.88 for patients with feeding artery aneurysms. Stapf and colleagues also demonstrated that borderzone AVMs fed by at least two arteries from the circle of Willis had a decreased risk of hemorrhage (27% vs. 60%, respectively).

Based on a cohort of 705 AVM patients, Nataf identified similar angiographic factors associated with hemorrhage risk: venous recruitment, venous stenosis, venous reflux, deep venous drainage, and intra- or juxta-nidal aneurysms. A classification scheme incorporating these factors demonstrated increasing hemorrhage risk with grade.

Despite these insights, most estimates of untreated AVM rupture risk are crude at best. There are statistical estimates based on the multiplicative law of probability for the lifetime risk of hemorrhage: Rupture risk = 1 – (Risk of no hemorrhage)$^{(\text{life expectancy})}$. This formula assumes a constant yearly risk of hemorrhage with independent behavior over all years. This formulaic approach yields an estimate lifetime hemorrhage risk, but is not a practical bedside tool. Simplified formulas are more practical and popular: Rupture risk = 105 – Patient age. The use of simplified formulas and the lack of an accepted natural history grading system demonstrate that efforts to define the risks of observation have lagged behind efforts to define the surgical risks.

The importance of such a natural history grading system is clear. As the underlying biology of AVMs and AVM rupture is elucidated, this system will likely include the clinical and anatomic factors discussed above, but also genetic and hemodynamic factors that influence the ongoing inflammation and angiogenesis inside an AVM nidus. Studies of AVM hemodynamics have yielded important potential risk stratification tools, but need further development. Noninvasive magnetic resonance or perhaps other tomographic methods are likely to offer the greatest potential for routine use. Genetic variations, determined by genotyping for one of several candidate single nucleotide polymorphisms (SNPs), offer promise for risk stratification of hemorrhagic risk and can be easily implemented clinically. Some tantalizing findings suggest that variations in the genes coding for inflammatory mediators are associated with increased hemorrhagic risk, offering a way to identify patients with AVMs that are more likely to bleed and individualize recommendations for surgical intervention.

Conclusions

The decision to treat a patient's AVM is a complex process that must consider the individual's clinical presentation, anatomy, and biology. A treatment strategy is conceived that may involve one or multiple modalities, and the cumulative risks of the overall treatment strategy are estimated. Alternative treatments and strategies are also conceived and analyzed for risk. Grading systems are useful in making these estimations. The grading systems that stand the test of time are simple, applicable, and accurate. Other grading systems that are complex, cumbersome, or inaccurate are quickly discarded. Final recommendations are derived by comparing the therapeutic risks with the natural history risks. It is important not only to individualize recommendations for a particular patient, but also to individualize grading systems for a particular neurosurgeon and a particular institution. There is no value in quoting published results if they differ from one's own personal results at one's own institution. Ultimately, grading systems enable clinicians to make management recommendations, but patients have the final say. The decision to embark on AVM treatment is difficult and frightening to most patients, and their individual preferences and feelings should dictate the final decision. Guiding patients through this decision process is an art form that cannot be replaced by grades or outcome data. One of the hardest things for neurosurgeons to accept is their limitations, and grading systems remind us when to say no.

The current crop of grading systems is generally useful, but imperfect and evolving. As the pathophysiology of AVMs is elucidated through research, grading systems will incorporate these advances with genetic information and biological markers. Hemodynamic data may also become a defining element of rupture risk and future grading scales. Therefore, the work of developing AVM grading systems should be viewed as an ongoing process, and clinicians should be open to reshaping established, proven grading systems.

19 Multimodality Management Strategies and Treatment Selection

Despite the surgical focus of this book, current management of brain arteriovenous malformations (AVMs) involves other treatment modalities, namely endovascular embolization and stereotactic radiosurgery, as surgical adjuncts or as competitive alternatives. In some cases, conservative observation is the best option. Therefore, designing an individualized, multimodality management strategy that maximizes safety and efficacy remains a major challenge. In light of their significant hemorrhage risks, brain AVMs are treated with the goal of completely resecting or obliterating the AVM with acceptably low therapeutic risk, thereby avoiding neurologic deficits or deaths that come with hemorrhage. Other clinical symptoms such as seizures or progressive neurologic deficits, while not life-threatening, also warrant consideration for treatment.

Individually, the disciplines of neurosurgery, endovascular surgery, and radiosurgery have made technical advances, and, together, multidisciplinary approaches have improved AVM patient outcomes. Unlike other pathologies for which therapies from different disciplines may be competitive and management recommendations may be controversial, AVMs offer a unique opportunity for specialists to join together with integrated treatment strategies. Arteriovenous malformations foster collaboration between the neurosurgical subspecialties such as vascular and skull base surgery in exposing AVMs; among neurosurgeons, neurologists, and epidemiologists in examining hemorrhage risk and selecting patients for treatment; and between neurosurgeons and basic scientists in investigating the biology of AVMs. This chapter summarizes the multidisciplinary approach at my center for managing patients with brain AVMs (**Table 19.1**).

■ Single Modality Treatment

Single modality management of AVMs (surgical resection, embolization, or radiosurgery alone) is becoming less common with recognition of multimodality management's advantages, namely increased therapeutic efficacy, decreased risks, and improved patient outcomes. Concurrently, novel embolization agents, sophisticated radiosurgical devices, and more accurate radiosurgical target planning have not dramatically raised single modality cure rates. Therefore, multimodality management is the standard for the majority of AVMs, but single modality management is indicated in special circumstances.

Microsurgical Resection

Microsurgical resection alone without any adjunctive therapy is utilized in only 8% of all AVM patients and only 14% of my operated AVM patients. The most common indication is neurologic deterioration due to intracerebral hematoma that produces mass effect and increased intracranial pressure (ICP). In these patients, the immediate need to evacuate the hematoma and relieve ICP prevents preoperative embolization, which might delay surgery and compromise outcome. Microsurgery alone is also indicated with AVMs located distally in a vascular territory with poor endovascular access, and with AVMs fed by small arteries arising perpendicularly from parent arteries, such as lenticulostriate arteries, thalamoperforators, or brainstem perforators. Catheterization of perforating arteries is technically difficult, and their embolization is associated with the risk of retrograde escape of the embolic agent. In some cases, superficial feeding arteries, like those from cortical middle cerebral artery (MCA) branches, are accessible endovascularly, but easy surgical accessibility makes embolization unnecessary.

Older series where AVMs were not embolized preoperatively report rates of complete obliteration (80–83%), permanent neurologic morbidity (5–17%), and operative mortality (1–12%) that are inferior to contemporary series where AVMs were routinely embolized preoperatively. The beneficial effects of preoperative embolization, combined with low procedural morbidity rates, have made it a routine surgical adjunct except in these special situations.

Embolization

Embolization alone was utilized in just 5% of our patients. Embolization with complete, curative AVM occlusion is rare, typically between 10 and 15%. However, cure rates are drifting upward (15–50%) with increasing use of aggressive Onyx embolization and prolonged intranidal injection techniques. However, embolization with the intent to cure is associated with high rates of morbidity (4–38%) and mortality (0–7%)

Table 19.1 Summary of Multimodality AVM Management During the Author's 16-Year Experience

Management	*N*	%
Single modality therapy		
Embolization	50	5
Microsurgery	86	8
Radiosurgery	148	14
Multimodality therapy		
Embolization–microsurgery	445	41
Radiosurgery–microsurgery	45	4
Embolization–radiosurgery	67	6
Embolization–microsurgery–radiosurgery	24	2
Conservative observation	208	19
Total	1073	

due to arterial perforation, nidus perforation, dissection, hemorrhage, thromboembolism, and infarction, all of which can increase further with deep or large AVMs treated in multiple sessions. Curative obliteration is typically observed with small AVMs with a single feeding artery, often distally located away from other critical branch arteries. Pial arteriovenous fistulas can also be cured with endovascular embolization, but these lesions are rare.

Therefore, endovascular AVM obliteration is uncommon, and single modality therapy is often intended for other indications, like palliation of symptoms related to large, high-flow AVMs and cerebral steal (fluctuating neurologic deficit, seizures, and intractable headaches). In selected cases where surgical therapy is too risky, palliative embolization can reduce nidus flow or venous hypertension to improve symptoms, despite significant persistent arteriovenous shunting. It is worth emphasizing, however, that palliative embolization confers no protection against AVM hemorrhage, with some studies documenting no significant difference in hemorrhage rate or clinical outcomes in treated patients compared to natural history, and other studies documenting increased hemorrhage rates. Therefore, palliative embolization should be considered only with AVMs that have no other good treatment options and whose symptoms have become disabling.

The treatment of feeding artery or flow-related aneurysms is another indication for single modality endovascular therapy. These aneurysms are often remote from the circle of Willis and difficult to access surgically. In addition, the proximity of the AVM or its draining veins to the aneurysm can complicate an otherwise straightforward aneurysm clipping. In these cases, treatment consists of coiling the aneurysm and observing the AVM, particularly when the AVM is high-grade. In cases where the patient presents with subarachnoid hemorrhage rather than intracerebral hemorrhage, the aneurysm is usually the lesion responsible for the hemorrhage and aneurysm coiling alone may be appropriate.

With some ruptured AVMs that have intranidal aneurysms, endovascular occlusion of the intranidal aneurysm may be beneficial when a decision has been made not to resect the AVM. In these cases, which again are typically the high-grade AVMs with elevated surgical risks, embolization may reduce the risk of rehemorrhage.

Stereotactic Radiosurgery

Stereotactic radiosurgery alone without any adjunctive therapy was utilized in 14% of our patients, making it the most common of the three single modality treatments. Stereotactic radiosurgery refers to radiation delivered to the entire AVM nidus in a single treatment session. Hypofractionated stereotactic radiation and volume-staged radiosurgery involve more than one treatment session and are generally used for AVMs with diameters greater than 3 cm, or volumes greater than 10 cc. Radiosurgery can be performed with a variety of devices including a Gamma Knife unit, a linear accelerator, Cyber Knife, or particle beams. Gamma Knife, Cyber Knife, and linear accelerator units employing photon irradiation are the most commonly used radiosurgical devices, whereas particle beam facilities for clinical treatments are few in number and used uncommonly.

The indications for radiosurgery include small nidus size, surgical inaccessibility, and high surgical risk. Small AVMs are well suited to radiosurgery because therapeutic doses can be delivered effectively with high obliteration rates. In contrast, large AVMs have lower obliteration rates after radiosurgery and longer intervals from treatment to obliteration. A relationship was reported by Kjellberg for particle beam therapy and by Flickinger for other radiosurgical therapies between targeted nidus volume, radiation dose, and a fixed risk of permanent complications of 3%. For example, larger AVMs require lower radiation doses to keep the complication rate below this limit. Therefore, AVMs with a diameter less than 3 cm can be treated with 20- to 25-Gy doses and have obliteration rates between 65% and 95% at 3 years. In contrast, larger AVMs treated with 15- to 20-Gy doses have obliteration rates between 33% and 58% at 3 years. Lunsford reported a direct relationship between nidus volume and radiosurgical obliteration, with obliteration rates of 100% after 2 years in AVMs with volumes less than 1 cm^3, 85% in AVMs with volumes between 1 and 4 cm^3, and 58% in AVMs with volumes greater than 4 cm^3. Our series of large AVMs treated radiosurgically confirmed this relationship, with a 58% obliteration rate for volumes of 4 to 14 cc and a 23% for volumes greater than 14 cc. No AVM treated with a dose less than 14 Gy was obliterated. A similar direct relationship between radiation dose and radiosurgical obliteration has been observed, with obliteration rates of 50 to 57% with 15-Gy doses, 67 to 70% with 20-Gy doses, and 88% with 25-Gy doses.

Surgical inaccessibility is another important indication for radiosurgery, and AVM locations that are difficult to access include brainstem AVMs, those in the medial temporal-occipital region, and deep AVMs in thalamus and basal ganglia. The AVMs in these locations are surrounded by critical neural structures and have elevated surgical risks. Small size makes AVMs in these locations ideal radiosurgical targets.

Large, high-grade AVMs also have elevated surgical risks, and radiosurgery offers an alternative to conservative observation. For reasons discussed above, large AVMs are not well suited to standard radiosurgery and instead require volume-staged radiosurgery. With volume-staged radiosurgery, the nidus is divided into two or three components and each component is treated in separate sessions 3 to 6 months apart, thereby delivering therapeutic radiation doses for AVM obliteration while minimizing adverse effects. Our mean treatment volume was 34 cc and our median dose was 15 Gy for each session. Despite these large target volumes, one third of treated lesions were obliterated and nearly two thirds were reduced in size. The hemorrhage rate during the latency period was no different than the AVM's natural history risk (1.9% per year). Patients were more likely to have side effects with volume-staged radiosurgery than with conventional radiosurgery, with 78% of patients showing T2-weighted signal changes on magnetic resonance imaging (MRI) and 38% having symptoms. Volume-staged radiosurgery offers a strategy for high-risk, high-grade AVMs, beginning as a single modality treatment designed not to obliterate the AVM but to reduce its volume, and evolving into a multimodality treatment in cases of dramatic volume reduction or hemorrhage. In these cases, microsurgery could be reconsidered later if necessary and performed with lower associated risk.

Multimodality Treatment

In the absence of special circumstances that dictate single modality treatment, multimodality treatment of brain AVMs is routine because an integrated approach increases obliteration rates, decreases therapeutic risks, and improves patient outcomes. In our series, 67% of treated AVMs underwent multimodality therapy, which can consist of any combination of two modalities or all three, with variations in the sequence of therapies. The more common combinations consisted of embolization–microsurgical resection, embolization–radiosurgery, radiosurgery–microsurgery, and embolization–microsurgery–radiosurgery.

Embolization and Microsurgical Resection

Preoperative embolization with microsurgical resection was our most common multimodality management approach, used in 74% of the surgical patients and 41% of the overall cohort. Other cerebrovascular centers have reported a similar reliance on preoperative embolization. Preoperative embolization reduces blood flow to the AVM, which decreases its turgor and makes it more tolerant of surgical manipulation. Embolized feeding arteries are easier to coagulate, and intraluminal embolic agents differentiate feeding arteries that need to be occluded from normal arteries en passage that need to be preserved. Diminished AVM blood flow also reduces blood loss and operative times.

Embolization is particularly valuable with medium and large AVMs with high blood flow and cerebral steal, because the stepwise occlusion of large feeding arteries in different vascular territories redirects blood flow to dysautoregulated arteries in adjacent brain in a staged manner, rather than all at once during surgery. This strategy of staged embolization prior to surgical resection enables these dysautoregulated arteries to readjust to increases in blood flow and can reduce the risk of normal perfusion pressure breakthrough bleeding postoperatively. We typically limit embolizations to one vascular territory per day, meaning that larger lesions with, for example, feeding arteries from the MCA and anterior cerebral artery (ACA) require preoperative embolization in two separate sessions. The strategy of staged feeding artery occlusion is relevant for higher Spetzler-Martin grade AVMs and helps keep associated morbidity and mortality rates in an acceptable range.

Embolization is individualized to AVM anatomy and surgical approach, targeting significant feeding arteries that are deepest, most inaccessible surgically, or accessible only at the end of the dissection. Superficial and easily accessible feeding arteries may not require embolization, even when they are large. However, feeding arteries on the side opposite the surgical approach are preferentially embolized. Communication between the neurosurgeon and endovascular surgeon is critical in establishing these priorities. The timing between embolization and surgery varies at different centers, and there are arguments for both immediate surgery and delayed surgery. Some embolic agents like polyvinyl alcohol are occlusive for only 3 to 4 weeks, making it difficult to delay surgery further. Other embolic agents like cyanoacrylate glues are more permanent and enable delayed surgery. Lengthy delays can result in recanalization of the embolized arteries or angiogenic recruitment of new feeding artery supply. My team tends to perform embolization and surgery during the same hospitalization, frequently on sequential days.

Recent surgical series incorporating preoperative embolization report higher obliteration rates (94–100% for small AVMs less than 3 cm diameter) and lower morbidity and mortality rates (1.5–7.8% and 0–1.3%, respectively), compared to surgical resection or embolization alone. However, the decision to embolize an AVM preoperatively must be made after carefully weighing the surgical benefits against the added risks of embolization, which include arterial dissections, intraprocedural rupture, hemorrhage, venous occlusion, and infarction.

Embolization and Radiosurgery

Embolization and radiosurgery were performed together in only 6% of our patients. Pre-radiosurgical embolization might reduce the nidus size and arteriovenous shunting, which may enhance the efficacy of radiosurgery. However, the nidus increases in size on the subsequent angiogram performed for radiosurgical targeting in one third of these patients. In addition, a small percentage (10–15%) of embolized AVMs recanalize within a year. Recanalization of embolized and occluded portions of the AVM that may have been outside the radiosurgical target results in persistent arteriovenous shunting and treatment failure. Unlike postembolization microsurgery that removes an AVM within several weeks, postembolization radiosurgery takes 2 to 3 years to induce AVM obliteration, allowing sufficient time for recanalization of embolized arteries, recruitment of new feeding arteries, or AVM remodeling.

Results with embolization–radiosurgery have been poor, especially with higher grade AVMs. Low radiosurgical obliteration rates are reported in patients with Spetzler-Martin grade III to V AVMs and incomplete embolization, and pre-radiosurgical embolization has been identified as a negative predictor of AVM obliteration in some series. The AVM obliteration rates and neurologic outcomes associated with combined embolization–radiosurgery are comparable to those of radiosurgery alone. Furthermore, treatment provides no protection during the latency period, with a risk of AVM hemorrhage after combined embolization–radiosurgery comparable to that of the untreated AVMs. In short, the combination of embolization and radiosurgery offers no advantages over radiosurgery alone, and may have significant disadvantages. Results with radiosurgery after embolization with newer agents like Onyx may be better than those with other embolic agents, but data from these experiences have not been reported. In the meantime, embolization–radiosurgery is not recommended and not practiced at our institution.

Radiosurgery and Microsurgery

Microsurgery can be used as a salvage technique after radiosurgery in cases where radiosurgery fails to obliterate the AVM completely. This combination was used in 4% of our overall cohort and 8% of our surgical patients. Failed radiosurgery is due to poor target localization (36%), inadequate definition of the nidus (16%), re-expansion of the nidus (8%), recanalization after embolization (12%), large nidus volume (20%), suboptimal radiation dose (32%), radioresistance (12%), and intranidal fistula (12%). In our cases, radiosurgery resulted in partial obliteration of the nidus, reduction of blood flow, and/or shrinkage of nidus size, all of which facilitated surgery. In addition, arteries feeding the AVM and within the nidus frequently evidenced structural changes in response to radiation that thickened their walls and made them easier to coagulate. Some vessels or portions of the AVM were thrombosed. The brain surrounding the AVM was often gliotic and occasionally formed cysts, which also facilitated the dissection around the AVM. Therefore, microsurgical resection was made possible or easier by radiation-induced changes that tamed once formidable AVMs.

For patients with large AVMs who are initially poor candidates for surgery, volume-staged radiosurgery can partially obliterate their lesions and induce changes that make them eligible for safe surgical resection. This approach has been successful in selected patients with high-grade AVMs. More experience with this promising new strategy will surely demonstrate microsurgical results superior to those obtained without previous radiosurgery.

However, radiosurgery can also complicate microsurgical resection, as in patients who present with new AVM hemorrhage during the latency period. Surgery is no more difficult after the hemorrhage and, in fact, may be easier due to the presence of a new intraparenchymal hematoma that creates a route of access to the nidus, dissects a plane of separation between AVM and adjacent brain, and after evacuation, opens a cavity to the deep sides. Although hemorrhage creates these important surgical advantages, it also injures brain tissue and compromises outcomes. Radiosurgery is often selected over microsurgery when patients are neurologically intact and worried about new deficits. Therefore, hemorrhage during radiosurgery's latency period is disappointing at the very least and devastating at the very worst.

Recruitment of new feeding arteries is another complication of previous radiosurgery. As the nidus obliterates over time, adjacent arteries can enlarge to keep blood shunting through the AVM, and the margins of the AVM can become less sharply defined, almost transforming it into a diffuse nidus. Dilated feeding arteries are more difficult to coagulate than the large arteries that initially fed the AVM, and the diffuse margins distort the separation between brain and nidus. These unfavorable side effects of radiosurgery can make microsurgery more difficult.

Embolization, Microsurgery, and Radiosurgery

Complete AVM resection is one of two surgical objectives; preservation of neurologic function is the other. Sometimes, one must accept an incomplete resection as part of a conservative posture that prioritizes neurologic outcomes. Incomplete resections are more common with deep AVMs, particularly those that are unruptured and without associated neurologic deficits. These AVMs typically have deep feeding arteries that are difficult to coagulate, such as lenticulostriates coursing near the internal capsule or thalamoperforators coursing through the thalamus. Deep AVMs are critically eloquent, and the extent of resection must be determined by intraoperative monitoring and the neurosurgeon's intuition regarding the safety of further dissection. When these alarm bells go off, one must be willing to stop the resection and consider adding radiosurgery to the management plan. Incomplete resection, or circumferential dissection except for the deep plane, results in reduced arterial supply. These surgical changes could possibly facilitate radiosurgical obliteration. Radiosurgery is specifically targeted to the deep remnant or tip of the AVM adjacent to the internal capsule and thalamus. Our experience with this subgroup of patients is small, and our radiosurgical results are unknown at this time. This approach adds risk of hemorrhage postoperatively and during the latency period. Still, we prefer conservative surgery with a triple modality approach over aggressive and perhaps curative resection with greater associated morbidity.

The combination of all three modalities is used in only 4% of the surgical patients and 2% of the overall cohort. In some cases, the intent was to treat with embolization–microsurgery but the anatomy prevented complete resection safely. In other cases, the nidus proved to be too diffuse or the surgical exposure too limited. All three modalities are integrated as a planned strategy when it was possible to identify upfront those AVMs unlikely to succumb to embolization and microsurgery alone. This recognition is important because embolic agents can be chosen appropriately. An incompletely resected AVM must be embolized with durable agents like glue or Onyx that will last throughout the latency period. Among the deep AVMs, thalamic AVMs were least likely to achieve complete resection, with a 46% complete resection rate compared to 80% in both the basal ganglia and insular groups.

The circumdissection is carried as far as possible, interrupting the arterial inputs, preserving the draining veins, and leaving the nidus in situ. Importantly, an AVM that is left unresected must retain its drainage. The most dangerous part of the circumdissection is typically the deep surface where there is perforating artery supply, and this surface is avoided. Theoretically, the efficacy of radiosurgery should improve without the large, high-flow feeders and only smaller, more responsive perforators. Data supporting this approach are limited by small clinical experiences, but do show obliteration rates between 40 and 60% and morbidity rates around 2% with triple modality therapy for Spetzler-Martin grade III to V AVMs, and higher obliteration rates when compared to single modality therapy.

Summary of Multimodality AVM Management

The variety of ways that embolization, microsurgery, and radiosurgery can be used alone or in combination makes it challenging to develop management plans. When presented with an AVM patient, the neurosurgeon begins by evaluating the microsurgery option. Application of the Spetzler-Martin and supplementary grading systems provides a quick, bedside assessment. A supplemented Spetzler-Martin grade of ≤ 6 makes microsurgery a viable option.

The AVMs eligible for microsurgery are then evaluated for embolization. Those that can be embolized with clear benefit to the surgical resection and low associated risk are selected for double modality therapy. Those that cannot be embolized without significant risk or because of other clinical issues, like a hematoma and elevated ICP, are managed microsurgically without embolization.

The AVMs that are poor surgical candidates (supplemented Spetzler-Martin grade > 6) are considered for radiosurgery. Small and medium-sized AVMs are treated with conventional stereotactic radiosurgery, and large AVMs are treated with volume-staged radiosurgery without embolization. These patients are evaluated throughout and at the end of the 3-year latency period, and those with incompletely obliterated AVMs are reconsidered for microsurgery. Elements of the supplemented AVM grade may have changed, particularly AVM size, hemorrhage status, and diffuseness. Significant changes in these variables may make a patient newly eligible for microsurgery. In this case, embolization is considered as a preoperative adjunct.

After an AVM has been treated microsurgically, with or without preoperative embolization, angiography determines the adequacy of resection. Nothing short of complete angiographic obliteration is considered curative or protective against future hemorrhage. Patients with unexpected residual AVM are usually returned to the operating room for complete resection if feasible and safe. Patients with deliberate incompletely resected AVM are considered for radiosurgery as part of triple modality therapy.

Many AVMs that are candidates for microsurgery are also candidates for radiosurgery. In these cases, radiosurgery is presented as a viable treatment alternative. Discussion about microsurgical and radiosurgical treatment alternatives enables comparison of risks, advantages, and disadvantages, with particular emphasis on technical differences, surgical morbidity, radiosurgical morbidity, hemorrhage risk during the latency period, and relative efficacies of therapy.

With all medical decisions, conservative observation is always another alternative. Patients with AVMs that will be observed need to be evaluated for associated aneurysms on feeding arteries, intranidally, and in the circle of Willis. Aneurysms ≥ 7 mm in diameter and associated with high-flow AVMs or with dysplastic morphology are considered for treatment. Untreated aneurysms are monitored with serial imaging, and those that enlarge are treated.

Conclusion

I hope this book contributes to the microsurgical management of brain arteriovenous malformations (AVMs). I am astonished that the surgical experience discussed in this book exceeds the 414 patients of Dr. Gazi Yasargil's in his landmark book, *Microneurosurgery*. With help from many colleagues whose contributions were invaluable (see Suggested Readings), I sifted through the rubble of over 600 AVM cases, poring over films, photographs, videos, charts, and data in an effort to distill the essence of AVM surgery. In the end, the most important message is this: instead of seeing each AVM as unique, recognize it as one of the established subtypes. With this perspective, each AVM can be thoroughly deciphered and methodically attacked. I have laid out a basic strategy for AVM surgery that can be summarized as follows: (1) choose surgical patients wisely, relying on grading systems that are modified, supplemented, and evolving, and on a strong surgeon–patient relationship that considers the patient's condition, concerns, and expectations; (2) study the radiographic and angiographic anatomy carefully; (3) determine the AVM type and subtype; (4) know the strategic battle plan for AVM resection; 5) execute the battle plan methodically in steps from the exposure, to the subarachnoid dissection, to the identification of draining veins and feeding arteries, to the pial dissection, to the parenchymal dissection, to the ependymal dissection, to the resection, all while maintaining absolute hemostasis and control; and (6) be courageous.

Although this book may provide some clarity in conceptualizing AVM surgery, I will be the first to admit some elements are contrived. Arteriovenous malformations do not respect the boundaries and labels in classification schemes, and in fact, are an unruly lot with tremendous variety and overlap, extending across brain surfaces and lobes without regard for neat definitions. Overall, 7% of the AVMs in my series were mixed subtypes or outside the subtypes described. I have seen temporal AVMs that reside on both the lateral and basal surfaces, medial temporal AVMs that extend into the insula, rolandic AVMs on both sides of the central sulcus, and many more. This variability demonstrates that AVMs defy classification. For most of my career, I viewed each one as a unique mixture of feeding arteries, draining veins, nidus anatomy, and patient characteristics. However, this perspective did not facilitate my learning process or strategic planning for AVM resection. By rethinking AVMs as a finite collection of recurring AVM subtypes that can be defined, characterized, and identified clinically again and again, I have been able to analyze my own AVM experience and gain some insights. If others agree with and validate this new perspective, perhaps we can standardize our analysis of AVMs in ways that will enlighten and inform us. At the least, this perspective will help aspiring AVM neurosurgeons figure out AVM surgery, progress along their learning curve, and see the forest through the trees.

Courage is a quality rarely discussed with surgery. Arteriovenous malformation surgery is more than just the execution of technical steps with predictable outcomes. These operations can quickly take a turn for the worse with one simple mistake, inflicting morbidity on the patient and great difficulty on the neurosurgeon. Arteriovenous malformation surgery demands skill, attention, precision, cunning, and endurance. It calls for neurosurgeons who bravely accept the challenges, uncertainties, and risks. Having used a military metaphor in this book, it is fitting to end with one more example. Battle-tested veterans have the fortitude to fight and possibly sacrifice their lives to advance a cause or right an injustice, despite the horrors of war. In the same spirit, AVM surgeons have a warrior's mentality and a special fortitude to tackle this difficult pathology. As a resident, I observed Dr. Robert Spetzler battle some ferocious AVMs, intrigued by the strategic dual, astonished by the sudden explosions of bleeding, thrilled by the bluing of the draining vein, unaware of the passage of hours, and ultimately inspired by the victory. I did not always understand what I was seeing, but I knew that I wanted to become an AVM surgeon. Strangely, I liked that extra danger and intensity that excite some neurosurgeons and scare most others. For those who are attracted to AVM surgery, it takes skill development, inspirational mentoring, dedication, and a clear calling, but most of all, courage.

Finally, I wrote this book because I want neurosurgeons to do a good job in resecting AVMs. Arteriovenous malformations resection remains the treatment of choice if we collectively remove them safely and completely with good patient outcomes. Endovascular therapy will continue to improve with new embolic agents and increasing obliteration rates. Radiosurgery will continue to improve with better targeting and sensitizing agents that increase radiation's efficacy. A randomized, controlled trial like ARUBA (A Randomized trial of Unruptured Brain Arteriovenous malformations) will call into question any intervention for patients without bleeding AVMs. Therefore, neurosurgeons must strive to optimize their surgical results. This book is intended as a guide to learning, practicing, and mastering the art of AVM resection, in the hope that open surgical resection will continue to play a dominant role in AVM management.

Suggested Readings

Achrol AS, Kim H, Pawlikowska L, et al. Association of tumor necrosis factor-alpha-238G>A and apolipoprotein E2 polymorphisms with intracranial hemorrhage after brain arteriovenous malformation treatment. Neurosurgery 2007;61:731–739, discussion 740

Achrol AS, Pawlikowska L, McCulloch CE, et al; UCSF BAVM Study Project. Tumor necrosis factor-a-238G: a promoter polymorphism is associated with increased risk of new hemorrhage in the natural course of patients with brain arteriovenous malformations. Stroke 2006;37: 231–234

Atkinson RP, Awad IA, Batjer HH, et al; Joint Writing Group of the Technology Assessment Committee American Society of Interventional and Therapeutic Neuroradiology; Joint Section on Cerebrovascular Neurosurgery a Section of the American Association of Neurological Surgeons and Congress of Neurological Surgeons; Section of Stroke and the Section of Interventional Neurology of the American Academy of Neurology. Reporting terminology for brain arteriovenous malformation clinical and radiographic features for use in clinical trials. Stroke 2001;32:1430–1442

Bharatha A, Faughnan ME, Kim H, et al. Brain arteriovenous malformation multiplicity predicts the diagnosis of hereditary hemorrhagic telangiectasia: quantitative assessment. Stroke 2012;43:72–78

Chen W, Guo Y, Walker EJ, et al. Reduced mural cell coverage and impaired vessel integrity after angiogenic stimulation in the Alk1-deficient brain. Arterioscler Thromb Vasc Biol 2013;33:305–310

Chen Y, Fan Y, Poon KYT, et al. MMP-9 expression is associated with leukocytic but not endothelial markers in brain arteriovenous malformations. Front Biosci 2006;11:3121–3128

Chen Y, Hao Q, Kim H, et al. Soluble endoglin modulates aberrant cerebral vascular remodeling. Ann Neurol 2009;66:19–27

Chen Y, Pawlikowska L, Yao JS, et al. Interleukin-6 involvement in brain arteriovenous malformations. Ann Neurol 2006;59:72–80

Chen Y, Zhu W, Bollen AW, et al. Evidence of inflammatory cell involvement in brain arteriovenous malformations. Neurosurgery 2008;62: 1340–1349, discussion 1349–1350

Chi JH, Lawton MT. Posterior interhemispheric approach: surgical technique, application to vascular lesions, and benefits of gravity retraction. Neurosurgery 2006;59(1, Suppl 1)ONS41–ONS49, discussion ONS41–ONS49

Davies JM, Kim H, Young WL, Lawton MT. Classification schemes for arteriovenous malformations. Neurosurg Clin N Am 2012;23:43–53

Davies J, Tawk RG, Lawton MT. The contralateral transcingulate approach: operative technique and results with vascular lesions. Neurosurgery 2012;71(1, Suppl Operative)4–13, discussion 13–14

Davies JM, Yanamadala V, Lawton MT. Comparative effectiveness of treatments for cerebral arteriovenous malformations: trends in nationwide outcomes from 2000 to 2009. Neurosurg Focus 2012;33:E11

Du R, Dowd CF, Johnston SC, Young WL, Lawton MT. Interobserver variability in grading of brain arteriovenous malformations using the Spetzler-Martin system. Neurosurgery 2005;57:668–675, discussion 668–675

Du R, Hashimoto T, Tihan T, Young WL, Perry V, Lawton MT. Growth and regression of arteriovenous malformations in a patient with hereditary hemorrhagic telangiectasia. Case report. J Neurosurg 2007;106: 470–477

Du R, Keyoung HM, Dowd CF, Young WL, Lawton MT. The effects of diffuseness and deep perforating artery supply on outcomes after microsurgical resection of brain arteriovenous malformations. Neurosurgery 2007;60:638–646, discussion 646–648

Du R, McDermott MW, Dowd CF, Young WL, Lawton MT. Neurosurgery at the crossroads: integrated multidisciplinary management of 449 patients with brain arteriovenous malformations. Clin Neurosurg 2005;52:177–191

Du R, Young WL, Lawton MT. "Tangential" resection of medial temporal lobe arteriovenous malformations with the orbitozygomatic approach. Neurosurgery 2004;54:645–651, discussion 651–652

Englot DJ, Young WL, Han SJ, McCulloch CE, Chang EF, Lawton MT. Seizure predictors and control after microsurgical resection of supratentorial arteriovenous malformations in 440 patients. Neurosurgery 2012;71:572–580, discussion 580

Fan Y, Ye J, Shen F, et al. Interleukin-6 stimulates circulating blood-derived endothelial progenitor cell angiogenesis in vitro. J Cereb Blood Flow Metab 2008;28:90–98

Frenzel T, Lee CZ, Kim H, et al. Feasibility of minocycline and doxycycline use as potential vasculostatic therapy for brain vascular malformations: pilot study of adverse events and tolerance. Cerebrovasc Dis 2008;25:157–163

Fullerton HJ, Achrol AS, Johnston SC, et al; UCSF BAVM Study Project. Long-term hemorrhage risk in children versus adults with brain arteriovenous malformations. Stroke 2005;36:2099–2104

Gabarrós A, Young WL, McDermott MW, Lawton MT. Language and motor mapping during resection of brain arteriovenous malformations: indications, feasibility, and utility. Neurosurgery 2011;68: 744–752

Gabarrós Canals A, Rodríguez-Hernández A, Young WL, Lawton MT; UCSF Brain AVM Study Project. Temporal lobe arteriovenous malformations: anatomical subtypes, surgical strategy, and outcomes. J Neurosurg 2013;119:616–628

Gao P, Chen Y, Lawton MT, et al. Evidence of endothelial progenitor cells in the human brain and spinal cord arteriovenous malformations. Neurosurgery 2010;67:1029–1035

Guo Y, Saunders T, Su H, et al; University of California, San Francisco Brain Arteriovenous Malformation (UCSF bAVM) Study Project. Silent intralesional microhemorrhage as a risk factor for brain arteriovenous malformation rupture. Stroke 2012;43:1240–1246

Halim AX, Singh V, Johnston SC, et al; UCSF BAVM Study Project. Brain Arteriovenous Malformation. Characteristics of brain arteriovenous malformations with coexisting aneurysms: a comparison of two referral centers. Stroke 2002;33:675–679

Hasan DM, Amans M, Tihan T, et al. Ferumoxytol-enhanced MRI to image inflammation within human brain arteriovenous malformations: A pilot investigation. Transl Stroke Res 2012;3(Suppl 1): 166–173

Hashimoto T, Lam T, Boudreau NJ, Bollen AW, Lawton MT, Young WL. Abnormal balance in the angiopoietin-tie2 system in human brain arteriovenous malformations. Circ Res 2001;89:111–113

Hashimoto T, Lawton MT, Wen G, et al. Gene microarray analysis of human brain arteriovenous malformations. Neurosurgery 2004;54: 410–423, discussion 423–425

Hashimoto T, Matsumoto MM, Li JF, Lawton MT, Young WL; University of California, San Francisco, BAVM Study Group. Suppression of MMP-9 by doxycycline in brain arteriovenous malformations. BMC Neurol 2005;5:1

Hashimoto T, Mesa-Tejada R, Quick CM, et al. Evidence of increased endothelial cell turnover in brain arteriovenous malformations. Neurosurgery 2001;49:124–131, discussion 131–132

Hashimoto T, Wen G, Lawton MT, et al; University of California, San Francisco BAVM Study Group. Abnormal expression of matrix metalloproteinases and tissue inhibitors of metalloproteinases in brain arteriovenous malformations. Stroke 2003;34:925–931

Hashimoto T, Wu Y, Lawton MT, Yang GY, Barbaro NM, Young WL. Coexpression of angiogenic factors in brain arteriovenous malformations. Neurosurgery 2005;56:1058–1065, discussion 1058–1065

Hetts SW, Keenan K, Fullerton HJ, et al. Pediatric intracranial nongalenic pial arteriovenous fistulas: clinical features, angioarchitecture, and outcomes. AJNR Am J Neuroradiol 2012;33:1710–1719

Kim EJ, Halim AX, Dowd CF, et al. The relationship of coexisting extranidal aneurysms to intracranial hemorrhage in patients harboring brain arteriovenous malformations. Neurosurgery 2004;54:1349–1357, discussion 1357–1358

Kim H, Hysi PG, Pawlikowska L, et al. Common variants in interleukin-1-beta gene are associated with intracranial hemorrhage and susceptibility to brain arteriovenous malformation. Cerebrovasc Dis 2009; 27:176–182

Kim H, McCulloch CE, Johnston SC, Lawton MT, Sidney S, Young WL. Comparison of 2 approaches for determining the natural history risk of brain arteriovenous malformation rupture. Am J Epidemiol 2010; 171:1317–1322

Kim H, Pourmohamad T, Westbroek EM, McCulloch CE, Lawton MT, Young WL. Evaluating performance of the Spetzler-Martin supplemented model in selecting patients with brain arteriovenous malformation for surgery. Stroke 2012;43:2497–2499

Kim H, Sidney S, McCulloch CE, et al; UCSF BAVM Study Project. Racial/ethnic differences in longitudinal risk of intracranial hemorrhage in brain arteriovenous malformation patients. Stroke 2007;38: 2430–2437

Kim YB, Young WL, Lawton MT; UCSF BAVM Study Project. Parafalcine and midline arteriovenous malformations: surgical strategy, techniques, and outcomes. J Neurosurg 2011;114:984–993

Kobayashi S, Hongo K, Bhagwati SN, Rappaport ZH, Lawton MT, Spetzler RF. Management of arteriovenous malformations: Part II. Surg Neurol 1997;48:2–6

Lawton MT. Seven Aneurysms: Tenets and Techniques for Clipping. New York: Thieme Medical Publishers, 2010

Lawton MT; UCSF Brain Arteriovenous Malformation Study Project. Spetzler-Martin grade III arteriovenous malformations: surgical results and a modification of the grading scale. Neurosurgery 2003;52: 740–748, discussion 748–749

Lawton MT, Arnold CM, Kim YJ, et al. Radiation arteriopathy in the transgenic arteriovenous fistula model. Neurosurgery 2008;62:1129–1138, discussion 138–139

Lawton MT, Chun J, Wilson CB, Halbach VV. Ethmoidal dural arteriovenous fistulae: an assessment of surgical and endovascular management. Neurosurgery 1999;45:805–810, discussion 810–811

Lawton MT, Du R, Tran MN, et al. Effect of presenting hemorrhage on outcome after microsurgical resection of brain arteriovenous malformations. Neurosurgery 2005;56:485–493, discussion 485–493

Lawton MT, Hamilton MG, Spetzler RF. Multimodality treatment of deep arteriovenous malformations: thalamus, basal ganglia, and brain stem. Neurosurgery 1995;37:29–35, discussion 35–36

Lawton MT, Jacobowitz R, Spetzler RF. Redefined role of angiogenesis in the pathogenesis of dural arteriovenous malformations. J Neurosurg 1997;87:267–274

Lawton MT, Kim H, McCulloch CE, Mikhak B, Young WL. A supplementary grading scale for selecting patients with brain arteriovenous malformations for surgery. Neurosurgery 2010;66:702–713, discussion 713

Lawton MT, Lu DC, Young WL; University of California, San Francisco Brain Arteriovenous Malformation Study Project. Sylvian fissure arteriovenous malformations: an application of the Sugita classification to 28 surgical patients. Neurosurgery 2007;61:29–36, discussion 36–38

Lawton MT, Sanchez-Mejia RO, Pham D, Tan J, Halbach VV. Tentorial dural arteriovenous fistulae: operative strategies and microsurgical results for six types. Neurosurgery 2008;62(3, Suppl 1)110–124, discussion 124–125

Lawton MT, Shetter A, Shapiro W, Spetzler RF. Angiogenesis factors and their clinical applications. BNI Q 1993;9:46–54

Lawton MT, Shetter AG, Shapiro W, Spetzler RF. Angiogenesis: A neurosurgical perspective. Advances in Clinical Neurosciences 1994;4: 27–43

Lawton MT, Spetzler RF. Arteriovenous malformations: principles of treatment. In Bogouslavsky J, Ginsberg MD, eds. Cerebrovascular Disease: Pathophysiology, Diagnosis, and Management. Cambridge, MA: Blackwell Science Publications, 1998:1995–2004.

Lawton MT, Spetzler RF. Surgical management of acutely ruptured arteriovenous malformations. In Welch KMA, Caplan L, Reis D, Seisjo B, Weir B, eds. Primer on Cerebrovascular Diseases. New York: Academic Press, 1997:234–243

Lawton MT, Stewart CL, Wulfstat AA, Derugin N, Hashimoto T, Young WL. The transgenic arteriovenous fistula in the rat: an experimental model of gene therapy for brain arteriovenous malformations. Neurosurgery 2004;54:1463–1471, discussion 1471

Leblanc GG, Golanov E, Awad IA, Young WL; Biology of Vascular Malformations of the Brain NINDS Workshop Collaborators. Biology of vascular malformations of the brain. Stroke 2009;40:e694–e702

Mikhak B, Weinsheimer S, Pawlikowska L, et al, for the BAVM Study Project. Angiopoietin-like 4 (ANGPTL4) gene polymorphisms and risk of brain arteriovenous malformations. Cerebrovasc Dis 2011;31: 338–345

Pawlikowska L, Poon KYT, Achrol AS, et al. Apolipoprotein E epsilon 2 is associated with new hemorrhage risk in brain arteriovenous malformations. Neurosurgery 2006;58:838–843, discussion 838–843

Pawlikowska L, Tran MN, Achrol AS, et al; UCSF BAVM Study Project. Polymorphisms in transforming growth factor-b-related genes ALK1 and ENG are associated with sporadic brain arteriovenous malformations. Stroke 2005;36:2278–2280

Pawlikowska L, Tran MN, Achrol AS, et al; UCSF BAVM Study Project. Polymorphisms in genes involved in inflammatory and angiogenic pathways and the risk of hemorrhagic presentation of brain arteriovenous malformations. Stroke 2004;35:2294–2300

Potts MB, Chang EF, Young WL, Lawton MT; UCSF Brain AVM Study Project. Transsylvian-transinsular approaches to the insula and basal ganglia: operative techniques and results with vascular lesions. Neurosurgery 2012;70:824–834, discussion 834

Potts MB, Young WL, Lawton MT; UCSF Brain AVM Study Project. Deep arteriovenous malformations in the basal ganglia, thalamus, and insula: microsurgical management, techniques, and results. Neurosurgery 2013;73:417–429

Quiñones-Hinojosa A, Auguste KI, Lawton MT. Unusual venous drainage of an arteriovenous malformation. Case illustration. J Neurosurg 2003;98:642

Racine CA, Lawton MT, Hetts SW, Josephson SA. Neuropsychological profile of reversible cognitive impairment in a patient with a dural arteriovenous fistula. Neurocase 2008;14:231–238

Rhoton AL, Jr: Cranial Anatomy and Surgical Approaches. Baltimore: Lippincott Williams & Wilkins, 2003.

Rodríguez-Hernández A, Kim H, Pourmohamad T, Young WL, Lawton MT; University of California, San Francisco Arteriovenous Malformation Study Project. Cerebellar arteriovenous malformations: anatomic subtypes, surgical results, and increased predictive accuracy of the supplementary grading system. Neurosurgery 2012;71:1111–1124

Rodríguez-Hernández A, Lawton MT. Anatomical triangles defining surgical routes to posterior inferior cerebellar artery aneurysms. J Neurosurg 2011;114:1088–1094

Rodríguez-Hernández A, Rhoton AL Jr, Lawton MT. Segmental anatomy of cerebellar arteries: a proposed nomenclature. Laboratory investigation. J Neurosurg 2011;115:387–397

Sanai N, Mirzadeh Z, Lawton MT. Supracerebellar-supratrochlear and infratentorial-infratrochlear approaches: gravity-dependent variations of the lateral approach over the cerebellum. Neurosurgery 2010;66(6, Suppl Operative)264–274, discussion 274

Sanchez-Mejia RO, Chennupati SK, Gupta N, Fullerton H, Young WL, Lawton MT. Superior outcomes in children compared with adults after microsurgical resection of brain arteriovenous malformations. J Neurosurg 2006;105(2, Suppl)82–87

Sanchez-Mejia RO, McDermott MW, Tan J, Kim H, Young WL, Lawton MT. Radiosurgery facilitates resection of brain arteriovenous malformations and reduces surgical morbidity. Neurosurgery 2009;64:231–238, discussion 238–240

Singh V, Smith WS, Lawton MT, Halbach VV, Young WL. Risk factors for hemorrhagic presentation in patients with dural arteriovenous fistulae. Neurosurgery 2008;62:628–635, discussion 628–635

Smyth MD, Sneed PK, Ciricillo SF, et al. Stereotactic radiosurgery for pediatric intracranial arteriovenous malformations: the University of California at San Francisco experience. J Neurosurg 2002;97:48–55

Su H, Kim H, Pawlikowska L, et al. Reduced expression of integrin alphavbeta8 is associated with brain arteriovenous malformation pathogenesis. Am J Pathol 2010;176:1018–1027

Vates GE, Hashimoto T, Young WL, Lawton MT. Angiogenesis in the brain during development: the effects of vascular endothelial growth factor and angiopoietin-2 in an animal model. J Neurosurg 2005;103:136–145

Vates GE, Lawton MT. Arteriovenous malformations. In Way LW, Doherty GM, eds. Current Surgical Diagnosis and Treatment, 11th ed. New York: Lange Medical Books/McGraw-Hill Companies, 2003:943–947

Vates GE, Lawton MT, Wilson CB, et al. Magnetic source imaging demonstrates altered cortical distribution of function in patients with arteriovenous malformations. Neurosurgery 2002;51:614–623, discussion 623–627

Vates GE, Quiñones-Hinojosa A, Halbach VV, Lawton MT. Conus perimedullary arteriovenous fistula with intracranial drainage: case report. Neurosurgery 2001;49:457–461, discussion 461–462

Waldron JS, Lawton MT. The supracarotid-infrafrontal approach: surgical technique and clinical application to cavernous malformations in the anteroinferior basal ganglia. Neurosurgery 2009;64(3, Suppl) ons86–ons95, discussion ons95

Walker EJ, Su H, Shen F, et al. Arteriovenous malformation in the adult mouse brain resembling the human disease. Ann Neurol 2011;69:954–962

Westbroek EM, Pawlikowska L, Lawton MT, McCulloch CE, Young WL, Kim H. Brain-derived neurotrophic factor Val66Met polymorphism predicts worse functional outcome after surgery in patients with unruptured brain arteriovenous malformation. Stroke 2012;43:2255–2257

Weinsheimer S, Brettman AD, Pawlikowska L, et al. G protein-coupled receptor 124 (GPR124) gene polymorphisms and risk of brain arteriovenous malformation. Transl Stroke Res 2012;3:418–427

Weinsheimer S, Kim H, Pawlikowska L, et al. EPHB4 gene polymorphisms and risk of intracranial hemorrhage in patients with brain arteriovenous malformations. Circ Cardiovasc Genet 2009;2:476–482

Weinsheimer SM, Xu H, Achrol AS, et al. Gene expression profiling of blood in brain arteriovenous malformation patients. Transl Stroke Res 2011;2:575–587

Wilson CB, Stein BM: Intracranial Arteriovenous Malformations. Baltimore: Williams & Wilkins, 1984.

Yao JS, Zhai W, Fan Y, et al. Interleukin-6 upregulates expression of KDR and stimulates proliferation of human cerebrovascular smooth muscle cells. J Cereb Blood Flow Metab 2007;27:510–520

Yasargil M. G.: Microneurosurgery: AVM of the Brain, History, Embryology, Pathological Considerations, Hemodynamics, Diagnostic Studies, Microsurgical Anatomy (Volume IIIA). New York: Thieme Medical Publishers, Inc, 1988.

Yasargil M. G.: Microneurosurgery: AVM of the Brain, Clinical Considerations, General and Special Operative Techniques, Surgical Results, Nonoperatied Cases, Cavernous and Venous Angiomas, Neuroanesthesia (Volume IIIB). New York: Thieme Medical Publishers, Inc, 1988.

Young WL, Talke P, Lawton MT. Anesthetic considerations for surgical resection of brain arteriovenous malformations. In Cottrell JE, Young WY, eds. Cottrell and Young's Neuroanesthesia, 5th ed. New York: Mosby Elsevier, 2009:264–277

Zador Z, Lu DC, Arnold CM, Lawton MT. Deep bypasses to the distal posterior circulation: anatomical and clinical comparison of pretemporal and subtemporal approaches. Neurosurgery 2010;66:92–100, discussion 100–101

Zhu Y, Lawton MT, Du R, et al. Expression of hypoxia-inducible factor-1 and vascular endothelial growth factor in response to venous hypertension. Neurosurgery 2006;59:687–696, discussion 687–696

ZhuGe Q, Zhong M, Zheng WM, et al. Notch-1 signalling is activated in brain arteriovenous malformations in humans. Brain 2009;132(Pt 12):3231–3241

Index

Note: Page references followed by *f* indicate figures; page references followed by *t* indicate tables.

C

U

V

W